Essentials of Audiology
second edition

Essentials of Audiology
second edition

Stanley A. Gelfand, Ph.D.

Professor
Department of Linguistics and Communication Disorders
Queens College of the City University of New York
Flushing, New York
and
Ph.D. Program in Speech and Hearing Sciences
Graduate Center of the City University of New York
New York, New York

with 320 illustrations

2001
Thieme
New York • Stuttgart

Thieme Medical Publishers, Inc.
333 Seventh Avenue
New York, NY 10001

Essentials of Audiology, 2nd edition
Stanley A. Gelfand, Ph.D.

Library of Congress Cataloging-in-Publication Data

Gelfand, Stanley A., 1948–
 Essentials of audiology/Stanley A. Gelfand.—2nd ed.
  p. cm.
 Includes bibliographical references and index.
 ISBN 1-58890-017-7
 1. Audiology. I. Title.

RF290.E73 2001
617.8—dc21   00-054511

Printed in the United States of America.

5 4 3 2 1

TMP ISBN 1-58890-017-7
GTV ISBN 3-13-103632-X

This book is lovingly dedicated to
Janice, Michael, Joshua, and Jessica.

Contents

Preface

Audiology is the scientific study of hearing and its disorders. As such, audiology may be defined as both the interdisciplinary study of audition in the broadest sense, as well as the independent clinical profession that deals with hearing and its disorders. When viewed as a body of scientific information and techniques, audiology is relevant and useful to a diverse number of scientists and professionals. Who are all of these people that could possibly be interested in hearing? Among others, they include speech-language pathologists; speech and hearing scientists; teachers of the deaf and hearing impaired; engineers; acousticians; industrial hygienists; musicologists; physicians; physiologists; psychologists; linguists; physicists; vocational counselors; and, of course, audiologists.

What is an audiologist? An audiologist is a practitioner of audiology as a clinical profession. Audiologists are principally concerned with the identification, evaluation, and management of patients with auditory disorders, as well as with the prevention of hearing impairment. The scope of audiological practice also includes such diverse areas as the evaluation of the vestibular system, noise assessment, and occupational and environmental hearing conservation; and a number of audiologists are involved in the physiological monitoring of various neurological functions during surgical procedures.

Similar to other respected professions, the proper education and training is necessary before individuals can practice audiology or call themselves audiologists. A person who is properly trained and entitled to practice the profession of audiology is identified by the Certificate of Clinical Competence in Audiology (CCC-A) issued by the American Speech-Language-Hearing Association (ASHA) and/or a state license in audiology. The designation Fellow of the American Academy of Audiology (FAAA) is granted by the American Academy of Audiology, and presupposes that the person is already ASHA certified and/or state licensed. The minimum training requirements for a career in audiology are in the midst of an evolutionary process which reflects rapidly unfolding advances in the profession. The current entry level requirements for the practice of audiology include a masters degree, a year of supervised postgraduate clinical experience called the Clinical Fellowship Year, and the successful completion of a nationally standardized examination. However, the required amount of graduate coursework will increase beginning in 2007; and as of 2012, the minimum requirements will include a doctoral degree, such as the Au.D., which stands for Doctor of Audiology, or the more familiar Ph.D.

Introductory audiology is an essential and fundamental aspect of the education of all students who are interested in the two related professions of speech-language pathology and audiology. This book is primarily intended to serve as a comprehensive introductory text for students who are preparing to enter both of these fields. As such, it attempts to address the needs of two rather different groups of students. Those who will follow the audiology route need a broad overview of the field and a firm understanding of its many basic principles so that they have a solid foundation for subsequent audiological training and clinical practice. The audiological needs of future speech-language pathologists are just as important, and go well beyond having the ability to understand audiological reports. Not only do speech-language pathologists often find themselves working hand-in-hand with their audiological colleagues; they also need to conduct certain audiological procedures themselves, especially where screening applications are involved; and they regularly make interpretations and referrals that are of audiological relevance. Moreover, speech-language pathologists often deal directly with hearing-impaired patients on an ongoing basis, and they frequently must explain the nature and management of auditory disorders to family members, teachers, and other professionals. This is especially true in school settings and long-term care facilities. What's more, cochlear implant and other multidisciplinary programs are enhancing the scope and depth of interactions among speech-language pathologists and audiologists, and are making a knowledge and understanding of audiology all the more important for budding speech-language pathologists. With considerations like these in mind, I hope that students who become speech-language pathologists will find this text useful as a reference source long after their audiology courses have been completed. (Of course, it would be less than forthright for me not to admit harboring the desire that at least a few speech-language pathology students will be attracted to a career in audiology by what they read here.)

This textbook attempts to provide a comprehensive overview of audiology at the introductory level; including such topics as acoustics, anatomy and physiology, sound perception, auditory disorders and the nature of hearing impairment, methods of measurement, screening, clinical assessment, and clinical management. It is mainly intended to serve as the core text for undergraduate speech and hearing students, and also to serve the needs of beginning level graduate students who need to learn or review the fundamentals of audiology. It is anticipated that the material will be covered in a one, two, or three term undergraduate sequence, depending on the curriculum at a given college or university. With these considerations in mind, I have tried to prepare a textbook that is extensive enough for professors to pick and choose material that provides the right depth and scope of coverage for a particular course. For example, text readings can be assigned to cover clinical masking at almost any level from simple to complex by selecting sections of Chapter 9. It is unlikely that all of that chapter will be assigned in a single undergraduate class. However, the material is there if needed for further study, to provide the groundwork for a term-paper or independent study report, or for future reference. Relatively extensive reference lists are provided for similar reasons.

The principal reasons for this second edition are to provide the beginning student with an up-to-date coverage of a field that is steadily developing, as well as to take advantage of experience to improve upon what is included and how it is presented. Many developments and changes have taken place in the few years since the first edition was introduced. Most of them are the slow and subtle—albeit important—advancements that occur over time in an active clinical science. Others have to do with changes in guidelines, expert position papers, and standards and regulations that affect clinical practices and technical matters. Then there are the astounding advances, such as the ones we have been seeing in areas like universal infant screening, early intervention, hearing aids, and cochlear implants. It often seems as though important changes are destined to occur just after a book is printed. Of course, this is one of the things that makes audiology so interesting.

Preparations to write the first edition of this text involved soliciting the opinions of many audiologists involved in clinical practice, teaching, and student supervision. Even greater effort was given to obtaining the insights of speech and hearing students who were taking, or recently completed, introductory audiology courses. The content and especially the style of the text was substantially influenced by this advice. A similar approach was used to prepare this second edition, concentrating on the reactions and suggestions of colleagues and students who used the first edition. The overall impact of these comments was to include updates and improvements to the text in a way that retains the fundamental character and approach of the original version. For example, the writing style has been kept as conversational and informal as possible; only classroom-proven examples and drawings are included; topics like clinical masking, acoustic immittance, and screening are covered in separate chapters; and the history of audiology has been omitted. The regular use of gender-specific terminology ("he," "she," "him," "her," etc.)—originally undertaken with great trepidation—has been very well received and has been continued. Its purpose is to maximize clarity for the benefit of the reader. The alternative was longer phrases and a more formal style, and would have detracted from the goal of providing the student with a textbook that is maximally reader-friendly (or at least minimally unfriendly). In addition, this style makes it possible to use different sexes for the clinician and patient when describing clinical procedures and interactions, which makes the material considerably easier to follow. Gender fairness is maintained by referring to both genders more-or-less equally throughout the text.

This book would not exist without the influence of many very special people. I am particularly indebted to my colleagues and students in the Department of Linguistics and Communication Disorders at Queens College, and the Doctoral Program in Speech and Hearing Sciences at the Graduate School of the City University of New York. I would also like to express my appreciation to the staff of Thieme Medical Publishers, who have been so helpful, cooperative, and supportive throughout the process of preparing this book, in spite of its demanding and dyslexic author. With sincere apologies to anyone inadvertently omitted, I am grateful to the following people for their influence, insights, advice, encouragement, assistance, support, and friendship: Moe Bergman, Arthur Boothroyd, Helen Cairns, Joseph Danto, Diane Ersepke, Lillian and Sol Gelfand, Phyllis Gold, Irving Hochberg, Gertrude and Oscar Katzen, Barbara Kurman, Harry Levitt, Ross Lumpkin, John Lutolf, Maurice Miller, Arlene Neuman, Neil Piper, Diane Sardini, Brian Scanlan, Teresa Schwander, Andrea Seils, Shlomo Silman, Carol Silverman, David Stewart, Helen, Harris and Gabe Topel, Anne Vinnicombe, Barbara Weinstein, and Mark Weiss.

Finally, my greatest appreciation is expressed to my wife and best friend, Janice, and our wonderful children, Michael, Joshua, and Jessica. Their love, encouragement, support, patience, and tolerance always exceed what can be imagined; and they make all the work worthwhile.

Stanley A. Gelfand

Acoustics and Sound Measurement

We begin our study of audiology by reviewing the nature of sound because, after all, sound is what we hear. The science of sound is called **acoustics**, which is a branch of physics, and relies on a number of basic physical principles.

Physical Quantities

The basic physical quantities are mass, time, and length (or distance). All other physical quantities are derived by combining these three basic ones, as well as other derived quantities, in a variety of ways. The principal basic and derived quantities are summarized in Table 1–1. These basic quantities are expressed in terms of conventional units that are measurable and repeatable. The unit of **mass (M)** is the **kilogram (kg)** or the **gram (g)**; the unit of **length (L)** is the **meter (m)** or the **centimeter (cm)**; and the unit of **time (t)** is the **second (sec or s)**. Mass is not really synonymous with weight even though we express its magnitude in kilograms. The mass of a body is related to its density, but its weight is related to the force of gravity. If two objects are the same size, the one with greater density will weigh more. However, even though an object's mass would be identical on the earth and the moon, it would weigh less on the moon where there is less gravity.

When we express mass in kilograms and length in meters, we are using the meter-kilogram-second or **MKS** system. Expressing mass in grams and length in centimeters constitutes the centimeter-gram-second or **cgs** system. These two systems also have differ-ent derived quantities. For example, the units of force and work are called newtons and joules in the MKS system, and dynes and ergs in the cgs system, respectively. We will emphasize the use of MKS units because this is the internationally accepted standard in the scientific community, known as the **System Internationale (SI)**. Equivalent cgs values will often be given as well because the audiology profession has traditionally worked in cgs units, and the death of old habits is slow and labored. These quantities are summarized with equivalent values in MKS and cgs units in Table 1–1. In addition, the correspondence between scientific notation and conventional numbers, and the meanings of prefixes used to describe the sizes of metric units are shown for convenience and ready reference in Tables 1–2 and 1–3.

Quantities may be scalars or vectors. A **scalar** can be fully described by its magnitude (amount or size), but a **vector** has both direction and magnitude. For example, length is a scalar because an object that is one meter long is always one meter long. However, we are dealing with a vector when we measure the distance between two coins that are one meter apart because their relationship has both magnitude and direction (from point x_1, to point x_2). This quantity is called **displacement (d)**. Derived quantities will be vectors if they have one or more components that are vectors; for example, velocity is a vector because it is derived from displacement, and acceleration is a vector because it involves velocity. We distinguish between scalars and vectors because they are handled differently when calculations are being made.

TABLE 1–1   Principal Physical Quantities

Quantity	Formula	MKS (SI Units)	cgs Units	Comments
Mass (M)	M	kilogram (kg)	gram (g)	$1 \text{ kg} = 10^3 \text{ g}$
Time (t)	t	second (s)	sec *or* s	
Area (A)	A	m^2	cm^2	$1 \text{ m}^2 = 10^4 \text{ cm}^2$
Displacement (d)	d	meter (m)	centimeter (cm)	$1 \text{ m} = 10^2 \text{ cm}$
Velocity (v)	$v = d/t$	m/s	cm/s	$1 \text{ m/s} = 10^2 \text{ cm/s}$
Acceleration (a)	$a = v/t$	m/s^2	cm/s^2	$1 \text{ m/s}^2 = 10^2 \text{ cm/s}^2$
Force (F)	$F = Ma$ $= Mv/t$	$kg \cdot m/s^2$ newton (N)	$g \cdot cm/s^2$ dyne	$1 \text{ N} = 10^5 \text{ dyne}$
Pressure (p)	$p = F/A$	N/m^2 pascal (Pa)	$dyne/cm^2$ microbar (μbar)	$2 \times 10^{-5} \text{ N/m}^2$ *or* μPa (reference value) $2 \times 10^{-4} \text{ dyne/cm}^2$ *or* μbar (reference value)
Work (W)	$W = Fd$	$N \cdot m$ joule	$dyne \cdot cm$ erg	$1 \text{ joule} = 10^7$
Power (P)	$P = W/t$ $= Fd/t$ $= Fv$	joule/s watt (w)	erg/s watt (w)	$1 \text{ w} = 1 \text{ joule/s}$ $= 10^7 \text{ erg/s}$
Intensity (I)	$I = P/A$	w/m^2	w/cm^2	10^{-12} w/m^2 (reference value) 10^{-16} w/cm^2 (reference value)

Velocity   Everyone knows that "55 miles per hour" refers to the speed of a car that causes it to travel a distance of 55 miles in a one-hour period of time. This is an example of **velocity (v)**, which is equal to the amount of displacement (d) that occurs over time (t):

$$v = \frac{d}{t}.$$

Displacement is measured in meters and time is measured in seconds (sec); thus, velocity is expressed in *meters per second (m/sec)*. Velocity is the vector equivalent of speed because it is based on displacement, which has both magnitude and direction. When we take a trip we usually figure out the distance traveled by making a mental note of the starting odometer reading and then subtracting it from the odometer reading at the destination (e.g., if we start at 10,422 miles and arrive at 10,443 miles, then the distance must have been 10,443 − 10,422 = 21 miles). We do the same thing to calculate the time it took to make the trip (e.g., if we left at 1:30 and arrived at 2:10, then the trip must have taken 2:10 − 1:30 = 40 minutes). Physical calculations involve the same straightforward approach. When an object is displaced, it starts at point x_1 and

time t_1 and arrives at point x_2 and time t_2. Its *average velocity* is simply the distance traveled $(x_2 - x_1)$ divided by the time it took to make the trip $(t_2 - t_1)$:

$$v = \frac{x_2 - x_1}{t_2 - t_1}.$$

TABLE 1–2   Expressing Numbers in Standard Notation and Scientific Notation

Standard Notation	Scientific Notation
0.000001	10^{-6}
0.00001	10^{-5}
0.0001	10^{-4}
0.001	10^{-3}
0.01	10^{-2}
0.1	10^{-1}
1	10^0
10	10^1
100	10^2
1,000	10^3
10,000	10^4
100,000	10^5
1,000,000	10^6
3,600	3.6×10^3
0.036	3.6×10^{-2}
0.0002	2×10^{-4}
0.00002	2×10^{-5}

TABLE 1–3   Examples of Prefixes Used to Express Metric Units

Prefix	Symbol	Definition	Multiply by	
			Standard Notation	Scientific Notation
micro	μ	millionths	1/1,000,000 *or* 0.000001	10^{-6}
milli	m	thousandths	1/1,000 *or* 0.001	10^{-3}
centi	c	hundredths	1/100 *or* 0.01	10^{-2}
deci	d	tenths	1/10 *or* 0.1	10^{-1}
deka	da	tens	10	10^{1}
hecto	h	hundreds	100	10^{2}
kilo	k	thousands	1,000	10^{3}
mega	M	millions	1,000,000	10^{6}

The term *instantaneous velocity* describes the velocity of a body at a *particular moment* in time. For the math-minded, it refers to the velocity when the displacement and time between one point and the next one approach zero, that is, the derivative of displacement with respect to time:

$$v = \frac{dx}{dt}.$$

Acceleration   Driving experience has taught us all that a car increases its speed to get onto a highway, slows down when exiting, and also slows down while making a turn. "Speeding up" and "slowing down" mean that the velocity is changing over time. The change of velocity over time is **acceleration (a)**. Suppose a body is moving between two points. Its velocity at the first point is v_1, and the time at that point is t_1. Similarly, its velocity at the second point is v_2 and the time at that point is t_2. *Average acceleration* is the difference between the two velocities $(v_2 - v_1)$ divided by the time interval $(t_2 - t_1)$:

$$a = \frac{v_2 - v_1}{t_2 - t_1}.$$

In more general terms, acceleration is written simply as

$$a = \frac{v}{t}.$$

Because velocity is the same as displacement divided by time, we can replace v with d/t, so that

$$a = \frac{d/t}{t},$$

which can be simplified to

$$a = \frac{d}{t^2}.$$

Consequently acceleration is expressed in units of *meters per second squared (m/sec^2)* in the MKS system. When measurements are made in cgs units, acceleration is expressed in centimeters per second squared (cm/sec^2).

Acceleration at a given moment is called *instantaneous acceleration*, and quantitatively oriented readers should note it is equal to the derivative of velocity with respect to time, or

$$a = \frac{dv}{dt}.$$

Because velocity is the first derivative of displacement, we find that acceleration is the second derivative of displacement:

$$a = \frac{d^2x}{dt^2}.$$

Force   An object that is sitting still will not move unless some outside influence causes it to do so, and an object that is moving will continue moving at the same speed unless some outside influence does something to change it. This commonsense statement is Newton's first law of motion. It describes the attribute of **inertia**, which is the property of mass to continue doing what it is already doing. The "outside influence" that makes a stationary object move, or causes a moving object to change its speed or direction, is called **force (F)**. Notice that force causes the moving object to change velocity or the motionless object to move, which is also a change in velocity (from zero to some amount). Recall that a change of velocity is acceleration. Hence, force is that influence (conceptually a "push" or "pull") that causes a mass to be accelerated. In effect, the amount of "push" or "pull" needed depends on how much mass you want to influence and the amount of acceleration you are trying to produce. In other words, force is equal to the product of mass times acceleration:

$$F = Ma.$$

Recalling that acceleration is the same as velocity over time (v/t), we can also specify force in the form:

$$F = \frac{Mv}{t}.$$

The quantity Mv is called **momentum**, so we may also say that force equals momentum over time.

The amount of force is measured in $kg \cdot m/s^2$ because force is equal to the product of mass (measured in kg) and acceleration (measured in m/s^2). The *unit of force* is the **newton (N)**, where one newton is the amount of force needed to cause a 1-kg mass to be accelerated by $1 \, m/s^2$, hence, $1 \, N = 1 \, kg \cdot m/s^2$. (This might seem very technical, but it really simplifies matters; after all, it is easier to say "one newton" than "one $kg \cdot m/s^2$"). It would take a 2-N force to cause a 1-kg mass to be accelerated by 2 m/s^2, or a 2-kg mass to be accelerated by $1 \, m/s^2$. A 4-N force is needed to accelerate a 2-kg mass by 2 m/s^2, and a 63-N force is needed to accelerate a 9-kg mass by 7 m/s^2. In the cgs system, the unit of force is called the **dyne**, which is the force needed to accelerate a 1-g mass by 1 cm/s^2; that is, 1 dyne = $1 \, g \cdot cm/s^2$. It takes 10^5 dynes to equal 1 newton.

Many different forces are usually acting upon an object at the same time. Hence, the force we have been referring to so far is actu-ally the **net** or **resultant force**, that is, the "bottom line" effect of all the forces that act upon an object. If a force of 3 N is pushing an object toward the right and a second force of 8 N is also pushing that object toward the right, then the net force would be 3 + 8 = 11 N toward the right. In other words, if two forces push a body in the same direction, then the net force would be the sum of those two forces. Conversely, if a 4-N force pushes an object toward the right at the same time that a 9-N force pushes it toward the left, then the net force is 9 − 4 = 5 N toward the left. Thus, if two forces push an object in opposite directions, then the net force is the difference between the two opposing forces, and it causes the object to accelerate in the direction of the greater force. If two *equal* forces push in *opposite* directions, then the net force is zero. Because the net force is zero it will not cause the motion of the object to change. The situation in which net force is zero is called **equilibrium**. In this case, a moving object will continue moving and an object that is **at rest** (i.e., not moving) will continue to remain still.

Friction   When an object is moving in the real world, it tends to slow down and eventually comes to a halt. For example, a bicycle that has been moving very quickly will slow down and stop if the rider allows it to coast in "neutral" on a level road. This happens because anything that is moving in the real world is always in contact with other bodies or mediums. For example, the coasting bicycle is in contact with the surrounding air and the roadway; in addition, its own parts (e.g., a wheel and axle) are sliding on each other. The sliding of one body on the other constitutes a force that opposes the motion, called **resistance** or **friction**.

The opposing force of friction or resistance depends on two parameters. The first factor is that the amount of friction depends on the nature of the materials that are sliding on one another. Simply stated, the amount of friction between two given objects is greater for "rough" materials than for "smooth" or "slick" ones, and is expressed as a quantity called the *coefficient of friction*. The second factor that determines how much friction occurs is easily appreciated by rubbing the palms of your hands back and forth on each other. First rub slowly and then more rapidly. The rubbing will produce heat, which occurs because friction causes some of the mechanical energy to be converted into heat. This notion will be revisited later, but for now we will use the amount of heat as an indicator of the amount of resistance. Your hands become hotter when they are rubbed together more quickly. This illustrates the notion that the amount of friction depends on the *velocity* of motion. In quantitative terms,

$$F = Rv,$$

where F is the force of friction, R is the coefficient of friction between the materials, and v is the velocity of the motion.

Elasticity and Restoring Force It takes some effort (an outside force) to compress or expand a spring; and the compressed or expanded spring will bounce back to its original shape after it is released. Compressing or expanding the spring is an example of deforming an object. The spring bouncing back to its prior shape is an example of elasticity. More formally, we can say that **elasticity** is the property whereby a deformed object returns to its original form. Notice the distinction between deformation and elasticity. A rubber band and saltwater taffy can both be stretched (deformed), but only the rubber band bounces back. In other words, what makes a rubber band *elastic* is not that it stretches, but rather that it bounces back. The more readily a deformed object returns to its original form, the more elastic (or stiff) it is.

We know from common experiences, such as using simple exercise equipment, that it is relatively easy to *begin* compressing a spring (e.g., a "grip exerciser"), but that it gets progressively harder to *continue* compressing it. Similarly, it is easier to *begin* expanding a spring (e.g., pulling apart the springs on a "chest exerciser") than it is to *continue* expanding it. In other words, the more a spring-

like material (an elastic element) is deformed, the more it *opposes* the applied force. The force that opposes the deformation of an elastic or spring-like material is known as the **restoring force**. If we think of deformation in terms of how far the spring has been compressed or expanded from its original position, we could also say that the restoring force increases with displacement. Quantitatively, then, restoring force (F_R) depends on the stiffness (S) of the material and the amount of its displacement as follows:

$$F_R = Sd.$$

Pressure Very few people can push a straight pin into a piece of wood, yet almost anyone can push a thumbtack into the same piece of wood. This is possible because a thumbtack is really a simple machine that concentrates the amount of force being exerted over a larger area (the head) down to a very tiny area (the point). In other words, force is affected by the size of the area over which it is applied in a way that constitutes a new quantity. This quantity, which is equal to force divided by area (A), is called **pressure (p)**, so

$$p = \frac{F}{A}.$$

Because force is measured in newtons and area is measured in square meters in MKS units, pressure is measured in newtons per square meter (N/m²). The unit of pressure is the **Pascal (Pa)**, so that 1 Pa = 1 N/m². In the cgs system, pressure is measured in dynes per square centimeter (dynes/cm²), occasionally referred to as **microbars (μbars)**.

Work and Energy As a physical concept, **work (W)** occurs when the force applied to a body results in its displacement, and the amount of work is equal to the product of the force and the displacement, or

$$W = Fd.$$

Because force is measured in newtons and displacement is measured in meters, work itself is quantified in newton-meters (N · m). For example, if a force of 2 newtons displaces a body by 3 meters, then the amount of work is $2 \times 3 = 6$ N · m. There can only be work if there is displacement. There cannot be work if there is no displacement (i.e., if $d = 0$) because work is the product of force and displacement, and zero times anything is zero. The MKS unit of work is the **joule (J)**. One joule is the amount of work that occurs when one newton of force effects one meter of displacement, or 1 J $= 1$ N · m. In the cgs system, the unit of work is called the erg, where 1 erg $= 1$ dyne · cm. One joule corresponds to 10^7 ergs.

Anyone who does crossword puzzles is aware that joules and ergs are also used with regard to an entity called energy. Hence, it is not surprising to find a close relationship between energy and work. Specifically, energy is defined as the capability to do work. The energy of a body at rest is **potential** energy and the energy of an object that is in motion is **kinetic** energy. The total energy of a body is the sum of its potential energy plus its kinetic energy, and work corresponds to the exchange between these two forms of energy. In other words, energy is not consumed when work is accomplished; it is converted from one form to the other. This principle is illustrated by the simple example of a swinging pendulum. The pendulum's potential energy is greatest when it reaches the extreme of its swing, where its motion is momentarily zero. On the other hand, the pendulum's kinetic energy is greatest when it passes through the midpoint of its swing because this is where it is moving the fastest. Between these two extremes, energy is being converted from potential to kinetic as the pendulum speeds up (on each down swing), and from kinetic to potential as the pendulum slows down (on each up swing).

Power   The rate at which work is done is called **power (P)**, so that power can be defined as work divided by time,

$$P = \frac{W}{t}.$$

The unit of power is called the **watt (w)**. One unit of power corresponds to one unit of work divided by one unit of time. Hence, one watt is equal to one joule divided by one second, or 1 w $= 1$ J/sec. Power is also expressed in watts in the cgs system, where work is measured in ergs. Since 1 J $= 10^7$ erg, we can also say that 1 w $= 10^7$ erg/sec.

Power can also be expressed in other terms. For example, because $W = Fd$, we can substitute Fd for W in the power formula, in order to arrive at

$$P = \frac{Fd}{t}.$$

We know that $v = d/t$, so we can substitute v for d/t and rewrite this formula as

$$P = Fv.$$

In other words, power is also equal to force times velocity.

Intensity   Consider a hypothetical demonstration in which one tablespoonful of oil is placed on the surface of a still pond. At that instant the entire amount of oil will occupy the space of a tablespoon. As time passes, the oil spreads out over an expanding area on the surface of the pond, and it therefore also thins out so that much less than all the oil will occupy the space of a tablespoon. The wider the oil spreads the more it thins out, and the proportion of the oil covering any given area gets smaller and smaller, even though the total amount of oil is the same. Clearly, there is a difference between the amount of oil, per se, and the concentration of the oil as it is distributed across (i.e., divided by) the surface area of the pond.

An analogous phenomenon occurs with sound. It is common knowledge that sound radiates outward in every direction from its source, constituting a sphere that gets bigger and bigger with increasing distance from the source, as illustrated by the concentric circles in Figure 1–1. Let us imagine that the sound source is a tiny pulsating object (at the center of the concentric circles in the figure), and that it produces a finite amount of power, anal-

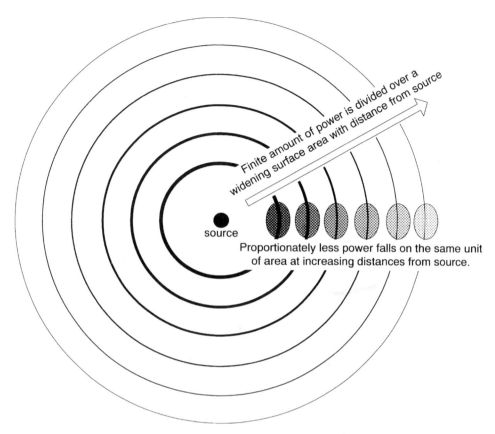

FIGURE 1–1 Intensity (power divided by area) decreases with distance from the sound source because a fixed amount of power is spread over an increasing area, represented by the thinning of the lines. Proportionately less power fans on the same unit area (represented by the lighter shading of the ovals) with increasing distance from the source.

ogous to the fixed amount of oil in the prior example. Consequently, the sound power will be divided over the ever-expanding surface as distance increases from the source, analogous to the thinning out of the widening oil slick. This notion is represented in the figure by the thinning of the lines at greater distances from the source. Suppose we measure how much power registers on a certain fixed amount of surface area (e.g., a square inch). As a result, a progressively smaller proportion of the original power falls onto a square inch as the distance from the source increases, represented in the figure by the lighter shading of the same-sized ovals at increasing distances from the source.

The examples just described reveal that a new quantity called **intensity (I)** develops when power is distributed over area. Specifically, intensity is equal to power per unit area, or power divided by area, or

$$I = \frac{P}{A}.$$

Because power is measured in watts and area is measured in square meters in the MKS system, intensity is expressed in watts per square meter (w/m^2). Intensity is expressed in watts per square centimeter (w/cm^2) in the cgs system.

Intensity decreases with increasing distance from a sound source according to a rule called the **inverse square law**. It states that the amount of intensity drops by one over the square of the change in distance. For example, doubling the distance from 1 meter to 2 meters causes the amount of intensity at 2 m to be 1/4 of what it was at 1 m (because $1/2^2 = 1/4$). Similarly, tripling the distance from 1 m to 3 m causes the intensity to fall to 1/9 of its prior value (because $1/3^2 = 1/9$).

The student has probably noticed that intensity and pressure are analogous concepts in the sense that intensity is power divided by area and pressure is force divided by area. An important relationship among these quantities is that power is equal to pressure squared,

$$P = p^2;$$

and pressure is equal to the square root of power,

$$p = \sqrt{P}.$$

In addition, intensity is proportional to pressure squared

$$I \propto p^2;$$

and pressure is proportional to the square root of intensity

$$p \propto \sqrt{I}.$$

This simple relationship makes it easy to convert between sound intensity and sound pressure, as we shall see.

The Nature of Sound

Sound is often defined as a form of vibration that propagates through the air in the form of a wave. This is correct, but what does it mean? Let us break down this definition so that it can make some sense. **Vibration** is nothing more than the to-and-fro motion (oscillation) of an object. Some examples include a playground swing, a pendulum, the floorboards under a washing machine, a guitar string, a tuning-fork prong, and air molecules. The vibration is usually called sound when it is transferred from air particle

to air particle (we will see how this happens later). The vibration air particles might have a simple pattern such as the tone produced by a tuning fork, or a very complex pattern such as the din heard in a school cafeteria. Most naturally occurring sounds are very complex, but the easiest way to understand sound is to concentrate on the simplest ones.

Simple Harmonic Motion

A vibrating tuning fork is illustrated in Figure 1–2. The initial force that was applied by striking the tuning fork is represented by the heavy arrow in frame 1. The progression of the drawings represents the motion of the prongs at selected points in time after the fork has been activated. Both prongs vibrate

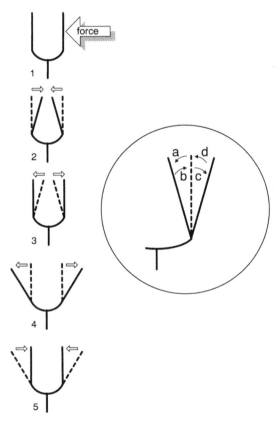

FIGURE 1–2 After being struck, a tuning fork vibrates or oscillates with a simple pattern that repeats itself over time. One replication (cycle) of this motion is illustrated going from frames 1 to 5. The arrows in the insert highlight the motion of one of the prongs.

as mirror images of each other, so that we can describe what is happening in terms of just one prong. The *insert* highlights the motion of the right prong. Here the center position is where the prong would be at rest. When the fork is struck the prong is forced inward as shown by arrow **a**. After reaching the leftmost position it bounces back (arrow **b**), accelerating along the way. The rapidly moving prong overshoots the center and continues rightward (arrow **c**). It slows down along the way until it stops for an instant at the extreme right, where it reverses direction again and starts moving toward the left (arrow **d**) at an ever-increasing speed. It overshoots the center again, and as before, the prong now follows arrow **a**, slowing down until it stops momentarily at the extreme left. Here it reverses direction again and repeats the same process over and over again. One complete round trip (or replication) of an oscillating motion is called a **cycle**. The number of cycles that occur in one second is called **frequency**.

This form of motion occurs when a force is applied to an object having the properties of inertia and elasticity. Due to its elasticity, the deformation of the fork caused by the applied force is opposed by a restoring force. In the figure the initial leftward force is opposed by a restoring force in the opposite direction, that is, toward the right. The rightward restoring force increases as the prong is pushed progressively toward the left. As a result, the movement of the prong slows down and eventually stops. Under the influence of its elasticity the prong now reverses direction and starts moving rightward. As the restoring force brings the prong back toward the center, we must also consider its mass. Because the prong has mass, inertia causes it to accelerate as it moves back toward its center resting position. In fact, the prong is moving at its maximum speed as it passes through the resting position. The force of inertia causes the prong to overshoot the center and continue moving rightward. The deformation process begins again once the prong overshoots its resting position. As a result, opposing elastic restoring forces

start building up again, now in the leftward direction. Just as before, the increasing (leftward) restoring force eventually overcomes the rightward inertial force, thereby stopping the prong's displacement at the rightmost point, and causing a reversal in the direction of its movement. Hence, the same course of events is repeated again, this time in the leftward direction; then rightward, then leftward, etc., over and over again. This kind of vibration is called **simple harmonic motion (SHM)** because the oscillations repeat themselves at the same rate over and over again.

We know from experience that the oscillations just described do not continue forever. Instead, they dissipate over time and eventually die out completely. The dying-out of vibrations over time is called **damping**, and it occurs due to resistance or friction. Resistance occurs because the vibrating prong is always in contact with the surrounding air. As a result, there will be friction between the oscillating metal and the surrounding air molecules. This friction causes some of the mechanical energy that has been supporting the motion of the tuning fork to be converted into heat. In turn, the energy that has been converted into heat is no longer available to maintain the vibration of the tuning fork. Consequently, the sizes of the oscillations dissipate and eventually die out altogether.

A diagram summarizing the concepts just described is shown in Figure 1–3. The curve in the figure represents the tuning fork's motion. The amount of displacement of the tuning fork prong around its resting (or center) position is represented by distance above and below the horizontal line. These events are occurring over time, which is represented by horizontal distance (from left to right). The initial displacement of the prong due to the original applied force is represented by the dotted segment of the curve. Inertial forces due to the prong's mass and elastic restoring forces due to the elasticity of the prong are represented by labeled arrows. Damping of the oscillations due to friction is shown by the decline in the displacement of the curve as time goes on. The curve in

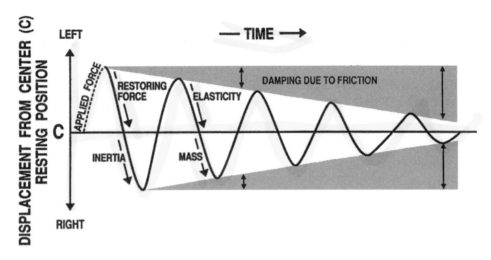

FIGURE 1–3   Diagrammatic representation of tuning fork oscillations over time. Vertical displacement represents the amount of the tuning fork prong displacement around its resting position. Distance from left to right represents the progression of time. From Gelfand (1998), p. 13, by courtesy of Marcel Dekker, Inc.

this diagram is an example of a **waveform**, which is a graph that shows displacement (or another measure of magnitude) as a function of time.

Sound Waves

Tuning fork vibrations produce sound because the oscillations of the prongs are transmitted to the surrounding air particles. When the tuning fork prong moves to the right, it displaces air molecules to its right in the same direction. These molecules are thus displaced to the right of their own resting positions. Displacing air molecules toward the right pushes them closer to the air particles to their right. The pressure that exists among air molecules that are not being disturbed by a driving force (like the tuning fork) is known as *ambient* or *atmospheric pressure*. We can say that the rightward motion of the tuning fork prong exerts a force on the air molecules that pushes them together relative to their undisturbed, resting situation. In other words, forcing the air molecules together causes an increase in air pressure relative to the ambient pressure that existed among the undisturbed molecules. This state of positive air pressure is called **compression**. The amount of compression

increases as the prong continues displacing the air molecules rightward. A maximum amount of positive pressure occurs when the prong and air molecules reach their greatest rightward displacement.

The tuning fork prong then reverses direction, overshoots its resting position, and proceeds to its leftmost position. The compressed air molecules reverse direction along with the prong. This occurs because air is an elastic medium, so the particles compressed to the right develop a leftward restoring force. Small as they are, air particles do have mass. Therefore, inertia causes the rebounding air particles to overshoot their resting positions and to continue toward their extreme leftward positions. As the particles move leftward, the amount of compression decreases and is momentarily zero as they pass through their resting positions. As they continue to move to the left of their resting positions, the particles are now becoming increasingly further from the molecules to their right (compared to when they are in their resting positions). We now say that the air particles are rarefied compared to their resting states, so that the air pressure is now below atmospheric pressure. This state of lower than ambient pressure is called

rarefaction. When the air particles reach the leftmost position they are maximally rarefied, which means that the pressure is maximally negative. At this point, the restoring force instigates a rightward movement of the air molecules. This movement is enhanced by the push of the tuning fork prongs that have also reversed direction. The air molecules now accelerate rightward, so that the amount of rarefaction decreases, overshoot their resting positions, and continue to the right, and so on. The tuning fork vibrations have now been transmitted to the surrounding particles, which are now also oscillating in simple harmonic motion. Sounds that are associated with simple harmonic motion are called **pure tones**.

Let us consider one of the air molecules that has already been set into harmonic motion by the tuning fork. This air particle now vibrates to-and-fro in the same direction that was originally imposed by the vibrating prong. When this particle moves toward its right it will cause a similar displacement of the particle that is located there. The subsequent leftward motion is also transmitted to the next particle, etc. Thus, the oscillations of one air particle are transmitted to the molecule next to it. The second particle is therefore set into oscillation, which in turn initiates oscillation of the next one, and so forth down the line. In other words, each particle vibrates back and forth around its own resting point, and causes successive molecules to vibrate back and forth around their own resting points, as shown schematically in Figure 1–4. Notice that each molecule vibrates "in place" around its own average position; it is the vibratory pattern that is transmitted through the air.

This propagation of vibratory motion from particle to particle constitutes the sound wave. This wave appears as alternating compressions and rarefactions radiating from

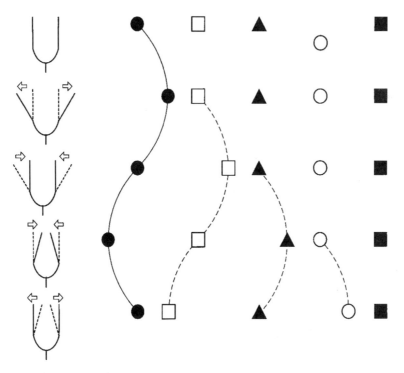

FIGURE 1–4 Sound is initiated by transmitting the vibratory pattern of the sound source to nearby air particles, and then the vibratory pattern is passed from particle to particle as a wave. Notice how it is the pattern of vibration that is being transmitted, whereas each particle oscillates around its own average location.

the sound source in all directions, as already suggested in Figure 1–1. The transmission of particle motion along with the resulting variations in air pressure with distance from the source are represented in Figure 1–5. Most people are more familiar with the kinds of waves that develop on the surface of a pond when a pebble is dropped into the water. These are **transverse waves** because the particles are moving at right angles to the direction that the wave is propagating. That is, the water particles oscillate up and down (vertically) even though the wave moves out horizontally from the spot where the pebble hit the water. This principle can be demonstrated by floating a cork in a pool, and then dropping a pebble in the water to start a wave. The floating cork reflects the motions of the water particles. The wave will move out horizontally, but the floating cork bobs up and down (vertically) at right angles to the wave. In contrast, sound waves are **longitudinal waves** because each air particle oscillates in the same direction in which the wave is propagating (Fig. 1–5). Although sound waves are longitudinal, it is more convenient to draw them with a transverse rep-

resentation, as in Figure 1–5. In such a diagram the vertical dimension represents some measure of the size of the signal (e.g., displacement, pressure, etc.), and left to right distance represents time (or distance). For example, the waveform in Figure 1–5 shows the amount of positive pressure (compression) above the baseline, negative pressure (rarefaction) below the baseline, and distance horizontally going from left to right.

The Sinusoidal Function

Simple harmonic motion (SHM) is also known as **sinusoidal motion**, and has a waveform that is called a **sinusoidal wave** or a **sine wave**. Let us see why. Figure 1–6 shows one cycle of a sine wave in the center, surrounded by circles labeled to correspond to points on the wave. Each circle shows a horizontal line corresponding to the horizontal baseline on the sine wave, as well as a radius line (r) that will move around the circle at a fixed speed, much like a clock hand but in a counterclockwise direction.

Point **a** on the waveform in the center of the figure can be viewed as the "starting

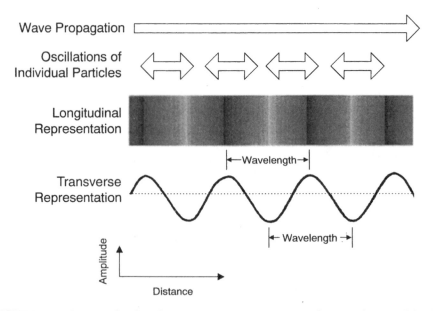

FIGURE 1–5 Longitudinal and transverse representations of a sound wave. Wavelength (λ) is the distance covered by one replication (cycle) of a wave, and is most easily visualized as the distance from one peak to the next.

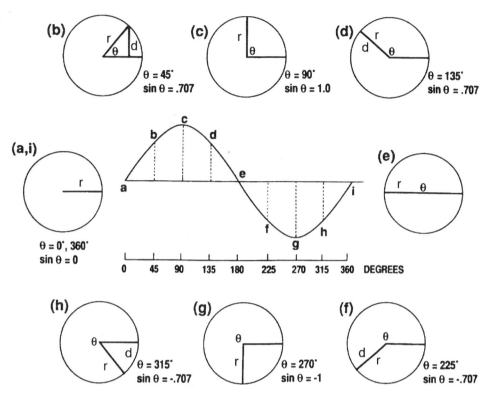

FIGURE 1–6 Sinusoidal motion (θ, phase angle; d, displacement). Adapted from Gelfand (1998), p. 17, by courtesy of Marcel Dekker, Inc.

point" of the cycle. The displacement here is zero because this point is *on* the horizontal line. The radius appears as shown in circle **b** when it reaches 45° of rotation, which corresponds to point **b** on the sine wave. The angle between the radius and the horizontal is called the **phase angle (θ)**, and is a handy way to tell location going around the circle and on the sine wave. In other words, we consider one cycle (one "round trip" of oscillation) to be the same as going around a circle one time. Just as a circle has 360°, we also consider one cycle to have 360°. Since 45/360 = 1/8, a phase angle (θ) of 45° is the same as one-eighth of the way around a circle or one-eighth of the way into a sine wave. Returning to the circle, the vertical displacement from the horizontal to the point where r intersects the circle is represented by a vertical line labeled **d**. This vertical line corresponds to the displacement of point **b** on the sine wave, where the displacement of the air particle is represented by the height of the point above

the baseline. Notice that we now have a right triangle in the circle, where r is the hypotenuse, θ is an angle, and d is the leg opposite that angle. Recall from high school math that the sine of an angle equals the length of the opposite leg over the length of the hypotenuse. Here, $\sin θ = d/r$. If we conveniently assume that the length of r is 1, then displacement d becomes the sine of angle θ, which happens to be 0.707. In other words, displacement is determined by the sine of the phase angle, and displacement at any point on the sine wave corresponds to the sine of θ. This is why it is called a sine wave.

The peak labeled **c** on the sine wave corresponds to circle **c**, where the rotating radius has reached the straight-up position. We are now one-fourth of the way into the wave and one-fourth of the way around the circle. Here, θ = 90° and the displacement is the largest it can be (notice that d = r on the circle). Continuing the counterclockwise rotation of r causes the amount of displacement from the horizontal to decrease, exemplified by point **d** on the sine wave and circle **d**, where θ is 135°. The oscillating air particle has already reversed direction and is now moving back toward the resting position. When it reaches the resting position there is again no displacement, as shown by point **e** on the sine wave and by the fact that r is now superimposed on the horizontal at θ = 180° in circle **e**. Notice that 180° is one-half of the 360° round trip, so we are now halfway around the circle and halfway into the cycle of SHM. In addition, displacement is zero at this location (180°).

Continuing the rotation of r places it in the lower left quadrant of circle **f**, corresponding to point **f** on the wave, where θ = 225°. The oscillating particle has overshot its resting position and the displacement is now increasing in the other direction, so that we are in the rarefaction part of the wave. Hence, displacement is now drawn in the negative direction, indicating rarefaction. The largest negative displacement is reached at point **g** on the wave, where θ = 270°, corresponding to circle **g** in which r points straight down.

The air particle now begins moving in the positive direction again on its way back toward the resting position. At point **h** and circle **h** the displacement in the negative direction has become smaller as the rotating radius passes through the point where θ = 315° (point **h** on the wave and circle **h**). The air particle is again passing through its resting position at point **i**, having completed one round trip or 360° of rotation. Here, displacement is again zero. Having completed exactly one cycle, 360° corresponds to 0°, and circle **i** is the same one previously used as circle **a**.

Recall that r rotates around the circle at a fixed speed. Hence, how fast r is moving will determine how many degrees are covered in a given amount of time. For example, if one complete cycle of rotation takes 1 second, then 360° is covered in 1 second; 180° is covered in 1/2 second; 90° takes

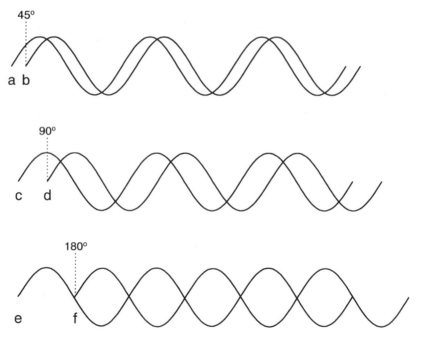

FIGURE 1–7 Each frame shows two waves that are identical in every way except they are displaced from one another in terms of phase. Waves **a** and **b** are 45° apart, waves **c** and **d** are displaced from one another by 90°, and waves **e** and **f** are 180° apart. (The dotted vertical guidelines are referred to in the text.)

1/4 second; 270° takes 3/4 second, etc. Hence, the phase angle also reflects the elapsed time from the onset of rotation. This is why the horizontal axis in Figure 1–6 can be labeled in terms of phase. As such, the phase of the wave at each of the points indicated in Figure 1–6 is 0° at **a**, 45° at **b**, 90° at **c**, 135° at **d**, 180° at **e**, 225° at **f**, 270° at **g**, 315° at **h**, and 360° at **i**, which is also 0° for the next cycle.

Phase is often used to express relationships between two waves that are displaced relative to each other, as in Figure 1–7. Waves **a** and **b** are identical except that they do not line up exactly along the horizontal (time) axis. Notice that wave **b** is displaced from wave **a** so that wave **a** is at 45° at the same time that **b** is at 0° (shown by the dotted vertical guideline in the figure). In other words, waves **a** and **b** are 45° apart or *out-of-phase*. Similarly, waves **c** and **d** are displaced from each other by 90° because wave **c** is at 90° when wave **d** is at 0° (at the dotted vertical guideline). Hence, **c** and **d** are 90° out-of-phase. Waves **e** and **f** are 180° out-of-phase. Here, wave **e** is at its 90° (positive) peak at the same time that wave **f** is at its 270° (negative) peak. The difference between them is 270° − 90° = 180° Notice that these two otherwise identical waves are exact mirror images of each other when they are 180° out-of-phase.

Parameters of Sound Waves

We now have enough information to outline the remaining principal parameters of sound waves. We already know that a **cycle** is one complete replication of a vibratory pattern. For example, two cycles are shown for each sine wave in the upper frame of Figure 1–8, and four cycles are shown for each sine wave in the lower frame. Each of the sine waves in this figure is said to be **periodic** because it repeats itself exactly over time. Sine waves are the simplest kind of periodic wave because simple harmonic motion is the simplest form of vibration. Later we will address complex periodic waves.

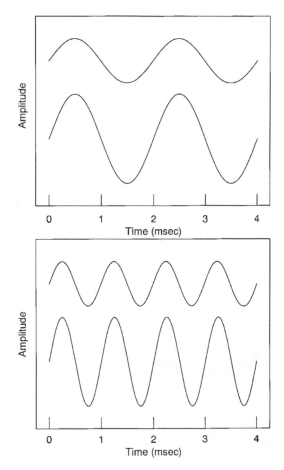

FIGURE 1–8   Each frame shows two sine waves that have the same frequency but different amplitudes. Compared to the upper frame, twice as many cycles occur in the same amount of time in the lower frame, thus the period is half as long and the frequency is twice as high.

The duration of one cycle is called its **period**. The period is expressed in time (t) because it refers to the amount of time that it takes to complete one cycle (i.e., how long it takes for one round trip). For example, a periodic wave that repeats itself every one-hundredth of a second has a period of 1/100 sec, or t = 0.01 sec. One-hundredth of a second is also ten-thousandths of a second (milliseconds), so we could also say that the period of this wave is 10 msec. Similarly, a wave that repeats itself every one-thousandth of a second has a period of 1 msec or 0.001 sec; and the period would be

2 msec or 0.002 sec if the duration of one cycle is two-thousandths of a second.

The number of times a waveform repeats itself in one second is its frequency (f), or the number of **cycles per second (cps)**. We could say that frequency is the number of cycles that can fit into one second. Frequency is expressed in units called **Hertz (Hz)**, which means the same thing as cycles per second. For example, a wave that is repeated 100 times per second has a frequency of 100 Hz; the frequency of a wave that has 500 cycles per second is 500 Hz; and a 1000 Hz wave has 1000 cycles in one second.

If frequency is the number of cycles that occur each second, and period is how much time it takes to complete one cycle, then frequency and period must be related in a very straightforward way. Let us consider the three examples that were just used to illustrate the relationship of period and frequency:

Period (t)	Frequency (f)
0.01 sec	100 Hz
0.002 sec	500 Hz
0.001 sec	1000 Hz

Now, notice the following relationships among these numbers:

1/100 = 0.01	and	1/0.01 = 100
1/500 = 0.002	and	1/0.002 = 500
1/1000 = 0.001	and	1/0.001 = 1000

In each case the period corresponds to 1 over the frequency, and the frequency corresponds to 1 over the period. In formal terms, frequency equals the reciprocal of period,

$$f = \frac{1}{t},$$

and period equals the reciprocal of frequency,

$$t = \frac{1}{f}.$$

Each wave in the upper frame of Figure 1–8 contains two cycles in 4 msec, and each wave in the lower frame contains four cycles in the 4 msec. If two cycles in the upper frame last 4

msec, then the duration of one cycle is 2 msec. Hence, the period of each wave in the upper frame is 2 msec (t = 0.002 sec), and the frequency is 1/0.002, or 500 Hz. Similarly, if four cycles last 4 msec in the lower frame, then one cycle has a period of 1 msec (t = 0.001), and the frequency is 1/0.001, or 1000 Hz.

Figure 1–8 also illustrates differences in the amplitude between waves. **Amplitude** denotes size or magnitude, such as the amount of its displacement, power, pressure, etc. The larger the amplitude at some point along the horizontal (time) axis, the greater its distance from zero on the vertical axis. With respect to the figure, each frame shows one wave that has a smaller amplitude and an otherwise identical wave that has a larger amplitude.

As illustrated in Figure 1–9, the **peak-to-peak amplitude** of a wave is the total vertical distance between its negative and positive peaks, and **peak amplitude** is the distance from the baseline to one peak. However, neither of these values reflects the overall, ongoing size of the wave because the amplitude is constantly changing. At any instant an oscillating particle may be at its most positive or most negative displacement from the resting position, or anywhere between these two extremes, including the resting position itself, where the displacement is zero. The magnitude of a sound at a given instant (**instantaneous amplitude**) is true only for that moment, and will be different at the next moment. Yet we are usually interested in a kind of "overall average" amplitude that reveals the magnitude of a sound wave throughout its cycles. A simple average of the positive and negative instantaneous amplitudes will not work because it will always be equal to zero. A different kind of overall measure is therefore used, called the **root-mean-square (RMS)** amplitude. Even though measurement instruments provide us with RMS amplitudes automatically, we can understand RMS by briefly reviewing the steps that would be used to calculate it manually: (1) All of the positive and negative values on the wave are squared, so that all values are positive (or zero for values on the resting position

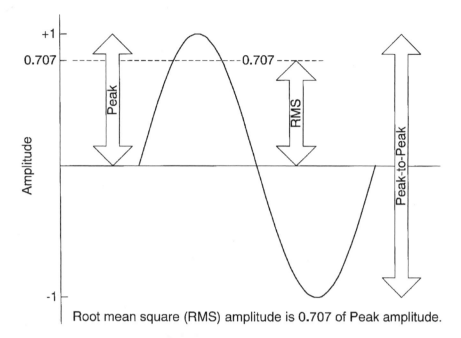

Root mean square (RMS) amplitude is 0.707 of Peak amplitude.

FIGURE 1–9   Peak, peak-to-peak, and root-mean-square (RMS) amplitude.

itself). (2) A mean (average) is calculated for the squared values. (3) This average of the squared values is then rescaled back to the "right size" by taking its square root. This is the RMS value. The RMS amplitude is numerically equal to 70.7% of (or 0.707 times) the peak amplitude (or 0.354 times peak-to-peak amplitude). Even though these values technically only apply to sinusoids, for practical purposes RMS values are used with all kinds of wave forms.

Referring back to Figure 1–5, we see that the distance covered by one cycle of a propagating wave is called its **wavelength (λ)**. We have all seen water waves, which literally appear as alternating crests and troughs on the surface of the water. Using this common experience as an example, wavelength is simply the distance between the crest of one wave and the crest of the next one. For sound, wavelength is the distance between one compression peak and the next one, or one rarefaction peak and the next one, that is, the distance between any two successive peaks in Figure 1–5. It is just as correct to use any other point, as long as we measure the distance between the same point on two suc-

cessive replications of the wave. The formula for wavelength is

$$\lambda = \frac{c}{f},$$

where f is the frequency of the sound and c is the speed of sound (about 344 m/sec in air). This formula indicates that wavelength is inversely proportional to frequency. Similarly, frequency is inversely proportional to wavelength:

$$f = \frac{c}{\lambda}.$$

These formulas show that wavelength and frequency are inversely proportional to each other. In other words, low frequencies have long wavelengths and high frequencies have short wavelengths.

Complex Waves

When two or more pure tones are combined, the result is called a complex wave. Complex waves may contain any number of frequencies from as few as two up to an infinite number of them. **Complex periodic waves** have waveforms that repeat themselves over time. If the waveform does not repeat itself over time, then it is an **aperiodic wave**.

COMBINING SINUSOIDS

The manner in which waveforms combine into more complex waveforms involves algebraically adding the amplitudes of the two waves to each other at every point along the horizontal (time) axis. Consider two sine waves that are to be added. Imagine that they are drawn one above the other on a piece of graph paper so that the gridlines can be used to identify similar moments in time (horizontally) for both waves, and their amplitudes can be determined by simply counting boxes vertically. The following exercise is done at every point along the horizontal time axis: (1) Determine the amplitude of each wave at that point by counting the boxes in the positive and/or negative direction. (2) Add these two amplitudes *algebraically* (e.g., +2 plus +2 is +4; −3 plus −3 is −6, and +4 plus −1 is +3, etc.). (3) Plot the algebraic sum just obtained on the graph paper at the same point along the horizontal time axis. After doing this for many points, drawing a smooth line through these points will reveal the combine wave.

Several examples of combining two sinusoids are illustrated in Figure 1–10. This figure shows what occurs when two sinusoids being combined have exactly the same frequencies and amplitudes. The two sinusoids being combined in Figure 1–10a are in phase with each other. Here, the combined wave looks like the two identical components, but has an amplitude twice as large. This case is often called complete **reinforcement** for obvious reasons. The addition of two otherwise identical waves that are 180° out-of-phase is illustrated in Figure 1–10b. In this case, the first wave is equal and opposite to the second wave at every moment in time, so that algebraic addition causes the resulting amplitude to be zero at every point along the horizontal (time) axis. The result is complete **cancellation**.

When the sinusoids being combined are identical but have a phase relationship that is any value other than 0° (in-phase) or 180° (opposite phase), then the appearance of the

resulting wave will depend on how the two components happen to line up in time. Figure 1–10c shows what happens when the two otherwise identical sinusoids are 90° out-of-phase. The result is a sinusoid with the same frequency as the two (similar) original waves but it differs in phase and amplitude.

COMPLEX PERIODIC WAVES

The principles used to combine any number of similar or dissimilar waves is basically the same as that just described for two similar waves: Their amplitudes are algebraically summed on a point-by-point basis along the horizontal (time) axis, regardless of their individual frequencies and amplitudes or their phase relationships. However, combin-

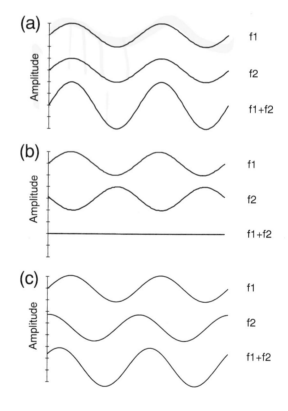

FIGURE 1–10 Combining sinusoids that have the same frequency and amplitude when they are (a) in-phase (showing complete reinforcement); (b) 180° out-of-phase (showing cancellation); (c) 90° out-of-phase.

ing unequal frequencies will not produce a sinusoidal result. Instead, the combined waveform depends on the nature of the particular sounds being combined. For example, consider the three different sine waves labeled f1, f2, and f3 in Figure 1–11. Wave f1 has a frequency of 1000 Hz, f2 is 2000 Hz, and f3 is 3000 Hz. The lower waveforms show various combinations of these sinusoids. The combined waves (f1 + f2, fl + f3, and f1 + f2 + f3) are no longer sinusoids, but they are periodic because they repeat themselves at regular intervals over time. In other words, they are all complex periodic waves.

Notice that the periods of the complex periodic waves in Figure 1–11 are the same as the period of f1, which is the lowest component for each of them. The lowest frequency component of a complex periodic wave is called its **fundamental frequency**. The fundamental frequency of each of the complex periodic waves in the figure is 1000 Hz because f1 is the lowest component in each of them. The period (or the time needed for one complete replication) of a complex periodic wave is the same as the period of its fundamental frequency. **Harmonics** are whole number or integral multiples of the fundamental frequency. In other words, the fundamental is the largest whole number common denominator of its harmonics, and the harmonics are integral multiples of the fundamental frequency. In fact, the fundamental is also a harmonic because it is equal to one times itself. In the case of wave f1 + f2 + f3, 1000 Hz is the fundamental (first har-

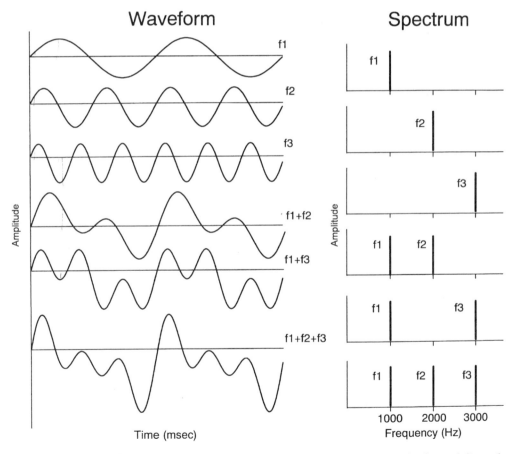

FIGURE 1–11 Three harmonically related sine waves of frequencies f1, f2, and f3; and complex periodic waves resulting from the in-phase addition of f1 + f2, f1 + f3, and f1 + f2 + f3. Notice that the fundamental frequency is f1 for all of these complex periodic waves.

monic), 2000 Hz is the second harmonic, and 3000 Hz is the third harmonic.

Another example of combining sinusoids into a complex periodic wave is given in Figure 1–12. Here, the sine waves being added are odd harmonics of the fundamental (1000 Hz, 3000 Hz, 5000 Hz, etc.), and their amplitudes get smaller with increasing frequency. The resulting complex periodic wave becomes squared-off as the number of odd harmonics is increased, and is called a **square wave** for this reason.

Waveforms show how amplitude changes with time. However, the frequency of a pure tone (sine wave) is not directly provided by its waveform, and the frequencies in a complex sound cannot be determined by examining its waveform. In fact, the same frequencies can result in dramatically different-looking complex waveforms if their phase relationships are changed. Hence, another kind of

graph is needed when we want to know what frequencies are present. This kind of graph is a **spectrum**, which shows amplitude on the y-axis as a function of frequency along the x-axis. Several examples are given in Figure 1–12. The frequency of the pure tone is given by the location of a vertical line along the horizontal (frequency) axis, and the amplitude of the tone is represented by the height of the line. According to Fourier's **theorem** complex sounds can be mathematically dissected into their constituent pure-tone components. The process of doing so is called **Fourier analysis**, which results in the information needed to plot the spectrum of a complex sound. The spectrum of a complex periodic sound has as many vertical lines as there are component frequencies. The locations of the lines show their frequencies, and their heights show their amplitudes, as illustrated in Figure 1–12.

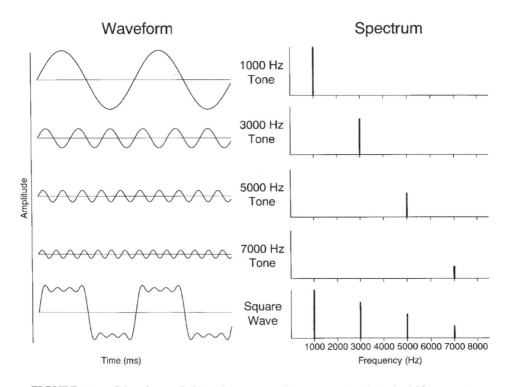

FIGURE 1–12   Waveforms (left) and corresponding spectra (right) of odd harmonics combined to form a square wave (bottom). Notice that the spectrum of a pure tone has one vertical line, whereas the spectrum of a complex periodic sound has a separate vertical line for each of its components.

APERIODIC WAVES

Aperiodic sounds are made up of components that are not harmonically related and have waveforms that do not repeat themselves over time, which is why they are called aperiodic. The extreme cases of aperiodic sounds are transients and random noise. A **transient** is an abrupt sound that is extremely brief in duration. It is aperiodic by definition because its waveform is not repeated (Fig. 1–13a). **Random noise** has a completely random waveform (Fig. 1–13b) so that it contains all possible frequencies at the same average amplitude over the long run. Random noise is also called **white noise** in analogy to white light because all possible frequencies are represented.

The spectrum of white noise is depicted in Figure 1–14a. Individual vertical lines are not drawn because there would be an infinite number of them. It is more convenient to draw a continuous line over their tops and leave out the vertical lines themselves. This kind of spectrum is used for most aperiodic sounds and is called a **continuous spectrum**. *Random noise* has a *flat* continuous spectrum because the amplitudes are the same, on average, for all frequencies. An ideal *transient* also has a *flat spectrum*.

Most aperiodic sounds do not have flat spectra because they have more amplitude concentrated in one frequency range or the other. This notion is demonstrated by a simple experiment: Tap or scratch several different objects. The resulting noises will sound different from one another because they have energy concentrations in different frequency ranges. This is exactly what is represented on the spectrum. For example, different continuous spectra might show concentrations of aperiodic sounds with greater amounts of amplitude at higher frequencies (Fig. 1–14b), at lower frequencies (Fig. 1–14c), or within a particular band (range) of frequencies (Fig. 1–14d).

Standing Waves and Resonance

The frequency(ies) at which a body or medium vibrates most readily is called its **natural** or **resonant frequency(ies)**. Differences in resonant frequency ranges enable different devices or other objects to act as filters by transmitting energy more readily for certain frequency ranges than for others. Examples of the frequency ranges that are transmitted by high-, low-, and band-pass filters are illustrated in Figure 1–14b, c, and d.

Vibrating Strings   Consider what happens when you pluck a guitar string. The waves initiated by the pluck move outward toward the two tied ends of the string. The waves are then reflected back and they propagate in opposite directions. The result is a set of waves that are moving toward each other, a situation that is sustained by continuing reflections from the two ends. Being reflections of one another, all of these waves will have the same frequency, and they will, of course, be propagating at the same velocity. Recall that waves interact with one another so that their instantaneous displacements add algebraically. As a result, the net displacement of the string at any point along its length will be due to the way in which the superimposed waves, interact. The resulting combined wave appears as a pattern that is standing still even though it is derived from

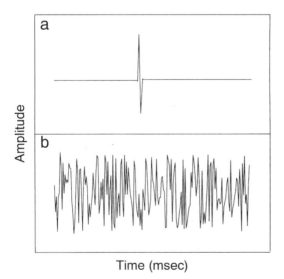

FIGURE 1–13 Artist's conceptions of the waveforms of (a) a transient and (b) random (white) noise.

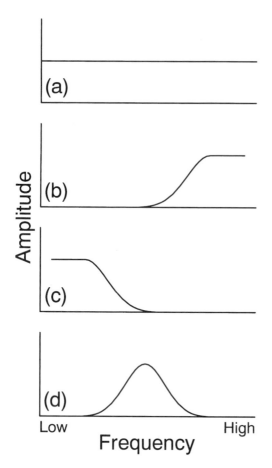

FIGURE 1–14 Idealized continuous spectra showing (a) equal amplitude at all frequencies for a transient or white noise; (b) greater amplitude in the higher frequencies (also a high-pass filter); (c) greater amplitude in the lower frequencies (also a low-pass filter); (d) amplitude concentrated within a certain band of frequencies (also a band-pass filter).

the interaction of waves, which themselves are propagating. Consequently, the points of maximum displacement (peaks of the combined wave pattern) and no displacement (baseline crossings of the combined wave pattern) will occur at fixed locations along the string. This pattern is called a **standing wave**.

Places along the string where there is zero displacement in the standing wave pattern are called **nodes**, and the locations where

maximum displacement occurs are called **antinodes**. The string is tied down at its two ends so that it cannot move at these locations. In other words, the displacement must always be zero at the two ends of the string. This means that the standing wave pattern must have nodes that occur at the two ends of the string. Just as no displacement occurs at each end of the string because it is most constrained at these points, the greatest displacement occurs in the middle of the string where it is least constrained, and therefore has the most freedom of motion. In other words, the standing wave pattern will have a node at each end of the string and an antinode at the center of the string. This pattern is illustrated in Figure 1–15a. Notice that the antinode occurs halfway between the nodes just as peaks (at 90° and 270°) alternate with zero displacements (at 0° and 180°) in a cycle of a sine wave.

The standing wave pattern that has a node at each end and an antinode in the center is not the only one that can occur on a given string; rather, it is just the *longest* one. This longest standing wave pattern is called the **first mode** of vibration. This standing wave pattern goes from no displacement to a peak and back to no displacement, which is analogous to going from 0° to 180° on a wave cycle. In other words, the pattern comprises exactly half of a cycle. Because we are dealing with displacement as a function of *distance* along the string (rather than over time), the parameter of the cycle with which we are dealing here is its wavelength (λ). In other words, the length of the longest standing wave pattern is the length of the whole string, and this length corresponds to one half of a wavelength ($\lambda/2$). Of course, if we know $\lambda/2$, then we can easily figure out λ. Now, a given wavelength is associated with a particular frequency because $f = c/\lambda$ (recall that c is the speed of sound). Consequently, the first mode of vibration is equal to half the wavelength ($\lambda/2$) of some frequency, which will, in turn, be its frequency of vibration. This will be the lowest **resonant frequency** of the string, which is its *fundamental frequency*. Finding this frequency is a matter of substituting what we know into

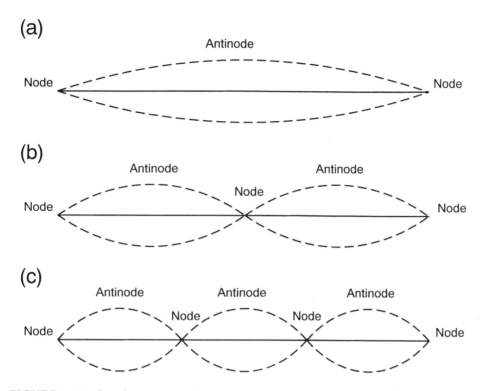

FIGURE 1–15 Standing wave patterns corresponding to the (a) first, (b) second, and (c) third modes of a vibrating string.

the formula $f = c/\lambda$. We know the length of the string (L), and we also know that $L = \lambda/2$. Therefore, $\lambda = 2L$. Substituting 2L for λ, the string's lowest resonant frequency is found with the formula $f = c/2L$. [In reality, the speed of sound (c) is different for a vibrating string than it is for air. For the benefit of the math-minded student, the value of c for a string equals the square root of the ratio of its tension M to its mass (M), so that the real formula for the string's resonant frequency is $f = 1/L \cdot \sqrt{T/M}$].

Other standing waves can also develop, provided they meet the requirement that there must be a node at both ends of the string. For this criterion to be met, the string must be divided into exact halves, thirds, fourths, etc., as illustrated in Figure 1–15. These standing wave patterns are called the second, third, fourth, etc., modes of vibration. Because the segments of the second mode are exactly half of the length of first mode, they produce a frequency that is

exactly twice the fundamental. If we call the fundamental the first harmonic, then the second mode produces the second harmonic. Similarly, the segments of the third mode are exactly one-third the length of the first mode, so that they produce a third harmonic that is exactly three times the fundamental. The same principles apply to the fourth mode and harmonic, and beyond.

Vibrations in Tubes The column of air inside a tube can be set into vibration by various means, such as blowing across the tube's open end. If this is done with different-sized tubes we would find that (1) shorter tubes are associated with higher pitches than longer ones, and (2) the same tube produces a higher pitch when it is open at both ends compared to when it is open at one end and closed at the other.

When a column of air is vibrating in a tube that is open at both ends, the least amount of particle displacement occurs in the center of the tube where the pressure is greatest. The greatest amount of displacement occurs at the two open ends where the pressure is lowest. Hence, there will be a standing wave that has a displacement node in the middle of the tube and antinodes at the two ends, as illustrated in Figure 1–16a. This standing wave pattern involves one-half of a cycle in the sense that going from one end of the tube to the other end involves going from a displacement peak to a zero crossing to another peak. This trip would cover 180° (half of a cycle) on a sine wave, and thus a distance corresponding to half of a wavelength. Because this longest standing wave involves half of a wavelength ($\lambda/2$), the tube's lowest resonant (fundamental) frequency must have a wavelength that is twice the length of the tube (where $\lambda = 2L$). For this reason, tubes open at both ends are **half-wavelength resonators**. In other words, the lowest resonant frequency of a tube open at both ends is determined by the familiar formula, $f = c/2L$. We could also say that the longest standing wave pattern is the first mode of vibration for the tube and that it is related to its fundamental frequency (lowest harmonic). As for the vibrating string, each successive higher mode corresponds to exact halves, thirds, etc., of the tube length, as illustrated in Figure 1–16a. In turn, these modes produce harmonics that are exact multiples of the fundamental frequency. Harmonics will occur at each multiple of the fundamental frequency for a tube open at both ends.

Air particles vibrating in a tube that is closed at one end and open at the other end are restricted most at the closed end. As a result, their displacement will be least at the closed end, where the pressure is the greatest. Thus, in terms of displacement, there must be a node at the closed end and an antinode at the open end, as illustrated in Figure 1–16b. This pattern is analogous to the distance from a zero crossing to a peak, which corresponds to one-quarter of a cycle (0° to 90°), and a distance of one-quarter of a wavelength ($\lambda/4$). Because the length of the tube corresponds to $\lambda/4$, its lowest resonant frequency has a wavelength that is four times the length of the tube (4L). Hence,

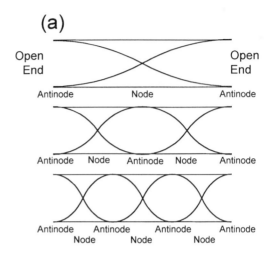

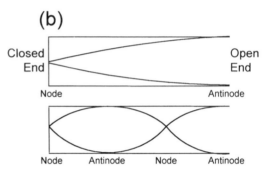

FIGURE 1–16 Standing wave patterns in (a) a tube open at both ends (a half-wavelength resonator), and (b) a tube open at one end and closed at the other end (a quarter-wavelength resonator).

$f = c/4L$. For this reason, a tube that is open at one end and closed at the other end is a **quarter-wavelength resonator**. Because a node can occur at only one end, these tubes have only odd modes of vibration and produce only odd harmonics of the fundamental frequency (e.g., f_1, f_3, f_5, f_7, etc.), as illustrated in the figure.

Immittance

Immittance is the general term used to describe how well energy flows through a system. The *opposition* to the flow of energy is called **impedance (Z)**. The inverse of impedance is called **admittance (Y)**, which is the *ease* with which energy flows through a system.

The concept of impedance may be understood in terms of the following example. (Although this example only considers mass, we will see that immittance actually involves several components.) Imagine two metal blocks weighing different amounts. Suppose you repetitively push and pull the lighter block back-and-forth across a smooth table top with a certain amount of effort. This is a mechanical system in which a sinusoidally alternating force (the pushing and pulling) is being applied to a mass (the block). The effort with which you are pushing (and pulling) the block is the amount of applied force, and the velocity of the block reflects how well energy flows through this system in order to effect motion. A particular block will move at a certain velocity given the amount of effort you are using to push (and pull) it. If the *same* amount of *effort* was used to push and pull the *heavier* block, then it would move slower than the first one. In other words, the heavier block (greater mass) moves with less velocity than the lighter block (smaller mass) in response to the same amount of applied force. We can say that the flow of energy is opposed more by the heavier block than by the lighter one. For this reason, the heavier block (greater mass) has more impedance and less admittance than the lighter block (smaller mass).

This example shows that impedance and admittance are viewed in terms of the relationship between an applied force and the resulting amount of velocity. In effect, higher impedance means that more force must be applied to result in a given amount of velocity, and lower impedance means that less force is needed to result in a given amount of velocity. For the mathematically oriented, we might say that impedance (Z) is the ratio of force to velocity:

$$Z = \frac{F}{v}.$$

The amount of impedance is expressed in ohms (Ω). The larger the number of ohms, the greater the opposition to the flow of energy.

Admittance (Y) is the reciprocal of impedance:

$$Y = \frac{1}{Z},$$

and is therefore equal to the ratio of velocity to force:

$$Y = \frac{v}{F}.$$

As we might expect, the unit of admittance is the inverse of the ohm, and is therefore called the **mho**. The more mhos, the greater the ease with which energy flows. The admittance values that we are concerned with in audiology are very small, and are thus expressed in **millimhos (mmhos)**.

Impedance involves the complex interaction of three familiar physical components: mass, stiffness, and friction. In Figure 1–17

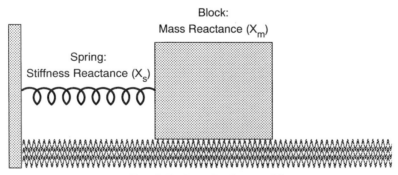

FIGURE 1–17   The components of impedance are (1) mass reactance (X_m), represented by the block; (2) stiffness reactance (X_s), represented by the spring; and (3) resistance (R), represented by the rough surface under the block.

mass is represented by the block, stiffness (or compliance) by the spring, and friction by the rough surface under the block. Let's briefly consider each of these components. Friction dissipates some of the energy being introduced into the system by converting it into heat. This component of impedance is called resistance (R). The effect of resistance occurs in-phase with the applied force (Fig. 1–18). Some amount of friction is always present. Opposition to the flow of energy due to mass is called **mass (positive) reactance (X_m)** and is related to inertia. The opposition due to the stiffness of a system is called **stiffness (negative) reactance (X_s)**, and is related to the restoring force that develops when an elastic element (e.g., a spring) is displaced.

Mass and stiffness act to oppose the applied force because these components are out-of-phase with it. They oppose the flow of energy by storing it in these out-of-phase components before effecting motion. First, consider the mass all by itself. At the same point in time (labeled 1) the applied force

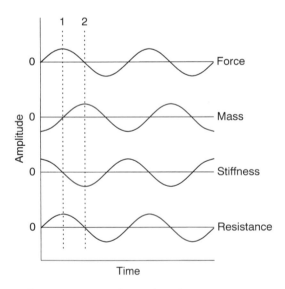

FIGURE 1–18 Relationship between a sinusoidally applied force (top), and the velocities associated with mass, stiffness, and resistance. The dotted lines labeled 1 and 2 show two moments in time (see text). Resistance is in-phase with the applied force (F). Mass and stiffness are 90° out-of-phase with force, and 180° out-of-phase with each other.

is maximal (in the upward direction) and the velocity of the block is zero (crossing the horizontal line in the positive direction). One-quarter of a cycle later, at the time labeled 2, the applied force is zero and the velocity of the mass is now maximal (in the upward direction). Hence, a sinusoidally applied force acting on a mass and the resulting velocity of the mass are a quarter-cycle (90°) out-of-phase. To appreciate this relationship, hold a weight and shake repetitively back and forth from right to left. You will feel that you must exert the most effort (maximal force) at the extreme right and left points of the swing, where the direction changes. Notice that the weight is momentarily still (i.e., its velocity is zero) at the extreme right and left points because this is where it changes direction. On the other hand, the weight will be moving the fastest (maximum velocity) as it passes the midpoint of the right-left swing, which is also where you will be using the least effort (zero force).

Now consider the spring all by itself at the same two times. At time 1, when the applied force is maximal (upward), the velocity of the spring is zero (crossing the horizontal line in the negative direction). One quarter-cycle later, at time 2, the applied force is zero, and the velocity of the spring is now maximal (downward). Hence, a sinusoidally applied force acting on a spring and the resulting velocity of the spring are a quarter-cycle (90°) out-of-phase. This occurs in the opposite direction of what we observed for the mass (whose motion is associated with inertia) because the motion of the spring is associated with restoring force. You can appreciate this relationship by alternately compressing and expanding a spring. You must push or pull the hardest (maximum applied force) at the moment when the spring is maximally expanded (or compressed), which is also when the spring is not moving (zero velocity) because it is about to change direction. Similarly, you will exert no effort (zero applied force) and the spring will be moving the fastest (maximum velocity) as it moves back through its "normal" position (where it is neither compressed nor expanded).

Notice that the mass and stiffness reactances are 180° out-of-phase with each other (Fig. 1–18). This means that the effects of mass reactance and stiffness reactance oppose each other. As a result, the **net reactance (X_{net})** is the difference between them; so that

$$X_{net} = X_s - X_m$$

when stiffness reactance is larger, or

$$X_{net} = X_m - X_s$$

when mass reactance is larger. For example, if X_s is 850 ohms and X_m is 140 ohms, then X_{net} will be 850 − 140 = 710 ohms of stiffness reactance. If X_m is 1000 ohms and the X_s is 885 ohms, then X_{net} will be 1000 − 885 = 115 ohms of mass reactance.

The overall impedance is obtained by combining the resistance and the net reactance. This cannot be done by simple addition because the resistance and reactance components are out-of-phase. (Recall here the difference between scalars and vectors mentioned at the beginning of the chapter.) The relationships in Figure 1–19 show how impedance is derived from resistance and reactance. The size of the resistance component is plotted along the x-axis. Reactance is plotted on the y-axis, with mass (positive) reactance represented upward and stiffness (negative) reactance downward. The net reactance here is plotted downward because X_s is greater than X_m, so that X_{net} is negative. Notice that R and X_{net} form two legs of a right triangle, and that Z is the hypotenuse. Hence, we find Z by the familiar Pythagorean theorem ($a^2 + b^2 = c^2$); which becomes $Z^2 = R^2 + X_{net}^2$. Removing the squares gives us the formula for calculating impedance from the resistance and reactance values:

$$Z = \sqrt{R^2 + X_{net}^2}.$$

Resistance tends to be essentially the same at all frequencies. However, reactance depends on frequency (f) in the following way: (1) mass reactance is proportional to frequency,

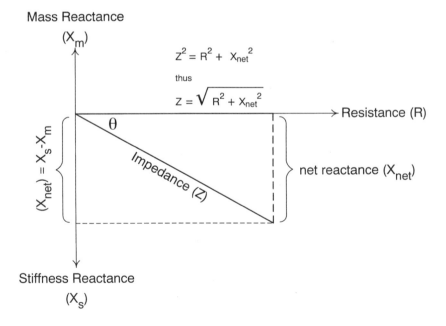

FIGURE 1–19 Impedance (Z) is the complex interaction of resistance (R) and the net reactance (X_{net}, which is equal to $X_s - X_m$). Notice the impedance value is determined by the vector addition of the resistance and reactance. The angle (θ) between the horizontal leg of the triangle (resistance) and its hypotenuse (impedance) is called the phase angle.

$$X_m = 2\pi fM,$$

where M is mass; and (2) stiffness reactance is inversely proportional to frequency,

$$X_s = \frac{S}{2\pi f},$$

where S is stiffness. In other words, X_m gets larger as frequency goes up, and X_s gets larger as frequency goes down. Because of these frequency relationships, impedance also depends on frequency:

$$Z = \sqrt{R^2 + \left(\frac{S}{2\pi f} + 2\pi fM\right)^2}.$$

In addition, there will be a frequency where X_m and X_s are equal, and thus cancel. This is the resonant frequency, where the only component that is opposing the flow of energy is resistance.

Admittance is the reciprocal of impedance:

$$Y = \frac{1}{Z},$$

and the components of admittance are the reciprocals of resistance and reactance: **Conductance (G)** is the reciprocal of resistance:

$$G = \frac{1}{R};$$

stiffness (compliant) susceptance (B_s) is the reciprocal of stiffness reactance:

$$B_s = \frac{1}{X_s};$$

and **mass susceptance (B_m)** is the reciprocal of mass reactance:

$$B_m = \frac{1}{X_m}.$$

Stiffness susceptance is proportional to frequency (B_s increases as frequency goes up), and mass susceptance is inversely proportional to frequency (B_m decreases as frequency goes up). Net susceptance (B_{net}) is the difference between B_s and B_m. The formula for admittance is

$$Y = \sqrt{G^2 + B_{net}^2},$$

where B_{net} is ($B_s - B_m$) when B_s is bigger and ($B_m - B_s$) when B_m is larger.

Up to this point we have discussed immittance in mechanical terms. **Acoustic immittance** is the term used for the analogous concepts when dealing with sound. The opposition to the flow of sound energy is called **acoustic impedance (Z_a)**, and its reciprocal is **acoustic admittance (Y_a)**. Thus,

$$Z_a = \frac{1}{Y_a}$$

and

$$Y_a = \frac{1}{Z_a}.$$

When dealing with acoustic immittance, we use **sound pressure (p)** in place of force, and velocity is replaced with the velocity of sound flow, called **volume velocity (U)**. Thus, acoustic impedance is simply the ratio of sound pressure to volume velocity,

$$Z_a = \frac{p}{U},$$

and acoustic admittance is the ratio of volume velocity to sound pressure,

$$Y_a = \frac{U}{p}.$$

The components of acoustic immittance are based on the acoustic analogies of friction, mass, and stiffness (compliance). Friction develops between air molecules and a mesh screen, which is thus used to model **acoustic resistance (R_a)**. **Mass (positive) acoustic reactance ($+X_a$)** is represented by a slug of air in an open tube. Here an applied sound pressure will displace the slug of air as a unit, so that its inertia comes into play. A column of air inside a tube open at one end and closed at the other end represents **compliant (negative) acoustic reactance ($-X_a$)**

because sound pressure compresses the air column like a spring. The formulas and relationships for acoustical immittance are the same as those previously given, except that the analogous acoustical values are used. For example, acoustic impedance is equal to

$$Z_a = \sqrt{R_a^2 + X_a^2},$$

where X_a is the net difference between compliant acoustic reactance ($-X_a$) and mass acoustic reactance ($+X_a$). Similarly, the formula for acoustic admittance is

$$Y_a = \sqrt{G_a^2 + B_a^2},$$

where B_a is the net difference between compliant acoustic susceptance ($+B_a$) and mass acoustic susceptance ($-B_a$).

Expressing Values in Decibels

It is extremely cumbersome to express sound magnitudes in terms of their actual intensities or pressures for several reasons. To do so would involve working in units of watts/m² (or watts/cm²) and newtons/m² (or dynes/cm²). In addition, the range of sound magnitudes with which we are concerned in audiology is enormous; the loudest sound that can be tolerated has a pressure that is roughly ten million times larger than the softest sound that can be heard. Even if we wanted to work with such an immense range of cumbersome values on a linear scale, we would find that it is hard to deal with them in a way that has relevance to the way we hear. As a result, these absolute physical values are converted into a simpler and more convenient form called **decibels (dB)** to make them palatable and meaningful.

The decibel takes advantage of ratios and logarithms. Ratios are used so that physical magnitudes can be stated in relation to a reference value that has meaning to us. It makes sense to use the *softest sound that can be heard by normal people* as our **reference value**. This reference value has an *intensity* of

$$10^{-12}\,\text{w/m}^2$$

in MKS units, which corresponds to

$$10^{-16}\,\text{w/cm}^2$$

in the cgs system. The same softest audible sound can also be quantified in terms of its *sound pressure*. This reference pressure is

$$2 \times 10^{-5}\,\text{N/m}^2$$

or

$$20\ \mu\text{Pa}$$

in the MKS system.[1] In cgs units this reference pressure is

$$2 \times 10^{-4}\ \text{dynes/cm}^2,$$

which the student will often find written as 0.0002 dynes/cm² in the older audiological literature.[2] The appropriate reference value (intensity or pressure, MKS or cgs) becomes the denominator of our ratio, and the intensity (or pressure) of the sound that is actually being measured or described becomes the numerator. As a result, instead of describing a sound that has an intensity of 10^{-10} w/m², we place this value into a ratio so we can express it in terms of how it compares to our reference value (which is 10^{-12} w/m²). Hence, this ratio would be

$$\frac{10^{-10}\ \text{w/m}^2}{10^{-12}\ \text{w/m}^2}.$$

This ratio reduces to simply 10^2.

Regardless of what this ratio turns out to be, it is replaced with its common logarithm because equal ratios correspond to different distances on a linear scale, but equal ratios correspond to equal distances on a logarithmic scale. In other words, the linear distance between two numbers with the same ratio relationship (e.g., 2 to 1) is small for small

---

[1] One pascal is 1 N/m², so 10^{-6} N/m² is 1 micropascal (μPa). Hence, 10^{-5} N/m² is 10 μPa, and 2×10^{-5} N/m² is also 20 μPa.

[2] Occasionally reported as 2×10^{-4} μbar or 0.0002 μbar, especially in the older literature.

numbers and large for large numbers, but the logarithm of that ratio is always the same. For example, all of the following pairs involve 2/1 ratios. Even though the linear distance between the numbers in the pairs gets wider as the absolute sizes of the numbers get larger, the logarithm of all of the ratios stays the same (2/1 = 2, and log 2 is always 0.3):

Pairs of numbers with 2:1 ratios	Distances between the absolute numbers get wider	Logarithms of all 2:1 ratios are the same
2/1	1	0.3
8/4	4	0.3
20/10	10	0.3
100/50	50	0.3
200/100	100	0.3
2000/1000	1000	0.3

The general decibel formula is expressed in terms of *power* as follows:

$$PL = 10 \log \frac{P}{P_0}.$$

Here, PL stands for **power level** (in dB), P is the power of the sound being measured, and P_0 is the reference power to which the former is being compared. The word *level* is added to distinguish the raw physical quantity (power) from the corresponding decibel value (which is a logarithmic ratio about the power). Similarly, intensity expressed in decibels is called **intensity level (IL)** and sound pressure expressed in decibels is called **sound pressure level (SPL)**.

Most sound measurements are expressed in terms of intensity or sound pressure, with the latter being the most common. The formula for decibels of **intensity level** is

$$IL = 10 \log \frac{I}{I_0},$$

where IL is intensity level in dB, I is the intensity of the sound in question (in w/m^2), and I_0 is the reference intensity (10^{-12} w/m^2). If the value of I is 10^{-10} w/m^2, then

$$IL = 10 \log \frac{10^{-10} \, w/m^2}{10^{-12} \, w/m^2}$$

$$= 10 \log \frac{10^{-10}}{10^{-12}}$$

(notice that w/m^2 cancels out)

$$= 10 \log 10^{(-10)-(-12)}$$

$$= 10 \log 10^2$$

$$= 10 \times 2$$

$$= 20 \, dB \quad re: 10^{-12} \, w/m^2$$

Consequently, an absolute intensity of 10^{-10} w/m^2 has an intensity level of 20 dB re: 10^{-12} w/m^2, or 20 dB IL. The phrase "re: 10^{-12} w/m^2" is added because the decibel is a dimensionless quantity that only has real meaning when we know the reference value, that is, the denominator of the ratio.

The formula for decibels of **sound pressure level (dB SPL)** is obtained by replacing all of the intensity values with the corresponding values of *pressure squared* (because $I \propto p^2$):

$$SPL = 10 \log \frac{p^2}{p_0^2}$$

Here, p is the measured sound pressure (in N/m^2) and p_0 is the reference sound pressure (2×10^{-5} N/m^2, or 20 µPa). This form of the formula is cumbersome because of the squared values, which can be removed by applying the following steps:

$$SPL = 10 \log \frac{p^2}{p_0^2}$$

$$= 10 \log \left(\frac{p}{p_0} \right)^2$$

$$= 10 \times 2 \log \left(\frac{p}{p_0} \right)$$

(because $\log x^2 = 2 \log x$)

$$= 20 \log \left(\frac{p}{p_0} \right)$$

Therefore, the commonly used simplified formula for decibels of SPL is

$$SPL = 20 \log \frac{p}{p_0},$$

where the multiplier is 20 instead of 10 as a result of removing the squares from the unsimplified version of the formula.

Let us go through the exercise of converting the absolute sound pressure of a sound into dB SPL. We will assume that the sound being measured has a pressure of 2×10^{-4} N/m². Recall that the reference pressure is 2×10^{-5} N/m². The steps are as follows:

$$SPL = 20 \log \frac{2 \times 10^{-4} N/m^2}{2 \times 10^{-5} N/m^2}$$

$$= 20 \log \frac{10^{-4}}{20^{-5}}$$

(notice that N/m² cancels out)

$$= 20 \log 10^{(-4)-(-5)}$$

$$= 20 \log 10^1$$

$$= 20 \times 1$$

$$= 20 \ dB \quad re: 2 \times 10^{-5} N/m^2 \text{ (or } 20 \,\mu Pa)$$

Hence, a sound pressure of 2×10^{-4} N/m² corresponds to a sound pressure level of 20 dB re: 2×10^{-5} N/m² (or 20 μPa), or 20 dB SPL.

What is the decibel value of the reference itself? In other words, what would happen if the intensity (or pressure) being measured is equal to the reference intensity (or pressure)? In terms of intensity, the answer is found by using the reference value (10^{-12} w/m²) as both the numerator (I) and denominator (I_0) in the dB formula; so that

$$IL = 10 \log \frac{10^{-12} w/m^2}{10^{-12} w/m^2}$$

$$= 10 \log 1$$

(anything divided by itself equals 1)

$$= 10 \times 0$$

$$= 0 \, dB \quad re: 10^{-12} w/m^2$$

Consequently, the intensity *level* of the reference intensity is 0 dB IL. Similarly, 0 dB SPL

means that the measured sound pressure corresponds to that of the reference sound:

$$SPL = 20 \log \frac{10^{-5} N/m^2}{10^{-5} N/m^2}$$

(anything divided by itself equals 1)

$$= 20 \log 1$$

$$= 20 \times 0$$

$$= 0 \, dB \quad re: 2 \times 10^{-5} N/m^2 \text{ (or } 20 \,\mu Pa)$$

Notice that 0 dB IL and 0 dB SPL mean the sound being measured is equal to the reference value; they do not mean "no sound." It follows that negative decibel values indicate that the magnitude of the sound is lower than the reference; for example, −10 dB means that the sound in question is 10 decibels below the reference value.

Sound Measurement

The magnitude of a sound is usually measured with a device called a **sound level meter (SLM)**. This device has a high-quality microphone that picks up the sound and converts it into an electrical signal that is analyzed by an electronic circuit, and then displays the magnitude of the sound on a meter in decibels of sound pressure level (dB SPL). An example of an SLM is shown in Figure 1–20. Sound level meters are used to calibrate or establish the accuracy of audiometers and other instruments used to test hearing, as well as to measure noise levels for such varied purposes as determining whether a room is quiet enough for performing hearing tests or identifying potentially hazardous noise exposures. Sound level meters or equivalent circuits that perform the same function are also found as components of other devices, such as hearing aid test systems.

The characteristics of sound level meters are specified in ANSI standard S1.4 (1997). The accuracy of the measurements produced by an SLM is established using a compatible acoustical calibrator, which is a device that produces a known precise signal that is directed into the SLM microphone. For

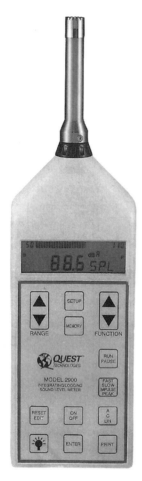

FIGURE 1–20 An example of a sound level meter with a measuring microphone attached. Courtesy of Quest Technologies, Inc.

example, if the calibrator produces a signal that is exactly 114 dB SPL, then the SLM is expected to read this amount when it is connected to the calibrator (within certain tolerances allowed in the ANSI standard). If the meter reading deviates from the actual value of 114 dB SPL, then its controls are adjusted to reset the meter to the right value, or it might be necessary to have the SLM repaired and recalibrated by the manufacturer or an instrumentation service company.

The microphone of an SLM picks up all sounds that are present at all frequencies within its operating range. At its **linear setting** the SLM measures the overall SPL for all of the sounds picked up by the microphone. In addition to the linear setting, SLMs also have weighting filters that change the emphasis given to certain parts of the spectrum, and may also have octave-band or third-octave-band filters, which measure only certain ranges of frequencies. We all know that turning up the bass control on a home stereo system makes the low pitches more pronounced, whereas turning the bass down makes the lows less noticeable. In other words, the bass control determines whether the low frequencies will be emphasized or de-emphasized. The treble control does the same thing for the high frequencies. The **weighting filters** or networks on a sound level meter do essentially the same thing, mainly by de-emphasizing the low frequencies. Figure 1–21 shows the three weighting networks found on the

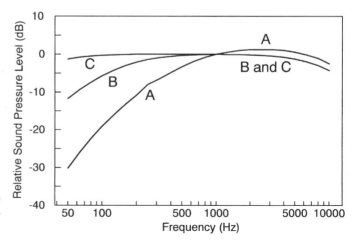

FIGURE 1–21 Frequency response curves for the A-, B-, and C-weighting networks.

SLM. The y-axis is relative level in decibels, and may be thought of as showing how the weighting network changes the sound that originally entered the SLM through the microphone. A horizontal line at 0 dB refers to how the sound would be without the weighting network. In other words, 0 dB here means "unchanged," which corresponds to the linear setting of the SLM. The negative decibel values tell the amount by which the sound level is de-emphasized at each frequency.

The **A-weighting** network considerably de-emphasizes the low frequencies, as shown by its curve, which gets progressively more negative as frequency decreases below 1000 Hz. For example, the curve shows that the A-weighting network de-emphasizes sounds by about 4 dB at 500 Hz, 11 dB at 200 Hz, 19 dB at 100 Hz, and 30 dB at 50 Hz. This is analogous to turning the bass all the way down on a stereo system. The **B-weighting** network also de-emphasizes the lower frequencies, but not as much as the A-weighting. For example, the amount of reduction is only about 6 dB at 100 Hz. The **C-weighting** is barely different from a linear response. Sound level measurements made with these networks are expressed as decibels of A-, B-, or C-weighted sound pressure levels, or as dBA, dBB, and dBC, respectively. Measurements in dBA are commonly used when it is desirable to exclude the effects of the lower frequencies, and are especially useful in noise level measurements. Measurements in dBC are also

commonly employed in noise level measurements. However, the B-scale is rarely used.

Sound level meters often have a set of built-in or attached **octave-band filters**, which is simply a group of filters that allows the SLM to "look at" a certain range of frequencies instead of all of them. In other words, the octave-band analyzer separates the overall frequency range into narrower ranges, which are each one octave wide, as illustrated in Figure 1–22. For example, the range from 355 to 710 Hz is an octave band because 710 = 2 × 355, and the bandwidth from 2800 to 5600 Hz is also an octave because 5600 = 2 × 2800. An octave band is named according to its center frequency, although the center is defined as the geometric mean of the upper and lower cutoffs rather than the arithmetic midpoint between them. Hence, the 500-Hz octave band goes from 355 to 710 Hz, and the 4000-Hz octave band includes 2800 to 5600 Hz. The center frequencies and the upper and lower cutoff frequencies of the octave bands typically used in acoustical measurements are listed in Table 1–4.

Measuring a noise on an octave-band by octave-band basis is called **octave-band analysis** and makes it possible to learn about the spectrum of a sound instead of just its overall level. An even finer level of analysis can be achieved by using **third-octave band filters**, in which case each filter is one-third of an octave wide. For example, the 500-Hz

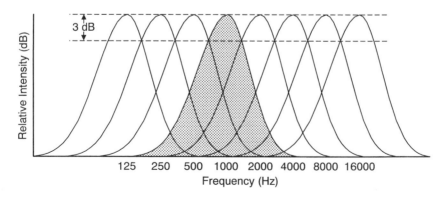

FIGURE 1–22 A series of octave-bands representing those typically used in octave-band analysis. Notice the bands overlap at their 3-dB down points. The 1000-Hz octave-band is highlighted for clarity.

TABLE 1-4   Examples of Octave-Band Center Frequencies, and Lower and Upper Cutoff Frequencies

Center Frequency (Hz)	Lower Cutoff (Hz)	Upper Cutoff (Hz)
31.5	22.4	45
63	45	90
125	90	180
250	180	355
500	355	710
1,000	710	1,400
2,000	1,400	2,800
4,000	2,800	5,600
8,000	5,600	11,200
16,000	11,200	92,400

third-octave filter includes the frequencies between 450 and 560 Hz, and the 4000-Hz third-octave band goes from 3550 to 4500 Hz. Octave-band and third-octave band filters are useful when we want to concentrate on the sound level in a narrow frequency range without contamination from other frequencies. For example, it is usually better to measure the level of a 1000 Hz tone while using a filter centered around 1000-Hz than to do the same thing at the linear setting of the SLM because the filter excludes other frequencies, thus the results are not contaminated.

Even though we cannot get the spectrum of a noise from overall sound level measurements, we can combine **octave-band levels (OBLs)** or **1/3-OBLs** to arrive at the overall level of a sound. There are two ways to combine OBLs into overall SPL. The simpler approach involves adding the OBLs in successive pairs using the rules for adding decibels shown in Table 1–5. It is very easy to use this table. First, find the difference in decibels between the two sounds being combined. For example, if one sound is 80 dB and the other is 76 dB, then the difference between them is 4-dB. Then find the increment that corresponds to the difference. According to the table, the increment for a 4-dB difference is 1.4 dB. Now, just add this increment to the larger of the original two sounds. The larger value in our example is 80 dB, so we add the

1.4-dB increment to 80 dB (80 + 1.4 = 81.4). Hence, combining 80 and 76 dB results in a total of 81.4 dB. To combine octave bands into an overall level, simply arrange their OBLs from largest to smallest, and combine pairs successively using the increments in the table. A complete example is shown in Appendix A.

The more precise method for combining octave-band levels into an overall SPL is to use the following formula for logarithmic addition:

$$L = 10 \log \sum_{i=1}^{n} 10^{Li/10}.$$

In this formula L is the overall (combined) level in dB SPL; n is the number of bands being combined; i is the ith band; and $L_i =$ is the OBL of the ith band. An example showing how this formula is used may be found in Appendix A.

The same methods can be used to combine octave-band levels into an A-weighted sound level (dBA), except a correction factor is

TABLE 1–5   Combining Decibels: Find the Difference in Decibels Between the Two Sounds, and then Add the Corresponding Decibel Increment to the Larger Original Decibel Value

Difference in dB (between original sounds)	Increment in dB (add to larger original sound)
0	3.0
1	2.6
2	2.2
3	1.8
4	1.4
5	1.2
6	1.0
7	0.8
8	0.6
9	0.5
10	0.4
11	0.35
12	0.3
13	0.25
14	0.2
15	0.15
16	0.1

TABLE 1–6   Corrections (dBA Weightings) to Convert Linear Octave-Band Levels into A-Weighted Octave-Band Levels

Octave-Band Center Frequency (Hz)	dBA Weighting
31.5	−39.4
63	−26.2
125	−16.1
250	−8.6
500	−3.2
1000	0
2000	+1.2
4000	+1.1
8000	−1.1

applied to each OBL. This correction factor is the amount by which the A-weighting de-emphasizes the level of the sounds within each octave-band. Table 1–6 shows the corrections (dBA weightings) that can be used to convert linear octave band levels into A-weighted octave-band levels. For example, dBA de-emphasizes the 125-Hz octave band by 16.1 dB. Thus, if the 125-dB OBL is 60 dB, we correct it to its dBA value by subtracting: 60 − 16.1 = 43.9 dB. A full example is shown

in Appendix A. The formula for more precisely converting OBLs into dBA is as follows:

$$L_A = 10 \log \sum_{i=1}^{n} 10^{(Li+ki)/10}.$$

The symbols here are the same as in the previous formula except L_A is now the overall (combined) level in dBA, and ki is the correction factor that must be applied to the OBL of the ith band to convert it into its equivalent value in dBA (which is the reason for the term Li + ki in the equation). Appendix A shows an example of how this formula is used.

REFERENCES

American National Standards Institute (ANSI). 1997. ANSI-S1.4-1983 (R1997). *American National Standard Specification for Sound Level Meters.* New York: ANSI.

Beranek LL. 1986. *Acoustics.* New York: American Institute of Physics.

Gelfand SA. 1998. *Hearing: An Introduction to Psychological and Physiological Acoustics,* 3rd ed. New York: Marcel Dekker.

Hewitt P. 1974. *Conceptual Physics.* Boston: Little, Brown.

Kinsler LE, Frey AR, Coppens AB, Sanders JB. 1982. *Fundamentals of Acoustics,* 3rd ed. New York: Wiley.

Peterson APG, Gross EE. 1972. *Handbook of Noise Measurement,* 7th ed. Concord, MA: General Radio.

Sears FW, Zemansky MW, Young HD. 1982. *University Physics,* 6th ed. New York: Addison Wesley.

2

Anatomy and Physiology of the Auditory System

General Overview

Hearing and its disorders are intimately inter-twined with the anatomy and physiology of the auditory system, which is composed of the ear and its associated neurological path-ways. The auditory system is fascinating, but learning about it for the first time means that we must face many new terms, relationships, and concepts. For this reason it is best to be-gin with a general bird's-eye view of how the ear is set up, and how a sound is converted from vibrations in the air to a signal that can be interpreted by the brain. A set of self-explanatory drawings illustrating commonly used anatomical orientations and directions is provided in Figure 2–1 for ready reference.

Figure 2–2 shows how the structures of the hearing system are oriented within the head. The major parts of the ear are shown in Figure 2–3. One cannot help but notice that the externally visible auricle, or pinna, and the ear canal (external auditory meatus) ending at the eardrum (tympanic membrane) make up only a small part of the overall auditory system. This system is divided into several main sections: The *outer ear* includes the auri-cle and ear canal. The air–filled cavity behind the eardrum is called the *middle ear*, also known as the tympanic cavity. Notice that the middle ear connects to the pharynx by the Eustachian tube. Medial to the middle ear is the *inner ear*. Three tiny bones (malleus, incus, and stapes), known as the ossicular chain, act

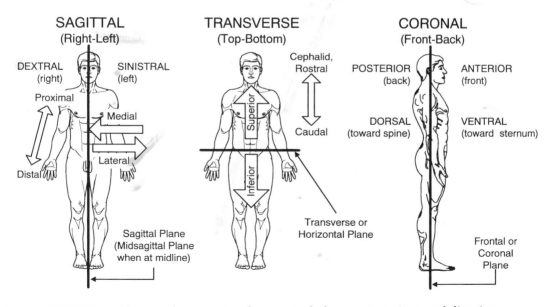

FIGURE 2–1 Commonly encountered anatomical planes, orientations, and directions.

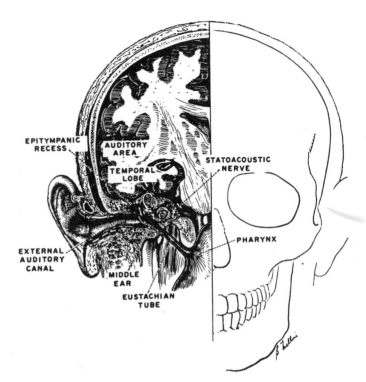

FIGURE 2–2 The auditory system in relation to the brain and skull. Courtesy of Abbott Laboratories.

as a bridge from the eardrum to the oval window, which is the entrance to the inner ear.

The inner ear contains the sensory organs of hearing and balance. Our main interest is with the structures and functions of the hearing mechanism. Structurally, the inner ear is composed of the vestibule, which lies on the medial side of the oval window,

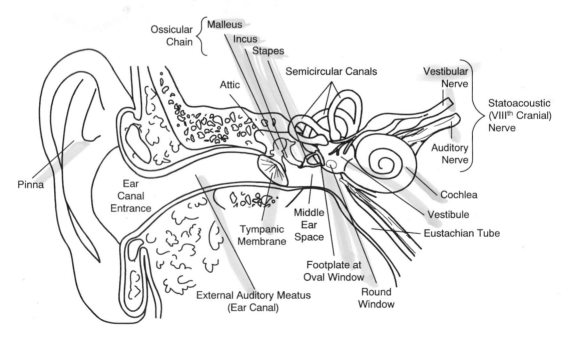

FIGURE 2–3 The major parts of the peripheral ear.

the snail-shaped cochlea anteriorly, and the three semicircular canals posteriorly. The entire system may be envisioned as a complex configuration of fluid-filled tunnels or ducts in the temporal bone, which is descriptively called the labyrinth. The labyrinth, which courses through the temporal bone, contains a continuous membranous duct within it, so that the overall system is arranged as a duct within a duct. The outer duct contains one kind of fluid (perilymph) and the inner duct contains another kind of fluid (endolymph). The part of the inner ear concerned with hearing is the cochlea. It contains the organ of Corti, which in turn has hair cells that are the actual sensory receptors for hearing. The balance (vestibular) system is composed of the semicircular canals and two structures contained within the vestibule, called the utricle and saccule.

The sensory receptor cells are in contact with nerve cells (neurons) that make up the eighth cranial (statoacoustic) nerve, which connects the peripheral ear to the central nervous system. The auditory branch of the eighth nerve is often called the auditory or cochlear nerve, and the vestibular branches are frequently referred to as the vestibular nerve. The eighth nerve leaves the inner ear through an opening on the medial side of the temporal bone called the internal auditory meatus (canal), and then enters the brainstem. Here, the auditory portions of the nerve go to the cochlear nuclei and the vestibular parts of the nerve go to the vestibular nuclei.

The hearing process involves the following series of events. Sounds entering the ear set the tympanic membrane into vibration. These vibrations are conveyed by the ossicular chain to the oval window. Here, the vibratory motion of the ossicles is transmitted to the fluids of the cochlea, which in turn stimulate the sensory receptor (hair) cells of the organ of Corti. When the hair cells respond, they activate the neurons of the auditory nerve. The signal is now in the form of a neural code that can be processed by the nervous system.

The outer and middle ear are collectively called the **conductive system** because their most apparent function is to bring (conduct)

the sound signal from the air to the inner ear. The cochlea and eighth cranial nerve compose the **sensorineural system**, so named because it involves the physiological response to the stimulus, activation of the associated nerve cells, and the encoding of the sensory response into a neural signal. The aspects of the central nervous system that deal with this neurally encoded message are generally called the **central auditory nervous system**.

Temporal Bone

To be meaningful, a study of the ear must begin with a study of the **temporal bone**. Most of the structures that make up the ear are contained within the temporal bone (Fig. 2–2). In fact, the walls of these structures and all of the bony aspects of the ear, except for the ossicles, are actually parts of the temporal bone itself. Recall from your anatomy class that the skeleton of the head is composed of 8 cranial bones and 14 facial bones. The right and left temporal bones compose the inferior lateral aspects of the cranium. Beginning posteriorly and moving clockwise, the temporal bone articulates with the occipital bone behind, the parietal bone behind and above, the sphenoid and zygomatic bones to the front, and the mandible anteriorly below. All of these connections, except for the articulation with the mandible, are firmly united, seam-like fibrous junctions called sutures. The articulation with the mandible is via the highly mobile **temporomandibular joint**.

Lateral and medial views of the temporal bone are shown in Figure 2–4. The lateral surface of the bone faces the outside of the head and the medial surface faces the inside of the head. The temporal bone is composed of five sections, including the mastoid, petrous, squamous and tympanic parts, and the styloid process.

The **squamous part** is a very thin, fan-shaped portion on the lateral aspect of the bone. It articulates with the parietal bone posteriorly and superiorly, and with the sphenoid bone anteriorly. The prominent zygomatic process runs anteriorly to join with the

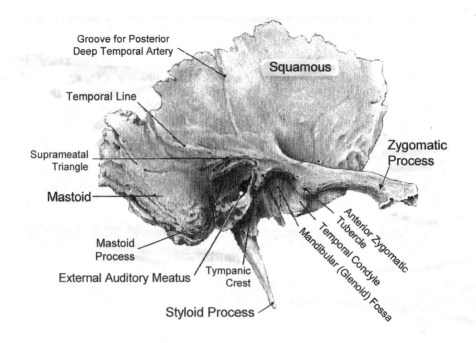

Lateral Aspect of the Right Temporal Bone

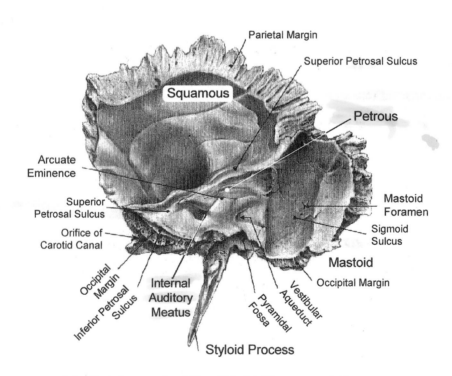

Medial Aspect of the Right Temporal Bone

FIGURE 2–4   Lateral and medial views of the left temporal bone. Adapted from Proctor (1989), with permission.

zygomatic bone, forming the zygomatic arch. Just below the base of the zygomatic process is a depression called the **mandibular fossa**, which accepts the condyle of the mandible to form the temporomandibular joint just anterior to the ear canal.

The **petrous part** is pyramid-shaped and medially oriented so that it forms part of the base of the cranium. This extremely hard bone contains the inner ear and the internal auditory meatus through which the eighth cranial nerve travels on its way to the brainstem, so that much of the discussion pertaining to the inner ear is also a discussion of this part of the temporal bone.

The **mastoid part** composes the posterior portion of the temporal bone. It extends posteriorly from the petrous part, below and behind the squamous part. The mastoid articulates with the occipital bone posteriorly and with the parietal bone superiorly. It has an inferiorly oriented, cone-shaped projection below the skull base called **mastoid process**. The mastoid contains an intricate system of interconnecting air cells that vary widely in size, shape, and number. These are connected with an anterosuperior cavity called the **tympanic antrum**, which is located just behind the middle ear cavity. An opening called the **aditus ad antrum** connects the antrum with the attic or upper part of the middle ear cavity. The roof of the antrum (and the middle ear) is composed of a thin bony plate called the **tegmen tympani**, which separates them from the part of the brain cavity known as the middle cranial fossa. Its medial wall separates it from the lateral semicircular canal of the inner ear. Notice the middle ear, antrum, and air cells compose a continuous, air-filled system. Hence, it is not hard to imagine how an untreated middle ear infection can spread to the mastoid air cell system and beyond.

The tympanic part is inferior to the squamous and petrous parts and anterior to the mastoid. The tympanic part forms the inferior and anterior walls of the ear canal, as well as part of its posterior wall.

The **styloid process** is an anteroinferior pillar-like projection from the base of the temporal bone that widely varies in size. It does not contribute to the auditory structures but is of interest to us as the origin of several muscles involved in the speech mechanism.

Outer and Middle Ear

The **outer ear** is composed of the pinna and the ear canal, ending at the eardrum. The **tympanic membrane** is generally considered to be part of the **middle ear** system, which includes the middle ear cavity and its contents, and "ends" where the ossicles transmit the signal to the inner ear fluids at the oval window.

Pinna

The externally visible aspect of the ear is an odd-shaped appendage called the **pinna** or **auricle**. The internal structure of the pinna is composed principally of elastic cartilage (except for the earlobe). It also contains some undifferentiated intrinsic muscle tissue, as well as a number of extrinsic muscles, although these are vestigial structures in humans. However, these muscles are not vestigial in many lower animals that are able to orient their pinnas with respect to the location of a sound source.

The major landmarks of the pinna are highlighted in Figure 2–5. Notice that the pinna is not symmetrical. For example, and most obviously, it has a flap-like extension that angles away from the skull in the backward direction, so that the pinna overlaps the side of the head posteriorly, superiorly, and inferiorly, but not anteriorly. It also has an intricate arrangement of ridges, bumps, and furrows. The entrance to the ear canal is at the bottom of a large, cup-shaped depression called the concha, and is partially covered by a posteriorly directed projection or ridge called the tragus. The ridged rim along most of the perimeter of the pinna is the **helix**. Starting at the very top of the pinna, the helix courses anteriorly and downward, making a hook-like turn in the posterior direction to form a shelf above the concha, which is the **crus of the helix**. Again, beginning at the top of the pinna, the helix courses downward along the posterior perimeter,

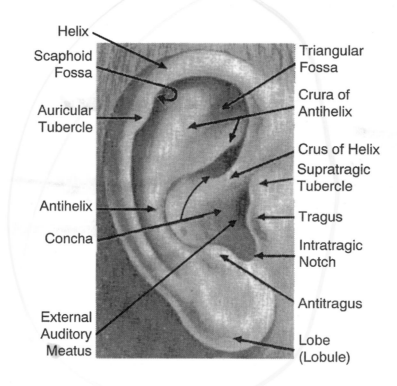

FIGURE 2–5   Major landmarks on the pinna.

reaching the **earlobe**, or **lobule**, at the bottom. The scaphoid fossa is the furrow just anterior to the helix as it courses down the posterior rim of the pinna. The ridge anterior to the scaphoid fossa is called the **antihelix**. The antihelix runs parallel with the helix, and splits superiorly into the two **crura of the antihelix**. The splitting of the antihelix into two crura creates a triangle-shaped depression called the **triangular fossa**. If we follow the antihelix downward, it widens at the bottom to form the **antitragus**, an upward pointing mound that is located posteroinferior to the tragus and superior to the earlobe. The space or angle between the tragus and the antitragus is the **intertragic incisure**.

EXTERNAL AUDITORY MEATUS

The ear canal is more formally called the **external auditory meatus (canal)**. On average, it is about 9 mm high by 6.5 mm wide,

and is roughly 2.5 cm to 3.5 cm long. The ear canal is not quite a straight tube, but has two curves forming a slightly S-like pathway. These curves usually make it difficult to get an unobstructed view of the eardrum, so that it is usually necessary to straighten the canal before looking inside with an otoscope. An otoscope is the familiar instrument used for examining the ear (Fig. 2–6). The ear canal is straightened by gently pulling up and back on the pinna, as illustrated in Figure 2–7.

The external auditory meatus is lined with tight-fitting skin. However, the outer third of the canal is different from the inner two-thirds in a number of ways. The underlying material is cartilage in the outer third and bone for the remainder of its length. The bony portion of the canal is derived from (1) the tympanic part of the temporal bone, which forms the floor and anterior wall, as well as the inferoposterior wall; (2) the squamous part, making up the roof and part of the posterior wall; and (3) the con-

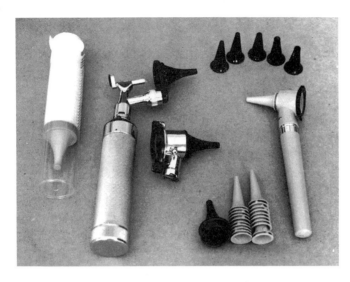

FIGURE 2–6 Examples of otoscopes used for examining the ear, along with reusable and disposable specula. The speculum is the cone-shaped attachment that is inserted into the ear canal.

dyle of mandible, which contributes to the inferoanterior wall at the temporomandibular joint. The cartilaginous portion contains hairs as well as a plentiful distribution of **sebaceous (oil)** and **ceruminous (wax) glands**, although this is not the case for the bony portion of the canal. Sebaceous glands are also present in the concha. These secretions serve lubricating and antimicrobial functions, and also help to keep the canal free of debris and even some foreign bodies and insects.

TYMPANIC MEMBRANE

The external auditory meatus ends at the **tympanic membrane** or **eardrum**, which is tilted at an angle of about 55° to the canal. The tympanic membrane is firmly attached to the **tympanic sulcus**, a groove in the bony canal wall, by a ring of fibrocartilaginous connective tissue called the **tympanic annulus**. The ring has a deficiency at the top due to a tiny interruption in the tympanic sulcus known as the **notch of Rivinus**. The eardrum is a smooth, translucent, and sometimes almost transparent membrane with an average thickness of only about 0.074 mm. It is slightly taller (about 0.9 to 1.0 cm) than it is wide (about 0.8 to 0.9 cm), and it is concave out-

ward rather than flat. The peak of the cone-like inward displacement is called the **umbo**. Structurally, the eardrum is often described as having three layers, although more correctly there are four of them. The most lateral layer of the tympanic membrane is continuous with the skin of the ear canal, and the most medial layer is continuous with the mucous

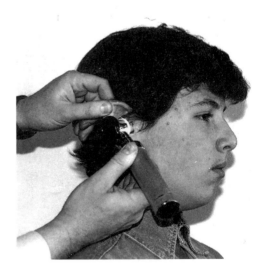

FIGURE 2–7 The ear canal is straightened to facilitate otoscopic inspection by gently pulling up and back on the pinna.

membrane of the middle ear. Sandwiched between them are two fibrous layers. One of them is composed of radial fibers reminiscent of the spokes of a wheel, and the other layer is made of essentially concentric circular fibers.

The tympanic membrane is connected to the malleus, which is the first of the three middle ear bones. Specifically, a long, lateral process of the malleus called the **manubrium** attaches almost vertically to the eardrum, with its tip at the umbo and continuing upward toward the position of 1 o'clock in the right ear and 11 o'clock in the left ear. This attachment of the manubrium of the malleus forms the **malleal prominence**. Ligamentous bands called the **anterior** and **posterior malleal folds** run from both sides of the malleal prominence to the notch of Rivinus, forming a triangular area between them on the eardrum. The largest part of the tympanic membrane lies *outside* or below the malleal folds, and is called the **pars tensa** ("tense part") because it contains all the four layers described above. The superior area of the eardrum between the malleal folds *is missing* the fibrous layers, and is called the pars flaccida ("flaccid area") for this reason. It is also known as **Shrapnell's membrane**.

Figure 2–8 shows some of the major landmarks that are identified when looking at the eardrum through an otoscope. In addition to the landmarks already mentioned, notice that the light from the otoscope is reflected back in a characteristic way, called the **cone of light** or **light reflex**. This reflection is seen as a bright area on the anteroinferior surface of the eardrum, radiating from the tip of the manubrium to the 5 o'clock position in the right ear and the 7 o'clock position in the left ear. It is often possible to identify one or more middle ear landmarks, especially when viewing relatively transparent eardrums.

MIDDLE EAR

The cavity in the temporal bone behind the tympanic membrane is called the **middle ear, tympanum,** or **tympanic cavity**. The posterosuperior portion of the middle ear space is usually viewed as an "attic room" above the main tympanic cavity, and is called the **epitympanic recess** or the **attic**. This space accommodates the more massive portions of the two larger ossicles, the incus and the malleus. Using a certain amount of artistic license, Figure 2–9 depicts the middle ear space as a box-shaped room. Keep in mind, however, that this box is only an analogy used to describe *relative* directions and relationships. The tympanic membrane forms the

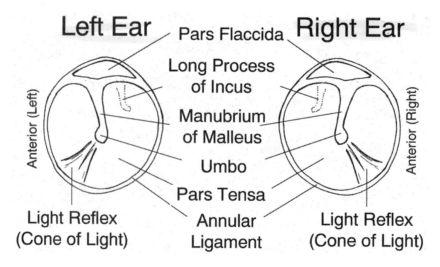

FIGURE 2–8 Major otoscopic landmarks of the tympanic membrane.

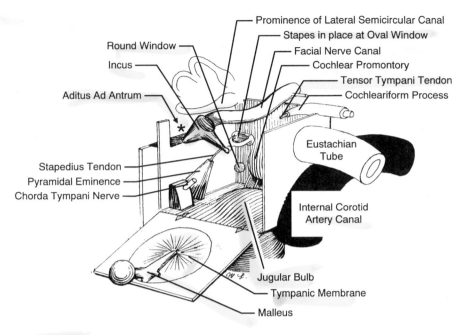

Prominence of Lateral Semicircular Canal
Stapes in place at Oval Window
Facial Nerve Canal
Cochlear Promontory
Tensor Tympani Tendon
Cochleariform Process
Round Window
Incus
Aditus Ad Antrum
Eustachian Tube
Stapedius Tendon
Pyramidal Eminence
Chorda Tympani Nerve
Internal Corotid Artery Canal
Jugular Bulb
Tympanic Membrane
Malleus

FIGURE 2–9 An artist's conceptualization of the middle ear cavity as a room, with the lateral wall (including the eardrum and attached malleus) folded down to reveal the inside. The stapes is shown in place in the oval window. Adapted from Proctor (1989), with permission.

lateral wall, and is shown folded downward to reveal the inside of the "room" in the figure. The middle ear really has irregularly shaped curved surfaces as in the other figures, *not* flat walls with right-angled corners. The floor of the tympanic cavity separates it from the **jugular bulb** below. The ceiling is the **tegmen tympani**, which is the thin bony plate that separates the tympanic cavity from the brain cavity above. Low down on the anterior wall (about 3 mm up from the floor) is the opening of the **Eustachian tube** (sometimes called the **auditory tube**). The **internal carotid artery canal** is located on the other side of (i.e., anterior to) the anterior wall, just below the Eustachian tube. Just above the Eustachian tube is the **tensor tympani semicanal,** which contains the **tensor tympani muscle**. The tensor tympani semicanal and Eustachian tube are separated by a bony shelf or septum. There is a curved bony projection on the anterior/medial wall that points into the middle ear space, called the **cochleari-**

form process. The tendon of the tensor tympani muscle bends around the cochleariform process and proceeds in the lateral direction on its way to the malleus.

The prominent bulge on the medial wall is the **promontory** of the basal turn of the cochlea. The **oval window** of the cochlea (with its attachment to the stapes) is located posterosuperior to the promontory, and the **round window** of the cochlea is posteroinferior to it. The **facial nerve canal prominence** is situated superior to the oval window.

The posterior wall separates the tympanic cavity from the mastoid. The **aditus ad antrum** is an opening located superiorly on the rear wall, and provides communication between the epitympanic recess of the middle ear cavity and the antrum of the mastoid air cell system. The **pyramidal eminence** or **pyramid** is a prominence on the posterior wall that contains the body of the **stapedius muscle**. The **stapedial tendon** exits from the apex of the pyramid and proceeds to the stapes. The

fossa incubus is a recess on the posterior wall that accommodates the short process of the incus. The **chord tympani nerve** is a branch of the **facial (seventh cranial) nerve** that enters the middle ear from an opening laterally at the juncture of the posterior and lateral walls, runs just under the neck of the malleus, and leaves the middle ear cavity via the opening of the **anterior chordal canal (of Huguier)** that is anterior to the tympanic sulcus.

Ossicular Chain Three tiny bones known as the ossicles or the **ossicular chain** transmit the sound-induced vibrations of the tympanic membrane to the cochlea via the oval window (Fig. 2–10). The ossicles are the smallest bones in the body, and include the **malleus, incus**, and **stapes**. Instead of being attached to other bones, the ossicular chain is suspended within the middle ear cavity by ligaments and tendons, as well as its attachments to the tympanic membrane and the oval window. The malleus ("hammer" or "mace") is approximately 8 to 9 mm long and weighs about 25 mg. Its **manubrium** (handle) is firmly embedded between the fibrous and mucous membrane layers of the eardrum, forming the lateral attachment of the ossicular chain. The neck of the malleus is a narrowing between its manubrium and head. Its lateral process produces a bulge on the eardrum that is often visible otoscopically. There is

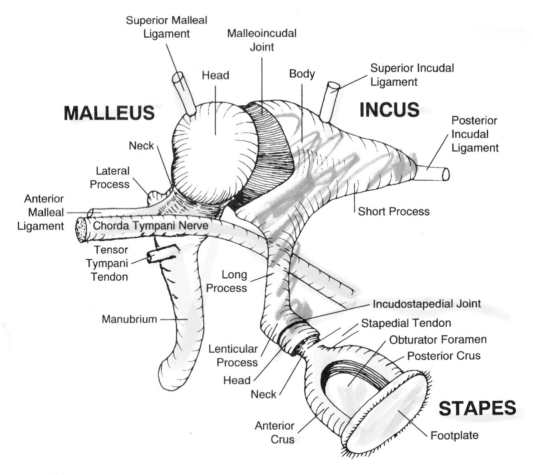

FIGURE 2–10 The ossicular chain in place within the middle ear. Adapted from Tos (1995), with permission.

also an **anterior process** near the junction of the neck and manubrium. The head of the malleus connects with the body of the incus by a diarthrodial or double-saddle joint, the **incudomallear articulation,** such that these two bones move as a unit.

The incus, which is about 7 mm long and weighs roughly 30 mg, is commonly called the "anvil" but looks more like a tooth with two roots. The **short process** is posteriorly oriented and is accommodated by the fossa incudis on the back wall of the middle ear. The **long process** descends from the body of the incus, parallel with the manubrium of the malleus, and then hooks medially to end at a rounded nodule called the **lenticular process**. In turn, the lenticular process articulates with the head of the stapes via a true ball-and-socket or enarthrodial joint called the **incudo-stapedial joint**.

The stapes bears a close resemblance to a "stirrup," which is its common name. Its head is connected via the neck to two strut-like processes called the **anterior** and **posterior crura**, which lead down to the oval-shaped **footplate**. The opening between the crura and footplate is called the **obturator foramen**. The stapes weighs only 3 to 4 mg. It is about 3.5 mm long, and the footplate has an area of roughly 3.2 mm². The footplate is attached to the oval window by the **annular ligament**, forming the medial attachment of the ossicular chain.

In addition to its lateral attachment to the tympanic membrane and its medial attachment at the oval window via the annular ligament, the ossicular chain is also supported by several ligaments and the tendons of the two middle ear muscles. The **superior malleal ligament** runs from the roof (tegmen tympani) of the attic down to the head of the malleus. The **anterior malleal ligament** goes from the anterior tympanic wall to the anterior process of the malleus. The **lateral malleal ligament** extends from the bony margin of the notch of Rivinus to the neck of the malleus. The **posterior incudal ligament** (actually a fold of mucous membrane rather than a ligament) runs from the fossa incudus to the short process of the incus.

Middle Ear Muscles   The **tensor tympani muscle** is innervated by the **trigeminal (fifth cranial) nerve**. It is housed within the tensor tympani semicanal in the anterior middle ear wall superior to the Eustachian tube. This muscle is about 25 mm long, and arises from the cartilage of the Eustachian tube, the walls of its semicanal, and the segment of sphenoid bone adjacent to the canal. The **tensor tympani tendon** bends around the cochleariform process and proceeds in the lateral direction to insert on the malleus at the top of the manubrium near the neck. Contraction of the tensor tympani pulls the malleus in the anteromedial direction, thereby stiffening the ossicular chain.

The **stapedius muscle** is the smallest skeletal muscle in the body, with an average length of only 6.3 mm. It is contained within the pyramidal eminence of the posterior wall of the tympanic cavity, and is innervated by the **facial (seventh cranial) nerve**. The **stapedius tendon** exists via the apex of the pyramidal eminence and runs anteriorly to insert on the posterior aspect of the neck of the stapes. Contraction of the stapedius pulls the stapes posteriorly. Even though the middle ear muscles pull in more or less opposite directions, they both exert forces that are perpendicular to the normal motion of the ossicles, and their contraction has the effect of stiffening the ossicular chain, thereby reducing the amount of energy that is delivered to the inner ear.

The **acoustic reflex** refers to the reflexive middle ear muscle contraction that occurs in response to high levels of sound stimulation (Gelfand, 1984, 1998). In humans this is at least principally a stapedius reflex, while the tensor tympani contracts as part of a startle reaction to very intense sounds, and also in response to certain kinds of nonacoustic stimulation such as an air jet directed at the eye. The acoustic reflex involves both muscles in some animals.

The fundamental aspects of the **acoustic (stapedius) reflex arc** are as follows (Borg, 1973; Wiley & Block, 1984): The sensory (afferent) pathway proceeds via the auditory nerve to the ventral cochlear nucleus, and then to the superior olivary complex on *both sides* of the brainstem (with the crossover to the opposite side by way of the trapezoid body). The motor (or efferent) pathway is followed bilaterally, and is from the motor nuclei of the **facial (seventh cranial) nerve** on both sides, and then via the facial nerves to the stapedius muscles. The motor pathway for tensor tympani activation goes from the **trigeminal (fifth cranial) nerve** nuclei to the tensor tympani muscles via the trigeminal nerves. Because contraction of the stapedius and tensor tympani muscles stiffens the middle ear system, the transmission of low frequencies is reduced (Simmons, 1959; Møller, 1965; Rabinowitz, 1976). This change has been observed as a decrease in hearing sensitivity or loudness for low-frequency sounds (Smith, 1946; Reger, 1960; Morgan & Dirks, 1975), although these effects are not always found (Morgan, Dirks, & Kamm, 1978).

The purpose of the acoustic reflex is not really known, although several theories have been proposed. The *protection theory* suggests the acoustic reflex protects the inner ear from potentially damaging sound levels. However, it is unlikely that this is its main purpose because the reflex has a delay (latency) that would make it an ineffective protection against sudden sounds, and the contraction adapts over time, limiting its protection against ongoing sounds. The *fixation theory* holds that the middle ear muscles maintain the appropriate positioning and rigidity of ossicles, and the *accommodation theory* states the muscles modify the characteristics of the conductive system so that the absorption of sound energy is maximized. Simmons (1964) suggested the acoustic reflex improves the audibility of environmental sounds by attenuating internal sounds. This enhancement of signal-to-noise ratio would improve the survival rates for both the fox who is hunting for dinner and the rabbit who is trying to avoid being the main course. Similarly, Borg (1976) proposed that one of the purposes of the reflex is to improve the listener's dynamic range by attenuating low frequency sounds. Discussions of these and other reflex theories may be found in several sources (Jepsen, 1963; Simmons, 1964; Borg, Counter, & Rosler, 1984).

EUSTACHIAN TUBE

The **Eustachian (auditory) tube** provides for the aeration and drainage of the middle ear system, and makes it possible for air pressure to be the same on both sides of the eardrum. It runs from the anterior middle ear wall to the posterior wall of the nasopharynx behind the inferior nasal turbinate, as illustrated in Figures 2–11 and 2–12. In adults the Eustachian tube follows a 3.5- to 3.8-cm-long course that is directed inferiorly, medially, and anteriorly, tilting downward at an angle of about 45°. However, it is important to be aware that the Eustachian tube is almost horizontal in infants and young children (see Fig. 6–5 in Chapter 6). The first third of the tube beginning at the middle

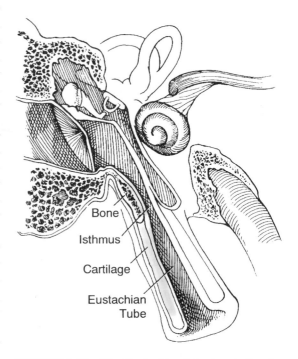

Bone

Isthmus

Cartilage

Eustachian Tube

FIGURE 2–11 The Eustachian tube in relation to the ear. Note that the bony portion of the tube meets the cartilaginous portion at the isthmus. Adapted from Hughes (1985), with permission.

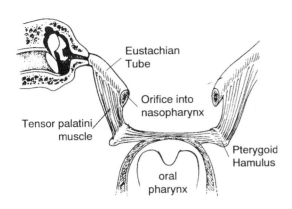

FIGURE 2–12 Relationship of the Eustachian tube to the tensor palatini muscle, highlighting the parts of the muscle that arise from the tubal cartilage, hook around the pterygoid hamulus of the sphenoid bone, and insert into the palate. Adapted from Hughes (1985), with permission.

ear is surrounded by bone and the remainder is surrounded by an incomplete ring of elastic cartilage. The meeting point of the **bony** and **cartilaginous portions** is called the **isthmus**. The lumen of the Eustachian tube is narrowest at the isthmus, where it is only 1 to 2 mm across compared to 3 to 6 mm in the remainder of the tube. A prominence on the pharyngeal wall, the **torus tubarius**, is formed by the cartilage of the Eustachian tube and other tissues (e.g., the salpingopalatine, salpingopharyngeous, and tensor palatini muscles).

The cartilaginous portion of the Eustachian tube is arranged as shown in Figure 2–13. Notice that the cartilage hooks around the tube from above, forming the incomplete ring alluded to above. A portion of the tensor palatini muscle is attached to the hooked segment of the cartilage (Figs. 2–12 and 2–13). At rest, the cartilage keeps the Eustachian tube closed (Fig. 2–13a). The lumen of the tube is opened when the cartilage is uncurled due to the pull exerted by the tensor palatini muscle (Fig. 2–13b). This occurs during swallowing, yawning, and other actions that cause the tensor palatini muscle to contract. Negative pressure develops in the

middle ear (compared to the outside, atmospheric pressure) when this mechanism fails to open the Eustachian tube frequently and effectively. We have all experienced this phenomenon as fullness in the ears that is (hopefully) alleviated when the tube "pops open" due to a swallow, yawn, or some other maneuver. Swelling and/or blockage by mucus due to colds or allergy, and obstruction of the pharyngeal orifice by hypertrophic (enlarged) adenoids, are just a few of the causes of a nonpatent Eustachian tube. The resulting negative pressure within the closed-off middle ear space often precipitates the development of clinically significant middle ear disease.

Functioning of the Conductive Mechanism

Sound entering the outer ear is picked up by the tympanic membrane. The vibrations of the eardrum are transmitted to the ossicular chain, which vibrates essentially in the right-left plane. This vibration is represented as a rocking motion of the stapes footplate in the

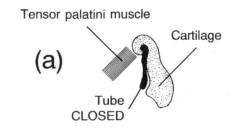

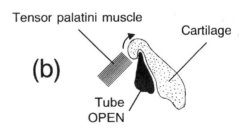

FIGURE 2–13 (a) The hook-shaped arrangement of the Eustachian tube cartilage keeps the tube in the normally closed state. (b) The tube is opened when the cartilage hook is uncurled by action of the tensor palatini muscle.

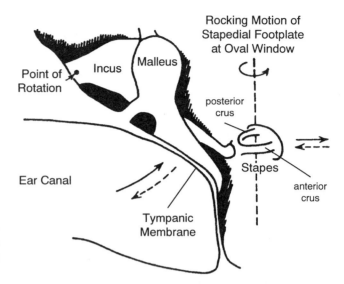

FIGURE 2–14 The middle ear transmits the signal to the cochlea via a rocking motion of the stapedial footplate at the oval window. After Bekesy (1941).

oval window, as shown in Figure 2–14. The resulting inward and outward displacements of the oval window are thus transmitted to the cochlear fluid. However, instead of just serving as an inert passageway that allows sound to travel to the cochlea from the surrounding air, the conductive mechanism actually modifies sound in several ways that have a direct bearing on how and what we hear.

HEAD-RELATED TRANSFER FUNCTION

Sounds reaching the eardrum are affected by the acoustics of the external auditory meatus, which operates as a quarter-wavelength resonator because it is essentially a tube with one open end and one closed end (at the tympanic membrane). Sounds entering the ear will be enhanced if they are close to the resonant frequency range, resulting in

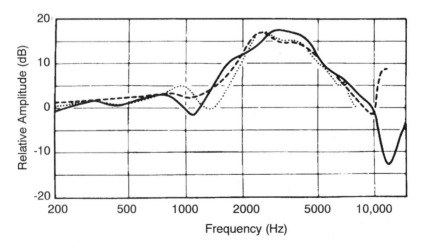

FIGURE 2–15 Average head-related transfer functions (sound level at the eardrum compared to outside of the ear) for sounds presented from a loudspeaker directly in front of the subjects. [Dotted line, Wiener & Ross (1946); dashed line, Shaw (1974); solid line, Mehrgardt & Mellert (1977).] From Mehrgardt & Mellert (1977), with permission of *J Acoust Soc Am*.

a boost in the sound pressure level (SPL) reaching the eardrum, called the **ear canal resonance effect**. To determine this boost in level (or gain) at the eardrum, the sound presented from a loudspeaker is monitored by a microphone outside the patient's ear and also by a special kind of microphone that monitors the sound level inside the subject's ear canal, very close to his eardrum. The difference between these two measurements is the amount of gain provided by the ear canal resonance, shown as a function of frequency in Figure 2–15. On this kind of graph, 0 dB means "unchanged," that is, that the SPL at the eardrum is the same as it is outside the person's ear. Positive values show the amounts of gain provided by the ear canal resonances (negative values mean that the level is lower at the eardrum than outside the ear). We see clearly that the resonance characteristics of the ear canal provide a sound level boost of as much as 15 to 20 dB in the frequency range from roughly 2000 to 5000 Hz. In addition, the middle ear has a resonant region between approximately 800 Hz and about 5000 or 6000 Hz (Zwislocki, 1975). The resonant responses of the conductive system affect our hearing sensitivity for sounds at different frequencies, as discussed in Chapter 3.

The graph in Figure 2–15 is technically called the **head-related transfer function (HRTF)** because it shows how the sound reaching the eardrum is affected by the direction of the sound source relative to the head. In other words, the HRTF shows how the spectrum is changed by the acoustical path from the loudspeaker to the eardrum. Thus, it is sometimes also called the **soundfield to eardrum transfer function**. The HRTF actually reflects the accumulated effect of all factors that influence the sound on the way from the loudspeaker to the tympanic membrane, including acoustical shadows, reflections, and diffraction due to the head and body, as well as the ear canal resonance. This is why the figure caption specifies the direction of the loudspeaker. These acoustical effects depend on the direction of the sound

and are important cues for directional hearing, or the ability to identify the location of a sound source and differences in locations between different sound sources.

Sound direction is described in terms of angles around the head (Fig. 2–16). The easiest way to describe the location of a sound source is to give its angle relative to the head (e.g., so many degrees to the right, so many degrees straight up from the front, etc.) The **horizontal plane** refers to horizontal directions around the head toward the right and toward the left. Horizontal directions

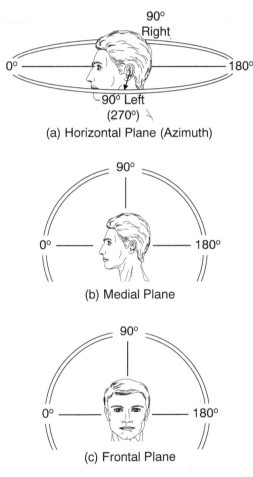

(a) Horizontal Plane (Azimuth)

(b) Medial Plane

(c) Frontal Plane

FIGURE 2–16 Directions around the head. The *horizontal plane* goes around the head horizontally from right to left; the *medial (median) plane* goes around the head vertically from front to back; the *frontal plane* goes around the head vertically in the right-left direction.

are usually called angles of **azimuth**. For example:

0° azimuth is *straight ahead* (in front of your nose);

90° azimuth is directly *to the right* (in front of your right ear);

180° azimuth is *straight back* (directly behind your head); and

270° azimuth is directly *to the left* (in front of your left ear).

Thus, an azimuth of 45° means 45° to the right, and 315° azimuth is the same as 45° to the left. By the way, it is perfectly fine to say "45° to the right" and "45° to the left." It is also acceptable (and often confusing) to use positive angles for one direction and negative values for the other, such as +60° azimuth for 60° to the right, and −60° azimuth for 60° to the left.

Azimuths of 0° and 180° are both dead center between the two ears. The same thing is true for elevations such as straight up above the center of the head, 45° upward from directly in front, 30° downward from directly in front, and 70° upward from straight back. These are examples of directions in the **medial (or median) plane**. The

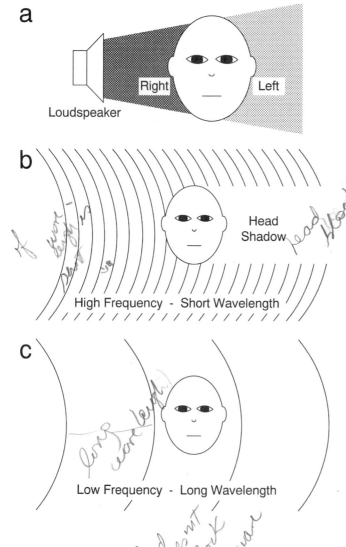

FIGURE 2–17 Sound coming from a loudspeaker off to the right side (a) arrives differently at the two ears. An acoustical shadow (the head shadow effect) occurs for high-frequency sounds because their wavelengths are small compared to the size of the head (b). Because of their large wavelengths, low-frequency sounds are not subjected to a head shadow because they are able to bend around the head (c).

medial plane is the same as going around the head vertically in the *midsagittal anatomical plane*, so that all locations on the medial plane are equidistant from the two ears. In the medial plane 0° is straight ahead, 90° is straight up, and 180° is straight back. To complete the picture, vertical directions around the head in an arc from right to left constitute the **frontal plane**. In this case, 0° is directly to the right, 90° is straight up, and 180° is straight to the left.

To appreciate how directional differences are represented acoustically at the ears, let us suppose that a loudspeaker is located at an azimuth of 45° to the right, as depicted in Figure 2–17a. Even though the original sound is the same, it reaches the left ("far") ear differently than the right ("near") ear. The far ear is subjected to an acoustical shadow when the head obstructs the path of the sound (Fig. 2–17b). As a result, the sound reaches the far ear at a softer level than it reaches the near ear. This level disadvantage at the far ear is called the head shadow effect. The head shadow occurs for frequencies that can be obstructed by the head. This occurs for sounds with wavelengths that are short compared to the size of the head. Recall that wavelength gets shorter as frequency increases. Hence, the head shadow affects relatively higher frequencies, especially those over about 1500 Hz. This level difference between the ears is called an **inter-ear (interaural) intensity difference**.

The result of these differences at the eardrum can be seen by comparing the ear canal transfer functions obtained when a loudspeaker is located at different locations around the head, and might be called the **azimuth effect**. Figure 2–18 illustrates the

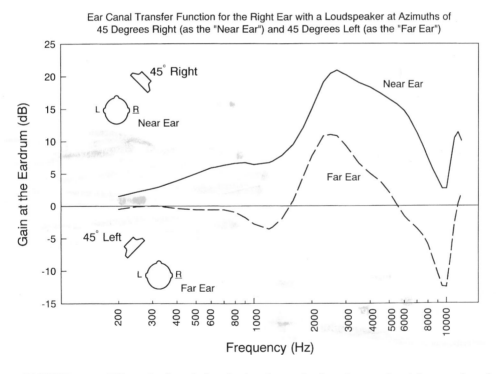

FIGURE 2–18 Effect of azimuth: head-related transfer functions at the right ear when the loudspeaker is located at azimuths of 45° to the right (a "near ear" situation) versus 45° to the left (a "far ear" situation). Based on data by Shaw (1974) and Shaw & Vaillancourt (1985).

azimuth effect by showing how the head-related transfer functions are different for the right ear when a loudspeaker is at an azimuth of 45° to the right compared to when it is 45° to the left (i.e., 45° versus 315°). The sound level at the right eardrum is greater when the sound comes from 45° to the right ("near ear") compared to when it comes from 45° to the left ("far ear"). Notice that the shape of the curve also changes depending on the azimuth. This graph shows the results at two representative azimuths. Curves obtained from many azimuths all around the head would reveal a continuum of these kinds of differences (Shaw, 1974).

Low frequencies have wavelengths that are long relative to the size of the head, so that diffraction can occur. In other words, they are able to bend around the head to the far ear with little if any loss of level (Fig. 2–17c). However, the sound will arrive at the near ear earlier than at the far ear, constituting an **inter-ear (interaural) time difference**. Interaural intensity and time differences provide the principal cues needed for directional hearing.

PINNA EFFECT

What does the pinna do for us? It has long been known that any amplification provided by the pinna is essentially negligible in spite of its funnel-like appearance, and that its main contribution to hearing is in the realm of sound source localization (Bekesy & Rosenblith, 1958). (To appreciate the importance of the pinna in directional hearing, one has only to watch a cat orient its pinnae toward a sound source.) The pinna provides sound localization cues because its asymmetrical and irregular shape, ridges, and depressions modify the spectrum of a sound in a way that depends on the direction of the source (Blauert, 1983). The simplest example is that sounds coming from the rear are obstructed by the pinna so that some of the high-frequency components of their spectra are attenuated compared to the same sounds

arriving from the front. These kinds of pinna-related spectral differences are particularly important when inter-ear sound differences are negligible or absent. This is the case for localizations in the medial plane and/or when trying to localize sounds with just one ear.

THE MIDDLE EAR TRANSFORMER

The sound signal that reaches the ear in the form of air vibrations must be transmitted to the cochlea, which is a fluid-filled system. The impedance of the cochlear fluids is much greater than the impedance of the air. As a result, most of the sound energy would be reflected back if airborne sound were to impinge directly on the cochlear fluids, and only about 0.1% of it would actually be transmitted. This situation is analogous to the reflection of airborne sound energy off the water's surface at the beach, which is why you cannot hear your friends talking when your head is under the water. The middle ear system overcomes this impedance mismatch by acting as a mechanical *transformer* that boosts the original signal so that energy can be efficiently transmitted to the cochlea.

The transformer function of the middle ear is accomplished by the combination of three mechanisms: (1) the area ratio advantage of the eardrum to the oval window, (2) the curved membrane buckling effect of the tympanic membrane, and (3) the lever action of the ossicular chain. The largest contribution comes from the **area advantage**. Here, the force that is exerted over the larger area of the tympanic membrane is transmitted to the smaller area of the oval window, just as the force applied over the head of a thumbtack is concentrated onto the tiny area of its point (Fig. 2–19). Pressure is force divided over area (p = F/A), so that concentrating the same force from a larger area of the eardrum down to a smaller area of the oval window results in a proportional boost in the pressure at the oval window.

The **curved membrane buckling** mechanism is illustrated in Figure 2–20. The ear-

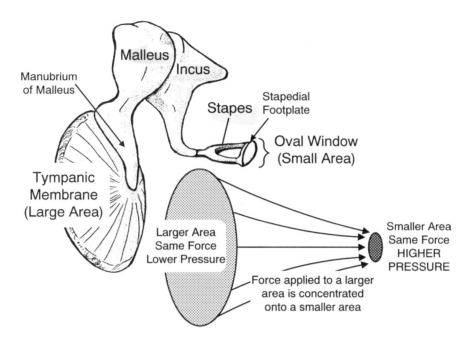

FIGURE 2–19   The area advantage involves concentrating the force applied over the tympanic membrane to the smaller area of the oval window.

drum curves from its rim at both ends to its attachment to the manubrium toward the middle. As a result, eardrum vibration involves greater displacement for the curved membranes and less displacement for the manubrium, which might be envisioned as a buckling effect. A boost in force accompanies the smaller displacement of the manubrium because the product of force and displacement must be the same on both sides of a lever ($F_1 \times D_1 = F_2 \times D_2$). The third and smallest contributor to the middle ear transformer mechanism is the lever **action of the ossicular chain**. Figure 2–21 shows how the malleus constitutes the longer leg of this lever and the incus is the shorter leg, as well as the axis of rotation.

How much of a boost does this transformer mechanism provide? To answer this question we can plug some representative values into the relationships just discussed. The area of the eardrum is roughly 85 mm²; however, only about two-thirds of this area vibrates effectively (Bekesy, 1960), so that the effective area of the eardrum is something

like 56.7 mm². The area of the oval window is roughly 3.2 mm. Hence, the area ratio is 56.7 to 3.2, or 17.7 to 1. The ossicular lever ratio is about 1.3 to 1. So far, the total advantage is $17.7 \times 1.3 = 23$ to 1. In terms of pressure the decibel value of this ratio would be $20 \times \log (23/1) = 27$ dB. However, if we add the curved membrane buckling advantage of 2 to 1, the ratio becomes $23 \times 2 = 46$ to 1. In decibels of pressure, the total advantage now becomes $20 \times \log (46/1) = 33$ dB. This is only an approximation; the actual size of the pressure advantage varies considerably with frequency (Nedzelnitsky, 1980).

Inner Ear

The Cochlea

Recall the inner ear is set up like a duct inside of a duct. The outer duct is called the **osseous or bony labyrinth** because its walls are made of the surrounding bone. The inside duct is made of membranous materials and is thus called the **membranous**

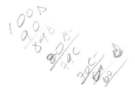

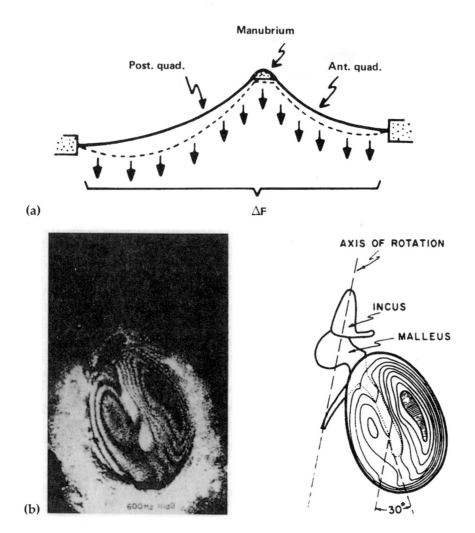

FIGURE 2–20   (a) The curved membrane buckling principle involves a boost in force at the manubrium because it moves with less displacement than the curved eardrum membrane. (b) Variations in the amount of displacement are shown by concentric contours in this photograph and corresponding drawing of the vibration pattern of the cat's eardrum at 600 Hz. The two areas of concentric contours on both sides of the manubrium show the eardrum's vibration pattern agrees with the curved membrane principle. From Tonndorf & Khanna (1970), with permission of *Ann Otol Rhinol Laryngol.*

labyrinth. The osseous and membranous labyrinths are represented in Figure 2–22.

It is useful to "build" a simple model of this apparently complicated system, as in Figure 2–23a. This model will represent the auditory part of the labyrinth, the cochlea. The outer, bony duct is represented by a steel pipe that is closed at the back end. The inner, membranous duct is represented by a pliable rubber hose (or a long balloon) with a closed-off end that is inserted almost all the way into the pipe. The left and right sides of the pliable hose are glued to the inner right and left sides of the pipe, forming

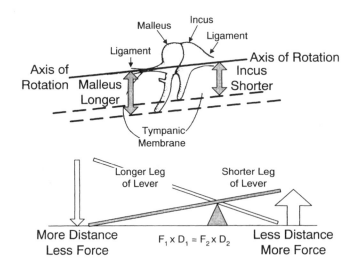

FIGURE 2–21 Axis of rotation and relative lengths of the longer (malleus) and shorter (incus) legs of the ossicular lever. Based in part on Bekesy (1941).

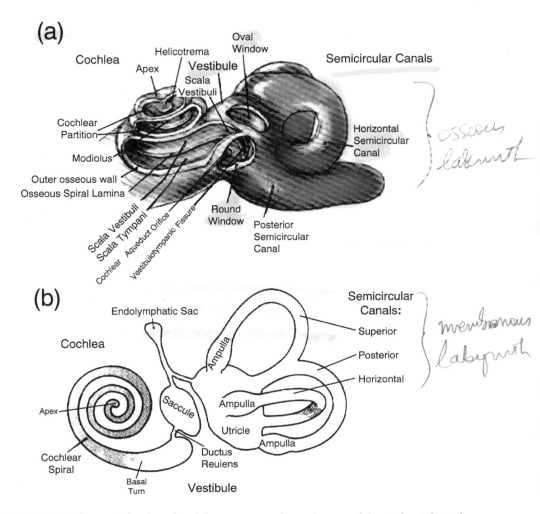

FIGURE 2–22 The major landmarks of the osseous and membranous labyrinths. Adapted from Proctor (1989), with permission.

three chambers. The middle chamber is completely enclosed by the rubber hose. The upper chamber is above the rubber hose and the lower chamber is below the rubber hose. We now pour water that contains blue food coloring into the rubber hose. Hence, the middle chamber contains blue water. Then we pour water that contains red food coloring into one of the outer chambers, and we find that the red water fills both of the outer chambers. This occurs because the rubber hose does not extend all the way to the far end of the pipe, so that the two outer chambers are jointed at that end. We then close off the open ends of the ducts with transparent plastic so that the water does not leak out. We now have a model of a duct inside of a duct. It has two outer chambers filled with

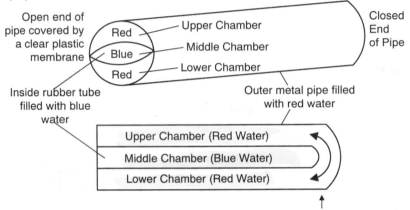

(a) "Pipe model" of the uncurled cochlea.

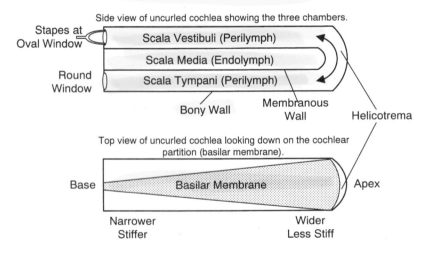

(b) Schematic views of the uncurled cochlea.

FIGURE 2–23 (a) A model made of a rubber hose glued within a steel pipe to represent an uncurled cochlea (see text). (b) Conceptual drawing of an uncoiled cochlea.

red water that are separated by an inner chamber filled with blue water. In addition, the outer chambers are continuous at the back end of the pipe.

Notice the similarities between our pipe model in Figure 2–23a and an artist's representation of a cochlea (Fig. 2–23b) that has been "uncurled" from its snail shell configuration. Here the upper duct is called the scala vestibuli and the lower duct is called the scala tympani. They are separated by a middle duct, called the scala media. A liquid called **endolymphatic fluid** or **endolymph** fills the scala media, whereas the two outer ducts are filled with a different liquid called **perilymphatic fluid** or **perilymph**. The two outer ducts meet at the far end of the tube at an opening called the **helicotrema**. The stapes at the oval window is at the base of scala vestibuli, and the round window is at the basal end of the scala tympani. The scala media is separated from the scala vestibuli above it by Reissner's membrane, and from the scala tympani below it by the **basilar membrane**. Notice that the basilar membrane is narrowest at the base and becomes progressively wider toward the apex.

Perilymph is similar to most extracellular fluids in the sense that it contains a large concentration of sodium. On the other hand, endolymph is virtually unique among extracellular fluids because it contains a high concentration of potassium. The same fluids are contained in the balance portion of the inner ear, as discussed below. The membranous labyrinths of the hearing and balance systems are connected by a tiny duct called the **ductus reuniens**, forming one continuous endolymph-filled system. Another conduit called the **endolymphatic duct** leads from the membranous labyrinth in the vestibule to the **endolymphatic** sac partly located in a niche in the petrous part of the temporal bone and between the layers of dura in the posterior cranial fossa. In addition, the **cochlear aqueduct** leads from an opening in the scala tympani to the subarachnoid space.

The cochlear duct is about 35 mm long and is coiled in the form of a cone-shaped spiral staircase. The resulting arrangement looks like a 5 mm high snail shell that is 9 mm wide at its base and tapers toward the apex (Fig. 2–22a). The superstructure of the spiral duct is a bony shelf called the **osseous spiral lamina** that makes about 2¾ turns around a central core called the **modiolus**, as shown in Figure 2–24. Figure 2–24a also shows that the medial side of the membranous duct (scala media) is attached to the lateral lip of the bony shelf, and follows it from base to apex. (Inside the cochlea, "medial" means toward the center core of the spiral, and "lateral" means toward the outer perimeter of the spiral, or away from the center core.) Figure 2–24b shows how the cochlea would appear if cut down the center and opened to reveal the inside arrangement. Here we see several cross-sectional views of the cochlear duct going around the modiolus. The osseous spiral lamina forms a shelf that divides each section of the duct into an upper and lower part. The section of each duct above the shelf is the scala vestibuli and the section below the shelf is the scala tympani. The membranous duct that is attached to the lip of the shelf in Figure 2–24a is not shown in Figure 2–24b; however, it would continue across the duct to form the middle chamber, the scala media. The osseous spiral lamina is actually composed of two plates separated by a space that serves as a passageway for nerve fibers. In addition, the core of the modiolus itself is hollow and leads to the **internal auditory meatus** (Fig. 2–24b), providing a conduit for the auditory nerve and blood supply to the cochlea.

Figure 2–25 is a cross section of one part of the cochlear duct, showing the scala media between the scala vestibuli above and the scala tympani below, as well as auditory nerve cells coursing through the osseous spiral lamina toward the modiolus. A close-up view emphasizing the structures inside the scala media is shown in Figure 2–26. Both of these figures are oriented so that the modiolus is toward the left (medial) and the outer wall of the cochlea is toward the right (lateral). The outer wall of the cochlear duct is covered with a band of fibrous connective

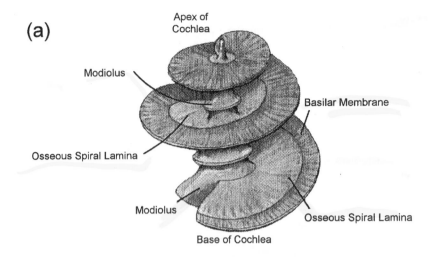

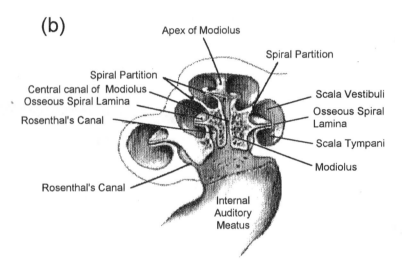

FIGURE 2–24   (a) The superstructure of the cochlea is a bony shelf called the osseous spiral lamina that spirals around a central core called the modiolus. (b) Cross section through the cochlea showing the cochlear duct coiling around the modiolus. The center of the modiolus is hollow and leads to the internal auditory meatus. Adapted from Proctor (1989), with permission.

tissue called the **spiral ligament**. The top of the osseous spiral lamina is covered by a thickened band of periosteum called the **limbus**. The **basilar membrane** is a fibrous membrane that runs horizontally from the osseous spiral lamina to the spiral ligament. Reissner's membrane is a thin membrane that goes from the top of the medial aspect of the limbus to the spiral ligament at an upward angle of about 45°. The endolymph-filled scala media is contained within these borders, with the perilymph-filled scalae vestibuli and tympani above and below, respectively.

The rounded space formed by the concave lateral side of the limbus is called the **internal spiral sulcus**. The **organ of Corti** is the

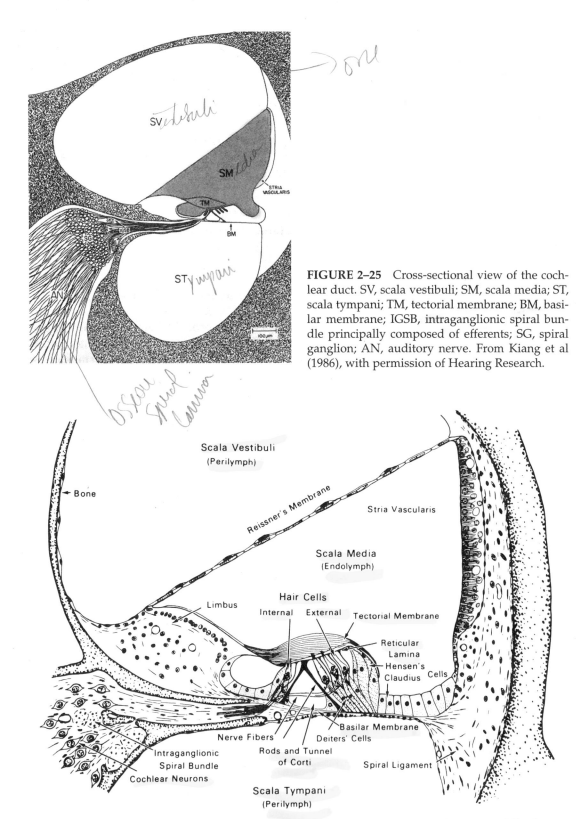

FIGURE 2–25 Cross-sectional view of the cochlear duct. SV, scala vestibuli; SM, scala media; ST, scala tympani; TM, tectorial membrane; BM, basilar membrane; IGSB, intraganglionic spiral bundle principally composed of efferents; SG, spiral ganglion; AN, auditory nerve. From Kiang et al (1986), with permission of Hearing Research.

FIGURE 2–26 Cross-sectional view of the cochlear duct emphasizing the organ of Corti in the scala media. Adapted from Davis (1962), with permission of *J Acoust Soc Am*.

61

sensory organ for hearing, and sits on the basilar membrane lateral to the internal spiral sulcus. The **tectorial membrane** arises from the upper lip of the limbus and forms the overlying membrane of the organ of Corti. The tectorial membrane is mainly composed of collagen fibers that give it considerable tensile strength and make it quite compliant (Zwislocki, Chamberlain, & Slepecky, 1988). The lateral margin of the tectorial membrane attaches via a net of fibers to the lateral supporting cells of the organ of Corti. Attached to the spiral ligament is a rich network of capillaries called the **stria vascularis** that maintain the chemical environment of the scala media.

The organ of Corti is a complex arrangement of sensory hair cells along with various accessory cells and structures. The conspicuous upside-down Y seen roughly in the center of the organ of Corti composes the **pillars or rods of Corti**. These pillar cells enclose a triangular space called the **tunnel of Corti**. The thin lines running across the tunnel are auditory nerve fibers (discussed later). Medial to the tunnel of Corti is a single row of **inner hair cells (IHCs)** and lateral to it are three rows of **outer hair cells (OHCs)**. These cells are called hair cells because they are topped by tufts of microscopic hairs called stereocilia. The stereocilia extend upward from the **cuticular plate**, which is a thickening on the top of the hair cell. Only one inner hair cell and three outer hair cells are shown in Figure 2–26 because this drawing cuts across the cochlear tube, whereas these rows of cells (along with all of the organ of Corti) course up the length of the duct. A variety of supporting cells are also identified in the figure, although it is not necessary to address them individually in an introductory discussion. Auditory nerve cells or fibers from the hair cells enter the osseous spiral lamina through openings called the **habenula perforata**.

An impervious layer called the **reticular lamina** is formed by the tops (cuticular plates) of the hair cells, as well as by the upper ends of the tunnel cells and other supporting cells. The reticular lamina isolates the underlying structures of the organ of Corti from the rest of the scala media above them. Moreover, the fluid in the spaces below the reticular lamina is similar to the perilymph of scala tympani,[1] and provides the sodium-rich environment needed for the functioning of the hair cells and unmyelinated nerve fibers in the organ of Corti. In addition, endolymph must be kept out because it is toxic to the hair cells.

Figure 2–27 shows the upper surface of the reticular lamina. Here we can easily see the three rows of outer hair cells topped by a W- or V-shaped cluster of stereocilia. The tops of the inner hair cells are identified by the row of stereocilia bunches located toward the right side of the figure. The stereocilia on top of the IHCs have a very wide W shape even though they seem to form a straight line at first glance. The tectorial membrane overlays the reticular lamina. The stereocilia of the OHCs are firmly attached to the undersurface of the tectorial membrane. On the other hand, it appears that the stereocilia of the IHCs are not attached to the tectorial membrane.

Electrical voltage differences called **resting potentials** exist between different parts of the cochlea. The perilymph is usually considered to be the reference point, so that its voltage is 0 millivolts (mV). Compared to the perilymph, the endolymph has polarity of about +100 mV and is called the **endocochlear potential** (Peak, Sohmer, & Weiss, 1969). The electrical potential inside the hair cells is called the **intracellular potential**, and is about –40 mV in the IHCs and –70 mV in the OHCs (Dallos, 1986).

Hair Cells   There are about 3500 inner hair cells and 12,000 outer hair cells in each ear. Schematic representations of the two kinds of cochlear hair cells are shown in Figures 2–28a,b. The IHCs are flask-shaped, whereas the OHCs are tube-like. Both types have rows

---

[1] It was previously thought to be a separate fluid known as *cortilymph*.

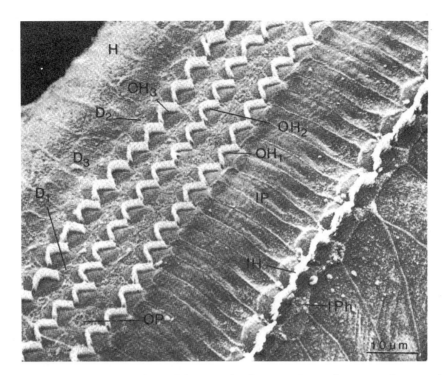

FIGURE 2–27 The upper surface of the reticular lamina. Notice the stereocilia extending upward from the single row of inner hair cells (IH) and the three rows of outer hair cells (OH1, OH2, OH3). The cilia are white in the figure. This picture is oriented so that the medial side of the duct (modiolus) is toward the right and the lateral or outer side (spiral ligament) is toward the left. [DI–3, Deiters' cells; OP and IP, outer and inner pillar cells; IPh, inner phalangeal cells; H, Hensen's cells.] From Lim (1986a), with permission of *Hearing Research*.

of different-sized stereocilia protruding from the cuticular plates at their top ends. There is also a noncuticular area containing another kind of cilium called the **basal body** or **rudimentary kinocilium** just beyond the tallest row of stereocilia. In spite of the similarities between inner and outer hair cells, one cannot help notice their many differences. We have already seen that the inner and outer hair cells differ substantially in number, occupy different locations in the organ of Corti, and relate differently to the tectorial membrane. We shall see that they have different neural connections, as well. Notice in the drawings that the distribution of cellular structures is also different for the two types of cells. The inner hair cells have concentrations of Golgi apparatus, mitochondria, and other organelles associated with the extensive metabolic activity needed to support the sensory reception process. The outer hair cells contain **contractile proteins** and a number of structural characteristics that are usually associated with muscle cells. In fact, the OHCs are able to shorten and lengthen (both pull and push) in response to neural signals and chemical agents. Their **motility** is important for the normal operation of the cochlea. The interested student will readily find several more detailed explanations of this and related issues elsewhere (Lippe, 1986; Dallos, 1988; Pickles, 1988; Brownell, 1990; Gelfand, 1998).

The hair cells are activated when their stereocilia are bent toward the basal body. The basal body is at the base of the W- or V-shaped arrangement

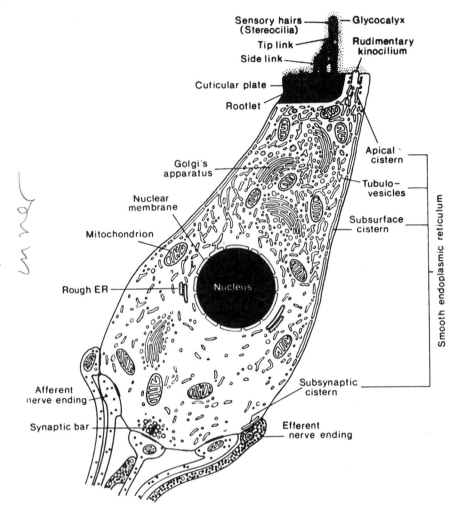

FIGURE 2–28a Schematic drawing of the inner hair cells. From Lim (1986b), with permission.

of the stereocilia, which is oriented toward the spiral ligament on the outer wall of the cochlear duct, that is, away from the modiolus (Fig. 2–27). Thus, *hair cells respond when their stereocilia are caused to bend toward the lateral wall of the duct, or away from the modiolus.* The reason why the hair cell responds when the stereocilia bend in a particular direction requires a closer look at the stereocilia themselves. Figure 2–29 shows a close-up of a representative bunch of stereocilia. Notice that there are various kinds of tiny filaments or **cross-links** between the stereocilia.

Figure 2–30 highlights the kind of filament that goes *upward* from the top of a shorter cilium to the side of a taller one, known as an upward-pointing or tip-to-side cross-link. The mechanism of hair cell activation is based on this relationship (Pickles, Comis, & Osborne, 1984; Hudspeth, 1985; Pickles & Corey, 1992), and is illustrated in Figure 2–31. Bending of the stereocilia in the direction just described pulls or stretches the upward-pointing cross-link, as in the figure panel labeled *excitation*. Pulling the filament opens a **pore** (analogous to a trap door) on

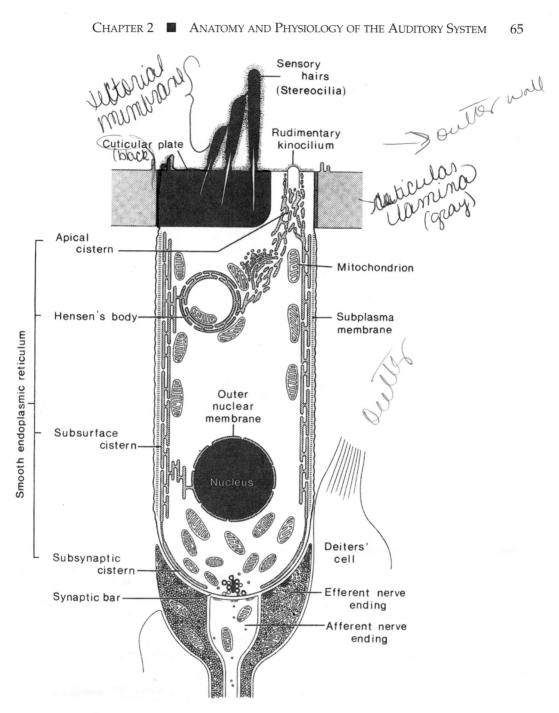

FIGURE 2–28b Schematic drawing of the outer hair cells. From Lim (1986b), with permission.

the top of the shorter cilium, which permits ions to flow through it, thereby activating the cell. Bending of the stereocilia in the opposite direction compresses the filaments so that the pore is closed, as shown in the figure panel labeled *inhibition*. This appears to be the mechanism by which mechanical-to-electrochemical transduction occurs in the hair

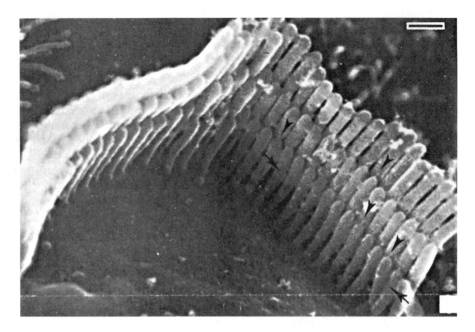

FIGURE 2–29   Cross-linking filaments between stereocilia. Arrows show *side-to-side* cross-links between adjacent stereocilia. Arrowheads show *upward-pointing* or *tip-to-side* cross-links that go from the top of a shorter cilium upward to the side of another cilium in the next taller row. From Furness & Hackney (1986), with permission of *Hearing Research*.

cells. The resulting response of the hair cell is then transmitted to the adjoining auditory neurons.

INNERVATION OF THE COCHLEA

The cochlear hair cells are connected to the auditory nervous system by their synapses with auditory nerve fibers within the organ of Corti. These nerve fibers go through the habenula perforata leading to their cell bodies to form the **spiral ganglia** located in **Rosenthal's canal** of the modiolus, and then proceed into the internal auditory meatus (Figs. 2–24b, 2–25, and 2–26). The neural fibers twist like the fibers of a rope to form the auditory nerve. In general, neurons originating from the apex of the cochlea are arranged toward the core of the nerve trunk and those from the base of the cochlea spiral are closer to the outside. The innervation of the cochlea involves both afferent and efferent neurons. The **afferent** nerve supply is made up of *ascending sensory* neurons that send sig-

nals from the cochlea to the nervous system. The **efferent** nerve supply includes a much smaller population of *descending* neurons that send signals from the nervous system to the cochlea.

Afferent Innervation   The afferent auditory nerve supply is unequally distributed between the inner and outer hair cells and involves two different kinds of neurons (Spoendlin, 1969, 1978, 1986; Kiang, Rho, Northrop, Liberman, & Ryugo, 1982; Liberman, 1982a). These relationships are shown in Figures 2–32 and 2–33. Approximately 95% of the afferent auditory neurons supply the inner hair cells and the remaining 5% go to the outer hair cells. Each IHC exclusively receives about 20 nerve fibers that come to it directly in the radial direction from the habenula perforata. The wiring diagram is much different for the much smaller number of afferent fibers that supply the OHCs. These neurons bypass the IHCs, cross under the tunnel of Corti (Fig. 2–26), turn and travel about 0.6 mm along

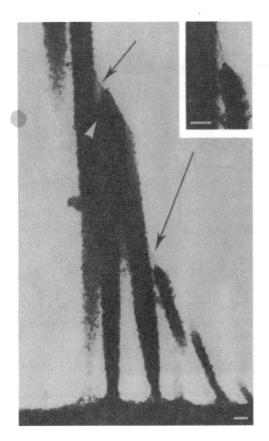

FIGURE 2–30 Upward-pointing (tip-to-side) cross-links going from the top of a shorter cilium upward to the side of a taller one are shown by arrows and the close-up in the insert. A row-to-row cross-link is also shown (white arrowhead). From Pickles, Comis, & Osborne (1984), with permission of *Hearing Research*.

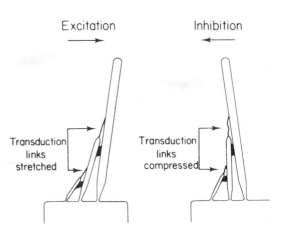

FIGURE 2–31 Bending of the stereocilia in one direction leads to excitation by stretching upward-pointing cross-links, thereby opening a pore which permits ions to flow. Bending in the opposite direction causes inhibition because the pore closes. From Pickles, Comis, & Osborne (1984), with permission of *Hearing Research*.

the spiral toward the base of the cochlea, and then send collateral fibers to about 10 *different* OHCs. In addition, each OHC receives collateral fibers from several different neurons. Because of the paths that they follow, the neurons that go to the IHCs are called **inner radial fibers** and the ones that go to the OHCs are called **outer spiral fibers**. All of these fibers are unmyelinated while they are inside the organ of Corti.

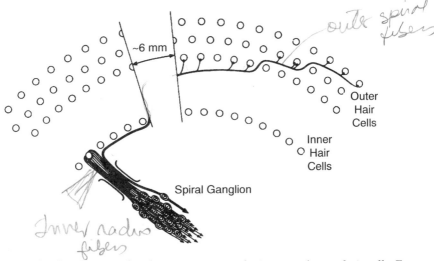

FIGURE 2–32 The distribution of auditory neurons to the inner and outer hair cells. From Spoendlin H, 1978, The afferent innervation of the cochlea, in Naunton RF, Fernandez C (Eds.): *Electrical Activity of the Auditory Nervous System* by Academic Press.

After exiting the organ of Corti, the inner radial fibers from the IHCs continue in the modiolus as type I auditory neurons. These fibers are large in diameter, myelinated, bipolar sensory neurons. A bipolar neuron has a cell body located somewhere along the axon as opposed to being at one end. Outer radial fibers from the OHCs continue as type II auditory neurons, which are unmyelinated, small in diameter, and pseudomonopolar rather than bipolar. Type I and type II auditory neurons are illustrated just below the spiral ganglion in Figure 2–33. Most if not all of what we know about the functioning of auditory nerve fibers is derived from the type I neurons. In summary: (1) the IHCs are innervated by inner radial fibers that continue outside the organ of Corti as type I auditory neurons; and (2) the OHCs are innervated by outer spiral fibers that continue outside the organ of Corti as type II auditory neurons.

Efferent Innervation   The cochlea receives efferent signals from the nervous system via the **olivocochlear bundle (Rasmussen's bundle)**, which is a series of descending pathways that go from the superior olivary complex to the cochlea. Approximately 1600 efferent neurons from the olivocochlear bundle enter the temporal bone along with the vestibular branch of the eighth nerve, and then split off to enter the cochlea where they are then distributed to the hair cells. The endings of the efferent neurons have vesicles containing the chemical neurotransmitter acetylcholine, and they communicate differently with the inner and outer hair cells.

The distribution of efferent fibers is the opposite of that for the afferents, that is, most of them go to the outer hair cells. The attachments of the efferent neurons are also different for the two groups of hair cells (Fig. 2–34). Efferent neurons synapse *directly* with OHCs.

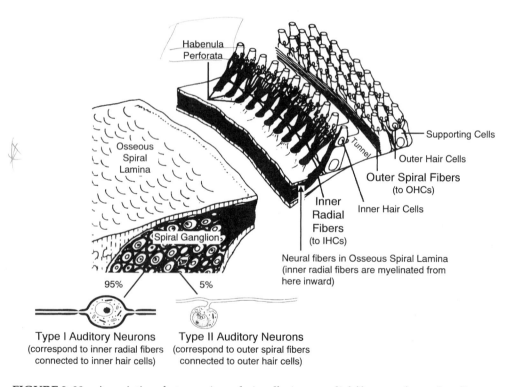

FIGURE 2–33   Associations between inner hair cells, inner radial fibers, and type I auditory neurons in the spiral ganglion, and outer hair cells, outer spiral fibers, and type II auditory neurons. Based on Spoendlin H, The afferent innervation of the cochlea, in *Electrical Activity of the Auditory Nervous System* (RF Naunton & C Fernandez, Eds.), © 1978 by Academic Press.

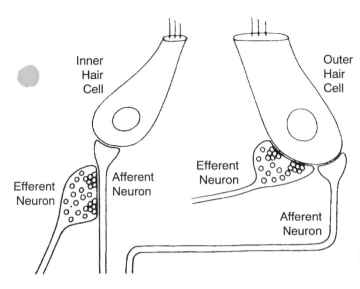

FIGURE 2–34 Efferent neurons synapse directly with outer hair cells and the afferent neurons of inner hair cells. Adapted from Spoendlin (1986), with permission.

As a result, efferent neurons act on OHCs before they synapse with their afferent neurons (presynaptically). However, this is not the case for the inner hair cells. Here, the efferent fiber synapses with the *afferent neurons that are associated with the inner hair cells*, so that their effect is postsynaptic. In other words, the efferent neuron acts directly on an outer hair cell, but for inner hair cells the efferent fiber acts on the afferent neuron downstream of its synapse with the hair cell.

Vestibular Organs and Innervation

The sensory receptor organs of the vestibular system share the bony and membranous labyrinths with the cochlea (Fig. 2–22). The balance end-organs are located posterior to the cochlea and include the **utricle** and **saccule**, which are within the vestibule, as well as the **semicircular canals**.

Each ear contains three semicircular canals that respond to angular acceleration, that is, circular motions such as turning one's head. These canals are at right angles to each other so that they can respond to angular motion in any direction. Each canal has an **ampulla**, which is a widening anteriorly where it joins the vestibule, as shown in Figure 2–35. The ampulla contains a receptor organ called the

crista. The base of the crista contains the **vestibular hair cells** and their supporting cells. These hair cells are very similar to cochlear hair cells, except that they have a large **kinocilium** instead of a basal body. The top portion of the crista is the **cupula**, a mound-shaped gelatinous mass that blocks the flow of endolymph in the canal, much like a swinging door. The stereocilia of the hair cells extend into the cupula. The vestibular hair cell synapses with vestibular neurons below it, which are part of the eighth cranial nerve.

The operation of the semicircular canals is quite straightforward. First, consider a simple experiment with a bowl of water that illustrates the concept. If you quickly revolve the bowl clockwise, you will notice the motion of the water lags behind the motion of the bowl. This occurs because of the inertia of the water (due to its mass), as well as the ability of the water to move within the bowl. In relative terms, the lagging behind of the water when the bowl moves clockwise is the same as if the bowl had stood still and the water moved counterclockwise. In this experiment the bowl represents the head and the water represents the endolymph within a semicircular canal. Similarly, the endolymph in the semicircular canals will lag behind when the head turns, which is the same as the motion of the endolymph in the opposite direction. For example, turning the head to the right causes a relative motion of the endolymph to the left in the horizontal (lateral) semicircular canals.

Recall that the cupula crosses the ampulla of the canal like a swinging door. Thus, the flow of the endolymph in the semicircular canals will deflect the cupula. Because the hair cell cilia extend into the cupula, deflection of the cupula also bends the cilia, thereby stimulating the hair cells, which in turn transmits their response to the underlying neurons. As Figure 2–35 shows, the response of the hair cells is excitatory (the neurons fire faster)

when the stereocilia bend toward the kinocilium, and inhibitory (the neurons fire slower) when they bend away from it. As illustrated in the left panel of the figure, the hair cells are oriented in the horizontal (lateral) canal so that the endolymph flow deflecting the cupula toward the utricle (utriculopedal flow) is excitatory, whereas endolymph flow away from the ampulla (utriculofugal flow) is inhibitory. The right panel in the figure shows that the opposite arrangement exists in the two vertical semicircular canals.

The utricle and saccule respond to gravity and linear acceleration, which means motion

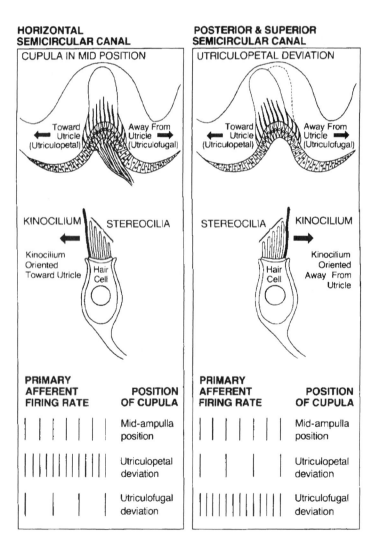

FIGURE 2–35 Head turning in one direction causes endolymph flow in the opposite direction within the semicircular canals, which deflects the cupula and in turn bends the hair cell cilia. From McGee (1986), Electronystagmography in peripheral lesions. *Ear Hear 7*, 167–175, with permission.

in a straight line (such as front-back, right-left, or up-down). The sensory receptor organs of the utricle and saccule are called the **maculae**. Each macule contains vestibular hair cells that synapse with the eighth nerve neurons. Their cilia project up into a gelatinous material called the **otolith membrane**, on top of which are found calcium carbonate crystals called **otoliths**. For this reason, the utricle and saccule are also called the **otolith organs**. The hair cells are stimulated when the otolith bears down on the otolith membrane, thereby deflecting the cilia. This can be caused by gravity or by linear acceleration, in which case the inertia of the otoliths causes them to lag behind the movement of the head. The otolith organs can respond to gravity or linear acceleration in any direction because of their orientation inside the vestibule and the way in which the hair cells are arranged along each macule. The saccule is approximately vertical and the utricle is roughly horizontal. In addition, hair cells are organized with opposite orientations on each side of a curved "line" (the **striola**) along each macule. Consequently, motion in any direction will cause some hair cells to be stimulated (i.e., their stereocilia will bend toward the kinocilium).

Functioning of the Sensorineural Mechanism

Stimulation is transmitted to the cochlear fluids by the in-and-out motions of the stapedial footplate at the oval window at the base of the cochlea. The oval window leads into the upper chamber (scala vestibuli). Hence, a given inward motion will cause the fluids to be displaced downward, pushing downward on the basilar membrane, and a given outward motion will displace the fluids and basilar membrane upward. The trick is to translate this vibratory stimulation into the bending of the hair cell stereocilia in the right direction, which we already know is necessary to activate the sensory process. In addition, the mechanism for accomplishing this activity must account for our ability to hear different pitches.

Historically, two kinds of classical theories have attempted to explain how basilar membrane vibrations are converted into neural signals that distinguish between different frequencies. In the **resonance place theory**, Helmholtz (1895) proposed that the basilar membrane was constructed of segments that resonated in response to different frequencies, and that these segments were arranged according to location (place) along the length of the basilar membrane. To achieve this tuning, the segments at different locations would have to be under different degrees of tension. (We all know that changing the tension on a guitar string changes its pitch, and that musicians adjust this tension to tune the instrument.) According to resonance theory, a sound entering the cochlea causes the vibration of the segments that are tuned to (resonate at) the frequencies that it contains. Because these resonators are laid out according to place, the locations of the vibrating segments signal which frequencies are present. In contrast, **temporal** (or **frequency**) **theories** of hearing, like Rutherford's (1896) "telephone theory," claimed that the entire cochlear responds as a whole to all frequencies instead of being activated on a place-by-place basis. Here, all aspects of the stimulus waveform would be transmitted to the auditory nerve (like a telephone receiver connected to the telephone wire), and then the frequency analysis is accomplished at higher levels in the auditory system.

The resonance theory had several significant problems, two of which will be mentioned. Sharply tuned resonators damp very slowly, so they would have to continue vibrating long after the stimulus is gone. This after-ringing would be like a never-ending echo that does not exist, and would preclude useful hearing if it did. In addition, this theory cannot explain why we hear a pitch corresponding to 100 Hz when we are presented with a stream of clicks at a rate of 100 per second, or when we are presented with several harmonics of 100-Hz (e.g., 1200, 1300, and 1400 Hz). After all, how can the 100-Hz segment of the basilar membrane respond when a 100-Hz signal is not physically present?

Temporal theory had its own problems. For example, damage to a certain part of the cochlea results in a hearing loss for certain frequencies but not for others (e.g., basal damage causes high-frequency hearing loss). Yet temporal theory says that location and frequency are unrelated. In addition, the auditory nerve must be able to carry all the information in the sound wave. Neurons code information in the form of individual all-or-none neural discharges (described later in this chapter). There is an *absolute refractory period* of about 1 msec between discharges during which they cannot fire, no matter how powerful the stimulus might be. It would be no problem for a neuron to fire 410 times per second for a 410-Hz signal, or 873 times per second for an 873-Hz signal, but the 1-msec refractory period limits the maximum firing rate to roughly 1000 times per second. Hence, temporal theory could not explain how we hear the frequencies well above about 1000 Hz.

The resonance model of place theory and the old temporal theories that denied place coding in the cochlea were both wrong. Place coding is very much real, but it operates according to the **traveling wave** model (Bekesy, 1960), discussed later. Temporal coding also exists. Even though neurons cannot respond to all of the individual cycles, it has been shown they can follow the periodicity of a sound for frequencies as high as about 5000 Hz on a probability basis, even though they actually fire in response to relatively few individual cycles (e.g., Kiang, 1965). In other words, even though a particular neuron may not discharge very often, when it does fire it will do so in synchrony with a certain phase of the stimulus. The synchronous nature of neural discharges to a certain phase of the signal is called **phase locking**.

The **volley principle** (Wever, 1949) proposed that several neurons operating *as a group* could fire in response to each cycle of a high-frequency sound, even though none of them can do so individually. This is possible if one neuron fires in response to one cycle, and another neuron fires in response to the next cycle (while the first nerve cell is still in its refractory period), etc. The **place-volley theory** (Wever & Lawrence, 1954) involves the combined operation of both place and temporal mechanisms. Low frequencies are handled by temporal coding, high frequencies by place, and an interaction of the two mechanisms occurs for the wide range of frequencies between the two extremes.

TRAVELING WAVE THEORY

Bekesy's (1960[2]) **traveling wave theory** describes how frequency is coded by place in the cochlea. Contrary to resonance theory, Bekesy found that the basilar membrane is not under any tension, but that its elasticity is essentially uniform. Because the basilar membrane gets wider going toward the top, the apex, the result is a *gradation of stiffness* along its length, going from *stiffest at the base* (near the stapes) to *least stiff at the apex* (near the helicotrema). As a result of this stiffness gradient, sounds transmitted to the cochlea develop a special kind of wave pattern on the basilar membrane that always travels from the base up toward the apex, called **the traveling wave**.

The characteristic traveling wave pattern is shown in Figure 2–36. In this diagram, the x-axis represents the distance in millimeters up the basilar membrane from the stapes. In the figure the base of the cochlea would be toward the left and the apex of the cochlea would be toward the right. The y-axis represents the relative amount of basilar membrane displacement. The outer dashed lines represent the *envelope* of the traveling wave displacement pattern along the basilar membrane. It shows the traveling wave involves a displacement pattern that (1) gradually increases in amplitude as it moves up the basilar membrane, (2) reaches a peak at a cer-

---

[2] Bekesy's work on the traveling wave is largely reproduced in his book, *Experiments in Hearing* (1960). For simplicity, the book is cited here as a general reference for this body of work; however, the figures cite the original sources.

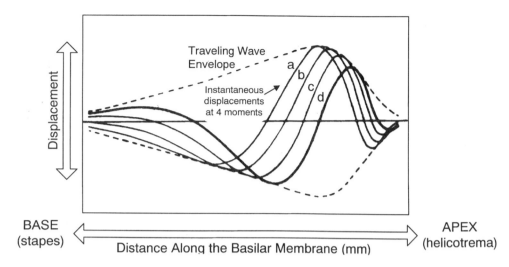

FIGURE 2–36   Characteristics of the traveling wave (see text). This particular traveling wave was generated by a 200-Hz stimulus, and peaked at a distance of about 29 mm from the base of the cochlea. Based on Bekesy (1953).

tain location, and (3) decays in amplitude rather quickly just beyond the peak. The four solid lines inside the envelope represent the *instantaneous displacements* of the basilar membrane at four phases of the wave cycle. In other words, the instantaneous displacement of the basilar membrane changes from moment to moment, proceeding from **a** to **b** to **c** to **d**, and so on. If these four instantaneous displacement curves were expanded into a complete set, then they would fill the shape of the traveling wave envelope. Imagine a movie in which each successive frame contains one of the instantaneous displacements, arranged in order. The resulting movie image would be a wave that travels up the cochlea (from left to right in the figure) with the overall shape of the traveling wave envelope indicated by the dashed lines.

The location (place) of the traveling wave peak along the basilar membrane depends on the frequency of the sound. In other words, the traveling wave is the mechanism that translates signal frequency into place of stimulation along the basilar membrane. High frequencies are represented toward the base of the cochlea, and successively lower frequencies are represented closer and closer to the apex, as illustrated in Figure 2–37. The

traveling wave brings the stimulus to the appropriate location for a given frequency, which involves motion *along* the length of cochlear duct. However, the stereocilia must be bent away from the modiolus in order for the hair cells to respond. In other words, the traveling wave moves *along* the cochlear duct (in the longitudinal direction) but the stereocilia must be bent *across* the duct (in the *radial* direction). This would be a problem if the basilar membrane was free on both sides so that its displacement would generate forces only in the *longitudinal* direction, as in Figure 2–38a, but this is not the case. The basilar membrane is actually attached along both sides, at the osseous spiral lamina medially and at the spiral ligament laterally. As a result, the traveling wave will also cause a *radial* force to be applied *across* the duct near the traveling wave peak, as in Figure 2–38b. (This type of effect can be approximated by jiggling the free end of a bed sheet when its sides are tucked under the sides of the mattress.)

This radial force near the traveling wave peak causes the stereocilia to bend away from the modiolus, thereby activating the hair cells by the following mechanism (Davis, 1958): The medial attachment of the basilar

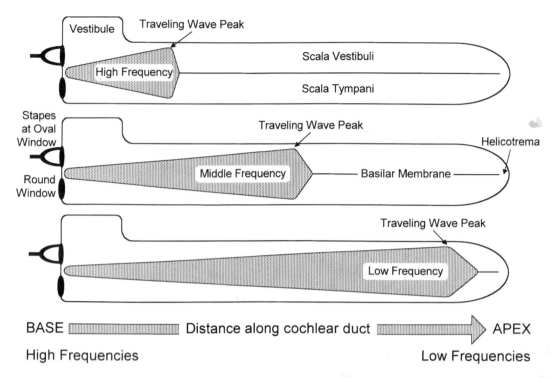

BASE ▨▨▨▨▨▨ Distance along cochlear duct ▨▨▨▨▨ ➤ APEX

High Frequencies   Low Frequencies

FIGURE 2–37   The traveling wave is the place coding mechanism of the cochlea. This artist's conceptualization shows that the traveling wave peak occurs toward the *base* of the cochlea for *high* frequencies and toward the *apex* for *low* frequencies.

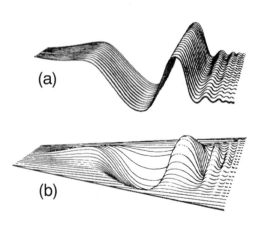

FIGURE 2–38   (a) Imagined basilar membrane vibration pattern if it was not fixed along its sides. (b) Actual basilar membrane vibration pattern, with forces in the radial direction in the vicinity of the traveling wave peak. From Tonndorf (1960), with permission of *J Acoust Soc Am*.

membrane is at the tip of the osseous, the spiral lamina. Hence, up or down motions will cause the basilar membrane to pivot around this point. The hair cells and reticular lamina also follow this motion. On the other hand, the tectorial membrane is attached at the lip of the limbus, so that it has a different pivot point than the reticular lamina. As a result of these different pivot points, upward and downward deflections will cause the reticular lamina and the tectorial membrane to move relative to one another. The stereocilia extend between these two differently hinged membranes, and are therefore subjected to a **shearing** action or shearing force when displacement of the duct causes these two membranes to move relative to each other. This shearing action bends the cilia away from the modiolus when the cochlear duct is displaced upward, as illustrated in Figure 2–39. The OHC cilia are sheared be-

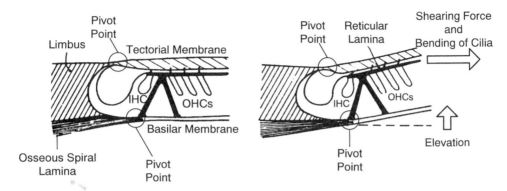

FIGURE 2–39 Relative motion between the basilar and tectorial membranes places a shearing force on the stereocilia so they are bent away from the modiolus when the cochlear duct is displaced upward. Based on Davis (1958).

cause they are attached to the tectorial membrane, and the IHC cilia are sheared because of the drag imposed on them by the surrounding fluid when the membranes are displaced (Dallos, Billone, Durrant, Wang, & Raynor, 1972). The result is activation of the hair cells leading to the excitation of their associated auditory neurons. [Shearing can sometimes occur with downward deflections because the flexibility of the tectorial membrane allows it to bend over the internal sulcus (e.g., Steel, 1983).]

The electrochemical activity involved in the hair cell response activity produces electrical signals called **receptor potentials**, which can be monitored with electrodes. One of these receptor potentials is an AC (alternating current) signal that faithfully represents the stimulus waveform, called the **cochlear microphonic**. The other receptor potential is the **summating potential**, which appears as a deviation or shift in the DC (direct current) baseline.

The Cochlear Amplifier   Recall that the outer hair cells are directly connected to the tectorial membrane, receive neural signals from the olivocochlear bundle, and have the capability of motility. These characteristics constitute an active, micromechanical system that sensitizes and fine tunes the responsiveness of the cochlea, known as the **cochlear amplifier** (Davis, 1983). In other words, the cochlear

amplifier enhances the signal received by the inner hair cells so they can be activated by faint sound levels and respond faithfully to narrow frequency ranges. This mechanism accounts for the sensitivity needed to hear soft sounds and the ability to hear fine frequency distinctions. Figure 2–40 shows an example of the sharply tuned response (tuning curve) of a normal cochlea that is seen only in live animals with healthy cochleas (Russell & Sellick, 1977; Khanna & Leonard, 1982; Sellick, Patuzzi, & Johnstone, 1982). In particular, the sharp peak is particularly dependent on the integrity of the outer hair cells (e.g., Kiang, Liberman, Sewell, & Guinan, 1986). Notice that the sharp peak is missing for the other curve in the figure, representing a situation where these conditions have not been met. The stria vascularis appears to be the source of metabolic energy for the cochlear amplifier. These active processes also appear to be responsible for the ability of the cochlea to *produce* sounds called **otoacoustic emissions** that can be picked up by sensitive microphones in the ear canal (Chapter 11).

AUDITORY NERVE RESPONSES

Neurons produce *all-or-none electrical discharges* called **action potentials**, which are recorded as **spikes**, as illustrated in Figure 2–41. The number of spikes per second is called the **firing** or **discharge rate**. Auditory

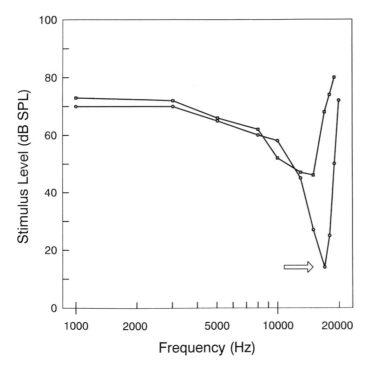

FIGURE 2–40 The sharply peaked curve reveals the very narrow, mechanical tuning of the basilar membrane in a completely healthy cochlea (arrow). The sharp peak is lost when the integrity of the cochlea is compromised, or post-mortem, as shown by the other curve. Idealized curves based on findings by Sellick et al (1982).

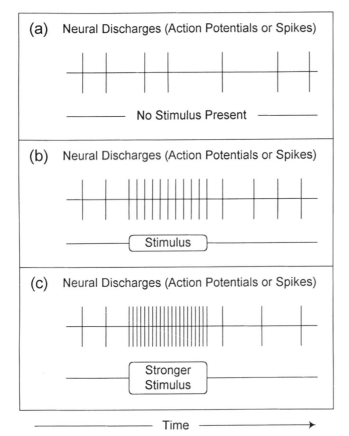

FIGURE 2–41 Idealized firing rates of an auditory neuron (a) in the absence of stimulation (spontaneous rate); (b) with a relative weaker stimulus; and (c) with a relatively stronger stimulus.

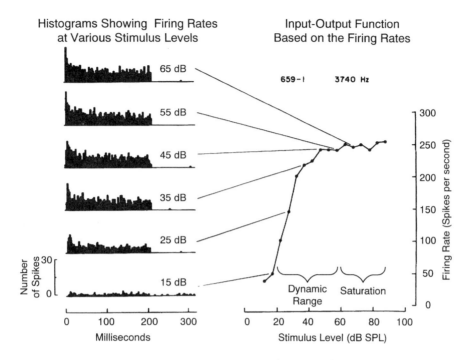

FIGURE 2–42 The firing rate of an auditory neuron increases as the stimulus intensity increases within its dynamic range, and eventually plateaus. Left: Histograms showing firing rates. (Notice that the discharge pattern has an initial peak followed by an ongoing firing rate that continues during the stimulus.) Right: Input-out function. Adapted from Salvi, Henderson, & Hamernik (1983). Physiological bases of sensorineural hearing loss, in Tobias, Shubert (Eds.): *Hearing Research and Theory, Vol. 2* by Academic Press.

neurons have a certain ongoing firing rate even when they are not being stimulated, called the **spontaneous firing rate** (Fig. 2–41a). Stimulation causes the firing rate to increase (Fig. 2–41b), and raising the stimulus level causes the neuron to fire even faster (Figure 2–41c), at least within certain limits. The faintest sound level that induces a response from a neuron is called its **threshold**.[3]

Figure 2–42 show that an auditory neuron has a **dynamic range** over which its firing rate increases with stimulus level, after which the firing rate **saturates** or stops growing as the stimulus level increases further.

Auditory neurons vary in threshold over a range of about 60 dB or more, and their dynamic ranges are about 25 dB wide for some groups of auditory neurons and about 40 dB or more for others (e.g., Sachs & Abbas; Liberman, 1988). These gradations of thresholds and dynamic ranges contribute to the ability of the auditory nerve to represent a wide range of sound intensities.

Auditory neurons represent frequency information by both place and temporal coding. The place coding mechanism is represented by the tuning curves in Figure 2–43 (Kiang, 1965). Each tuning curve shows the range of frequencies to which a given nerve fiber responds at different levels of stimulation. A given curve was obtained here by finding the threshold for a particular neuron for many different frequencies. Let us concentrate on the curve highlighted by the

---

[3] Auditory neurons often respond with a reduction in firing rate from the spontaneous rate at bare-threshold levels, above which increasing stimulus levels result in an increasing firing rate.

arrow because it shows a complete set of thresholds over a wide range of frequencies. The narrow part of the curve shows that the neuron responds to a very limited range of frequencies at relatively soft levels (downward on the y-axis). The peak of the curve shows the lowest threshold of the neuron, and the frequency where this occurs is its **characteristic frequency (CF)**. The CF is 5000 Hz for the highlighted curve. The orderly arrangement of CFs reflects the places along the length of the cochlea where the neurons are connected (e.g., Liberman, 1982b). The neuron responds to a slightly wider range of frequencies around its CF as the stimulus level is raised (upward on the y-axis). If the stimulus is raised high enough, then the neuron will respond to a wide range of frequencies extending well below its characteristic frequency. This phenomenon appears as the "tail" on the low-frequency side of the curve. However, the neuron is not responsive to much higher frequencies even when they are presented at very intense stimulus levels.

Another way to look at how auditory neurons respond to stimuli is illustrated by the graphs in Figure 2–44. They show responses from four neurons that have characteristic frequencies of 540, 1170, 2610, and 2760 Hz. They were tested by presenting a click and then measuring how many times each neuron fires as a function of time since the onset of the click. Such a time delay is called a **latency**. This is done many times, and the number of spikes is then tallied for each latency. On each graph, latency is shown along the x-axis, and the number of spikes is shown vertically, as indicated in the insert. These graphs are called **post-stimulus time (PST) histograms** because tallies are shown on a histogram, and the histograms are arranged according to the time since ("post") the stimulus. The peaks show that the neurons tended to fire at certain latencies but not at other times. The latencies to the first peak get shorter as the characteristic frequency gets higher. This occurs because it takes less time for the traveling wave to reach high-

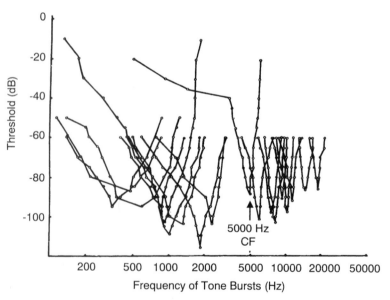

FIGURE 2–43 Tuning curves of auditory neurons with a variety of characteristic frequencies. The y-axis shows signal intensity as decibels below some maximum value (0 dB indicates the most intense sound used, and –100 dB is 100 dB below that most intense sound). The *arrow* refers to material in the text. Reprinted from *Discharge Patterns of Single Fibers in the Cat's Auditory Nerve* by NYS Kiang, with permission of The MIT Press, Cambridge, MA © 1965, p. 87.

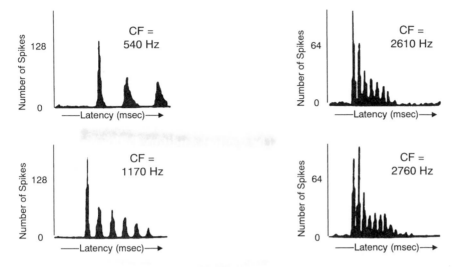

FIGURE 2–44 Selected post-stimulus time (PST) histograms showing the number of spikes (vertically) at different latencies since the onset of the click (horizontally). The PST histograms are shown for four nerve fibers with characteristic frequencies of 540, 1170, 2610, and 2760 Hz. Adapted from *Discharge Patterns of Single Fibers in the Cat's Auditory Nerve* by NYS Kiang, with permission of The MIT Press, Cambridge, MA © 1965, p. 28.

frequency locations near the base of the cochlea and more time for it to reach low-frequency places near the apex. The latencies between the successive peaks in each graph are equal to the period of each neuron's characteristic frequency (or 1/CF). The peaks alternate with times when there is little, if any, neural firing, which reveals temporal coding for individual cycles of the tone; spikes are timed to the upward deflections of the basilar membrane and spaces (inhibition) occur when it is deflected downward. [For neurons with higher CFs (not shown), the later peaks clump together because the time between them (1/CF) gets very short; they eventually disappear when the neuron cannot fire fast enough due to its refractory period.]

Temporal coding for tones is revealed by the **period histogram**, which is a graph that shows the timing of neural firings during the presentation of a pure tone. The four period histograms in Figure 2–45 show the firing patterns produced by the same neuron during the presentation of pure tones at 412, 600, 900, and 1000 Hz. In each graph, the number

of spikes is shown on the y-axis, and time during a tone is shown along the x-axis. Each x-axis is labeled with dots that are spaced at intervals equal to the period of the pure tone (2427 μsec for 412 Hz, 1667 μsec for 600 Hz, 1111 μsec for 900 Hz, and 1000 μsec or 1 msec for 1000 Hz). In each case, notice that the neural firing peaks line up with the periods of the tones (the dots), revealing a temporal representation of the signal frequency in the neuron's firing pattern.

Neural representations of the signal can also be viewed by measuring the overall response of the auditory nerve as a whole. In this case, we present a click or some other brief sound that can cause a very large number of neurons to fire at more or less the same time (synchronously). The result is the auditory nerve's **compound** or whole-nerve **action potential (AP)**. An idealized example is shown in Figure 2–46a. This kind of waveform is really the average of many individual responses, and is obtained with techniques regularly used in clinical practice (discussed in Chapter 11). The compound AP has a

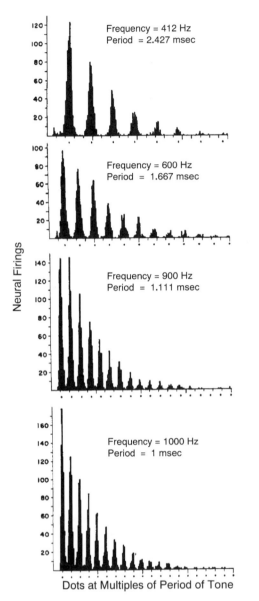

Neural Firings

Frequency = 412 Hz
Period = 2.427 msec

Frequency = 600 Hz
Period = 1.667 msec

Frequency = 900 Hz
Period = 1.111 msec

Frequency = 1000 Hz
Period = 1 msec

Dots at Multiples of Period of Tone

FIGURE 2–45 Selected period histograms showing that neural firing during a pure tone is timed to the period of the tone. Dots along each x-axis correspond to the multiples of the period of the tone. Adapted from Rose, Brugge, Anderson, & Hind (1967), with permission of *J Neurophysiol.*

major negative peak called **N1** that is usually followed by a second peak (**N2**), and often by a third peak as well (**N3**, not shown). It is quantified in terms of the amplitude and latency of the N1 peak. These parameters are shown as a function of stimulus level on an amplitude-latency function such as the one shown in Figure 2–46b. Notice that the amplitude of N1 increases and its latency decreases as the level of the click stimulus increases. In other words, raising the intensity of the stimulus causes the AP to become bigger and occur sooner.

The Central Auditory Pathways

In this section we will track the major aspects of the ascending central auditory nervous system, as well as briefly overview the olivo-cochlear pathways and the central connections of the vestibular system.

AFFERENT AUDITORY PATHWAYS

The major pathways of the **central auditory nervous system** from the cochlea to the auditory cortex are depicted in Figure 2–47. Notice that the auditory pathway is quite *redundant*. Information originating from each ear is carried by pathways on both sides of the brain. The neural connections have what might be called a "series-parallel" wiring diagram. This is simpler than it sounds. A series circuit is like a string of cheap Christmas lights and a parallel circuit is like a string of expensive Christmas lights. The cheap string of lights has a single set of wires that go from bulb to bulb to bulb. We all know what happens if even one of the bulbs breaks: it interrupts the flow of electricity down the line so that all the lights go out. This does not happen with an expensive string of lights because the electricity goes to each bulb without passing through the preceding ones. Hence, if three bulbs blow in a string of 12, the remaining nine bulbs will still light up. The term "series-parallel" is used because *both arrangements exist together* in the central auditory pathways. For example, points A and C are connected by many neural fibers ("wires"); some of them go from A to B to C, and others bypass B on their way from A to C. As a result of the redundant pathways, a given lesion (analogous to a cut wire or a blown bulb) that occurs *within* the *central* auditory pathway rarely causes a loss of hearing *sensitivity* because the signal is usu-

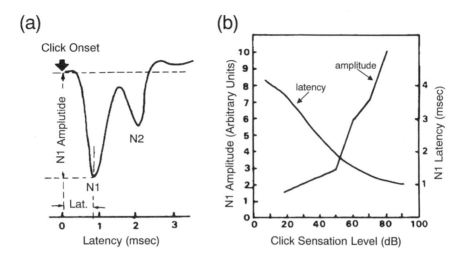

FIGURE 2–46 (a) Idealized auditory nerve compound action potential. (b) Typical amplitude-latency function of the compound action potential based on Yoshie (1968). From Gelfand (1998), p. 205, by courtesy of Marcel Dekker, Inc.

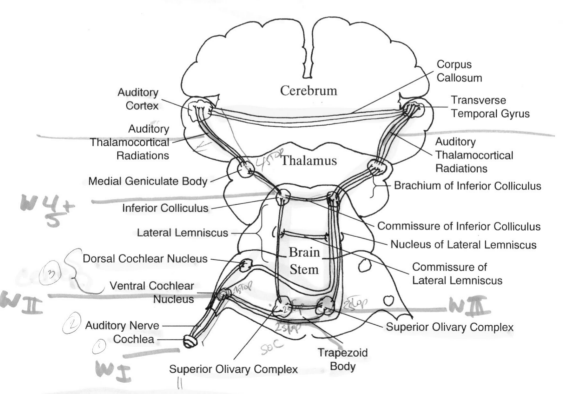

FIGURE 2–47 The major nuclei and pathways of the central auditory nervous system (see text).

ally also represented along an alternative route. However, this does *not* mean that a central lesion does not cause auditory impairments. On the contrary, significant disturbances are caused by central lesions because they affect the processing of auditory information that allows you to determine sound locations, differentiate among sounds and background noises, and interpret speech.

What are the major pathways of the ascending auditory system? The auditory nerve exits the temporal bone through the internal auditory meatus and enters the brainstem at a location called the **cerebellopontine angle**, which is a term that describes the relationship of the pons and cerebellum in this area. The auditory nerve fibers, constituting the **first-order neurons** of the auditory pathway, terminate at either the **ventral cochlear nucleus** or the **dorsal cochlear nucleus**, where they synapse with the next level of nerve cells, called **second-order neurons**. Some second-order neurons go to the **superior olivary complex** on the same (ipsilateral) side of the brainstem, but a majority will decussate (cross to the opposite side) via the **trapezoid body** and proceed along the contralateral pathway. The fibers that cross over will either synapse with the opposite superior olivary complex or ascend in the contralateral **lateral lemniscus**. As a result, each superior olivary complex receives information from both ears, so that **bilateral representation** exists as of this low level in the auditory nervous system.

Third-order neurons arise from the superior olivary complex and rise via the lateral lemniscus. Fibers also originate from the nuclei of the lateral lemniscus. Notice here that the pathway rising out of the lateral lemniscus contains neurons that originated from several different levels. Neurons ascending from this point may synapse at the **inferior colliculus** or may bypass the inferior colliculus on their way to the next level. Neurons originating from the inferior colliculus and those that bypass it ascend via the **brachium of the inferior colliculus** to terminate at the medial geniculate body of the **thalamus**. This is the last subcortical way station in the audi-

tory pathway, and all ascending neurons that reach the medial geniculate body will synapse here. Neurons from the medial geniculate then ascend along a pathway called the **auditory radiations (auditory geniculocortical** or **thalamocortical radiations**) to the **auditory cortex** located in the transverse **temporal (Heschl's) gyrus**.

Recall that crossovers between the two sides of the brain occur beginning with second-order neurons from the cochlear nuclei, so that **bilateral** representation exists as low as the superior olivary complex. **Commissural tracts** also connect auditory nuclei on the two sides at the levels of the lateral lemniscus (via the **commissure of Probst**), the inferior colliculus (via the **commissure of the inferior colliculus**), and the auditory cortex (via the **corpus callosum**). However, communication does not occur between the medial geniculate bodies on the two sides.

FINAL

FUNCTIONING OF THE CENTRAL AUDITORY SYSTEM

The central auditory pathways include a variety of different kinds of neurons, and we find many different kinds of firing patterns as well. Several examples are shown in Figure 2–48, where the *on-response* that is typical of auditory nerve fibers is identified as *primary-like*. The other examples are descriptively named according to their appearance as *choppers*, *build-up* units, *onset* units, and *pausers*. These are not the only types of firing patterns found in the central auditory system. For example, there are also fibers that respond to stimulus offset, and others have discharge patterns that decay exponentially over time. Neurons in the auditory cortex generally do not respond more than a few times to ongoing stimuli, but are more receptive to novel stimuli. For example, they might respond only at the beginning and end of a stimulus; only to sounds that rise, fall, or modulate in frequency; only to sounds coming from a certain direction; or only to moving sound sources.

The responses of central auditory neurons depend on the origin of the signal, as well as on the nature of the signal. Recall that infor-

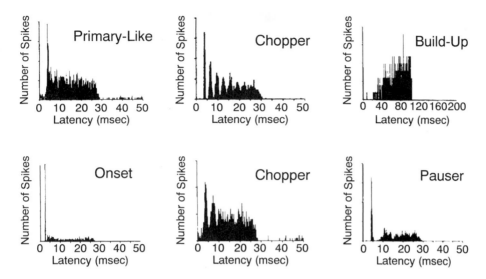

FIGURE 2–48 Examples of several kinds of firing patterns observed in central auditory neurons (obtained from neurons in the cochlea nucleus). Adapted from Rhode (1985), with permission of *J Acoust Soc Am*.

mation from both ears is represented in the pathways on both sides of the head as low as the superior olivary complex, and that there are commissural pathways between the two sides at all levels through the cortex, except for the medial geniculates. Nerve cells that receive inputs originating from the two sides are excited and/or inhibited in a manner that depends on the interaction of the two inputs. Figure 2–49 shows how cells in the superior olivary complexes on each side of the head receive signals from the cochlear nuclei on both sides of the head. In this diagram, ipsilateral (same side) signals are inhibitory and contralateral (opposite side) signals are excitatory; however, just about all excitatory/inhibitory combinations actually exist. This kind of arrangement allows the cells in various nuclei at all levels, including the cortex, to respond to the inter-ear time and intensity differences discussed earlier, and underlies much of our directional hearing ability and other binaural perceptions.

The systematic organization of frequency by location is called **tonotopic organization**, and is seen at every level of the auditory system from the cochlea up to and including the cortex. Tonotopic relationships are

determined by measuring the characteristic frequencies of many individual cells for each nucleus, and have been reported for the auditory nerve (e.g., Liberman, 1982b; Keithley & Schreiber, 1987), cochlear nuclei (e.g., Rose, Galambos, & Hughes, 1959), superior olivary complex (e.g., Tsuchitani & Boudreau, 1966), lateral lemniscus (e.g.,

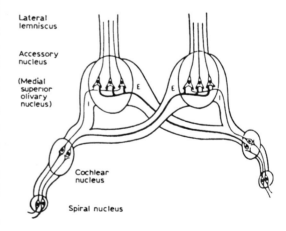

FIGURE 2–49 Schematic diagram of binaural (ipsilateral and contralateral) inputs to cells in the superior olivary complex. From van Bergeijk (1962), with permission of *J Acoust Soc Am*.

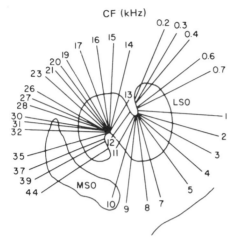

FIGURE 2–50 Tonotopic organization in the S-shaped lateral superior olive (cat). Adapted from Tsuchitani & Boudreau (1966), with permission of *J Neurophysiol.*

Aitkin, Anderson, & Brugge, 1970), inferior colliculus (e.g., Rose, Greenwood, Goldberg, & Hind, 1963), medial geniculate bodies (e.g., Aitkin & Webster, 1971), and the cortex (e.g., Woolsey, 1960). For example, Figure 2–50 shows the frequency map for the S-shaped lateral superior olive of the cat, and Figure 2–51 is a composite summary picture showing the layout of frequencies by place for various areas of the cortex.

EFFERENT AUDITORY PATHWAYS

The efferent neurons that communicate with the organ of Corti are derived from the superior olivary complexes on both sides of the brainstem, constituting the **olivocochlear bundle (OCB),** also known as Rasmussen's bundle (Rasmussen, 1946; Warr, 1978). The major aspects of the OCB are depicted in Figure 2–52, where we readily see that there are two systems rather than one. The **uncrossed olivocochlear bundle (UOCB)** is the olivocochlear pathway derived from the same side of the head as the cochlea in question. Most of its fibers are from the area of the **lateral superior olive (LSO)** and terminate at the afferent fibers of the *inner* hair cells, and some of its fibers are from the vicinity of the **medial superior olive (MSO)** and go to the *outer* hair cells. The opposite arrangement exists for the **crossed olivocochlear bundle (COCB),** whose neurons originate on the opposite side of the brainstem and cross along the floor of the fourth ventricle to the side of the cochlea in question. Here, most of the fibers are from the MSO and go to the *outer* hair cells, while a much smaller number come from the LSO and terminate at the *inner* hair cells. In other words, the uncrossed olivocochlear bundle extends mainly from the LSO to the afferent neurons of the IHCs, and the crossed olivo-

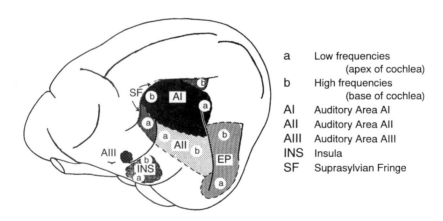

a	Low frequencies (apex of cochlea)
b	High frequencies (base of cochlea)
AI	Auditory Area AI
AII	Auditory Area AII
AIII	Auditory Area AIII
INS	Insula
SF	Suprasylvian Fringe

FIGURE 2–51 Composite diagram of the tonotopic organization of the cerebral cortex. Adapted from Woolsey (1960), in *Neural Mechanisms of the Auditory and Vestibular System* (GL Rasmussen and WF Windel, Eds.). Courtesy of C.C. Thomas, Publisher.

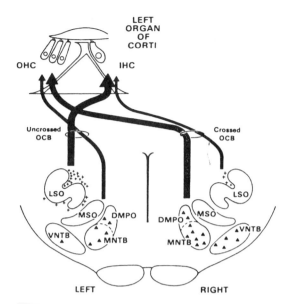

FIGURE 2–52 The crossed and uncrossed olivocochlear bundles. Thicker arrows show that most of the fibers from the crossed olivocochlear bundle (OCB) go from the medial superior olive (MSO) to outer hair cells, and most of the fibers from the uncrossed OCB go from the lateral superior olive (LSO) to inner hair cells. MNTB, medial nucleus of the trapezoid body; VNTB, ventral nucleus of the trapezoid body; DMPO, dorsal perolivary nucleus. Adapted from Warr, WB, The olivocochlear bundle: Its origins and terminations in the cat, in *Electrical Activity of the Auditory Nervous System* (RF Naunton & C Fernandez, Eds.), © 1978 by Academic Press.

cochlear bundle extends mainly from the MSO to the OHCs.

The olivocochlear bundle is by no means the only descending neural pathway in the auditory system. We have already seen that efferent signals influence the transmission system of the middle ear by innervating the stapedius and tensor tympani muscles. In addition, higher centers exert influences over lower ones at many levels of the auditory system, with some efferents going to the ear and others going to lower centers within the nervous system itself (e.g., Harrison & Howe, 1974; Winer, Diamond, & Raczkowksy, 1977). For example, some of these efferent connections descend to lower levels from the cortex,

lateral lemniscus, and inferior colliculus, and are received by various central auditory centers such as the medial geniculates and the inferior colliculi.

Central Vestibular Pathways

The vestibular neurons join to compose the *vestibular branch* of the eighth (statoacoustic) nerve, with the **vestibular (Scarpa's) ganglia** in the internal auditory meatus. After entering the brainstem at the cerebellopontine angle, the vestibular nerve goes to the **vestibular nuclei** on the same side, and also sends a branch directly to the cerebellum. There are actually four (the superior, inferior, lateral, and medial) vestibular nuclei on each side. The details of the central vestibular pathways are beyond the scope of an introductory text, but the beginning student should be aware of the breadth of these connections, if only to appreciate the multiplicity of factors that contribute to our ability to maintain balance and body orientation in space. The vestibular nuclei communicate with the nuclei of the nerves that control eye movements while the head is turning, most notably with the **third (oculomotor)** and **sixth (abducens) cranial nerves**. These connections compose the **medial longitudinal fasciculus**, which coordinates eye motion with vestibular activity. The vestibular nuclei also communicate with the vestibulospinal tracts, which influence skeletal muscle tone and antigravity muscle reflexes, as well as the cerebellum, cerebral cortex, and the vestibular nuclei on the other side of the brain.

Hearing by Bone-Conduction

Hearing usually involves receiving a sound in the form of vibrating air particles. This "regular route" is called air-conduction. It is also possible to hear by **bone-conduction**, which means that the sound is transmitted via vibrations of the bones of the skull. Bone-conduction can be initiated by air-conducted sounds that are intense enough to set the bones of the skull into vibration, or by directly activating the bones of the skull with a vibrator made for this purpose. In clinical audiology, air-conduction signals are presented from earphones or loudspeakers, and bone-conduction stimuli are presented from a bone-conduction vibrator.

Air-conduction and bone-conduction result in the same cochlear activity, that is, the initiation of traveling waves and displacements of the hair cell cilia. Figure 2–53 shows how the skull vibrates when stimulated at different frequencies with a bone-conduction vibrator at the forehead (Bekesy, 1932). At 200 Hz the whole skull vibrates as a unit in the same (forward-backward) directions as the applied vibrations. It continues to vibrate in the forward-backward direction at 800 Hz, but the pattern changes so that the front and back of the skull vibrate out-of-phase with each other. By 1600 Hz the skull begins to vibrate in four segments, involving right-left as well as front-back displacements.

Skull vibrations activate the cochlea by three mechanisms, including inner ear, middle ear, and even outer ear components (Tonndorf et al, 1966). All three components are similarly important above approximately 1000 Hz, but the middle and outer ear mechanisms take on a dominant role in the lower frequencies (Tonndorf et al, 1966). The *inner ear component* of bone-conduction primarily involves a **distortional** mechanism, as illustrated conceptually in Figure 2–54. Vibrations of the temporal bone cause the cochlear capsule (the circle) to be distorted in a manner that is synchronized with the stimulus (represented by the flattened and elongated ovals). Because the scala vestibuli has a larger volume than the scala tympani, the distortions of the fluid-filled capsule result in compensatory upward and downward displacement of the basilar membrane (represented by the lines within the circle and ovals). The distortional mechanism is supplemented and modified by a **compressional** mechanism (Bekesy, 1932). Here, temporal bone vibrations alternately compress and expand the cochlear capsule. When compressed, the cochlear fluids push outward at the oval and round windows. The greatest amount of bulging occurs at the *round* window because it is much more compliant than the oval window. As a result the fluid is

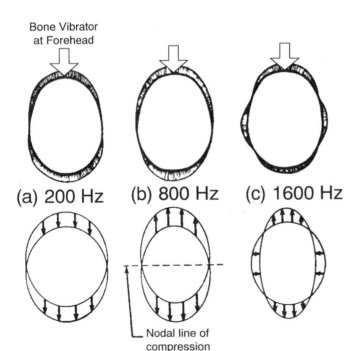

FIGURE 2–53 Skull vibration patterns initiated by bone-conduction stimulation applied to the forehead at (a) 200 Hz, (b) 800 Hz, and (c) 1600 Hz. Based on Bekesy (1932).

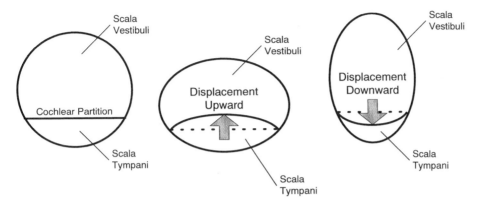

FIGURE 2–54   Basilar membrane displacements due to distortional bone-conduction (see text). Based on Tonndorf (1962).

displaced downward from the scala vestibuli toward the scala tympani and the round window, displacing the basilar membrane as well (Figure 2–55a). This displacement is enhanced because the total surface area of the scala vestibuli and the vestibule is larger than that of the scala tympani (Fig. 2–55b).

The *middle ear component* of bone-conduction is illustrated in Figure 2–56. The ossicles are represented by pendulums because they are essentially suspended within the middle

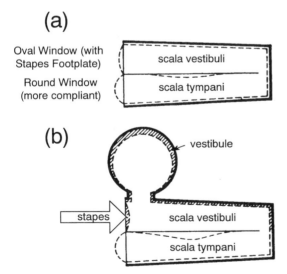

FIGURE 2–55   Principles of compressional bone-conduction (see text). Based on Bekesy (1932).

ear where they can move relative to the rest of the head. Notice that the pendulums (the ossicles) vibrate in the left-right direction. A bone-conduction vibrator at the mastoid process causes the skull to vibrate in the left-right direction, which will also induce left-right motions of the ossicles (Fig. 2–56a). However, the inertia of the suspended ossicular chain will cause its motion to lag behind the motion of the head, which means that the ossicles will be moving relative to the head. This relative movement effects a rocking motion of the stapedial footplate in the oval window, thereby transmitting the signal to the cochlear fluids. The middle ear contribution is called **ossicular-lag** or **inertial** bone-conduction for this reason. In contrast, a bone vibrator at the forehead would shake the head in the front-back direction. This vibration is at right angles to the motion of the ossicular chain, so that ossicular motion would not be initiated at low frequencies where the head moves only in the same plane as the vibrator (Fig. 2–56b).

The *outer ear component* of bone-conduction is due to **acoustical radiations**, and is sometimes called **osseotympanic** bone-conduction. The vibrations of the cartilaginous canal wall are radiated into the ear canal itself, and are then picked up by the tympanic membrane and transmitted to the cochlea via the air-conduction route. You can easily appreciate the outer ear component of

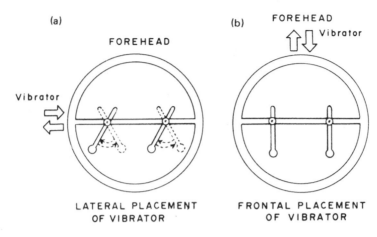

(a) FOREHEAD

Vibrator

LATERAL PLACEMENT
OF VIBRATOR

(b) FOREHEAD

Vibrator

FRONTAL PLACEMENT
OF VIBRATOR

FIGURE 2–56 Inertial or ossicular-lag bone-conduction occurs when a vibrator at the mastoid process shakes the skull in the same direction as ossicular chain motion (a), but not when a vibrator at the forehead shakes the skull perpendicular to it (b). Based on Barany (1938). From Gelfand (1998), p. 100, by courtesy of Marcel Dekker, Inc.

bone-conduction by clicking your teeth together, first without touching your ears and then while firmly (but gently) closing off your ear canals with the palms of your hands. The sound will be noticeably louder under the second, occluded, condition because it enhances the effect of the outer ear bone-conduction mechanism by preventing low frequencies from being lost.

This **occlusion effect** has a number of clinical ramifications that will become apparent in forthcoming chapters.

REFERENCES

Aitkin IM, Anderson DJ, Brugge JF. 1970. Tonotopic organization and discharge characteristics of single neurons in nuclei of the lateral lemniscus of the cat. *J Neurophysiol* 33, 421–440.

Aitkin IM, Webster WR. 1971. Tonotopic organization in the medial geniculate body of the cat. *Brain Res* 26, 402–405.

Anson BJ, Donaldson JA. 1967. *The Surgical Anatomy of the Temporal Bone and Ear.* Philadelphia: WB Saunders.

Barany E. 1938. A contribution to the physiology of bone conduction. *Acta Otolaryngol Suppl* 26, 1–223.

Bekesy G. 1932. Zur Theorie des Horens bei der Schallauftiahme durch Knochenleitung. *Ann Physik* 13, 111–136.

Bekesy G. 1941. Uber die Messung der Schwingungsamplitude der Gehörknöchelchen mittels einer kapazitiven Sonde. *Akust Zeits* 6, 1–16.

Bekesy G. 1947. The variation of phase along the basilar membrane with sinusoidal variations. *J Acoust Soc Am* 19, 452–460.

Bekesy G. 1953. Description of some mechanical properties of the organ of Corti. *J Acoust Soc Am* 25, 770–785.

Bekesy G. 1960. *Experiments in Hearing.* New York: McGraw-Hill.

Bekesy G, Rosenblith WA. 1958. The mechanical properties of the ear. In Stevens SS (Ed.): *Handbook of Experimental Psychology.* New York: Wiley, 1075–1115.

Blauert J. 1983. *Spatial Hearing: The Psychophysics of Human Sound Localization.* Cambridge, MA: MIT Press.

Borg E. 1973. On the neuronal organization of the acoustic middle ear reflex: A physiological and anatomical study. *Brain Res* 9, 101–123.

Borg E. 1976. Dynamic characteristics of the intraaural middle ear reflex. In Feldman AS, Wilber LA (Eds.): *Acoustic Impedance and Admittance—The Measurement of Middle Ear Function.* Baltimore: Williams & Wilkins, 236–299.

Borg E, Counter A, Rosler G. 1984. Theories of middle ear muscle function. In Silman S (Ed.): *The Acoustic Reflex: Basic Principles and Clinical Applications.* Orlando: Academic Press, 63–99.

Brownell WE. 1990. Outer hair cell electromotility and otoacoustic emissions. *Ear Hear* 11, 82–92.

Dallos P. 1986. Neurobiology of cochlear inner and outer hair cells: Intracellular recordings. *Hear Res* 22, 185–198.

Dallos P. 1988. Cochlear neurobiology: Revolutionary developments. *ASHA* 30, 50–56.

Dallos P, Billone MC, Durrant JD, Wang C-Y, Raynor S. 1972. Cochlear inner and outer hair cells: Functional differences. *Science* 177, 356–358.

Davis H. 1958. Transmission and transduction in the cochlea. *Laryngoscope* 68, 359–382.

Davis H. 1962. Advances in the neurophysiology and neuroanatomy of the cochlea. *J Acoust Soc Am* 34, 1377–1385.

Davis H. 1983. An active process in cochlear mechanics. *Hear Res* 9, 79–90.

Furness DN, Hackney CM. 1986. High-resolution scanning-electron microscopy of stereocilia using the osmium-thiocarbohydrazide coating technique. *Hear Res* 21, 243–249.

Gelfand SA. 1984. The contralateral acoustic reflex threshold. In Silman S (Ed.): *The Acoustic Reflex: Basic Principles and Clinical Applications.* Orlando: Academic Press, 137–186.

Gelfand SA. 1998. *Hearing: An Introduction to Psychological and Physiological Acoustics,* 3rd ed. New York: Marcel Dekker.

Harrison JM, Howe ME. 1974. Anatomy of the descending auditory system (mammalian). In Keidel WD, Neff WD (Eds.): *Handbook of Sensory Physiology,* Vol. 511. Berlin: Springer, 363–388.

Helmholtz H. 1895. *Die Lehre von der Tonempfindugen* (trans. by A. Ellis, *On the Sensation of Tones*).

Hudspeth AJ. 1985. The cellular basis of hearing; the biophysics of hair cells. *Science* 230, 745–752.

Hughes GB. (Ed.) 1985. *Textbook of Otology.* New York: Thieme-Stratton.

Jepsen O. 1963. The middle ear muscle reflexes in man. In Jerger J (Ed.): *Modern Developments in Audiology.* New York: Academic Press, 194–239.

Keithley EM, Schreiber RC. 1987. Frequency map of the spiral ganglion in the cat. *J Acoust Soc Am* 81, 1036–1042.

Khanna SM, Leonard DGB. 1982. Basilar membrane tuning in the cat cochlea. *Science* 215, 305–306.

Kiang NYS. 1965. *Discharge Patterns of Single Fibers in the Cat's Auditory Nerve.* Cambridge, MA: MIT Press.

Kiang NYS, Liberman MC, Sewell WF, Guinan JJ. 1986. Single unit clues to cochlear mechanisms. *Hear Res* 22, 171–182.

Kiang NYS, Rho JM, Northrop CC, Liberman MC, Ryugo DK. 1982. Hair-cell innervation by spiral ganglion cells in adult cats. *Science* 217, 172–177.

Liberman MC. 1982a. Single-neuron labeling in the cat auditory nerve. *Science* 216, 1239–1241.

Liberman MC. 1982b. The cochlear frequency map for the cat: Labeling auditory-nerve fibers of known characteristics frequency. *J Acoust Soc Am* 72, 1441–1449.

Liberman MC. 1988. Physiology of cochlear efferent and afferent neurons: Direct comparisons in the same animal. *Hear Res* 34, 179–192.

Lim DJ. 1986a. Functional structure of the organ of Corti. *Hear Res* 22, 117–146.

Lim DJ. 1986b. Effects of noise and ototoxic drugs at the cellular level in the cochlea: A review. *Am J Otolaryngol* 7, 73–99.

Lippe WR. (1986). Recent developments in cochlear physiology. *Ear Hear* 7, 233–239.

McGee ML. 1986. Electronystagmography in peripheral lesions. *Ear Hear* 7, 167–175.

Mehrgardt S, Mellert V. 1977. Transformation characteristics of the external human ear. *J Acoust Soc Am* 61, 1567–1576.

Møller AR. 1965. An experimental study of the acoustic impedance and its transmission properties. *Acta Otolaryngol* 60, 129–149.

Morgan DE, Dirks DD. 1975. Influence of middle ear muscle contraction on pure tone suprathreshold loudness judgments. *J Acoust Soc Am* 57, 411–420.

Morgan DE, Dirks DD, Kamm C. 1978. The influence of middle-ear muscle contraction on auditory threshold for selected pure tones. *J Acoust Soc Am* 63, 1896–1903.

Nedzelnitsky V. 1980. Sound pressure in the basal turn of the cat cochlea. *J Acoust Soc Am* 68, 1676–1689.

Peak WT, Sohmer HS, Weiss TF. 1969. Microelectrode recordings of intracochlear potentials. *MIT Res Lab Elect Q Rep* 94, 293–304.

Pickles JO. 1988. *An Introduction to the Physiology of Hearing,* 2nd ed. London: Academic Press.

Pickles JO, Comis SD, Osborne MP. 1984. Crosslinks between stereocilia in the guinea-pig organ of Corti, and their possible relation to sensory transduction. *Hear Res* 15, 103–112.

Pickles JO, Corey DP. 1992. Mechanoelectric transduction by hair cells. *Trends Neurosci* 15, 254–259.

Proctor B. 1989. *Surgical Anatomy of the Ear and Temporal Bone.* New York: Thieme.

Rabinowitz WM. 1976. Acoustic-reflex effects on the input impedance and transfer characteristics of the human middle-ear. Unpublished Ph.D. dissertation. Cambridge, MA: MIT.

Rasmussen GL. 1946. The olivary peduncle and other fiber projections of the superior olivary complex. *J Comp Neurol* 84, 141–219.

Reger SN. 1960. Effect of middle ear muscle action on certain psycho-physical measurements. *Ann Otol Rhinol Laryngol* 69, 1179–1198.

Rhode WS. 1985. The use of intracellular techniques in the study of the cochlear nucleus. *J Acoust Soc Am* 78, 320–327.

Rose JE, Brugge JF, Anderson DJ, Hind JE. 1967. Phase-locked response to low-frequency tones in single auditory nerve fibers of the squirrel monkey. *J Neurophysiol* 30, 769–793.

Rose JE, Galambos R, Hughes JR. 1959. Microelectrode studies of the cochlear nuclei of the cat. *Bull Johns Hopkins Hosp* 104, 211–251.

Rose JE, Greenwood DD, Goldberg JM, Hind JE. 1963. Some discharge characteristics of single neurons in the inferior colliculus of the cat: 1. Tonotopic organization, relation of spike-counts to tone intensity, and firing patterns of single elements. *J Neurophysiol* 26, 294–320.

Russell IJ, Sellick PM. 1977. Tuning properties of cochlear hair cells. *Nature* 267, 858–860.

Rutherford W. 1896. A new theory of hearing. *J Anat Physiol* 21, 166–168.

Sachs MB, Abbas PJ. 1974. Rate versus level functions for auditory nerve fibers in cats: Tone burst stimuli. *J Acoust Soc Am* 56, 1835–1847.

Salvi R, Henderson D, Hamernik R. 1983. Physiological bases of sensorineural hearing loss. In Tobias JD, Shubert ED (Eds.): *Hearing Research and Theory,* Vol. 2. New York: Academic Press, 173–231.

Sellick PM, Patuzzi R, Johnstone BM. 1982. Measurement of basilar membrane motion in the guinea pig using the Mossbauer technique. *J Acoust Soc Am* 72, 131–141.

Shaw EAG. 1974. Transformation of sound pressure level from the free field to the eardrum in the horizontal plane. *J Acoust Soc Am* 56, 1848–1861.

Shaw EAG, Vaillancourt MM. 1985. Transformation of sound-pressure level from the free field to the eardrum presented in numerical form. *J Acoust Soc Am* 78, 1120–1123.

Simmons BF. 1959. Middle ear muscle activity at moderate sound levels. *Ann Otol Rhinol Laryngol* 68, 1126–1143.

Simmons BF. 1964. Perceptual theories of middle ear function. *Ann Otol Rhinol Laryngol* 73, 724–740.

Smith HD. 1946. Audiometric effects of voluntary contraction of the tensor tympani muscles. *Arch Otolaryngol* 38, 369–372.

Spoendlin H. 1969. Innervation of the organ of Corti of the cat. *Acta Otolaryngol* 67, 239–254.

Spoendlin H. 1978. The afferent innervation of the cochlea. In Naunton RF, Fernandez C (Eds.): *Electrical Activity of the Auditory Nervous System*. London: Academic Press, 21–41.

Spoendlin H. 1986. Neuroanatomical basis of cochlear coding mechanisms. *Audiology* 14, 383–407.

Steel KP. 1983. The tectorial membrane in mammals. *Hear Res* 9, 327–359.

Tonndorf J. 1960. Shearing motion in scala media of cochlear models. *J Acoust Soc Am* 32, 238–244.

Tonndorf J. 1962. Compressional bone conduction in cochlear models. *J Acoust Soc Am* 34, 1127–1132.

Tonndorf J, et al. 1966. Bone conduction: Studies in experimental animals; A collection of seven papers. *Acta Otolaryngol Suppl* 213, 1–132.

Tonndorf J, Khanna SM. 1970. The role of the tympanic membrane in middle ear transmission. *Ann Otol Rhinol Laryngol* 79, 743–753.

Tos M. 1995. *Manual of Middle Ear Surgery: Vol. 2, Mastoid Surgery and Reconstructive Procedures*. Stuttgart: Thieme.

Tsuchitani C, Boudreau JD. 1966. Single unit analysis of cat superior olivary S segment with tonal stimuli. *J Neurophysiol* 29, 684–697.

van Bergeijk WA. 1962. Variation on the theory of Bekesy: A model of binaural interaction. *J Acoust Soc Am* 34, 1431–1437.

Warr WB. 1978. The olivocochlear bundle: Its origins and terminations in the cat. In Naunton RF, Fernandez C (Eds.): *Electrical Activity of the Auditory Nervous System*. London: Academic Press, 43–65.

Wever EG. 1949. *Theory of Hearing*. New York: Dover.

Wever EG, Lawrence M. 1954. *Physiological Acoustics*. Princeton: Princeton University Press.

Wiener FM, Ross DA. 1946. The pressure distribution in the auditory canal in a progressive sound field. *J Acoust Soc Am* 18, 401–408.

Wiley TL, Block MG. 1984. Acoustic and nonacoustic reflex patterns in audiologic diagnosis. In Silman S (Ed.): *The Acoustic Reflex: Basic Principles and Clinical Applications*. New York: Academic Press, 387–411.

Winer JA, Diamond IT, Raczkowsky D. 1977. Subdivisions of auditory cortex of the cat, the retrograde transport of horseradish peroxidase to medial geniculate body, and posterior thalamic nuclei. *J Comp Neurol* 176, 387–418.

Woolsey CN. 1960. Organization of cortical auditory system: A review and a synthesis. In Rasmussen GL, Windel WF (Eds.): *Neural Mechanisms of the Auditory and Vestibular System*. Springfield, IL: Charles Thomas.

Yoshie N. 1968. Auditory nerve action potential responses to clicks in man. *Laryngoscope* 78, 198–213.

Zwislocki J. 1975. The role of the external and middle ear in sound transmission. In Tower DB, Eagles EL (Eds.): *The Nervous System: Vol. 3, Human Communication and Its Disorders*. New York: Raven Press, 45–55.

Zwislocki J, Chamberlain SC, Slepecky NB. 1988. Tectorial membrane: I. Static mechanical properties in vivo. *Hear Res* 33, 207–222.

3

Measurement Principles and the Nature of Hearing

Physical attributes such as a person's height, body temperature, or blood sugar can be measured directly. This is not so for sensory and perceptual capabilities such as hearing. To find out about what a person can hear and how these sounds are perceived we must, in effect, ask her. In other words, hearing assessment relies for the most part on *presenting a stimulus and measuring the response* to that stimulus. Raising one's hand when a sound is heard, repeating a test word, judging which of two sounds is louder than the other, and even the electrical activity of the nervous system ("brain waves," so to speak) elicited by a sound are all responses. The trick is to contrive the stimulus-response situation in a way that is (1) **valid**, which means that we are really testing what we think is being tested, and (2) **reliable**, which means that the same results will be obtained if the test is repeated.

We must also be aware of the nature of the measurement being made and its limitations. For example, there is a major difference between whether a person can hear a sound presented at one particular intensity, as opposed to what is the smallest intensity that she needs to just barely hear the presence of that sound. The first test classifies a person according to whether she falls into the group of people who can hear that sound or the group that cannot hear it; the second test classifies her hearing along a continuum. Finally, we need to know that how a person responds is affected by more than whether she did or did not hear the stimulus sound. Responses are often affected by confounding influences that are built into the testing

approach (e.g., how the last response affects the next one) and the criteria employed by the person taking the test (e.g., how sure she must be before saying "yes").

Scales and Measurements

Scales of Measurement

Most tests and other measures of hearing can be viewed in terms of the classic nominal, ordinal, interval, and ratio scales of measurement described by Stevens (1975). In a **nominal scale**, subjects or observations are simply categorized into different groups, but there is *no* order or hierarchy among the groups. Some examples include grouping people according to gender (male/female) or eye color (brown/blue/hazel), or classifying paintings by subject type (landscape/portrait/still life). On the other hand, if there is also some hierarchy or order among the observations or categories, then we have an **ordinal scale**. For example, we might ask subjects to specify their relative preferences for different kinds of paintings, or to organize the paintings according to relative price. Here, there is an orderly progression from group to group, but the spacing between groups is different. For example, several paintings might be rank ordered according to their prices, which are $10, $25, $100, $150, and $175. Because we know the relative order of the observations, the information on ordinal scales can be described in terms of medians and percentiles.

An ordinal scale becomes an **interval scale** when the spacing between categories or

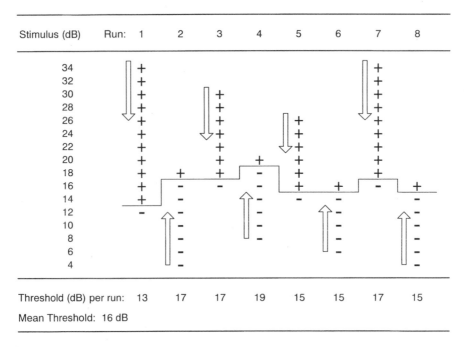

FIGURE 3–1 Eight "runs" being used to find the threshold of hearing with the method of limits. From Gelfand (1998), p. 247, by courtesy of Marcel Dekker, Inc.

observations is equal, such as the hours on a clock or degrees of temperature in Fahrenheit or Celsius. Notice that the spacing is the same between any successive two points on the scale: There is 1 hour from 6 AM to 7 AM and there is also 1 hour from 10 PM to 11 PM; and there is one degree from 30°C to 31°C and also from 99°C to 100°C. An interval scale allows us to use most kinds of calculations so information can now be described in terms of means (averages) and standard deviations. However, ratios may not be used because there is no true zero point. **Ratio scales** have all the characteristics of interval scales plus a true zero point (an inherent origin). Length and temperature on the Kelvin scale (where 0 is absolute zero) are typical examples of ratio scales, as are loudness in *sones* and pitch in *mels*, described later in this chapter. All mathematical calculations can be used with ratio scale information, including the use of ratios, geometric means, and decibels.

Classical Measurement Methods

The classical techniques that have been used to measure hearing and other senses are the methods of limits, adjustment, and constants (or constant stimuli). Other testing methods are also available, such as the direct scaling approaches (discussed below) as well as the clinical techniques (discussed later). Sophisticated *adaptive testing methods* (see, e.g., Gelfand, 1998) are usually employed in research applications, but they have clinical uses as well. We will describe each of the methods of limits, adjustment, and constants in the context of a test to find the subject's **threshold** of hearing for a pure-tone signal, which is simply the lowest intensity level at which the subject is able to hear. However, these methods can also be used for other kinds of measurements, such as determining the smallest perceptible difference in intensity or frequency between two sounds.

The **method of limits** is illustrated in Figure 3–1. The subject is presented with one tone at a time, and he responds by indicating whether the stimulus was heard ("yes" or +) or not heard ("no" or −) after each presentation. The tester controls the level of the stimulus and changes it in fixed steps (e.g., 2 dB at a time) in one direction (ascending or descending) until the responses change from "yes" (+) to "no" (–), or from "no" (–) to "yes" (+). Each set of presentations is called a run. Eight runs are shown in the figure. Descending runs begin above the subject's expected threshold, and the stimulus level is lowered until the tone first becomes inaudible. Ascending runs start below the subject's threshold, and the level is raised until the tone is first heard. Notice that the crossover point varies from run to run, so the best estimate of the threshold is the average of several runs. Testing biases are minimized by averaging across an equal number of ascending and descending runs with different starting levels, as illustrated in the figure.

In the **method of adjustment**, the stimulus level changes continuously rather than in fixed steps, and is controlled by the subject herself. To find her threshold, the subject increases (or decreases) an unmarked level control until the tone first becomes audible (or inaudible). *Bracketing*, or increasing and decreasing the level alternately until a change point is reached, is a commonly employed modification of the methods of adjustment and limits.

The methods of limits and adjustment are sequential techniques because one presentation level depends on the response to the previous one. In contrast, the **method of constant stimuli (constants)** uses an equal number of stimuli at each of several predetermined levels, which are presented to the subject in random order. The "yes" (+) and "no" (–) responses are tallied for each of the levels used. The threshold is then obtained by calculating the level that corresponds to 50% from these tallies. Figure 3–2 shows an example in which the percentage of "yes" (+) responses is calculated on the basis of 50 random tone presentations at 11 levels from 0 dB to 10 dB sound pressure level (SPL). The tallies are converted into percentages, which are then plotted on a graph known as a **psychometric function**. The 50% point on the psychometric function is usually considered to be the threshold, which corresponds to 7.5 dB in this example. The method of constants is very accurate, but it can be inefficient because many presentations are "wasted" at levels well above and well below the threshold.

Direct Scaling

In direct scaling the subject directly establishes the correspondence between physical sounds and how they are perceived. The major approaches are partition scales and ratio or magnitude scales. The loudness (sone) and pitch (mel) scales discussed later

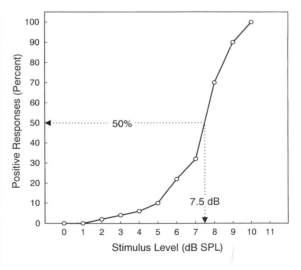

Data Tallies		
Stimulus Level in dB	Responses	
	Number	Percent
10	50	100
9	45	90
8	35	70
7	17	32
6	11	22
5	5	10
4	3	6
3	2	4
2	1	2
1	0	0
0	0	0

FIGURE 3–2 Illustration of the method of constant stimuli. The data tallies (left) are used to plot a psychometric function (right), on which the 50% point constitutes the threshold.

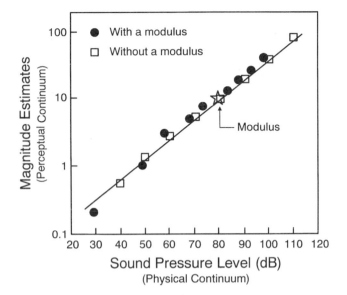

FIGURE 3–3 Magnitude estimates showing the perceptual values of a range of intensities. Notice that similar results are obtained with and without a modulus. Based on data by Stevens (1956).

in this chapter were developed using the magnitude and ratio scaling methods. With **partition scales** the subject is presented with a range of intensities or frequencies, and is asked to divide (partition) this range into equally spaced categories on the basis of how she perceives them.

Ratio scales are developed by ratio estimation or production. In **ratio estimation** the subject is presented with pairs of tones and describes (estimates) how they are related in the form of a ratio. For example, compared to the first one, the second tone might be twice as loud, half as loud, four times louder, etc; or its pitch might be half as high, one-quarter as high, twice as high, etc. The opposite approach is **ratio production**. Here, the subject is asked to adjust (produce) the intensity of a tone until it sounds twice or half as loud as another tone, or to change the frequency of a tone so that its pitch is one-quarter, half, or twice that of another tone.

Magnitude scales are similar to ratio scales, except they use numbers (magnitudes) instead of ratios or fractions. In **magnitude estimation** the subject is presented with stimuli along a continuum (e.g., intensity) and is asked to assign numbers to each

of them in a way that reflects the magnitude of the perception (e.g., loudness). The results show the relationship between physical stimuli and their perception, as in Figure 3–3. There are two major variations of the magnitude estimation method. In one approach the subject is presented with a "standard" tone called a **modulus** and is told that it has a magnitude of, say, "10." She then hears other tones at other intensities and is asked to describe (estimate) their magnitudes with numbers that are proportional to the modulus. A tone that is twice as loud as the modulus is rated 20; 40 means four times louder; and 2 means one-fifth as loud. The alternative approach is to omit the modulus. In this case the subject is asked to provide a rating for each sound using numbers that represent how they are perceived. Similar results are obtained with and without the modulus, as illustrated in the figure. The opposite of magnitude estimation is **magnitude production**. Here the subject is presented with numbers and must adjust the intensity (or frequency) to produce a tone with the corresponding loudness (or pitch).

Magnitude scales have been developed for a large number of sensations, and it is even possible to make **cross-modality matches**, that is, to express a perception from one sensory modality in terms of a different sense. Cross-modality matching can be useful audiologically by facilitating the ability to assess a patient's perception of loudness in terms of perceived line length (Hellman & Meiselman, 1988; Hellman, 1999).

The Nature of Normal Hearing

Audiology is concerned with the normal and abnormal aspects of hearing, its place in the communicative process, and the clinical evaluation and management of patients with auditory impairments. The area of science that deals with the perception of physical stimuli is called psychophysics. Hence, in addition to being an aspect of audiology, the science that deals with perception of sound is also known as **psychoacoustics**.

The Range of Hearing

MINIMAL AUDIBLE LEVELS

It is useful to conceive of a range of hearing that includes sounds that are audible and tolerable. The lower curves in Figure 3–4 show the faintest audible sounds or **thresholds** of normal people in decibels of sound pressure level (dB SPL) as a function of frequency. The striking feature of these curves is they are not flat. Instead, the SPL needed for a sound to be barely audible depends on its frequency to a major extent. Hearing thresholds are reasonably sensitive between approximately 100 and 10,000 Hz, and become poorer (i.e., more intensity is needed to reach threshold) as frequency increases and decreases above and below this range. In addition, hearing is most sensitive (i.e., the least amount of intensity is needed to reach threshold) in the 2000 to 5000 Hz range. The resonant responses of

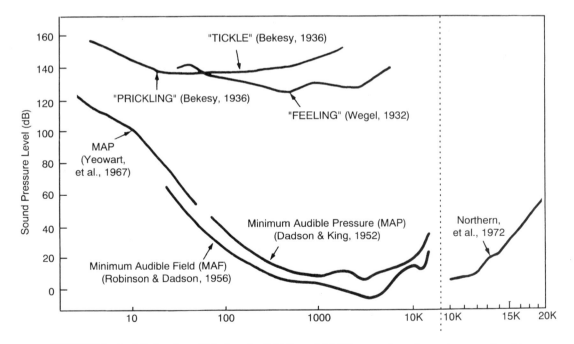

FIGURE 3–4 Minimal audible levels (MAP and MAP curves) and maximum tolerable levels in decibels of sound pressure level (dB SPL) as a function of frequency from selected studies cited in the figure. The frequency scale is expanded above 10,000 Hz for clarity. Adapted from Gelfand (1998), p. 283, by courtesy of Marcel Dekker, Inc.

the conductive system are largely responsible for the lower thresholds in this most sensitive frequency range (see Chapter 2).

The sound levels needed to achieve minimum audibility also depend on how they are obtained. Notice that the curve labeled "MAF" is about 6 to 10 dB lower (i.e., better or more sensitive) than the curves labeled "MAP." **Minimal audible pressure (MAP)** is based on monaural (one ear) thresholds that are obtained with earphones. First, the subject's threshold is obtained with an appropriate method. Then the sound pressure that corresponds to that threshold is measured as it actually exists under the earphone in the subject's ear canal. A commonly used alternative approach is to measure the sound in a 6-cc *coupler*, which is a special measurement cavity standardized for this purpose. We shall see that the latter method is used to calibrate audiological instruments. In contrast, **minimal audible field (MAF)** values are based on the binaural (two ear) thresholds of subjects listening to sounds presented from a loudspeaker in an echo-free (*anechoic*) room. After determining the threshold, the subject leaves the room and is replaced by a microphone that measures the sound as it exists in the same location previously occupied by the subject's head.

The discrepancy between the MAF and MAP thresholds has been known as the "missing 6 dB," and was a problematic issue for quite some time. However, it appears that the MAF-MAP difference is more apparent than real because it is accounted for by a combination of factors, including binaural versus monaural hearing, physiologic noise that masks stimuli presented under earphones, real ear versus coupler measurements, and other technical factors (Killion, 1978).

UPPER LIMITS OF HEARING

The upper levels of usable hearing depend on how they are defined. The threshold of *uncomfortable loudness* occurs at approximately 100 dB SPL (Hood & Poole, 1970). However, the threshold is much higher for sensations such as feeling, tickle, and pain. These un-

pleasant and potentially intolerable sensations are generally *tactile* rather than auditory in nature, and occur roughly between 120 and 140+ dB SPL, depending on the nature of the sensation. Several examples are shown in Figure 3–4. In contrast to the threshold sensitivity curves, the upper limits of hearing are relatively flat across the frequency range for both uncomfortable loudness and tactile sensations.

TEMPORAL SUMMATION

The threshold for a sound is not affected by its duration unless it becomes shorter than approximately one-third of a second. When a sound is shorter than about 300 msec, then its threshold increases when its duration decreases, and vice versa (Fig. 3–5a). In general, a ten-times increase in duration can be offset by a 10-dB decrease in intensity, and a ten-times (or decade) decrease in duration can be offset by a 10-dB increase in intensity. This phenomenon is called **temporal summation** or **temporal integration** and is illustrated by the following example: Suppose a subject's threshold is 18 dB for a 250-msec tone. Reducing the duration by ten times to 25 msec will cause the threshold to increase by 10 dB to 28 dB. Similarly, if the threshold of a 25-msec tone is 28 dB, then increasing its duration by ten times to 250 msec will cause the threshold to improve by 10 dB to 18 dB. The same relationship also applies to the loudness of a sound; for example, a 25-msec tone at 40 dB will sound as loud as a 50-dB tone if its duration is increased by ten times to 250 msec.

Temporal summation reflects the ear's ability to integrate energy within a time frame of roughly one-third of a second. The principle is illustrated in Figure 3–5b, where the area of each rectangle represents the amount of energy present. Notice that the area (energy) is the same regardless of whether the rectangle is (1) high and narrow (representing more intense and shorter in duration) or (2) short and wide (representing less intense and longer in duration). Students with some photographic experience will recognize that this phenomenon is similar to the trade-off between lens opening and shutter speed.

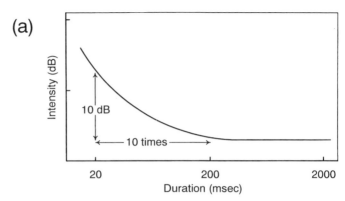

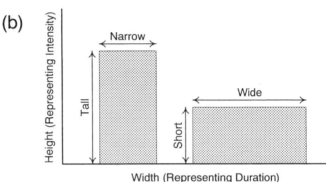

FIGURE 3–5 (a) Temporal summation involves a trade-off in which a ten-times change in duration can be offset by a complementary 10-dB intensity change. (b) The area of each rectangle represents the amount of energy that is present, and is the same regardless of whether it is (1) high and narrow (more intense and shorter in duration) or (2) short and wide (less intense and longer in duration).

Differential Sensitivity

The smallest perceptible difference between two sounds is called a **difference limen (DL)** or the **just noticeable difference (jnd)**. For example, the smallest intensity difference that can be distinguished between two sounds is the DL for intensity. Because *delta* (Δ) is the symbol for "change," the intensity DL is often called ΔI. If ΔI is the intensity difference needed to tell two sounds apart, then one of those sounds has an intensity of I and the other one has an intensity of $I + \Delta I$ (Fig. 3–6). Analogous terms apply to just noticeable differences for other aspects of sounds as well. For example, the difference limen for frequency, Δf, is the smallest discernible difference between the frequencies of two sounds, f and $f + \Delta f$.

The values of ΔI and Δf are *absolute* difference limens because they specify the actual physical difference needed to tell two sounds apart. However, common experience tells us that the physical size of a DL is not the same

under all conditions. For example, we all know that the additional illumination provided by a tiny night-light is very noticeable in the dark of night but is totally indiscernible during the day. In other words, the size of ΔI depends on the size of I. For this reason, we are, especially interested in the *relative* difference limen that considers both the DL as well as the starting value. The relative DL is equal to $\Delta I / I$ and is called the **Weber fraction**. The notion that the Weber fraction ($\Delta I / I$) is a constant value (k) is called **Weber's law**. In numerical terms, Weber's law says that $\Delta I / I = k$.

These principles become clear when we consider a classic, albeit hypothetical, experiment described by Hirsh (1952) that tries to answer the question: "If we already have a certain number of candles, how many more candles must be added in order for us to notice a difference in brightness?" The "results" are given in Table 3–1. The first column gives the original numbers of candles

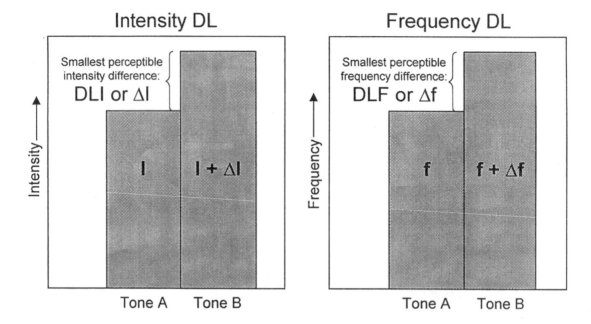

FIGURE 3–6 The difference limen (DL) is the smallest difference that can be discerned between two sounds. The intensity DL or ΔI is the smallest noticeable intensity difference between two sounds, I and I + ΔI. The frequency DL or Δf is the smallest perceptible frequency difference between two sounds, f and f + Δf.

(I), which might be 10, 100, 1000, 10,000, or even 100,000. The additional candles needed to tell a difference (the DL or ΔI) in each case are in the second column, and the new totals (I + ΔI) are in the third column. The fourth column, labeled "Weber fraction," shows the raw ratios of ΔI/I in each case, and the last column, labeled "Weber's law," shows the results of simplifying each of these fractions. The results are obvious: the more candles you

start with (I), the more candles you must add (ΔI) to tell a difference; but relative size of the increase (ΔI/I) is always the same (ΔI/I = k = 0.1).

DIFFERENCE LIMENS FOR INTENSITY AND FREQUENCY

The relative difference limen for intensity (ΔI/I) improves to some extent with increas-

TABLE 3-1   Illustration of the Weber fraction (ΔI/I) and Weber's Law (ΔI/I = k) with make-believe data showing how many candles must be added to a number of originally present candles (I) to produce a difference limen (ΔI) for brightness

Original Candles (I)	Additional Candles (ΔI)	New Total (I + ΔI)	Weber Fraction (ΔI/I)	Weber's Law (ΔI/I = k)
10	1	11	1/10	0.1
100	10	110	10/100	0.1
1,000	100	1,100	100/1,000	0.1
10,000	1,000	11,000	1,000/10,000	0.1
100,000	10,000	110,000	10,000/100,000	0.1

ing sensation level. **Sensation level (SL)** is simply the number of decibels above threshold, so that 0 dB SL means "at threshold" and 40 dB SL means 40 dB above threshold. For example, Jesteadt, Wier, and Green (1977a) found the values of AI/I are roughly 0.4 near threshold, 0.3 at 40 dB SL, 0.2 at 60 dB SL, and somewhat smaller at high intensities. Hence, there appears to be a "near miss to Weber's law" for the intensity difference limen in the sense that $\Delta I/I$ is not quite constant. The size of $\Delta I/I$ appears to be reasonably constant in the middle frequencies, but it is not clear whether this holds true for all audible frequencies.

The difference limen for frequency becomes larger (wider) as frequency increases and also as sensation level decreases (Wier, Jesteadt, & Green, 1977). At the readily audible and comfortable level of 40 dB SL, the size of Δf is approximately 1 Hz at 200 Hz and 400 Hz, and 2 Hz at 1000 Hz, 3 Hz at 2000 Hz, 16 Hz at 4000 Hz, and 68 Hz at 8000. In terms of the Weber fraction, $\Delta f/f$ is smallest (about 0.002) between 600 Hz and 2000 Hz, and gets larger for the frequencies below and above this range. All of these values become larger (poorer) as the intensity decreases toward threshold.

TEMPORAL DISCRIMINATIONS

The closest analogy in the time domain to the intensity and frequency DLs just discussed would be the difference limen for signal duration. Here the subject must determine which one of two signals lasted for a longer period of time. The difference limen for duration (Δt) becomes larger (longer) as the overall duration of the signal (t) increases, and the Weber fraction, $\Delta t/t$, is not constant (Abel, 1972; Dooley & Moore, 1988). However, this is by no means the only kind of time-related discrimination in hearing.

The shortest perceptible time interval or **temporal resolution** is typically on the order of 2 to 3 msec in young, normal individuals, and can be measured by gap detection as well as other approaches (e.g., Fitzgibbons & Wightman, 1982; Buus & Florentine, 1985;

Green, 1985; Fitzgibbons & Gordon-Salant, 1987). The stimulus used for **gap detection testing** is usually a pair of noises that are presented in rapid succession, separated by a very short break or gap. The duration of this gap is varied according to an appropriate method of measurement, and the subject's task is to determine whether a gap can or cannot be heard. The shortest discernible gap is the **gap detection threshold**. These principles are illustrated in Figure 3–7. The same results are obtained if the subject is asked whether she heard one continuous sound or two of them in succession. However, an interval of about 20 msec is needed if the subject must indicate which of two distinguishable signals came first, or **perceived order** (Hirsh, 1959).

Loudness and Pitch

Loudness and pitch refer to how we *perceive* the *physical attributes* of intensity and frequency, respectively. It may seem odd to make this distinction since everyone knows sounds with greater intensities are louder than sounds with smaller intensities, and higher frequencies have higher pitches. These generalities are true. However, we will see that there is far from a one-for-one relationship between the perceptual world of loudness and pitch and the physical world of intensity and frequency.

LOUDNESS

We have already seen that sounds of different frequencies are not equally audible (Fig. 3–4). In other words, different SPLs are needed to reach threshold at different frequencies; for example, 10 dB SPL may be audible at one frequency but not at another frequency. The same thing applies to loudness: even though tone A and tone B have the same intensity, one of them is likely to be louder than the other. In other words, loudness depends on frequency. We may now ask how much intensity is needed at each of two different frequencies for one tone to be perceived just as loud as the other tone. For

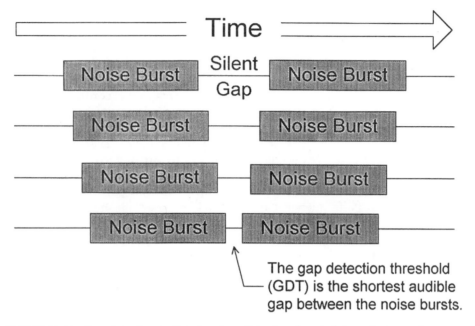

FIGURE 3–7 Gap detection testing involves listening for a brief gap between two sounds (noise bursts) presented in rapid succession. The gap detection threshold (GDT) is simply the shortest gap that can be heard.

example, how many decibels would it take for a 100-Hz tone to sound *equally loud* to a 1000-Hz tone at 40 dB SPL? To answer this question we may present a 1000-Hz tone at 40 dB alternately with various levels of a 100-Hz tone, and ask the subject whether each 100-Hz tone is louder, softer, or equally loud to the 1000-Hz *reference tone.* Alternatively, we might have the subject adjust the level of a 100-Hz tone until it sounds just as loud as a reference tone of 1000 Hz at 40 dB. The same procedure would then be repeated with other frequencies until we have developed a list of the SPLs at many different frequencies that all sound equally loud to the 40-dB 1000-Hz tone. It makes sense that if all of these sounds are equally loud to the 1000-Hz, 40-dB reference tone, then they are also equal in loudness to each other. We could then plot these equally loud SPLs as a function of frequency, and draw a smooth line through them.

The results look like the curve labeled "40" in Figure 3–8. Notice this curve corresponds

to an SPL of 40 dB *at* 1000 Hz, but that the SPLs are quite different at the other frequencies. For example, this curve tells us that all of the following tones *sound equally loud* even though their SPLs are different:

61 dB at 50 Hz,
45 dB at 100 Hz,
42 dB at 200 Hz,
38 dB at 500 Hz,
40 dB at 1000 Hz (the reference),
38 dB at 2000 Hz, and
36 dB at 5000 Hz.

Because all of these sounds are equally loud we say they have the same **loudness level**. The loudness level curve is called a **loudness level contour, equal loudness contour,** or **Fletcher-Munson curve.** The number 40 does not mean 40 dB. Instead, it refers to the loudness level of the sounds along the curve, that is, all of the SPLs at different frequencies that are perceived to be equally loud to a 1000-Hz reference frequency at 40 dB SPL. To avoid confusing loudness and intensity, the loudness level of this curve is said to be "40 phons" (as distinguished from decibels). The **phon** is the *unit of loudness level*. By convention, the number of phons corresponds to the number of decibels *at* 1000 Hz. As a result, an equal-loudness contour is also called a **phon curve**. Hence, we have been discussing the *40-phon curve*. The other phon curves in Figure 3-8 were obtained in the same manner used to generate the 40-phon curve, except that the loudness balances were made to different levels of the 1000-Hz reference tone (e.g., 1000 Hz at 20 dB for the 20-phon line, 80 dB for the 80-phon line, etc.).

The equal-loudness contours flatten as intensity increases, particularly for the lower frequencies. This is analogous to what we saw when we compared the effect of frequency on auditory thresholds versus maximum listening levels. As a result, the distance in decibels between a softer phon curve and a much louder phon curve is narrower for the low frequencies than for higher frequencies. For example, 10 phons corresponds to about 30 dB at 100 Hz and 10 dB at 1000 Hz, whereas

100 phons corresponds to about 103 dB at 100 Hz and 100 dB at 1000 Hz. As a result, the spread between 10 phons and 100 phons is 90 dB wide at 1000 Hz but only 73 dB wide at 100 Hz. In other words, a 73 dB increase at 100 Hz sounds like a 90-dB increase at 1000 Hz.

These curves are not just some esoteric effect confined to the laboratory. It is an experience familiar to anyone who has ever changed the volume control on a stereo system: a musical selection that has a natural sound when it is being played softly will become "boomy" when the volume is increased, and a natural-sounding loud selection begins to sound "tinny" when the volume is decreased. This is one of the reasons why there are *bass* (low pitch) and *treble* (high pitch) controls on stereo systems. We turn down the bass after raising the volume to counteract the disproportionate loudness boost in the low frequencies, which results when the intensity is increased. Similarly, we turn up the bass after lowering the volume to counteract the disproportionate drop in low-frequency loudness, which occurs when the intensity is decreased.

Phon curves show equally loud relationships among different sounds but they do not show how loudness is related to intensity. This would require a scale of loudness as a function of intensity of the type described in the earlier discussion of magnitude and ratio scales (e.g., as in Fig. 3–3). The loudness-intensity relationship based on methods of this type is called the **sone scale** (Stevens, 1975), and is illustrated in Figure 3–9. The *unit of loudness* is called the **sone**. By convention, the reference intensity for the sone scale is a 1000-Hz tone at 40 dB, and its loudness is 1 *sone*. The sone scale expresses loudness as ratios. Hence, the tone that is twice as loud as 40 dB (1 sone) would be 2 sones; the tone that is four times as loud is 4 sones; and the tone that is half as loud would be 0.5 sone; etc. Notice the distinction between *loudness in sones* and *loudness level in phons*. At other frequencies than 1000 Hz the level of the sound would be expressed in phons (which are uniformly equivalent to

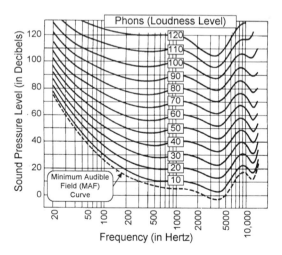

FIGURE 3–8 Loudness-level or phon curves [based on data by Robinson & Dadson (1956) and ISO (1961)]. The loudness level in phons is shown in the box at 1000 Hz for each contour. The "0 phon line" corresponds to the minimum audibility (MAF) curve.

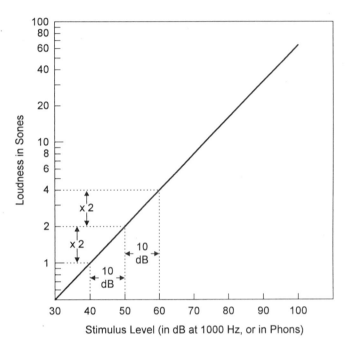

FIGURE 3–9 The sone scale of loudness (idealized). Notice that a doubling or halving of loudness in sones corresponds to a 10-dB (or 10-phon) increase or decrease in level (dotted lines). (More precisely, the function actually curves downward at low sound levels.)

decibels only at 1000 Hz). Comparing dotted lines in the figure reveals that a level increase of about 10 dB (or 10 phons) results in a doubling of loudness (e.g., 1 to 2 sones, 2 to 4 sones, etc.), and a 10-dB decrease results in a halving of loudness (e.g., 2 to 1 sone; 1 to ½ sone).

The sone scale is shown as a straight line in the figure, and both axes of the graph are logarithmic. The logarithmic scale is clearly indicated on the y-axis, and is implicit for the x-axis because decibels are logarithmic values. A straight line on a log-log graph indicates an exponential or power relationship. Consequently, we can say that loudness (L) is a *power function* of intensity (I), or $L = k I^e$. The exponent **e** describes the slope of the line that relates loudness to intensity (it will suffice to say k is a constant). This relationship is **Stevens' power law** (1975), which more generally states that the magnitude of a perception is equal to a power (exponent) of the

magnitude of the stimulus. The slope of the loudness function is approximately 0.6, so that $L = I^{0.6}$. A slope (exponent) of 1.0 means that the perception has a one-to-one relationship to the size of the stimulus. The slope of 0.6 means that loudness increases at a slower rate than intensity increases. Other perceptions such as brightness also have exponents that are less than 1.0. On the other hand, exponents greater than 1.0 are encountered for percepts that increase faster than the physical stimulus level; electric shock is a noteworthy example.

The Critical Band   Loudness is related to the bandwidth of the sound. Suppose we have a sound made up of two frequencies that are just 10 Hz apart (e.g., 995 Hz and 1005 Hz). We then slowly move these two tones further apart in frequency so that the separation between them increases. We will find that the loudness of this sound stays the same until

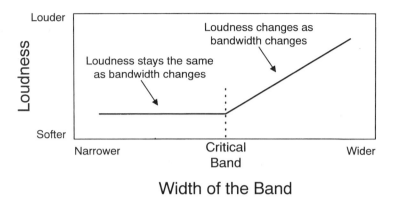

FIGURE 3–10 Loudness increases when the bandwidth of a sound becomes wider than the critical band.

the separation reaches a certain critical width. Beyond this, making the separation between the two frequencies any wider will cause the sound to become louder even though the intensity is still the same; the wider the separation, the louder the sound becomes. The same phenomenon occurs using a band of noise that starts out narrow and gets wider and wider: the loudness stays the same until a certain bandwidth is reached, but it becomes louder as the bandwidth widens beyond that point, as illustrated in Figure 3–10. This bandwidth, where perceptual changes occur, is called the **critical band** (Scharf, 1970) and is one of several indicators of the frequency-selective nature of the ear. The critical bandwidth becomes broader as the center frequency gets higher above approximately 1000 Hz, as shown in Figure 3–11. However, the student should avoid the

FIGURE 3–11 Width of the critical band [Δf (Hz)] and the masking critical ratio as a function of center frequency. Adapted from Zwicker, Flottorp, & Stevens (1957), with permission of *Journal of the Acoustical Society of America*.

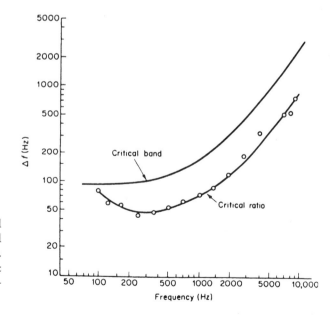

trap of thinking of a fixed series of individual bands that are arranged one next to the other. Instead, critical bands may be conceived of as overlapping on a smooth continuum, so that there would be a critical bandwidth no matter what the center frequency might be.

PITCH

Even though we can detect sound frequencies as low as about 2 Hz, the lowest frequency that is associated with "tonality" or a perceptible pitch is about 20 Hz. There is also a minimum duration necessary before a sound takes on a tonal quality, which is about 10 msec for frequencies above 1000 Hz. Lower frequency sounds must be on long enough for us to hear several cycles (periods)

in order for tonality to be perceived (e.g., 15 msec at 500 Hz and 60 msec at 50 Hz).

Just as the sone scale relates intensity and loudness, the relationship between pitch and frequency is depicted by the **mel scale**, in which the *unit of pitch* is the **mel** (Stevens, 1975). The reference point for the mel scale is a 1000-Hz tone at 40 phons, which has a pitch of 1000 *mels*. Following what we know about the nature of ratio scales, 2000 mels is twice as high as (twice the pitch of) 1000 mels; 500 mels is half as high, etc. An idealized example of the mel scale is shown in Figure 3–12.

Notice the relation between frequency and pitch is somewhat S-shaped rather than linear, and that the frequency range of 16,000 Hz is "compressed" into a pitch range of only about 3300 mels. (This point is high-

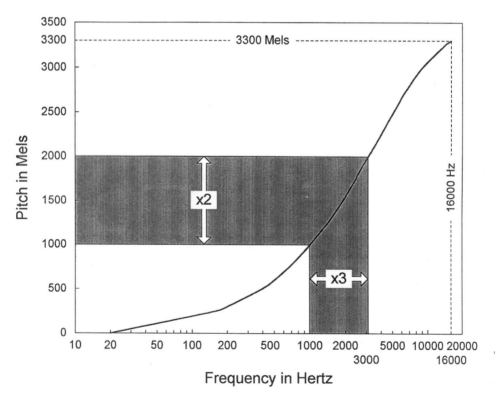

FIGURE 3–12   The mel scale of pitch is shown here by an idealized curve based on data tabulations by Beranek (1988). It shows the relationship between pitch in mels and frequency in Hertz (see text).

lighted by the dashed lines labeled 16,000 Hz and 3300 mels extending to the upper right hand end of the curve.) Let's see what this means. A doubling of pitch from 1000 mels to 2000 mels corresponds to a tripling of frequency from 1000 Hz to roughly 3000 Hz, as illustrated by the guidelines and shaded region in the figure. In other words, doubling the frequency from 1000 Hz to 2000 Hz results in *less than* a doubling of the pitch. We would expect that doubling the pitch again from 2000 mels should bring us to 4000 mels. However, this does not happen. Instead, the maximum pitch that is attainable within the entire audible frequency range is less than about 3500 mels.

There is disagreement between the musical pitch scale and the psychoacoustic pitch scale in mels, even though neither of them is wrong. For example, the range from 100 to 200 Hz and the range from 1000 to 2000 Hz are both musical octaves. An **octave** is a two-to-one ratio. However, these two doublings of frequency (on the x-axis) do not correspond to equal distances in mels (on the y-axis). You can see this for yourself by drawing vertical pencil lines from 100, 200, and 2000 Hz on the x-axis up to the curve, and then extending them horizontally to the y-axis, just like the dotted lines already printed at 1000 Hz and about 3000 Hz. The distance in mels on the y-axis between the 100- and 200-Hz lines will be smaller than the distance between the 1000- and 2000-Hz lines.

PITCH OF COMPLEX TONES

The pitch of complex tones depends to a large extent upon the perception of the harmonics in the sound as opposed to the place of maximal displacement along the cochlear spiral. This phenomenon is demonstrated most dramatically by the perception of the **missing fundamental** or **residue pitch** (Seebeck, 1841; Schouten, 1940). In this case, a subject is presented with a complex periodic sound composed of only the *high* frequency harmonics of some fundamental but *without*

any energy present at the fundamental frequency itself. For example, the sound might be composed of components at only 1800 Hz, 2000 Hz, 2200 Hz, and 2400 Hz. These are all harmonics of 200 Hz, but the spectrum of the sound does not contain 200 Hz. In this case, the subject perceives the pitch associated with 200 Hz (the missing fundamental) even though the absence of any energy at 200 Hz makes it impossible for that location on the basilar membrane to be activated. The hypothetical spectrum of this sound is shown in Figure 3–13, where the location of the perceived but absent 200-Hz component (the missing fundamental or residue pitch) is represented by the shaded bar. The perception of the missing fundamental appears to depend upon pattern recognition of some aspect of the harmonics within the auditory nervous system.

A related phenomenon is the perception of **periodicity** or **repetition pitch**, which is the perception of a pitch when a sound is pulsed on and off. For example, if a subject listens to a high-frequency tone that is interrupted every 10 milliseconds (which is the period of a 100 Hz tone), then she will perceive a pitch corresponding to 100 Hz (Thurlow & Small, 1955). Perceptions of this type are not surprising because the auditory system is equipped with mechanisms for coding frequency information on the basis of temporal factors as well as place.

Audible Distortions

It is possible to hear frequencies that are not actually present in the stimulus. These responses are called **distortion products** that are produced by **nonlinear distortions** in the cochlea. A distortion product is any signal that is present at the output of a system (in this case, what we hear) that was not present at the input to the system (the sound entering the ear). To understand the concept of a nonlinear response and distortion products, consider what happens when you hold a flexible ruler at one end and shake it. The motion of the free

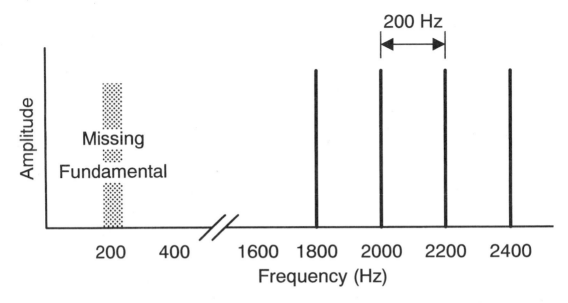

FIGURE 3–13 A missing fundamental or residue pitch of 200 Hz is perceived (represented by the shaded bar) when we are presented with a complex tone composed of just the harmonics of 200 Hz.

end of the ruler (the output) will include several frequencies above and beyond the rate at which you are shaking it (the input), which is understandable because the flexibility of the ruler causes it to bounce and wobble when shaken. These extra frequencies in the motion of the free end are distortion products.

The simplest distortion products occur when tones are presented at high levels, resulting in the generation of **aural harmonics** that are heard by the subject. For example, an original or "primary" tone presented at 500 Hz may cause the ear to generate signals at multiples (harmonics) of 500 Hz, so that the person will hear 500 Hz plus 1000 Hz, 1500 Hz, etc. Figure 3-14 shows two examples of aural harmonics. The primary tone at 800 Hz (labeled one) produced the aural harmonic at 1600 Hz ($2 \times f_1$). Similarly, the primary tone at 1000 Hz (f_2) generated the aural harmonic at 2000 Hz ($2 \times f_2$).

If two primary tones that are *close together* in frequency (e.g., $f_1 = 1000$ Hz and $f_2 = 1005$ Hz) are presented simultaneously, then their representations in the cochlea will be cyclically in-phase and out-of-phase, so that the combination alternates between reinforcement and cancellation. The result is a tone that waxes and wanes, or modulates, at a rate equal to the difference between the two tones, as illustrated in Figure 3–15. For example, primary tones of 1000 Hz and 1005 Hz will be heard as a 1000 Hz that modulates or beats at a rate of five times per second (because $1005 - 1000 = 5$ Hz).

Two primary tones (f_1 and f_2) that are relatively far apart in frequency will be heard as two separate tones; however, they may interact with each other to produce audible **combination tones**. Several examples of combination tones are shown in Figure 3–14, where the primary tones are 800 Hz (f_1) and 1000 Hz (f_2). A **difference tone** is often heard when the primary tones are presented at relatively high sensation levels. As its name implies, this distortion product occurs at the frequency equal to the difference between the two primaries ($f_2 - \times f_1$), which is $1000 - 800 = 200$ Hz in this example. It is sometimes possible to hear a **summation tone** at the fre-

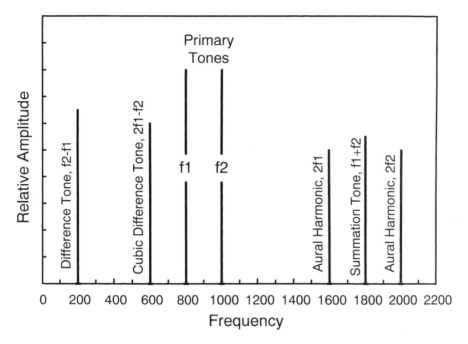

FIGURE 3–14 Examples of distortion products produced by 800 Hz and 1000 Hz tones (see text).

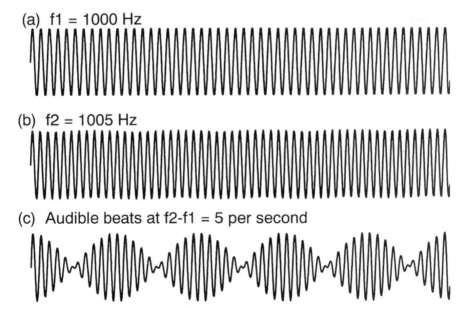

FIGURE 3–15 The interaction of two similar tones, (a) $f_1 = 1000$ Hz and (b) $f_2 = 1005$ Hz, results in the perception of (c) audible beats at a rate of $f_2 - f_1 = 5$ times per second.

quency equal to the sum of the two primaries ($f_1 + f_2$), which is 1800 Hz in the figure. Another distortion product is the **cubic difference tone** that occurs at the frequency corresponding to $2f - f_2$. For primaries of 800 Hz and 1000 Hz, the cubic difference tone occurs at $2(800) - 1000 = 600$ Hz, as shown in the figure. The cubic difference tone is audible even when the primary tones are relatively soft, and is of particular interest in audiology because of its applications in otoacoustic emissions assessment (Chapter 11).

Masking

We are all familiar with some variation of the expression, "I didn't hear you because the water was running." This is masking. More formally, **masking** is the interference with the ability to hear one sound (the **signal**) because of the presence of a second sound (the **masker**). In other words, an otherwise audible signal is rendered inaudible by the presence of the masker. The typical masking procedure involves a few simple steps:

1. Find the threshold for a signal, such as a tone.
2. Add a masker, such as a noise.
3. Find the threshold of the tone again, this time in the presence of the masking noise.

The second threshold obtained in the presence of the masker will be higher, revealing that the noise has masked the tone. In fact, comparing the second threshold to the first one tells us how much of an effect the noise had on the audibility of the tone.

Suppose the threshold of a signal is 8 dB when it is presented alone, or "in quiet," as represented by the **unmasked threshold** in Figure 3–16. Retesting the signal's threshold in the presence of a masking noise results in a **masked threshold** of 22 dB. In other words, the level of the tone had to be increased by 14 dB in order to be heard over the noise. The amount by which the masked threshold is elevated or "shifted" is called a **threshold shift**. Hence, the masking noise caused a 14-dB threshold shift from 8 dB to 22 dB. The size of the threshold shift shows the *amount of masking* caused by the noise. In other words, there

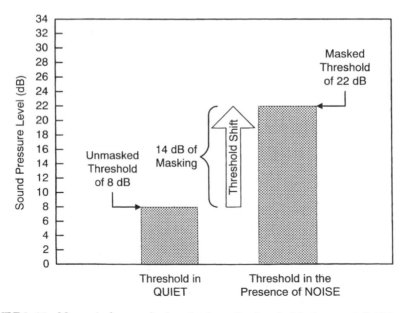

FIGURE 3–16 Numerical example showing how the threshold of a tone is 8 dB in quiet and 22 dB in the presence of a masking noise, revealing the noise has caused 14 dB of masking.

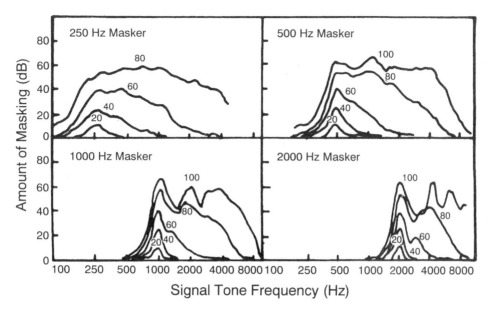

FIGURE 3–17 Masking patterns showing the amount of masking (threshold shift) as a function of signal frequency produced by 250-Hz, 500-Hz, 1000-Hz, and 2000-Hz maskers. The numbers near each individual curve correspond to the levels of the masker. Adapted from Ehmer (1959a), with permission of *Journal of the Acoustical Society of America*.

was 14 dB of masking because the noise caused the threshold of the tone to shift by 14 dB.

The frequency and intensity of a masker determines which signals it will mask and how much masking it will produce. To see the effects of the masker's frequency, it must be either a narrow band of noise or pure tone. For example, a 1000-Hz *masker* could be either a 1000-Hz *tone* or a *narrow band* of noise that is centered around 1000 Hz. Similar masking patterns are obtained either way (Wegel & Lane, 1924; Egan & Hake, 1950; Ehmer, 1959a,b).

Figure 3–17 shows the masking effects produced by various intensities of four different masker frequencies—250 Hz, 500 Hz, 1000 Hz, and 2000 Hz. The masker frequency is indicated at the top of each frame, and the number next to each curve shows the level of the masker (in dB SPL) that produced it. These are called **masking patterns**. The frequencies of the *test signals* are shown along the abscissa, and the *amount of masking* (threshold shift) produced by a masker is shown on the ordinate. In other words, the decibel values on the y-axis show how much the signal threshold was shifted by the masker: if the height of a curve is 25 dB at 1000 Hz, this means that the masker caused 25 dB of masking at 1000 Hz. In other words, the 1000-Hz threshold was raised 25 dB above its unmasked threshold due to the noise. Similarly, if the curve is at 0 dB at 500-Hz, this means that the 500-Hz threshold in the presence of the noise is the same as it was with no noise at all (i.e., there was no masking at this frequency).

These masking patterns tell us a lot about the nature of masking. First, the amount of masking increases (the curves get higher) as the masker level increases. Second, more masking is produced at frequencies close to the frequency of the masker than at more distant frequencies. For example, the curve for a 500-Hz masker has a peak at 500 Hz, indicating that it produces more masking at 500 Hz than it does above and below this frequency; and the 1000-Hz masker produces the most masking at 1000 Hz. Third, the masking pattern produced by a low-level masker (e.g.,

20 dB) tends to be narrow and essentially symmetrical around the masker frequency. As the intensity of the masker increases, the range of frequencies that it masks becomes wider and extends asymmetrically upward in frequency. For example, an intense 1000-Hz masker is able to mask frequencies higher than 1000 Hz but it has very little effect at frequencies below 1000 Hz. In addition, comparing one frame to the other in the figure reveals that masking patterns are quite wide for low-frequency maskers and become progressively narrower for higher-frequency maskers. The notion that masking extends to frequencies that are higher than the masker, but not below it, is called **upward spread of masking**.

These masking patterns can be understood in terms of the excitation patterns of the signal and masker along the basilar membrane, as represented schematically in Figure 3–18. Recall the traveling wave envelope rises grad-

ually on the basal (high-frequency) side of its peak and then falls rapidly on the apical (low-frequency) side. In addition, the excitation pattern becomes larger as the intensity of a sound increases. As a result, the broad trailing part of the excitation pattern produced by a lower-frequency masker is able to encompass the excitation pattern of a higher frequency signal (Fig. 3–18a). However, the leading side of the excitation pattern produced by a higher-frequency masker is not able to envelop the excitation pattern of a lower-frequency signal (Fig. 3–18b).

Figure 3–19 shows the masking of tones by white noise (Hawkins & Stevens, 1950). Here, the lowest curve represents the unmasked thresholds of pure tones as a function of frequency, and the other curves show the masked thresholds produced by various levels of the noise, indicated by the numbers above each curve. Notice that increasing the masking noise level by 10 dB also causes the masked threshold to increase by 10 dB. In other words, the amount of masking is a linear function of masker level, as illustrated in Figure 3–20.

The noise levels in Figure 3–19 are expressed in spectrum level, which is the *level per cycle* of the noise. For the benefit of the mathematically oriented student, spectrum level (dB_{SL}) is obtained by applying the formula,

$$dB_{SL} = dB_O - 10\log BW,$$

where dB_O is the overall power of the noise and BW is its bandwidth. For example, if a noise that is 10,000 Hz wide has an overall power level of 95 dB, then its spectrum level is 55 dB, because:

$$dB_{SL} = dB_O - 10 \log BW$$
$$= 95 - 10 \log 10{,}000$$
$$= 95 - 10(4) = 95 - 40 = 55.$$

Notice that the bandwidth is converted into its decibel equivalent (10 log BW), which is then subtracted from the power level (the equivalent of dividing the power by the bandwidth) to arrive at the level per cycle or spectrum level.

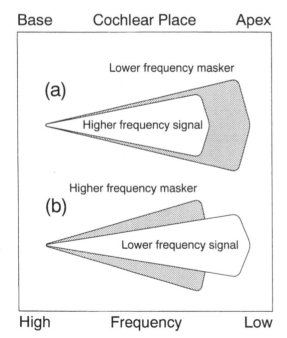

Base   Cochlear Place   Apex

Lower frequency masker

(a)

Higher frequency signal

Higher frequency masker

(b)

Lower frequency signal

High   Frequency   Low

FIGURE 3–18   (a) The cochlear excitation pattern of a lower-frequency masker is able to envelop that of a higher-frequency signal, but (b) the excitation pattern of a higher-frequency masker does not encompass that of a lower-frequency signal.

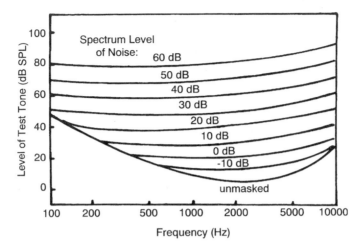

FIGURE 3–19 Masked thresholds in dB SPL of pure tones as a function of frequency for various levels of a white noise masker. The lowest curve shows unmasked thresholds. The amount of masking produced by a given noise level at a particular frequency can be found by subtracting the corresponding unmasked threshold (from the lowest curve) from the masked threshold. The masker levels near each curve are expressed in decibels of spectrum level (see text). Adapted from Hawkins & Stevens (1950), with permission of *Journal of the Acoustical Society of America*.

CRITICAL BAND FOR MASKING OR CRITICAL RATIO

Is all of the white noise actually needed to mask a particular tone, or is a particular frequency masked by only a certain range or bandwidth within the noise that is around it? Fletcher (1940) found that the masked threshold for a tone increases as the bandwidth of the masking noise around it gets wider. However, once a certain bandwidth is reached, then any further widening of the

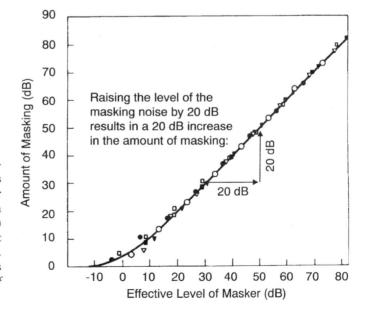

FIGURE 3–20 The amount of masking produced by a masker increases linearly with increases in masker level. Notice that a 10-dB increase in the level of the masker (x-axis) causes a 10-dB increase in the amount of masking for the signal (y-axis). Adapted from Hawkins & Stevens (1950), with permission of *Journal of the Acoustical Society of America*.

Raising the level of the masking noise by 20 dB results in a 20 dB increase in the amount of masking:

noise does not cause any more masking. Hence, only a certain **critical band** within the white noise is actually helping to mask the tone at the center of that band, whereas the parts of the noise above and below this range do not help to mask the tone (Fig. 3–21).

At the masked threshold, the power of the signal (S) is equal to the power of the noise (N) inside the critical band (CB), or S = CB × N (Fletcher, 1940). Consequently, the *critical band for masking* is actually a **critical ratio** because CB = S/N, or $dB_S - dB_N$ when expressed in decibels. For example, the 1000-Hz threshold is 58 dB when the masking noise is 40 dB, so that the critical ratio is 58 − 40 = 18 dB, which corresponds to 63.1 Hz when it is converted back to frequency (Hawkins & Stevens, 1950). In other words, when a white noise is used to mask a 1000-Hz tone, the only part of the noise that actually does the masking is a 63 Hz-wide band of the noise around 1000 Hz. The masking critical ratio is shown as a function of frequency in Figure 3–11, along with the critical band that was discussed earlier. In general, the critical band tends to be approximately 2.5 times wider than the critical ratio for masking (Scharf, 1970).

PSYCHOACOUSTIC TUNING CURVES

We have already seen that a masking pattern shows the *threshold shifts* at many different signal frequencies that are produced by a certain *fixed masker* (e.g., a 1000-Hz narrow band of noise at, say, 40 dB). We can also address masking in terms of finding what *masker levels* at different frequencies are needed to just mask a certain *fixed signal* (e.g., Cristovich, 1957; Small, 1959; Zwicker & Schorn, 1978). Figure 3–22 illustrates this concept and an example of typical results. The filled circle in the graph represents the frequency and intensity of a fixed test signal, which happens to be a 1000-Hz pure tone at 15 dB. Maskers at many different frequencies are then used to mask this fixed signal, and the resulting masker levels are then graphed as a function of frequency, shown by the curve in the figure. This kind of masking diagram is called a **psychoacoustic tuning curve (PTC)** because of its resemblance to auditory nerve fiber tuning curves; however, it is *not* the "perceptual replica" of a neuron's response area. Instead, the PTC takes on this shape because the closer the frequency of the masker gets to the frequency of the test tone,

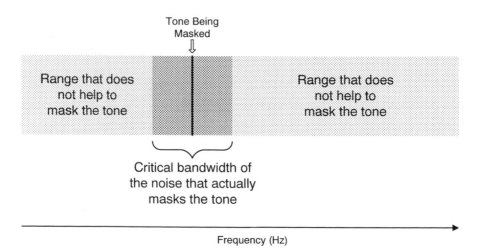

FIGURE 3–21   The critical band for masking is the limited bandwidth within a noise that actually contributes to masking a tone whose frequency is at the center of that band.

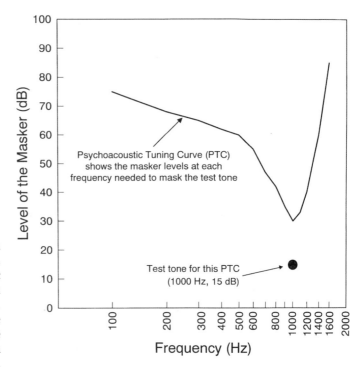

FIGURE 3-22 An example of a psychoacoustic tuning curve (PTC). This PTC shows the masker levels at each frequency needed to keep a 15-dB, 1000-Hz tone just masked. The frequency and level of the tone are represented by the filled circle for illustrative purposes. Based on material by Zwicker & Schorn (1978).

the lower its level has to be to mask that tone. As a result, the PTC provides a good representation of the ear's frequency selectivity.

CENTRAL AND TEMPORAL MASKING

Until now, we have been considering masking in terms of two sounds that are in the same ear at the same time, or **simultaneous monaural masking**. However, masking effects can also occur when one or both of these conditions are not met. **Central masking** refers to the masking of a sound in one ear due to a masker in the *other* ear, and is the result of interactions in the lower portions of the central auditory nervous system (e.g., Dirks & Norris, 1966; Zwislocki, Buining, & Glantz, 1968; Zwislocki, 1973). Overall, central masking occurs principally in the higher frequencies, and the threshold shifts that it produces are much smaller than what occurs by monaural masking.

Temporal masking occurs when the signal and masker are not presented at the same time (e.g., Pickett, 1959; Elliott, 1962a,b; Wilson & Carhart, 1971). Here, a very brief signal (often a click) is presented either before or after a brief masker, as illustrated in Figure 3-23. In **forward masking** the masker comes before the signal so that the masking effect operates forward in time. **Backward masking** occurs when the signal comes before the masker, so that the masking operates backward in time. Forward masking effects occur for intervals of up to roughly 100 msec between the masker and the signal, whereas backward masking is effective for intervals up to about 50 msec between the signal and masker. Temporal masking effects involve interactions between the representations of the signal and masker in the auditory nervous system, but there may be some overlapping of the excitation patterns within the cochlea when the intervals between the signal and masker are very brief.

Binaural Hearing

Binaural hearing is the general term used to describe the nature and effects of listening

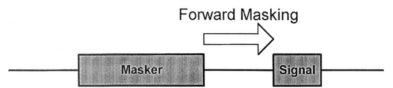

Forward Masking

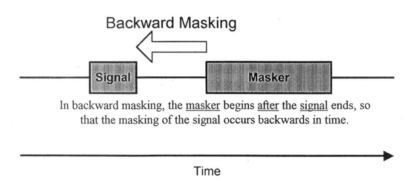

In forward masking, the <u>masker</u> ends <u>before</u> the <u>signal</u> begins,
so that the masking of the signal occurs forward in time.

Backward Masking

In backward masking, the <u>masker</u> begins <u>after</u> the <u>signal</u> ends, so
that the masking of the signal occurs backwards in time.

Time

FIGURE 3–23   Temporal masking occurs when the masker and signal do not overlap in time.

with two ears instead of just one. Every aspect of binaural hearing is fascinating, beginning with a phenomenon that is so fundamental to our perception of sound we actually fail to realize its existence. Specifically, we perceive *one world* through *two ears* (Cherry, 1961). This phenomenon is called **binaural fusion.** In formal terms, it means that the separate signals received by the two ears are perceived as a *single, fused auditory image.* Recall that similar sounds are rarely identical at the two ears. Instead, there are inter-ear differences in intensity, time, and spectrum. Binaural fusion occurs as long as there is some similarity between these two signals, particularly for the frequencies below approximately 1500 Hz. Under typical listening conditions the fused image is perceived as coming from a location outside of the head (extracranially); however, it is heard inside the head (intracranially) when the signals are presented through earphones. It is easy to experience extra- versus intracranial locations using a home stereo system by listening to a CD recording first from loudspeakers and then through earphones.

Earlier in this chapter, we learned that beats are heard when two tones of slightly different frequencies are presented to the same ear. **Binaural beats** can be heard when one of the tones is presented to the right ear and the other tone is presented to the left ear as long as the tones are relatively low in frequency (optimally between about 300 and 600 Hz). Unlike monaural beats, which are due to interactions in the cochlea, binaural beats result from interactions between the neural representations of the tones from the two ears within the central nervous system.

BINAURAL SENSITIVITY AND LOUDNESS

The threshold of hearing is approximately 3 dB lower (better) when listening with two ears compared with just one (e.g., Shaw, Newman, & Hirsh, 1947). This advantage is called **binaural summation.** In addition to more sensitive absolute thresholds binaurally than monaurally, binaural hearing also results in more acute differential sensitivity, that is, smaller difference limens, for intensity and frequency. For example, Jesteadt,

Wier, and Green (1977b) found that difference limens are larger (poorer) monaurally than binaurally by a factor of 1.65 to 1 for intensity and 1.44 to 1 for frequency.

Binaural summation also occurs for loudness, so that a given sound level is perceived to be twice as loud binaurally compared with its monaural loudness (Fletcher & Munson, 1933; Marks, 1978). For a monaural tone to sound as loud as a binaural tone, it must be raised by about 3 dB at near threshold levels. This binaural loudness advantage increases to about 6 dB at sensation levels of 35 dB and above (Caussé & Chavasse, 1942).

MASKING LEVEL DIFFERENCES

The binaural **masking level difference** occurs for abstract sounds such as tones as well as for speech (Hirsh, 1948; Licklider, 1948; Durlach, 1972). It is easily understood in terms of the following example: A 500-Hz tone is presented to one ear at a level well above threshold. A masking noise is then also presented to that ear and its level is adjusted until it just masks the tone. This is the typical situation in monaural masking and is illustrated in Figure 3–24a. Let's use the letter S to represent the signal (the tone), N to stand for the noise, and m to mean monaural. Using this shorthand, monaural masking is written as $S_m N_m$. The same masking outcome occurs if the tone is presented binaurally and the noise is also presented binaurally (Fig. 3–24b). Using o to mean "the same in both ears," the second situation would be called $S_o N_o$ because the signal is the same in both ears (S_o), and is being just masked by a noise that is the same in both ears (N_o).

Let us see what happens when we start with the $S_o N_o$ situation and simply *invert the phase of the signal in just one ear* (so that it is positive in the right ear whenever it is negative in the left ear, and vice versa). This situation is called $S_\pi N_o$, where 7π means "*antiphasic* (or 180° out-of-phase) at the two ears," and is illustrated in Figure 3–24c. Strangely, the tone becomes audible again with $S_\pi N_o$, even though the noise and signal levels are the same as they were for $S_o N_o$. In

other words, just changing the phase of the signal between the ears from $S_o N_o$ to $S_\pi N_o$ causes the tone to become *unmasked*. This unmasking effect will also occur if the noise is made antiphasic while keeping the tone the same at the two ears, written as $S_o N_\pi$. This *release from masking* relies upon binaural interactions as low as the superior olivary complex. Now that the tone has become audible, the noise must be raised even further to mask the tone again. The number of decibels that the noise must be raised to mask the tone again is called the **masking level difference (MLD)**. In other words, the MLD is the difference between (1) the noise level needed to

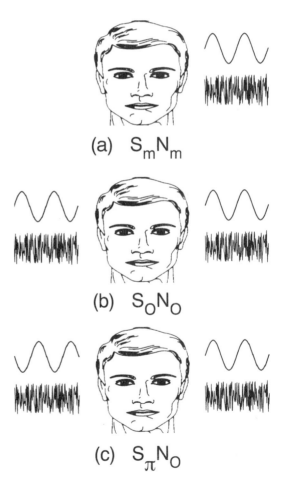

(a) $S_m N_m$

(b) $S_o N_o$

(c) $S_\pi N_o$

FIGURE 3–24 Masking level differences for the (a) $S_m N_m$, (b) $S_o N_o$, and (c) $S_\pi N_o$ conditions (see text).

mask the signal for $S_\pi N_o$ (or $S_o N_\pi$), and (2) the noise level needed to mask the signal for $S_o N_o$. In normal individuals this difference is approximately 13 to 15 dB for frequencies below about 500 Hz. The MLD provides us with a way to look at some of the binaural processes that make it possible for us to hear and communicate effectively in spite of noise and reverberant conditions.

DIRECTIONAL HEARING

Localization and Lateralization The notions of directional hearing, inter-ear (interaural) differences, and spectral cues were introduced in Chapter 2. In addition, it has already been mentioned that the binaurally fused image is **lateralized intracranially** when listening through earphones and **localized extracranially** when listening in a soundfield. The most fundamental explanation for how binaural hearing provides for directionality is known as the **duplex theory**. According to the duplex theory, the main cues for determining the direction of a sound source are **interaural intensity differences (IIDs)** and **interaural time differences (ITDs)**, with IIDs taking on the principal role for the high frequencies and ITDs predominating for the low frequencies. In other words, sound sources can be localized because slightly different signals reach the two ears, and the characteristics of these interaural differences depend on the direction of the sound source relative to the head. There are no interaural differences when the sound source is directly in front of or behind the listener, or elsewhere in the median plane, because these locations are equally distant from the two ears. As a result, median plane localizations depend upon the **spectral variations** that result from the effects of the pinna, head, and torso. It is no wonder that front-back confusions occur more often than other kinds of localization errors.

The Minimal Audible Angle In addition to sound localization, we must also be able to distinguish between two sound sources. Just as we express locations in degrees around the head, the separation between two sound sources is also given in degrees. The smallest

perceptible separation between two sound sources is called the **minimal audible angle (MAA)** and might be thought of as a difference limen for localization. We can distinguish between sound sources that are only 1° to 2° apart if they are directly in front of the head, but the MAA gets larger (poorer) as the two sounds move off to the side (Mills, 1972). In fact, there is an ambiguous zone called the "cone of confusion" on each side of the head, where a pair of sound source directions cannot be distinguished because both of them are facing the same ear. Along with front-back confusions, this cone of confusion highlights the importance of head movements for effective localization. The MAA is acute in front of the head because small changes in location here cause noticeable changes in inter-ear differences. This is not the case on the side of the head where interaural differences are already very large (favoring the near ear), so the two sound sources must be far apart (a large MAA) before there will be any distinguishable change in inter-ear differences.

An advanced note is in order here: there are actually two kinds of minimal audible angles, depending on whether the two sounds are *presented one after the other* (sequentially) or *at the same time* (concurrently). They both involve distinguishing locations, but the *concurrent* MAA also involves identifying the two sound sources. For this reason the concurrent MAA is also affected by spectral differences between the two sounds (Perrott, 1984).

The Precedence Effect Sounds are reflected back when they hit a surface, creating echoes. In rooms and other enclosures, there will be multiple echoes that cause the sound in the room to linger after the original or direct sound, called **reverberation**. As a result, we are often presented with multiple signals coming from different directions. Yet we are usually aware of just the original or direct sound, and we rarely have any difficulty telling the direction of its source. The perception of the direct sound and its correct direction is due to a principle known as the **precedence effect, first wavefront law**, or **Haas effect**. The precedence effect is illustrated most simply as follows:

Suppose a click is presented to both ears through earphones, but the click arrives at the right ear a few milliseconds prior to arriving at the left ear. Instead of hearing two separate clicks, the listener will hear a single fused image that appears to be coming from the leading right ear (Wallach, Newman, & Rosenzweig, 1949). Similarly, if a sound is presented from one of two separated loudspeakers followed by an "echo" coming from the other loudspeaker, then the listener will hear only one sound coming from the leading speaker (Haas, 1951). In other words, the direction of the first-arriving signal determines the perceived direction of the sound. This effect occurs for delays up to approximately 40 msec. Two separate signals are perceived by the time the delay reaches 50 msec, in which case a distinct echo is heard.

REFERENCES

Abel SM. 1972. Duration discrimination of noise and tone bursts. *J Acoust Soc Amer* 51, 1219–1223.

Bekesy G. 1936. Über die Hörschwelle und Fülgrenze langsamer sinusförmiger Luftdruckschwankungen. *Ann Physik* 26, 554–566.

Beranek, LL. 1988. *Acoustical Measurements,* revised edition. New York: Acoustical Society of America.

Buus S, Florentine M. 1985. Gap detection in normal and impaired listeners: The effect of level and frequency. In Michelsen A (Ed.): *Time Resolution in Auditory Systems.* New York: Springer, 159–179.

Caussé R, Chavasse P. 1942. Difference entree L'ecout binauriculaire et monauriculaire pour la perception des intensites supraliminaires. *Comp R Soc Biol* 139, 405.

Cherry EC. 1961. Two ears—but one world. In Rosenblith, WA (Ed.): *Sensory Communication.* Cambridge, MA: MIT Press, 99–117.

Cristovich LA. 1957. Frequency characteristics of masking effect. *Biophysics* 2, 708–715.

Dadson RS, King JH. 1952. A determination of the normal threshold of hearing and its relation to the standardization of audiometers. *Laryngol Otol* 46, 366–378.

Dirks DD, Norris JC. 1966. Shifts in auditory thresholds produced by pulsed and continuous contralateral masking. *J Acoust Soc Am* 37, 631–637.

Dooley GJ, Moore BCJ. 1988. Duration discrimination of steady and gliding tones: A new method for estimating sensitivity to rate of change. *J Acoust Soc Am* 84, 1332–1337.

Durlach NI. 1972. Binaural signal detection: Equalization and cancellation theory. In Tobias JV (Ed.): *Foundations of Modern Auditory Theory,* Vol. 2. New York: Academic Press, 369–462.

Egan JP, Hake HW. 1950. On the masking pattern of a simple auditory stimulus. *J Acoust Soc Am* 22, 622–630.

Ehmer RH. 1959a. Masking patterns of tones. *J Acoust Soc Am* 31, 1115–1120.

Ehmer RH. 1959b. Masking by tones vs. noise bands. *J Acoust Soc Am* 31, 1253–1356.

Elliott LL. 1962a. Backward masking: Monotic and dichotic conditions. *J Acoust Soc Am* 34, 1108–1115.

Elliott LL. 1962b. Backward masking: Monotic and dichotic conditions. *J Acoust Soc Am* 34, 1116–1117.

Fitzgibbons PJ, Gordon-Salant S. 1987. Temporal gap resolution in listeners with high-frequency sensorineural hearing loss. *J Acoust Soc Am* 81, 133–147.

Fitzgibbons PB, Wightman RL. 1982. Gap detection in normal and hearing impaired listeners. *J Acoust Soc Am* 72, 761–765.

Fletcher H. 1940. Auditory patterns. *J Acoust Soc Am* 12, 47–65.

Fletcher H, Munson MA, 1933. Loudness: Its definition, measurement and calculation. *J Acoust Soc Am* 5, 82–108.

Gelfand SA. 1998. *Hearing: An Introduction to Psychological and Physiological Acoustics,* 3rd ed. New York: Marcel Dekker.

Green DM. 1985. Temporal factors in psychoacoustics. In Michelsen A (Ed.): *Time Resolution in Auditory Systems.* New York: Springer, 122–140.

Haas H. 1951. Ober den Einfachechos auf die Horsamkeit von Sprache. *Acoustica* 1, 49–58. [1972. On the influence of a single echo on the intelligibility of speech. *J Audio Eng Soc* 20, 146–159.]

Hawkins JE, Stevens SS. 1950. The masking of pure tones and of speech by white noise. *J Acoust Soc Am* 22, 6–13.

Hellman RP. 1999. Cross-modality matching: A tool for measuring loudness in sensorineural hearing loss. *Ear Hear* 20, 193–213.

Hellman RP, Meiselman CH. 1988. Prediction of individual loudness exponents from cross-modality matching. *J Speech Hear Res* 31, 605–615.

Hirsh IJ. 1948. The influence of interaural phase on interaural summation and inhibition. *J Acoust Soc Am* 20, 536–544.

Hirsh IJ. 1952. *The Measurement of Hearing.* New York: McGraw-Hill.

Hirsh IJ. 1959. Auditory perception of perceived order. *J Acoust Soc Am* 31, 759–767.

Hood JD, Poole JP. 1970. Investigations upon the upper physiological limit of normal hearing. *Int Audiol* 9, 250–255.

International Standards Organization (ISO). 1961. Recommendation 226. Normal equal loudness contours for pure tones and normal thresholds of hearing under free-field listening conditions. Geneva: ISO.

Jesteadt W, Wier CC, Green DM. 1977a. Intensity discrimination as a function of frequency and sensation level. *J Acoust Soc Am* 61, 169–177.

Jesteadt W, Wier CC, Green DM. 1977b. Comparison of monaural and binaural discrimination of intensity and frequency. *J Acoust Soc Am* 61, 1599–1603.

Killion MC. 1978. Revised estimate of minimum audible pressure: Where is the "missing 6 dB"? *J Acoust Soc Am* 63, 1501–1508.

Licklider JCR. 1948. The influence of interaural phase relations upon the masking of speech by white noise. *J Acoust Soc Am* 20, 150–159.

Marks LE. 1978. Binaural summation of loudness of pure tones. *J Acoust Soc Am* 64, 107–113.

Mills AW. 1972. Auditory localization. In Tobias JV (Ed.): *Foundations of Modern Auditory Theory, Vol. 2*. New York: Academic Press, 301–348.

Northern JL, Downs MP, Rudmose W, Glorig A, Fletcher J. 1972. Recommended high frequency audiometric threshold levels (8000–18000 Hz). *J Acoust Soc Am* 52, 585–595.

Perrott DR. 1984. Concurrent minimal audible angle: A re-examination of the concept of auditory spatial acuity. *J Acoust Soc Am* 75, 1201–1206.

Pickett JM. 1959. Backward masking. *J Acoust Soc Am* 31, 1613–1715.

Robinson DW, Dadson RS. 1956. A re-determination of the equal loudness relations for pure tones. *Br J Appl Phys* 7, 166–181.

Scharf B. 1970. Critical bands. In Tobias JV (Ed.): *Foundations of Modern Auditory Theory*, Vol. 1. New York: Academic Press, 157–202.

Schouten JF. 1940. The residue, a new concept in subjective sound analysis. *Proc Kon Ned Akad* 43, 356–365.

Seebeck A. 1841. Beohchtungen über einige Bedingungen der Entstehung von Tonen. *Ann Phys Chem* 53, 417–436.

Shaw WA, Newman EB, Hirsh IJ. 1947. The difference between monaural and binaural thresholds. *J Exp Psychol* 37, 229–242.

Small AM. 1959. Pure tone masking. *J Acoust Soc Am* 31, 1619–1625.

Stevens SS. 1956. The direct estimation of sensory magnitudes-loudness. *Am J Psychol* 69, 1–25.

Stevens SS. 1975. *Psychophysics*. New York: Wiley.

Thurlow WR, Small AM. 1955. Pitch perception of certain periodic auditory stimuli. *J Acoust Soc Am* 27, 132–137.

Wallach H, Newman EB, Rosenzweig MR. 1949. The precedence effect in sound localization. *Am J Psychol* 57, 315–336.

Wegel RL. 1932. Physical data and physiology of the auditory nerve. *Ann Otol Rhinol Laryngol* 41, 740–779.

Wegel RL, Lane CE. 1924. The auditory masking of pure tone by another and its probable relation to the dynamics of the inner ear. *Physiol Rev* 23, 266–285.

Wier CC, Jesteadt W, Green DM. 1977. Frequency discrimination as a function of frequency and sensation level. *J Acoust Soc Am* 61, 178–184.

Wilson RH, Carhart R. 1971. Forward and backward masking: Interactions and additivity. *J Acoust Soc Am* 56, 957–962.

Yeowart NS, Bryan M, Tempest W. 1967. The monaural MAP threshold of hearing at frequencies from 1.5 to 100c/s. *J Sound Vib* 6, 335–342.

Zwicker E, Flottorp G, Stevens SS. 1957. Critical band width in loudness summation. *J Acoust Soc Am* 29, 548–557.

Zwicker E, Schorn K. 1978. Psychoacoustical tuning curves in audiology. *Audiology* 17, 120–140.

Zwislocki J. 1973. In search of physiological correlates of psychoacoustic characteristics. In Møller AJ (Ed.): *Basic Mechanisms in Hearing*. New York: Academic Press, 787–808.

Zwislocki J, Buining E, Glantz J. 1968. Frequency distribution of central masking. *J Acoust Soc Am* 43, 1267–1271.

4

The Audiometer and Test Environment

The Audiometer

The principal *tool* used in the process of evaluating a patient's auditory functioning is the **audiometer**. Fundamentally, the audiometer is nothing more than an electronic device that produces and delivers sounds to the patient. What makes the audiometer unique is that these sounds are very specific: we know precisely what is being presented to the patient, and we can be confident that these sounds will be consistent from audiometer to audiometer. A basic audiometer should make it possible to perform the most fundamental audiological tests, which involve determining how much intensity is needed for a patient to hear pure tones at different frequencies. The **pure-tone audiometer** must be able to produce pure tones at certain frequencies, precisely control the levels of these tones, and deliver them to the patient in the manner intended by the audiologist. A typical pure-tone audiometer is shown in Figure 4–1.

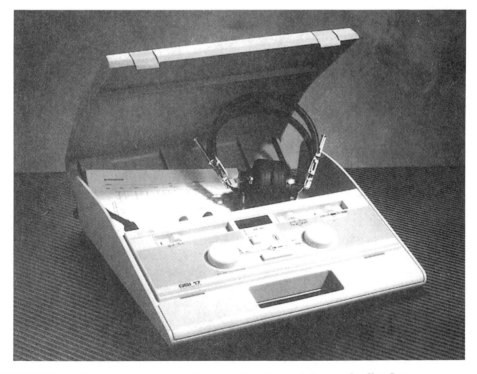

FIGURE 4–1 A basic pure-tone audiometer. Courtesy of Grason-Stadler, Inc.

The components of an audiometer are shown in Figure 4–2. The **power switch** controls the electrical supply to the instrument, and there is often a power indicator lamp to show whether it is on or off. Test tones are presented to the patient by turning them on and off with a button called the **interrupter**. The **frequency control** is used to select among the various test frequencies. Most audiometers include the frequencies 125, 250, 500, 750, 1000, 1500, 2000, 3000, 4000, 6000, and 8000 Hz. The pure tones themselves are produced by a circuit within the audiometer called a pure-tone oscillator. There is a **stimulus** or **tone mode switch** that allows the test tone to be presented either continuously on or pulsed on-and-off at a regular rate. Another mode produces a warble tone, which means that the frequency varies periodically (e.g., 1000 Hz ± 5%) rather than staying steady over time. This feature is not commonly found in basic audiometers. The intensity of the test signal is controlled by the **attenuator** or **Hearing Level control**. (*"Frequency dial," "attenuator or HL dial,"* and *"dial readings"*

are convenient terms that continue to be used even though many digital instruments have replaced dials with other kinds of controls.) Unlike common volume controls, attenuators are **calibrated**, which means that the markings on the attenuator refer to *specific physical values and increments*. Setting the attenuator to "45 dB HL" will cause the sound coming out of the earphone to have a sound pressure level (SPL) that actually corresponds to 45 dB HL; and changing the attenuator setting by 5 dB means the sound pressure level will really change by *5 dB*. Most audiometers have attenuators that are calibrated in 5-dB steps, and more sophisticated models also provide for testing in 1-dB, 2-dB, or other step sizes. The range of intensities that can be tested usually goes from as low as –10 dB HL up to 115 dB HL for air-conduction and about 70 dB for bone-conduction. The testable range varies for each type of signal and is indicated on the audiometer.

Finally, an **output selector** is used to direct the signal to the right or left earphones, or to the **bone-conduction vibrator**. Figure 4–3

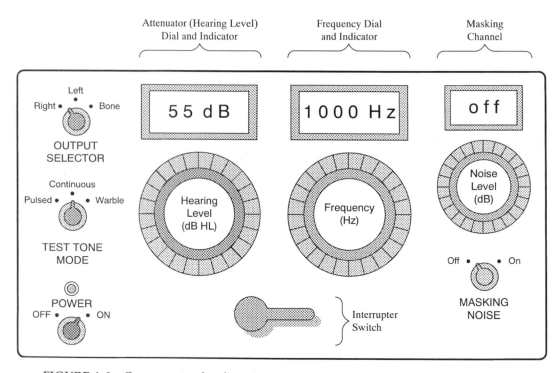

FIGURE 4–2   Components of audiometers.

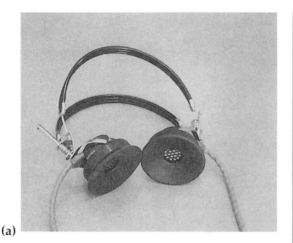

(a)

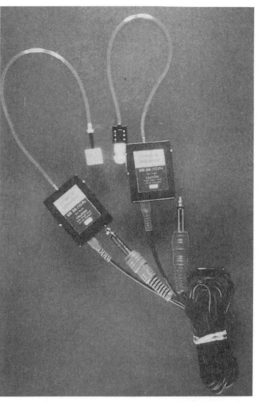

(b)

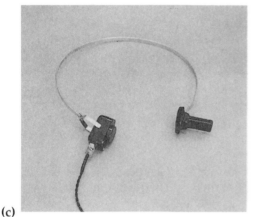

(c)

FIGURE 4–3 Examples of (a) standard supra-aural audiometric earphones, (b) insert receivers, and (c) a bone-conduction vibrator.

shows examples of typical audiometric earphones and a bone-conduction vibrator. The standard audiometric headset includes a headband that holds two earphones, each of which is surrounded by rubber cushions. They are often called supraaural earphones because the earphone/cushion combination is worn over the ear. This is in contrast to the less frequently used circumaural earphones, which have cushions that fit around the ears. **Insert earphones** have a pliable earpiece that is inserted into the external auditory canal, and are also used for various clinical purposes, as discussed in Chapters 5 and 9. A **bone-conduction vibrator** is usually held against the mastoid by a spring-like headband.

The audiometer described so far would be considered a single-channel instrument because it can produce only one signal. How-

ever, many pure-tone audiometers have a second channel that can produce a **masking noise**. The second channel has its own interrupter switch and attenuator. The noise signal is produced by a circuit inside the audiometer called a noise generator. It is premature to discuss masking at this point, except to say that we might need to put a masking noise into the left ear to prevent it from hearing the test tones that are being presented to the right ear.

Clinical audiometers such as the ones depicted in Figure 4–4 include all of the features of pure-tone audiometers, plus a wide array of features that enable them to perform sophisticated tests with tones and many other kinds of signals. These instruments also include microphones; inputs for tape and CD players that are used to present

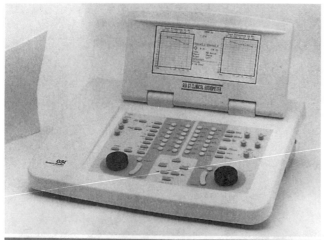

(a)

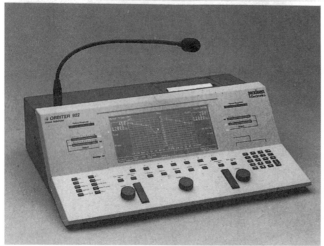

(b)

FIGURE 4–4 Examples of state-of-the-art clinical audiometers that are able to perform a wide variety of clinical tests. Photographs courtesy of (a) Grason-Stadler, Inc. and (b) Madsen Electronics, Inc.

recorded tests; patient response microphones; an intercom system; a patient response signal, computer interface; etc. Some instruments provide for testing in the 8000 to 16,000-Hz range, and are identified as **extended high frequency audiometers**. In addition, the output selectors of a clinical audiometer provide a wide choice of **output transducers**, such as (1) the right or left earphone, (2) the right or left insert receiver, (3) the bone-conduction vibrator, (4) loudspeakers, and (5) any *combination* of these. How many and which ones of these and other functions are provided varies by manufacturer and model. In fact, the term *"clinical audiometer"* is really professional jargon for

an instrument that is sufficiently versatile and accurate to meet the extensive clinical needs of an audiologist. Technically, audiometers are actually specified in terms of types based on standards for the functions they provide and the accuracy of these capabilities (ANSI S3.6-1996).

Hearing Level

Recall from Chapter 3 that our actual hearing sensitivity in decibels of sound pressure level (dB SPL re: 2×10^{-5} N/m^2 or 20 μPa) is not the same at every frequency. For example, the average normal person needs 26.5 dB SPL just to barely hear a 250-Hz tone, but only 7.5 dB SPL to just hear a 1000-Hz tone. Table 4–1 shows what the normal threshold SPLs are when using typical audiometric earphones. We consider these values to be **normal reference values**—more technically, **reference equivalent threshold sound pressure levels (RETSPLs)**—because they are the physical intensities needed by normal people to reach the threshold of hearing. In fact, when we say a person has a "hearing loss," we really mean that she requires higher SPLs than these values to just hear a sound; the more her thresholds deviate from these reference values, the worse is her hearing loss.

It is inconvenient to have different reference values at every frequency, particularly when they are "odd" numbers like 47.5, 13.5, 7.5, and 11. Life would be more pleasant if we could use the same number to represent the normal value at every frequency, especially if that reference could have a convenient value like zero. How can we make that happen?

Even though the reference values in Table 4–1 have different sound pressure levels, they are all just barely audible—and therefore equally audible. In other words, these different physical intensities are the *same* with respect to *hearing*. Hence, we can say that each of these different *sound pressure levels* has the same *hearing level*.

What is the **hearing level** of each of these threshold sounds? Because each of the SPLs in Table 4–1 is the softest sound that can be heard, it makes sense to say that they constitute the reference values for hearing. We already know that a reference has a decibel value of zero. In other words, each of these threshold SPL values corresponds to a *hearing level (HL) of 0 dB, or simply, 0 dB HL*. Now we can say it takes 26.5 dB SPL to reach 0 dB HL at 250 Hz, 7.5 dB SPL to reach 0 dB HL at 1000 Hz, and 10.5 dB SPL to reach 0 dB HL at 4000 Hz.

The circles in Figure 4–5 show these normal threshold reference values as a function of frequency in terms of both SPL (frame **a**) and hearing level (frame **b**). Notice that the SPL graph is read upward whereas the HL graph is read downward. The curved line in Figure 4–5a demonstrates these thresholds have different physical values in dB SPL, but they fall along a straight line at 0 dB HL in Figure 4–5b because they have the same hearing levels. We might say that hearing level considers each reference SPL value to be 0 dB HL. For illustrative purposes, the threshold curve of a person with a hearing loss at high frequencies is shown by the triangles in the figure. The hearing loss (triangles) is seen as a deviation from the normal values (the circles). Notice how much easier it is to think of "normal" as a straight line.

Let us now put the idea of hearing level together with the audiometer. The attenuator dial on the audiometer reads in decibels of hearing level (dB HL), and all of the reference values shown in Table 4–1 are built into the audiometer's circuitry. When the tester sets the attenuator dial to any value in dB HL, the audiometer automatically adds the reference value needed to produce the corresponding physical intensity. For example,

TABLE 4–1 Reference values [reference equivalent threshold sound pressure levels (RETSPLs)] for standard supraaural audiometric earphones expressed as the sound pressure levels (dB SPL in a 6-cc coupler, type NBA-9A) corresponding to 0 dB hearing level (HL)[a]

Frequency (Hz)	125	250	500	750	1000	1500	2000	3000	4000	6000	8000
TDH-49 and -50 earphones	47.5	26.5	13.5	8.5	7.5	7.5	11.0	9.5	10.5	13.5	13.0
TDH-39 earphones	45.0	25.5	11.5	8.0	7.0	6.5	9.0	10.0	9.5	15.5	13.0

[a] Adapted from ANSI S3.6-1996.

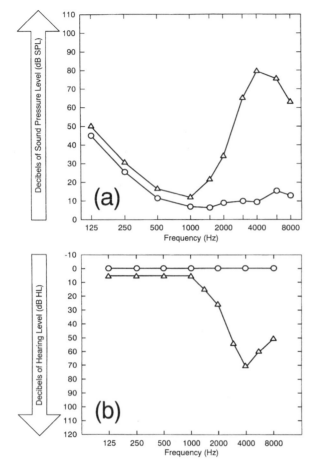

FIGURE 4–5 Normal hearing thresholds (circles) as a function of frequency appear as a curved line representing different physical values in dB SPL **(a)** and as a straight line representing the same hearing values in dB HL **(b)**. The triangles show the thresholds of a person who has a hearing loss in the higher frequencies in **(a)** dB SPL and **(b)** dB HL. Notice how intensity increases upward in frame **(a)** and downward in frame **(b)**. Adapted from Gelfand (1981), with permission.

when the frequency is set to 1000 Hz (where the reference value is 7.5 dB SPL) an attenuator setting of 0 dB HL causes the audiometer to produce a tone of

$$0 + 7.5 = 7.5 \text{ dB SPL,}$$

and an attenuator setting of 55 dB HL results in

$$55 + 7.5 = 62.5 \text{ dB SPL.}$$

If the frequency is set to 500 Hz (where the reference value is 13.5 dB SPL), then 0 dB HL yields

$$0 + 13.5 = 13.5 \text{ dB SPL,}$$

and 65 dB HL would result in a tone of

$$65 + 13.5 = 78.5 \text{ dB SPL.}$$

For most purposes, the SPLs are transparent to us and we deal only in terms of the hearing level values in dB HL.

Audiometer Calibration

We need to know what sound is actually being presented to the patient. For example, when the frequency dial says "1000 Hz" and the attenuator says "40 dB HL," the audiometer should actually be producing a 1000-Hz tone at 40 dB HL. For this reason, there are **national** and **international standards** that specify the physical characteristics of the sounds that are produced by an audiometer. These standards also specify the tolerances for these characteristics, which means how far the actual sounds are allowed to deviate from the standard values. Most of these requirements are contained in the *American National Standard Specifications for Audiometers (ANSI S3.6-1996)*. **Calibration** is the process of making sure that an instrument is really doing what it is supposed to be doing. In this case, it is the process of making sure the audiometer is in compliance with the applicable standards. When an audiometer is calibrated to the ANSI S3.6-1996 standard, it is said to be calibrated to **ANSI/ISO Hearing Level**, and we say that the values are expressed in *decibels of ANSI/ISO Hearing Level,* or *dB re: ANSI-1996* (or similar terminology). The term "ANSI/ISO" reflects the corresponding international standards (ISO 389-1–5,7, 1994a–f), as well as the ANSI standard.

Air-Conduction Calibration

An audiometer is calibrated with a **sound level meter** to ensure that the correct SPLs are being presented to the patient. More sophisticated calibration measurements employ other instruments, as well. For example, a **frequency counter** is used to determine whether the test frequencies are within acceptable limits. Other instruments such as **oscilloscopes** and **distortion analyzers** are used to determine the timing characteristics of the test signal and the types and amounts of distortions that might be present. An audiometer calibration system incorporating many of these components is illustrated in Figure 4–6.

Air-conduction calibration involves measuring the sounds produced by the earphones, and is done separately for each earphone. As shown in Figure 4–6, the earphone is placed on an **NBS-9A coupler**, which is a metal cavity having a volume of 6 cc. This coupler is used because it roughly approximates the acoustical characteristics of the ear, and is often called a **6-cc coupler** or an **artificial ear**. A high-quality microphone is located at the bottom of the coupler. The microphone is connected to the audiometer

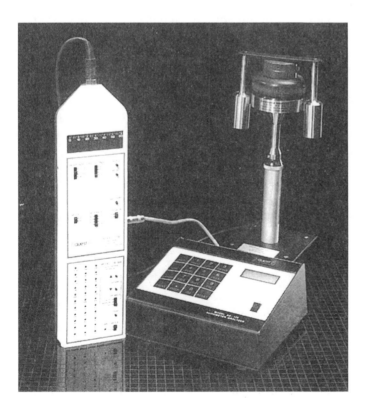

FIGURE 4–6 Air-conduction calibration using an audiometer calibration system. Notice that the audiometer's earphone is mounted on an artificial ear (6-cc coupler). Courtesy of Quest Technologies, Inc.

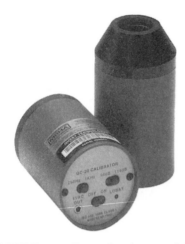

FIGURE 4–7 Example of a sound level calibrator used to confirm the accuracy of the sound level meter. The sound level meter's microphone is inserted into the depression at the end of the calibrator, which is then set to produce one or more precisely known test signals. Courtesy of Quest Technologies, Inc.

calibrator or sound level meter, which measures the actual sound pressure level being produced by the earphone. Notice that the microphone measures the sound coming from the audiometer earphone in a very specific way, as it exists within the 6-cc coupler. The accuracy of the sound level meter itself is often confirmed using a **sound level calibrator**, which is a device that produces a precisely controlled signal (Fig. 4–7).

Table 4–1 shows the reference values specified by the ANSI S3.6-1996 standard for TDH-39, TDH-49, and TDH-50 supraaural earphones. We will use the values for TDH-49 and TDH-50 earphones for the purpose of illustration because these are the values most commonly used. However, reference values will also be provided for other types of receivers, as well.

The reference values for Etymotic ER-3A and EARtone 3A insert receivers are shown in Table 4–2. The reference values for insert earphones are obtained using special types of **2-cc couplers** or **occluded ear simulators** instead of the 6-cc NBS-9A coupler described for use with standard audiometric earphones. Special measurement couplers are used because insert receivers are placed *into* the ear canal instead of being worn over the ear, and are used for many hearing aid measurements.

Extended high-frequency audiometry involves testing in the frequency range beyond 8000 Hz, and involves the use of circumaural earphones like the ones shown in Figure 4–8. Interim normal reference values for extended high-frequency audiometry are shown for two kinds of circumaural earphones in Table 4–3. Because of their shape, a *flat plate adapter* is used to couple these kinds of earphones to the artificial ear.

It is very simple to perform a *sound level calibration check* once we know the reference SPLs and the equipment has been set up as

TABLE 4–2 Reference values (RETSPLs) for Etymotic ER-3A and EARtone 3A insert receivers expressed as the sound pressure levels (in two kinds of measurement couplers used for this purpose) corresponding to 0 dB Hearing Level (HL)[a]

Frequency (Hz)	125	250	500	750	1000	1500	2000	3000	4000	6000	8000
dB SPL in HA-2 coupler	26.0	14.0	5.5	2.0	0.0	2.0	3.0	3.5	5.5	2.0	0.0
dB SPL in occluded ear simulator	28.0	17.5	9.5	6.0	5.5	9.5	11.5	13.0	15.0	16.0	15.5

[a] Adapted from ANSI S3.6-1996, which also provides RETSPLs for the HA-1 coupler and the details about how the insert receiver is attached to the measurement device in each case.

TABLE 4–3 Interim reference values (RETSPLs) at representative frequencies for Sennheiser HDA200 circumaural earphones expressed as the sound pressure levels (dB re: 20 μPa) corresponding to 0 dB Hearing Level (HL)[a]

Frequency (Hz)	500	1000	4000	6000	8000	9000	10,000	11,200	12,500	14,000	16,000
RETSPL (dB)	9.5	6.5	8.5	9.5	16.0	17.0	21.5	21.0	27.5	37.5	58.0

[a] Adapted from ANSI S3.6-1996.

shown in Figure 4–6. The following procedure is followed at each test frequency and for both earphones:

1. Select the frequency.
2. Set the attenuator to a convenient level, such as 70 dB HL. (We use a high level so that the intensity of the tone will be well above any noise levels in the room.)
3. Turn on the tone.
4. Read the meter on the audiometer calibrator (or sound level meter) to measure the actual sound pressure level that is produced by the earphone.
5. Compare the actual sound pressure level to what it is supposed to be.
6. Record any difference.

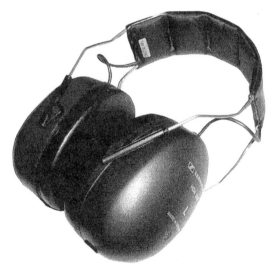

FIGURE 4–8 Circumaural earphones used for extended high-frequency audiometry. Courtesy of Sennheiser.

Using a calibration worksheet such as the one shown in Table 4–4 facilitates the procedure and also serves as a permanent record of the calibration and its results. Let us examine one of the measurements on this worksheet. The level of the 500-Hz tone should be 83.5 dB SPL, which is equal to the dial setting of 70 dB plus the 13.5 dB reference value (which is built into 0 dB HL). The calibrator meter showed that its level was actually only 81.3 dB for the right earphone. Thus, the 500-Hz tone produced by this audiometer and earphone was 2.2 dB less than it should have been. The ANSI S3.6-1996 standard requires that all sound pressure levels (and force levels for bone-conduction) should be within ±3 dB of their expected values up to 5000 Hz, and ±5 dB at and above 6000 Hz. Thus, our 2.2-dB difference is within the acceptable range of tolerances. The worksheet in Table 4–4 reveals that SPLs are within ±3 dB of the expected values for all of the other frequencies as well.

An audiometer is considered to be out of calibration if it deviates from the reference values in the standard by an amount that exceeds the allowable tolerances. There are three ways to handle this situation: (1) Its internal settings can be adjusted so that the audiometer's output is brought into calibration. (2) The instrument might have to be repaired. (3) A "correction chart" can be posted, which shows how to adjust test results before recording them.

It is also necessary for the attenuator (hearing level) dial to be calibrated for **linearity**. A linearity check is done by changing the attenuator setting throughout its entire range

TABLE 4–4   Example of a pure-tone air-conduction calibration worksheet

Right Ear

Frequency (Hz)	125	250	500	750	1000	1500	2000	3000	4000	6000	8000
Reference SPLs for 0 dB HL	47.5	26.5	13.5	8.5	7.5	7.5	11.0	9.5	10.5	13.5	13.0
Attenuator dial setting (dB HL)	70	70	70	70	70	70	70	70	70	70	70
Expected SPL at 70 dB HL dial setting	117.5	96.5	83.5	78.5	77.5	77.5	81.0	79.5	80.5	83.5	83.0
Actual SPL Measured	117.0	96.5	81.3	78.0	77.5	78.2	82.0	79.0	81.5	83.0	83.0
Calibration Error	−0.5	0	−2.2	−0.5	0	0.7	1.0	−0.5	1.0	−0.5	0

Left Ear

Frequency (Hz)	125	250	500	750	1000	1500	2000	3000	4000	6000	8000
Reference SPLs for 0 dB HL	47.5	26.5	13.5	8.5	7.5	7.5	11.0	9.5	10.5	13.5	13.0
Attenuator dial setting (dB HL)	70	70	70	70	70	70	70	70	70	70	70
Expected SPL at 70 dB HL dial setting	117.5	96.5	83.5	78.5	77.5	77.5	81.0	79.5	80.5	83.5	83.0
Actual SPL Measured	116.0	97.0	84.0	78.5	78.0	79.0	83.0	78.8	81.0	84.0	83.7
Calibration Error	−1.5	0.5	0.5	0	0.5	1.5	2.0	−0.7	0.5	0.5	0.7

HL, hearing level; SPL, sound pressure level.

to make sure that every 5-dB dial change actually results in a 5-dB change in SPL at the earphone. The standard requires the linearity of an audiometer's attenuator to be accurate within ±1 dB per 5-dB step.[1]

A frequency calibration is required to ensure each test frequency is within a certain percentage of the nominal value. The tolerance limits for frequency accuracy is between ±1% and ±3%, depending on the audiometer's type according to ANSI S36.-1996. Specifically, the frequency must be accurate within ±1% for type 1 and extended high-frequency audiometers, ±2% for type 2 audiometers, and ±3% for the type 3, 4, and 5 instruments. For example, if the dial is set to 1000 Hz, then the frequency must actually be between 990 and 1010 Hz for a type 1 audiometer, 980 and 1020 Hz for a type 2, and 970 and 1030Hz for types 3, 4, and 5. Sweep-frequency audiometers (in which the frequency increases continuously from low to high over a certain period of time) must be accurate within ±5% of the frequency indicated on the audiogram, so that the actual frequency must be between 950 and 1050 Hz when the audiogram reads 1000 Hz.

Other calibrations are also required, although these are usually done by a service technician because they require either a complete audiometric calibration system or a variety of special instruments. Some of these measurements involve determining the amount of harmonic distortion, rise and fall times, switching parameters, etc.

In addition to periodic electroacoustic calibrations such as the ones just described, it is desirable for **biological calibrations** to be done as frequently as possible. This is done by checking the thresholds of someone

---

[1] Although 5 dB is the typical step size, many audiometers provide for testing at smaller increments as well. Thus, to be very specific, the standard dictates that the tolerance for hearing level increments up to 5 dB must be accurate to within 1 dB or three-tenths of the interval, whichever is smaller.

whose hearing levels are already known. Biological calibrations should also include a general listening check, which is done to make sure that the instrument is working well overall, and to make sure that there is no static, extraneous noises, broken wires, or other apparent problems. For example, a broken earphone wire or contact is often discovered by listening to the test tone while wiggling the wires between the hands. It is far better to find out that the left earphone is intermittently dead during a five-minute listening check in the morning than to figure out you have a problem in the middle of a clinical evaluation.

Bone-Conduction Calibration

The bone-conduction system can be calibrated using an **artificial mastoid** or **mechanical coupler**, as shown in Figure 4–9. This type of measurement is usually done by a service technician because most clinical facilities do not own their own artificial mastoids. The basic concept is analogous to what is done with the earphone and artificial ear, but involves reference values in terms of the force needed to achieve 0 dB HL for bone conduction. Table 4–5 shows the

reference values used for bone-conduction calibration according to the ANSI S3.6-1996 standard. These values are called **reference equivalent threshold force levels (RETFLs)** because they show the force (in dB re: 1 μN) needed to achieve 0 dB HL with bone-conduction stimulation.

A useful method for biological bone-conduction calibration is based on the premise that air-conduction and bone-conduction thresholds are the same in patients who have sensorineural hearing losses (Chapter 5). The technique requires that the air-conduction system be properly calibrated, and requires access to patients who are known to have reliable sensorineural hearing losses. The biological calibration procedure is done at each frequency where bone-conduction testing is done (usually up to 4000 Hz), as follows: (1) Obtain and record the air-conduction threshold. (2) Obtain the bone-conduction threshold and record the number of decibels indicated on the attenuator dial. (3) Find the difference between the air-conduction hearing level and the bone-conduction dial reading. This is the amount by which the bone-conduction dial reading must be corrected to indicate the correct bone-conduction threshold. For example, if the air-

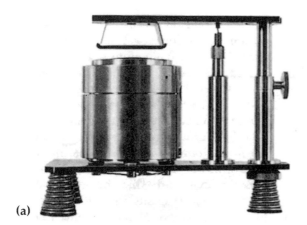
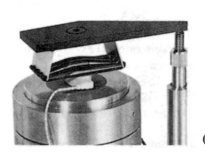

(a)

(b)

FIGURE 4–9   (a) An artificial mastoid used for the calibration of bone-conduction signals. (b) Close-up view of a bone-conduction vibrator being tested on the artificial mastoid. The output of the artificial mastoid is connected to a sound level meter. In effect, the artificial mastoid transduces the vibrations of the bone-conduction vibrator into an electrical signal that can be read on the sound level meter. Photographs courtesy of Brüel & Kjaer.

TABLE 4–5   Reference values for audiometric bone-conduction vibrators, expressed as reference equivalent threshold force levels (RETFLs) in dB re: 1 μN, when measured on an artificial mastoid (mechanical coupler)[a]

Frequency (Hz)	250	500	750	1000	1500	2000	3000	4000
At mastoid	67.0	58.0	48.5	42.5	36.5	31.0	30.0	35.5
At forehead	79.0	72.0	61.5	51.0	47.5	42.5	42.0	43.5

[a]Adapted from ANSI S3.6-1996.

conduction threshold is 40 dB and the dial reading of the bone-conduction threshold is 50 dB, then the difference is −10 dB. In other words, 10 dB needs to be subtracted from the bone-conduction dial reading in order for it to be correct (for this frequency and subject). (4) Correction values are obtained for several patients with sensorineural losses (using steps 1 to 3) to arrive at average corrections for each frequency, which are then posted on a correction chart. The more subjects used to establish the averages, the more confidence you can have in the correction factors.

The following example will show why the biological bone-conduction calibration method cannot validly be done with normal subjects. Suppose a subject responds at −10 dB HL for air-conduction and bone-conduction, which are the softest levels produced by the audiometer. It *seems* like both thresholds are −10 dB HL, but the reality might be that he could have heard one or both signals at an even lower level. This is a big problem if we are interested in knowing the difference between the two dial readings at threshold, which is the basis of the biological bone-conduction calibration.

Calibrating the Speech Signal

Many audiological procedures use various kinds of speech stimuli. These are either recordings that are directed into the audiometer, or may involve "live voice," which means the audiologist herself speaks into a microphone. Both types of signals involve using the audiometer's **VU meter**, which is similar to the VU meter found on almost

every stereo system and tape recorder. In effect, the VU meter tells whether the level of the incoming signal is appropriate. For the system to be calibrated, the input signal must achieve 0 dB VU. If the VU meter reads −3 dB, then the signal will be 3 dB less than the attenuator dial reading, and +2 dB means the signal will be 2 dB, greater than what the dial says. If the meter is "pinned" to the end on the plus side, then you have no idea of how high the signal is, and you can also assume it is being distorted. In the live-voice situation, the audiologist talks into the microphone while monitoring her speech on the VU meter, and adjusts an input level dial so that her average speech peaks fall at 0 dB on the VU meter. Hence, presenting speech in this way is called **monitored live-voice (MLV)** testing. Recorded speech tests usually have a 1000-Hz **calibration tone** on the recording. The level of the calibration tone corresponds to the average level of the speech peaks. The input level dial on the audiometer is adjusted so that this calibration tone is at 0 dB VU.

The reference level (RETSPL) for speech signals is 12.5 dB higher than the reference level (RETSPL) for a 1000-Hz pure tone. This relationship between the reference levels of the 1000-Hz tone and the speech signal is used because it results in agreement between the pure-tone thresholds and speech reception thresholds (Chapters 5, 8, and 14) in normal hearing listeners (Jerger, Carhart, Tillman, & Peterson, 1959). Table 4–6 shows these references levels for various kinds of audiometric transducers and testing conditions. For example, the 1000-Hz RETSPL is 7.5 dB SPL for TDH-49 and -50 earphones, so that

TABLE 4–6   Reference values for speech stimuli corresponding to 0 dB hearing level (HL) for various audiometric transducers[a]

Transducer	Reference Level in dB[b]
TDH-49 and -50 supraaural earphones	20.0
TDH-39 supraaural earphones	19.5
Insert receivers	
In HA1 or 2 coupler	12.5
In occluded ear simulator	18.0
Sennheiser HDA200 circumaural earphones	19.0
Bone vibrators	
At mastoid	55.0
At forehead	63.5
Soundfield	
Binaural at 0°	14.5
Monaural at 0°	16.5
Monaural at 45°	12.5
Monaural at 90°	11.0

[a] Adapted from ANSI S3.6-1996.

[b] RESPLs for earphones and loudspeakers; RETFLs for bone vibrators.

the reference level for speech is 20 dB SPL. For practical purposes, this reference actually refers to the level of the calibration tone on the speech test recording. It means that when the 1000-Hz calibration tone is adjusted to zero on the VU meter it will then have a magnitude of 20 dB SPL at the earphone when the attenuator dial is set to 0 dB HL.

The calibration procedure uses the recorded calibration tone the same way we calibrated the pure-tone system, except that the selectors are set to "speech" and the reference level is now 20 dB SPL (for a TDH-49 earphone): The attenuator is set to 70 dB HL and we turn on the speech recording to play the calibration tone. We expect the calibration tone to be measured as 70 + 20 = 90 dB SPL in the artificial ear.

Soundfield Calibration

Soundfield testing means that the test sounds are delivered into the test room by loud-speakers instead of through earphones or a bone-conduction vibrator. The signal from the loudspeaker is transmitted through the air and picked up by the microphone of the sound level meter, which is placed where the patient's head would normally be located.

Recall from Chapters 2 and 3 that hearing in a soundfield is affected by the head-related transfer function as well as by whether the individual is listening monaurally or binaurally. For these reasons, the ANSI S3.6-1996 standard provides different reference levels (RETSPLs) for soundfield testing for monaural and binaural listening when the loudspeaker is located directly in front of the patient (0° azimuth), as well as for monaural listening with loudspeakers at azimuths of 45° and 90° (i.e., to the side). These values are shown for commonly tested frequencies[2] in Figure 4–10 and for speech in Table 4–6. As with earphone calibration, a relatively high attenuator dial setting (e.g., 70 dB HL) is used so that the sound level measurements can be made well above any room noise.

The Test Environment and Ambient Noise

We know from experience that you must talk louder to be heard in a noisy room than in a quiet room. This occurs because of **masking**, whereby one sound interferes with the ability to hear other sounds. Consequently, we must be sure audiological testing is done in a room quiet enough so that the softest test sounds used will not be masked by any noise in the room. In practical terms, this means that the ambient noise level in the test room must be low enough to allow us to measure thresholds down to 0 dB HL at each audiometric test frequency by both air-conduction and bone-conduction, and in soundfield.

---

[2] Because of acoustical considerations, soundfield testing uses frequency-modulated tones or narrow-band noises centered around these audiometric frequencies instead of pure tones.

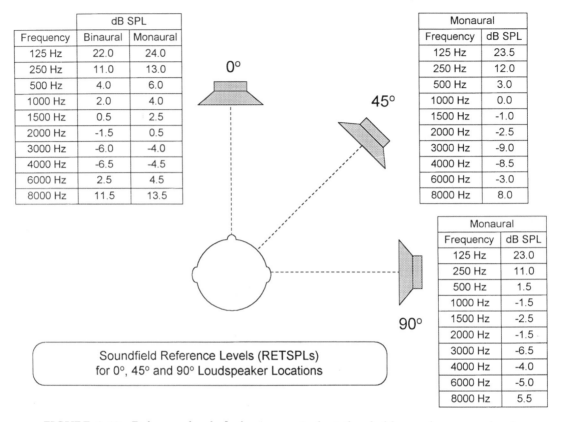

dB SPL		
Frequency	Binaural	Monaural
125 Hz	22.0	24.0
250 Hz	11.0	13.0
500 Hz	4.0	6.0
1000 Hz	2.0	4.0
1500 Hz	0.5	2.5
2000 Hz	-1.5	0.5
3000 Hz	-6.0	-4.0
4000 Hz	-6.5	-4.5
6000 Hz	2.5	4.5
8000 Hz	11.5	13.5

Monaural	
Frequency	dB SPL
125 Hz	23.5
250 Hz	12.0
500 Hz	3.0
1000 Hz	0.0
1500 Hz	-1.0
2000 Hz	-2.5
3000 Hz	-9.0
4000 Hz	-8.5
6000 Hz	-3.0
8000 Hz	8.0

Monaural	
Frequency	dB SPL
125 Hz	23.0
250 Hz	11.0
500 Hz	1.5
1000 Hz	-1.5
1500 Hz	-2.5
2000 Hz	-1.5
3000 Hz	-6.5
4000 Hz	-4.0
6000 Hz	-5.0
8000 Hz	5.5

Soundfield Reference Levels (RETSPLs)
for 0°, 45° and 90° Loudspeaker Locations

FIGURE 4–10 Reference levels [reference equivalent threshold sound pressure levels (RETSPLs)] for sound field testing at commonly tested audiometric frequencies for monaural listening at three loudspeaker locations 0°, 45° and 90° azimuth and for binaural listening with a loudspeaker at 0° azimuth (based on ANSI S3.6-1996).

Audiological Testing Rooms

In order to meet the need for an appropriately quiet environment, audiological testing is carried out in specially constructed, sound isolated rooms. These testing suites can be purchased from several manufacturers or can be locally constructed. Although we will describe only the commercial booths, the same goals must be addressed when testing rooms are constructed locally.

Commercial audiometric booths come as either single rooms (Fig. 4–11) or as two-room suites (Fig. 4–12). When single-room booths are used, the patient stays in the booth and the tester and equipment are located on the outside. Two-room suites include a patient room and a control room. The noise levels permitted in audiometric booths, which are outlined in the next section, actually apply to the patient room. However, the control room should be as quiet as possible, especially if any live-voice speech testing is done. Room size is a critical issue because money and space are always limited. The patient room should be as large as possible, especially for soundfield testing and/or pediatric evaluations. The tester's room must be large enough to comfortably accommodate the equipment, the tester, and an observer. In addition, space planning must account for at least the *outside* dimensions of the test suite, room for the doors to swing open, and wheelchair access. Stretcher access should also be taken into account, depending on the setting, and the space needed for wheelchairs and/or stretchers must consider whether turns must be made to enter and exit.

The walls, ceilings, floors, and doors are usually constructed of 4-inch-thick panels composed of metal sheets filled with sound-attenuating material. In order to minimize reverberation within the room the metal surfaces facing into the sound-treated chamber are covered with holes, giving the appearance of pegboard (except for the floor, which is typically carpeted). Single-walled booths are one panel thick. Double-walled booths are made of two layers of panels, usually with dead air space between them, and provide more sound isolation than single-walled rooms. The type of room construction is dictated by the amount of sound attenuation that is needed in light of the noise levels at the location in question.

Several other measures are taken to ensure that the acoustical isolation provided by the chamber is not compromised: the doors should close with tight seals; the windows between the patient and tester rooms are made of multiple panes of glass with dead air spaces between them; prewired jack panels are used so that holes do not have to be made to pass wires between the rooms. The test booth often "floats" on vibration isolators to minimize the transmission of vibrations through the structures of the building into the test booth. Air enters and leaves the booths via a sound-muffled ventilation system. It might be noted that vibration isolation and muffled ventilation systems are often problem areas with noncommercial booths that are constructed locally. It is preferable to use incandescent lights because they do not produce any noise; however, fluorescent lighting can be used if care is taken

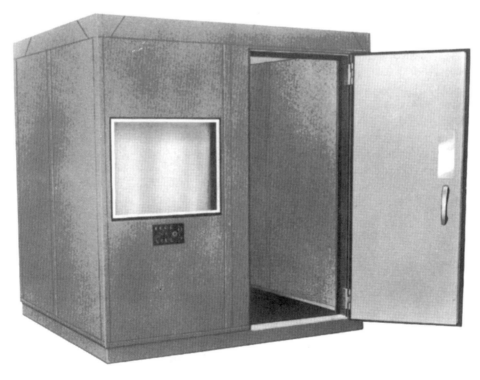

FIGURE 4–11 Example of a single-room audiological testing chamber. Photograph courtesy of Industrial Acoustics Corporation, Inc.

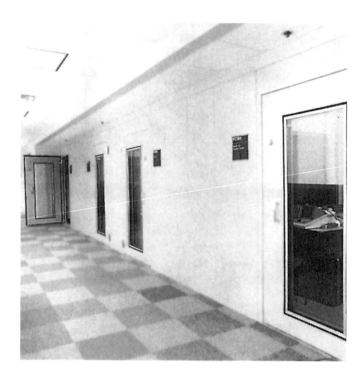

FIGURE 4–12 Two double-room audiological testing suites are shown. Instrumentation can be seen through the control room window of the closer suite. Photograph courtesy of Industrial Acoustics Company, Inc.

to mount their noisy ballasts or starters outside the booth.

Maximum Permissible Ambient Noise Levels

How quiet must it be in an audiological testing room? The ambient noise in the audiometric booth is measured with a sound level meter. We could measure this noise in overall SPL or in dB-A (see Chapter 1), but values such as these do not tell us how the room noise will affect *each* of the audiometric frequencies. It is more useful to determine how much noise exists in the vicinity of each audiometric testing frequency. (Recall from Chapter 3 that a given tone is masked most by noise that is close to it in frequency, and that lower frequency sounds can often mask higher frequency sounds.) To do this we must first specify a range of frequencies (a bandwidth) to be considered around each frequency. This is done in terms of **octave bands** and **third-octave bands**.[3] An octave

band is a range of frequencies that is an octave wide and a third-octave band is a frequency range that is one-third of an octave wide. These bandwidths are shown in Table 4–7. For example, the 500-Hz octave band includes the range of frequencies between 354 and 707 Hz. Here, we say 500 Hz is the center frequency, and that 354 and 707 Hz are the lower and upper cutoff frequencies, respectively. The range of frequencies between the lower and upper cutoffs is called the **bandwidth**. Similarly, the 500-Hz third-octave band has a bandwidth of 116 Hz between cutoff frequencies of 445 and 561 Hz. These bandwidths are used when specifying the maximum allowable room noise levels for each audiometric frequency.

To determine whether a given room is sufficiently quiet for audiological testing, the ambient noise levels in the room are measured with a sound level meter that has a set of octave band or third-octave band filters. The sound pressure level within an octave band is called an **octave band level (OBL)**, and the sound pressure level within a third-octave band is called a **third-octave band level (third-OBL)**. These ambient room

---

[3] The characteristics of bandwidths are specified in the ANSI S1.11-1986 (R1998) standard.

TABLE 4–7 Octave bands and third-octave bands for the audiometric test frequencies[a]

Center Frequency	Octave Bands			Third-Octave Bands		
	Lower	Upper	Bandwidth	Lower	Upper	Bandwidth
125	88	176	88	111	140	29
250	177	354	177	223	281	58
500	354	707	354	445	561	116
1000	707	1414	707	891	1122	232
1500	1061	2121	1061	1336	1684	347
2000	1414	2828	1414	1782	2245	463
3000	2121	4243	2121	2673	3367	695
4000	2828	5657	2828	3564	4490	926
6000	4243	8485	4243	5345	6735	1389
8000	5657	11,314	5657	7127	8980	1853

[a] All numbers are in Hz (calculations subject to rounding errors).

noise levels are then compared to the **maximum permissible ambient** noise levels specified by the ANSI S3.1-1991 standard. The maximum allowable room noise levels that apply when testing the frequencies between 250 and 8000 Hz are shown in Tables 4–8 and 4–9. Table 4–8 shows the octave band levels of the noise at center frequencies of 125 to 8000 Hz, and Table 4–9 shows the respective third-octave band levels. These two tables are used in the same way; the choice between them depends only on whether the room noise was measured using a sound level meter with octave versus third-octave filters. We will assume the use of a sound level meter with octave filters and refer only to Table 4–8; but the same principles apply to third-octave band levels and Table 4–9.

The octave band levels in Table 4–8 are the maximum ambient room noise levels that will

still allow a normal hearing patient to hear a tone presented as low as 0 dB HL. Two sets of maximum octave band levels are given for each frequency, one with "ears covered" and one with "ears uncovered." The higher maximum room noise levels for "ears covered" apply only when the patient is wearing earphones. The lower (stricter) maximum room noise levels apply whenever the test ear is not covered with an earphone, which occurs during bone-conduction and soundfield testing. Higher noise levels are allowed in the room when earphones are being worn because the earphones and their cushions act as earmuffs that reduce the amount of room noise reaching the eardrum. For example, the maximum room noise at 1000 Hz has an OBL of 14 dB with the ears uncovered and 26.5 dB with the ears covered. The allowable room noise is 12.5 dB higher with the ears covered because the earphone and cushion are expected to reduce

TABLE 4–8 Maximum *octave* band levels (OBLs) (in dB) allowed when testing in the 250- to 8000-Hz range[a,b] with ears covered and with ears uncovered (based on ANSI S3.1-1991); the ears uncovered values must be used if bone-conduction or soundfield tests are done

Center Frequency (Hz)	125	250	500	750	1000	1500	2000	3000	4000	6000	8000
Ears uncovered	32.5	18.5	14.5	12.5	14.0	10.5	8.5	8.5	9.0	14.0	20.5
Ears covered	36.5	22.5	19.5	21.5	26.5	26.5	28.0	33.5	34.5	38.0	43.5

[a] If 125 Hz is also tested, then the maximum allowable OBL at 125 Hz is lowered to 28 dB for ears uncovered and 34 dB for ears covered.

[b] If the *lowest* test frequency is 500 Hz, then the maximum allowable OBLs are raised to 42.5 dB at 125 Hz and 28.5 dB at 250 Hz for ears uncovered, and 47.5 dB at 125 Hz and 33.5 dB at 250 Hz for ears covered.

TABLE 4–9   Maximum *third-octave band* levels (in dB) allowed when testing in the 250- to 8000-Hz range[a,b] with ears covered and with ears uncovered (based on ANSI S3.1-1991); the ears uncovered values must be used if bone-conduction or soundfield tests are done

Center Frequency (Hz)	125	250	500	750	1000	1500	2000	3000	4000	6000	8000
Ears uncovered	27.5	13.5	9.5	7.5	9.0	5.5	3.5	3.5	4.0	9.0	15.5
Ears covered	31.5	17.5	14.5	16.5	21.5	21.5	23.0	28.5	29.5	33.0	38.5

[a] If 125 Hz is also tested, then the maximum allowable third-OBL at 125 Hz is lowered to 23 dB for ears uncovered, or 29 dB for ears covered.

[b] If the *lowest* test frequency is 500 Hz, then the maximum allowable third-OBLs are raised to 37.5 dB at 125 Hz and 23.5 dB at 250 Hz for ears uncovered, or 42.5 dB at 125 Hz and 28.5 dB at 250 Hz for ears covered.

(attenuate) the noise entering the ear by 12.5 dB. The noise level actually getting into the ear is 14 dB in either case.

The "ears uncovered" ambient noise standards should be met by all rooms where bone-conduction and/or soundfield testing are done. The less stringent "ears covered" standards are appropriate only when testing is limited to air-conduction measurements, such as screening programs and certain industrial testing settings. Perusal of the footnotes in Tables 4–8 and 4–9 reveals that higher noise levels become acceptable at low frequencies when the range of frequencies being tested changes from (a) 125 to 8000 Hz to (b) 250 to 8000 Hz to (c) 500 to 8000 Hz. Using the maximum noise levels for the 250- to 8000-Hz range is no problem (and is usually desirable) because (1) most clinical testing is limited to this 250- to 8000-Hz range, and (2) patients who need to be tested at 125 Hz usually have hearing losses that are so severe that ambient noise is not an issue for them anyway. However, even though limiting the testable range to ≥500 Hz is appropriate for screening and some industrial hearing conservation programs, it is not desirable for clinical purposes.

The maximum permissible ambient noise levels in Tables 4–8 and 4–9 must be met in order to obtain thresholds as low as 0 dB HL. The presence of higher noise levels will limit the kind of testing that can be done in the room. For example, if the actual noise in the test room exceeds the appropriate maximum allowable levels by 15 dB, then the lowest

measurable threshold in that room will be 15 dB HL. If the noise levels are 30 dB higher than the permissible maximum, then the lowest measurable threshold will be 30 dB HL. In addition, meeting the "ears covered" noise requirements but not meeting the "ears uncovered" standards can distort the comparison between air-conduction and bone-conduction thresholds, which is a fundamental diagnostic consideration in clinical audiology (see Chapter 5). Hence, ambient room noise is not just a technicality but is a primary limiting factor in clinical testing.

Unfortunately, compliance with room noise standards appears to be astonishingly poor. Frank and Williams (1993) studied the noise levels of 136 test rooms in a variety of different types of audiological facilities. Only 14% of the rooms met the standards for "ears uncovered" for either 125- to 8000-Hz or 250- to 8000-Hz ranges, and only 37% of the rooms met the standards for testing at 500 to 8000 Hz. Compliance with room noise requirements for "ears covered" was better but still quite disappointing, at 50% for testing either 125 to 8000 Hz and 250 to 8000 Hz, and 82% for testing 500 to 8000 Hz.

It is often necessary to do hearing screening tests in "quiet" rooms in schools or other buildings rather than in sound-isolated environments of the type we have been assuming thus far. Here the goal is to separate those who are *probably* normal from those who should be referred for complete evaluations. The general screening approach is to determine whether the patient can hear several pure tones at a fixed level, such as 25 dB HL, on a pass-fail basis. The screening level that is chosen must not only be adequate to separate probably normal from possibly impaired hearing, but it must also be appropriate for the room in which the testing is being done. For example, if the screening level is to be 25 dB HL, then the ambient room noise can be *no more than 25 dB* above those in Tables 4–8 and 4–9 (which apply to testing at 0 dB HL). In other words, the ambient noise levels in the room are as much of a limiting factor for screening tests as they are for clinical testing. These points apply equally to hearing screenings that are being done in therapy rooms as part of speech-language pathology or other evaluations.

REFERENCES

American National Standards Institute (ANSI). 1998. *American National Standard Specification for Octave-Band and Fractional-Band Analog and Digital Filters.* ANSI S1.11-1986 (R1998). New York: ANSI.

American National Standards Institute (ANSI). 1996. *American National Standard Specifications for Audiometers.* ANSI S3.6-1996. New York: ANSI.

American National Standards Institute (ANSI). 1991. *Maximum Permissible Ambient Noise Levels for Audiometric Test Rooms.* ANSI S3.1-1991. New York: ANSI.

Frank T, Williams DL. 1993. Ambient noise levels in audiometric rooms for clinical audiometry. *Ear Hear* 14, 414–422.

Gelfand, SA. 1981. *Hearing: An Introduction to Psychological and Physiological Acoustics.* New York: Marcel Dekker.

International Organization for Standardization (ISO). 1994a. *Acoustics—Reference Zero for Calibration of Audiometric Equipment—Part 1: Reference Equivalent Threshold Sound Pressure Levels for Pure Tone and Supraaural Earphones.* ISO 389-1. Geneva: ISO.

International Organization for Standardization (ISO). 1994b. *Acoustics—Reference Zero for Calibration of Audiometric Equipment—Part 2: Reference Equivalent Threshold Sound Pressure Levels for Pure Tone and Insert Earphones.* ISO 389-2. Geneva: ISO.

International Organization for Standardization (ISO). 1994c. *Acoustics—Reference Zero for Calibration of Audiometric Equipment—Part 3: Reference Equivalent Threshold Sound Pressure Levels for Pure Tone and Bone Vibrators.* ISO 389-3. Geneva: ISO.

International Organization for Standardization (ISO). 1994d. *Acoustics—Reference Zero for Calibration of Audiometric Equipment—Part 4: Reference Levels for Narrow-Band Masking Noise.* ISO 389-4. Geneva: ISO.

International Organization for Standardization (ISO). 1994e. *Acoustics—Reference Zero for Calibration of Audiometric Equipment—Part 5: Reference Equivalent Threshold Sound Pressure Levels for Pure Tones in the Frequency Range 8 kHz to 16 kHz.* ISO 389-5. Geneva: ISO.

International Organization for Standardization (ISO). 1994f. *Acoustics—Reference Zero for Calibration of Audiometric Equipment—Part 7: Reference Threshold of Hearing Under Free-Field and Diffuse-Field Listening Conditions.* ISO 389-7. Geneva: ISO.

Jerger J, Carhart R, Tillman TW, Peterson JL. 1959. Some relations between normal hearing for pure tones and for speech. *J Speech Hear Res* 2, 126–140.

5

Pure-Tone Audiometry

Hearing Threshold

We often conclude that someone has a hearing loss because we have to talk at a louder than normal level for that person to hear us. Even though we cannot directly experience the degree of that person's hearing loss, we can appreciate its magnitude in terms of how loud we must speak to be heard. This is certainly *not* the only manifestation of a hearing impairment, but it does highlight an important point: We can quantify the degree of a patient's hearing loss in terms of the magnitude of the stimulus needed for him to respond to it. The smallest intensity of a sound that a person needs to detect its presence is called his **threshold** for that sound. For clinical purposes, we define the threshold as the lowest intensity at which the patient responds to the sound at least 50% of the time.

The sounds used to test a person's hearing must be clearly specified so that his thresholds are both accurate and repeatable. The test sounds used to determine the degree of hearing loss are usually pure tones of different frequencies. Recall from Chapter 3 that the normal threshold value at each frequency is said to be 0 dB **Hearing Level (HL)**. Also recall the actual physical magnitude (in decibels of sound pressure level, dB SPL) needed to produce 0 dB HL is specified in the American National Standard Specifications for Audiometers (ANSI S3.6-1996), which corresponds to several international (ISO) standards (see Chapter 4). Hearing thresholds are thus given in **decibels of hearing level** or **dB HL**, which is more completely expressed as "dB HL re: ANSI-1996" or "dB HL re:

ANSI/ISO"; or "dB HL re: ANSI-1969" (because the original version was published in 1969).

In the most general terms, a person has "normal hearing" if his thresholds are close to the norm and a "hearing loss" if the tones must be presented at higher intensities for them to be heard. In other words, the amount of the hearing loss is expressed in terms of how many decibels above 0 dB HL are needed to reach the person's threshold. For example, when we say a patient has a hearing loss of 55 dB HL, we mean his ear problem has caused his threshold to be elevated to the extent that it is 55 dB higher than 0 dB HL.

Test signals can be presented by **air-conduction**, **bone-conduction**, or in **soundfield**. Thresholds are obtained by both air- and bone-conduction because a comparison between the two sets of results enables us to distinguish between different kinds of hearing losses, as will be explained later. Soundfield testing involves presenting signals from loudspeakers, and is discussed later in this chapter.

Air-Conduction Testing

Air-conduction testing usually involves presenting the test signals from standard audiometric (supraaural) earphones, as shown in Figure 5–1. Insert earphones can also be used for air-conduction testing. Recall from Chapter 4 that insert earphones go into the ear canals instead of being worn over the ears. They are useful when facing several problem situations, but the convenience of standard earphones makes them the method of choice under routine conditions.

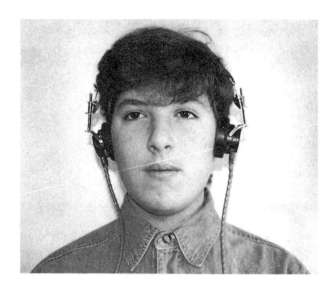

FIGURE 5–1   Arrangement of the earphones for air-conduction testing.

Earrings and most eyeglasses (except contact lenses) must be removed for both comfort and proper fitting of the earphones. It is also necessary to remove any other objects (e.g., headbands or other hair adornments) that could interfere with the placement of the headset (or the bone vibrator that will be used later). Hearing aids should be removed, turned off, and put away during the test. Chewing gum and candy must be disposed of. The audiologist should check to see whether putting pressure on the external ear seems to cause the ear canal to close. This is important because the pressure exerted by the earphones might similarly cause collapse of the ear canals, and give the false impression of a conductive hearing loss. We will return to the issue of ear canal collapse later in this chapter. Finally, the clinician gently places the headset on the patient, being careful that the earphone receivers are located over the entrances to the ear canals. It is not desirable to allow the patient to apply the headset because the fit may not be optimal. If the patient is allowed to do this, then the clinician must check the fit and make any necessary adjustments.

Bone-Conduction Testing

Bone-conduction is tested by applying a vibratory stimulus to the skull, which is trans-

mitted to the cochlea and heard as sound. To do this, a **bone-conduction vibrator** is placed on the mastoid process or forehead, and is held in place by a spring headband. Even though mastoid versus forehead placement of the bone vibrator is an arguable issue (see below), mastoid placement is recommended here and is the more commonly used method. Figure 5–2 illustrates the proper placement of

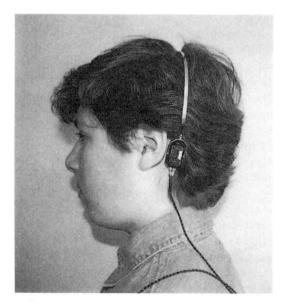

FIGURE 5–2 Arrangement of the bone-conduction vibrator at the mastoid process for bone-conduction testing.

a bone-conduction vibrator of the mastoid process.

The bone-conduction vibrator itself is encased in a small plastic shell as shown in Figure 4–3c of Chapter 4. The part that comes in contact with the skin is a disk with a flat surface having an area of 1.75 cm^2. Most American audiometers use the Radioear B-71 bone-conduction vibrator, which is the one in the figure. Radioear's model B-72 is also available but is less commonly used. The B-71 and B-72 vibrators have replaced the older B-70 model, which does not have a disk-shaped contact area.

Before putting the bone vibrator on the patient, one must identify any structural aberrations or other problems that would affect the proper placement. Common problems are hair under the vibrator, oily skin, and oddly shaped or narrow mastoids that make it hard to place the vibrator without slipping. Pathologies and surgically modified structures are less common but equally important. Earrings, glasses, hearing aids, etc., as well as gum and candy, should already have been removed prior to air-conduction testing. The vibrator is gently placed on the mastoid process on one side, and the other end of the spring band is placed gently on the opposite side of the head (usually just anterior to the opposite ear). The vibrator should be placed so that the surface of its disk sits flatly on the skin of the mastoid process without touching the pinna. The vibrator should be held to the head with a force corresponding to at least 400 grams in order to achieve adequate reliability (Dirks, 1964) and 5.4 newtons to meet ANSI S3.6-1996 standards.

Placement variations on the mastoid can result in threshold differences. For this reason, many audiologists have the patient listen to a readily audible 500-Hz bone-conduction tone while they shift the vibrator around on the mastoid. The vibrator is then kept in the location where the tone sounds loudest. In order to minimize the chances that the vibrator will shift once it has been placed, it is wise to instruct the patient to keep her head still and not to talk during bone-conduction testing. The patient should also be instructed to tell you if the vibrator moves in any way. It is also a good idea to provide a strain relief so that an unintentional tug on the wire will not dislodge the vibrator. This can be done with a small clip or by looping the wire under the patient's collar.

Occlusion Effect

We have been assuming that the ears are not being covered by the earphones while bone-conduction is being tested. This is the typical method, and the results obtained this way are called **unoccluded** bone-conduction thresholds. In contrast, **occluded** bone-conduction thresholds are obtained when one or both ears are covered with the earphones. A stronger signal reaches the cochlea when bone-conduction signals are presented with the ears occluded compared to unoccluded. This boost is called the **occlusion effect**. As a result, occluded bone-conduction thresholds are lower (better) than unoccluded ones, and a given bone-conduction signal will sound louder with the ears covered compared to when the ears are open. An occlusion effect occurs when the cartilaginous section of the ear canal is occluded, but not when the bony portion is blocked. It is also absent when there is a disorder of the conductive system. The occlusion effect can be used clinically to help determine whether a conductive impairment is present in the form of the Bing test (described later in this chapter), as well as to help determine how much noise is needed for masking during bone-conduction testing (Chapter 9). The occlusion effect is discussed further in Chapters 2 and 9.

The magnitude of the occlusion effect is found by simply comparing the bone-conduction thresholds obtained when the ears are occluded and unoccluded. Figure 5–3 shows the mean occlusion effects obtained at various frequencies by various studies. The figure shows that the occlusion effect occurs for frequencies up to about 1000 Hz, and that it is largest at lower frequencies. The size of the occlusion effect also varies considerably among individuals. This variability is reflected by the differences among the means shown in the figure.

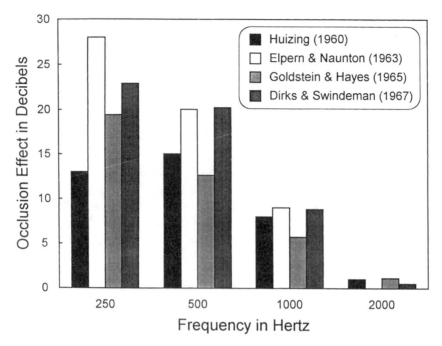

FIGURE 5–3   Mean occlusion effects at different frequencies from various studies.

Mastoid versus Forehead Bone-Conduction

There is a long-standing controversy about whether the best vibrator placement is at the forehead or at the mastoid, and it is not definitively resolved. Forehead placement has several advantages in terms of higher test-retest reliability and lower intersubject variability; however, the sizes of these benefits are probably too small to be of serious clinical significance (Studebaker, 1962; Dirks, 1964).

A practical forehead advantage has to do with the fact that mastoid vibrators can shift rather easily, and on rare occasions even pop off. In contrast, forehead placement is very stable, provided the vibrator is held in place with a holder that encircles the head.

Another advantage of forehead placement has to do with the middle ear component of bone-conduction provided by the inertial lag of the ossicular chain (Chapter 2). Recall that this component involves a relative movement of the ossicles in the right-left direction with respect to the head. At low frequencies, the side-to-side motion of the middle ear bones is

activated by the right-left vibrations produced by a mastoid bone vibrator, but not by the front-back vibration caused by a forehead bone vibrator. Thus, the middle ear component makes a bigger contribution to the normal bone-conduction threshold (which we call 0 dB HL) with mastoid placement than with forehead placement. By interfering with the ossicular lag mechanism, some conductive disorders can elevate bone conduction thresholds to the extent that they depend on the middle ear component. Hence, conductive pathologies have a bigger effect on bone-conduction thresholds with mastoid placement than at the forehead (Link & Zwislocki, 1951; Studebaker, 1962; Dirks & Malmquist, 1969). This is undesirable because we like to think of bone-conduction thresholds as testing the cochlea directly.

In spite of various forehead placement advantages, mastoid placement enjoys a practical advantage that is of overwhelming clinical relevance. The strength of the vibration that is needed to reach threshold is smaller when the vibrator is on the mastoid than on the forehead. This was shown in Table 4–5 of

Chapter 4, where the reference force levels were smaller for the mastoid than for the forehead. Because it takes less vibratory energy to reach threshold at the mastoid, the maximum hearing level produced by a bone vibrator will also be greater at the mastoid than on the forehead. For example, the highest testable bone-conduction threshold at some frequency might be 70 dB HL at the mastoid but only 55 dB HL at the forehead. Hence, a wider range of bone-conduction thresholds can be tested with mastoid placement. For this reason, we often say bone-conduction has a wider **dynamic range** at the mastoid than on the forehead.

A second advantage of mastoid placement has to do with the concept that there is no interaural attenuation (IA) for bone-conduction, so that the signal reaches both cochleae equally. This is really a half-truth. There is no IA for bone-conduction at the *forehead*, but the fact is that IA for *mastoid* bone-conduction is often as much as 15 dB at 2000 Hz and 4000 Hz (see Chapter 9). For example, suppose a patient has 4000-Hz air-conduction thresholds that are 50 dB HL in the right ear and 65 dB HL for the left. The *forehead* bone-conduction threshold will be 50 dB HL, reflecting the better sensitivity of the right cochlea, but there is still the possibility of a 15-dB air-bone-gap in the left ear. We shall see in Chapter 9 that this situation requires retesting with masking. On the other hand, it is quite possible that the bone-conduction thresholds will be 50 dB HL at the *right mastoid* and 65 dB HL at the *left mastoid*. Hence, the existence of IA for mastoid bone-conduction is an advantage for mastoid placement because it can avert the need for unnecessary masking under some conditions.

Some audiologists routinely test forehead bone-conduction while the patient is also wearing the air-conduction headset. This technique is called "forehead-occluded bone-conduction." One argument for this arrangement is that the dynamic range problem that comes with placing the vibrator at the forehead can be overcome by a boost in the bone-conduction signal that results from covering the ears with the earphones, due to the occlusion effect. However, the occlusion effect is simply too variable for this argument to be plausible. This approach does facilitate some aspects of testing because the patient is set up for all tests from the start, but it tends to be quite uncomfortable after a while.

Pretesting Issues and Considerations

Talk Before You Test   You want to establish a working rapport with the patient, but this is certainly not the only reason to talk to him before testing. A case history should be taken at this point. If a case history form was completed in advance, then this is the time to review it with the patient for clarification of pertinent details. Always ask if there have been any changes since the last time he was seen. This is also the time when the clinician observes the patient to develop a clinical picture of his auditory status, communicative strategies, and related behaviors. For example, does the patient favor one ear, watch the talker's face and lips, lean toward the talker, ask for repetition, respond as though a question was misheard, have aberrant speech or voice characteristics, or look to his wife for clarification? These are only a few of the questions that go through the clinician's mind during the pretest interview. The information gathered during the interview will be combined with the formal test results to reach a clinical audiologic impression, and will be important in planning the patient's aural rehabilitation. In addition, the impressions gathered here will be useful when giving the patient test instructions, and in making other decisions about test administration.

Look Before You Touch   The clinician should assess whether there are any apparent structural abnormalities and asymmetries of the head in general and the ears in particular, and perform an otoscopic inspection prior to testing. For example, is there evidence of active ear disease, eardrum perforations, atresia, exostoses, external ear abnormalities, or impacted cerumen (see Chapter 6)? Besides leading to appropriate referrals, this information may affect how testing is done and/or interpreted. Test procedures will have to be modified if there is a collapsing ear canal or a mastoid process that cannot properly support a bone-conduction vibrator.

Orientation of the Patient   The patient should be seated in a reasonably comfortable chair. Armrests are very desirable because they make almost every kind of response method (e.g., hand or finger raising) easier for the patient. Chairs that swivel or lean back should be avoided because the movements are noisy and distracting, and can pose a safety problem for some patients.

Whether the patient should be seated facing toward or away from the tester has always been a controversial question. Many audiologists prefer to have the patient seated with her back to the clinician so that she will not receive inadvertent clues about when test signals are being presented. The unintended cues might come from seeing (1) the tester's behavior (e.g., changes in facial expression or head position while presenting a tone), or (2) the reflections of indicator lamps on the audiometer that light up when the interrupter button is pressed.

The other point of view is that the patient should face the clinician for several reasons. (1) Subtle patient behaviors that can affect the test outcome can be observed. For example, the clinician can notice eye movements or the beginnings of incomplete finger motions when the tone is presented 5 dB lower than the level where the patient actually decides to raise her hand. This often means that the patient is being too strict about when to respond, and therefore she should be reinstructed. (2) Many patients need encouragement and/or retraining during the test. Reinforcing correct response behaviors and retraining the patient is more effective and more pleasant when you can see one another. (3) Most speech audiometric tests (Chapter 8) involve verbal responses spoken by the patient. This means that the accuracy of the audiologist's own hearing can affect the test results. Hence, being able to see the patient's lips and face makes it more likely that the results are due to the patient's hearing ability

and not due to errors made by the clinician. But what about inadvertent cues? The answer to this question is that indicator lights are easily covered (as is one's mouth if live-voice speech audiometry is being done), and that controlling one's own behavior is a valuable skill for clinicians to develop. Moreover, the ability to control the apparent cues provided by one's facial expressions can be a valuable clinical skill when dealing with patients who have functional hearing losses. Functional, or nonorganic, hearing impairments are discussed in Chapter 14.

As a compromise, the patient may be seated so that she faces the clinician at an angle between full face and profile. This permits the clinician to see the patient, but it limits the patient to a peripheral view of the clinician.

Patient Responses   The patient can indicate that she heard a tone by pushing a response button that causes a response lamp to light up on the audiometer, raising her hand or finger, or verbally (e.g., saying "yes" when a tone is heard). Modified and special modes of responding are often needed for young children and for difficult-to-test patients of various kinds. Among the routine response methods, hand (or finger) raising and pushing a button are desirable for two reasons: (1) They are clear-cut actions that give the tester an unambiguous indication of when the patient heard the tone. (2) They are silent responses that do not interfere with the ability to hear the test tones.

Verbal responses (e.g., saying "yes") should generally be avoided, if possible. The obvious reason for avoiding verbal responses is that test tones will be masked by the patient's own voice if she happens to respond while a tone is being presented. A second reason is that some patients do not limit themselves to saying "yes" when a tone is heard. Some patients occasionally say "no" when a tone has not been heard for a while. Others add comments like "I'm not sure" or "I think I hear it," thus increasing the chances that the patient will be talking while the tone is being presented. Comments such as these also force the tester to decide whether the tone was heard instead of keeping this decision with the patient.

Some clinicians have the patient indicate the ear in which the tone was heard, others consider this approach to be undesirable, and still others ask the patient to indicate laterality on an ad hoc basis. The simplest approach for routine cases is probably to avoid the issue of laterality when instructing the patient, and to give her the option of indicating sidedness if she asks. Having the patient indicate the sidedness of the tone in an appropriate manner is often useful in special cases and with children.

Test Instructions The patient must know exactly what to do during the test. For this reason, test instructions should be explicit and clear. However, they also must be appropriate to the patient, which means that the same set of instructions cannot be given to every patient. Always remember that patients are calmer and more cooperative when they understand what is going on, what to expect, and what they have to do. With these points in mind, the following is a typical set of instructions for pure-tone, air-conduction testing:

> The idea of this test is to find out the softest sounds you can hear. You're going to hear tones from these earphones. There will be many tones, one at a time. Some of the tones will be loud, but most of them will be very faint, and many of them will be too soft to hear. Your job is to raise your hand every time you hear a tone, no matter how faint it is, and to put your hand down whenever you don't hear any tones. We will test one ear and then the other one. Remember, raise your hand every time you hear a tone, no matter how faint it is. Do you have any questions?

Determining the Pure-Tone Threshold

A number of techniques to obtain pure-tone thresholds are accepted by the audiological community, such as the Carhart-Jerger (1959) modification of the Hughson-Westlake (1944) approach, and the ANSI (1997) and ASHA (1978) testing guidelines. That these respected

methods are not identical highlights the point that there is no one method that is the singularly "right" way to test pure-tone thresholds. However, these methods agree on the most important issues, and their similarities reveal a consensus of general approach within the audiological community.

Testing begins by familiarizing the patient with the test tone and making a ballpark guestimate of where the threshold might be. One technique is to present the patient with discrete tones at certain levels. The Carhart-Jerger (1959) method does this by first presenting to the patient a test tone lasting 1 to 2 seconds at about 30 dB HL if the patient seems to be normal, or at 70 dB HL if he appears to have a hearing impairment. If the patient does not respond to the first tone, then its level is raised in 15-dB steps until the tone is heard.

The clinical threshold for a tone is generally defined as the lowest hearing level at which it can be heard for at least 50% of the presentations on ascending runs. In addition to this, the Carhart-Jerger and ASHA methods require at least three responses at this level, whereas the ANSI approach requires at least two, therefore taking less time. The two- and three-response rules appear to yield essentially the same results (Harris, 1979; Tyler & Wood, 1980).

The ANSI (1997) and ASHA (1978) methods start with a 30 dB HL presentation, which is followed by 50 dB HL if the initial level was inaudible. If the patient still does not hear the 50 dB HL tone, then its level is raised in 10-dB steps until the patient responds. The threshold search procedure is then begun, which uses the following strategy:

1. The tone is adjusted to a level that is below the patient's threshold. This is done so that the threshold can then be approached from below. The procedure is to simply lower the tone to 10 to 15 dB below where the patient responded in the first phase, and then to present it to him. The tester continues to lower the tone in 10- to 15-dB steps until it becomes inaudible to the patient.
2. The level of the tone is then raised in 5-dB steps until the patient responds.

3. The tone is now decreased by 10 dB (or 15 dB) and presented again, in which case it should again be inaudible. This is done so that the threshold can again be approached from below. [Sometimes a patient will respond at this lower level. When that happens the tone is decreased another 10 dB (or 15 dB) and presented, and so on, until it is inaudible.]

4. The level of the tone is then raised in 5-dB steps until the patient responds.

Steps 3 and 4 are repeated until the clinical threshold criterion is achieved. In other words, the clinician *lowers* the level of the next tone by 10 dB after every "yes" response, and *raises* the level of the next tone by 5 dB after every "no" response. The tone presentations should be reasonably irregular in their timing rather than following any rhythmic pattern.

In summary, the pure-tone testing procedure can be thought of as having two parts. First, we raise or lower the intensity of the tone in fairly large steps (often 15 dB) to quickly find the ballpark location of the threshold. Once we know the general location of the threshold, we switch to a more formal threshold determination strategy in which the threshold is approached from below in 5-dB steps. This involves two tactics, which are illustrated in Figure 5–4: (1) Whenever the patient does not hear the tone (−), we *increase* the level of the next tone by 5 dB ("up 5" after a "no"). (2) Whenever the patient hears the tone (+), we *decrease* the level of the next tone by 10 dB ("down 10" after a "yes"). It is no wonder this is known as the "*up-5 down-10*" technique.

A Step-by-Step Example

The threshold search procedure itself is easily understood by going through a typical example. The example shows how to do the procedure and also reveals why it works. We will illustrate only one "threshold search." However, the student should remember that a separate threshold is needed for every test frequency for both ears, and for both air- and bone-conduction. The threshold search procedure is therefore carried out many times for each patient. The example is portrayed in Figure 5–5. The numbers along the abscissa represent each of the individual presentations of the test tone, or trials. The ordinate shows the hearing levels of the tones presented to the patient. It is assumed that all of the necessary preliminary procedures have been done, and that we are ready to begin the actual testing process.

We begin by presenting the tone at 30 dB HL. The patient does not respond, implying that 30 dB was not heard. This situation is indicated by the − for trial 1 at 30 dB HL.

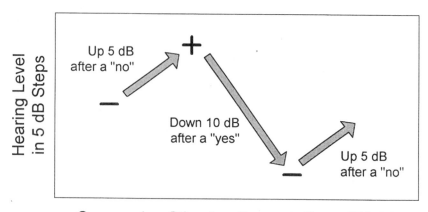

Successive Stimulus Presentations (Trials)

FIGURE 5–4 Conceptual illustration of the "*up-5 down-10*" technique typically used in pure-tone audiometry.

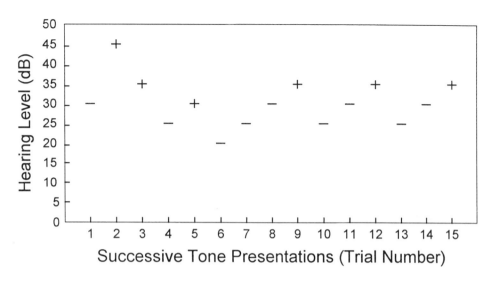

FIGURE 5–5 Hypothetical threshold search for a patient whose threshold is 35 dB HL. A + indicates the patient heard the presentation, and a – shows the patient did not hear the tone. Notice that the hearing level of a trial is raised by 5 dB following a – (the "up-5" rule) and is lowered by 10 dB following a + (the "down-10" rule), which causes the tester to search for responses in a series of ascending runs.

Clearly, 30 dB HL is below threshold, so we increase the level of the tone to 45 dB HL for the next trial. This time the patient does respond, indicated by the + for trial 2 at 45 dB HL. We now know that the threshold is between 30 and 45 dB HL. If the patient did not hear the 45 dB HL tone, we would have raised the level in 15 dB steps until he did. On the other hand, if the patient heard the tone at the initial level of 30 dB HL, we would have lowered it until he could no longer hear the tone. In either case, the idea is to rapidly find the approximate range of the threshold, so that we do not waste any effort.

Having established the ballpark range, we proceed to make our threshold estimate using the "up-5 down-10" method. Because the tone was heard at 45 dB HL in trial 2, the tone will be lowered by 10 dB and will be presented at 35 dB HL in trial 3 (*"down 10" after a "yes"*).

The patient hears the tone (+) at 35 dB in trial 3, so we again drop its level by 10 dB and present it at 25 dB HL in trial 4.

The patient does not hear the tone (–) at 25 dB HL in trial 4, suggesting that this level is below the patient's threshold. The rule now tells us to raise the level by 5 dB for the next

presentation (*"up 5" after a "no"*). The response is + at 30 dB HL in trial 5, so that trial 6 is presented at 20 dB HL (*"down 10" after a "yes"*).

The tone is not heard at 20 dB HL in trial 6 (–). Hence, the tone is presented 5 dB higher in trial 7. The patient does not hear the 25 dB tone in trial 7 (–), and so trial 8 is presented at 30 dB HL. Similarly, the 30 dB HL tone in trial 8 was also not heard (–). Thus, the "up 5" rule calls for trial 9 to be presented at 35 dB HL, which is heard (+) by the patient. Notice how trials 6 through 9 constitute an "ascending run" that ends in a "yes" (+) response for trial 9. In other words, we have approached the response from below.

The + response at 35 dB HL in trial 9 means that the tone must be presented 10 dB lower, at 25 dB HL, in trial 10 (*"down 10" after a "yes"*).

The patient does not hear the tone at 25 dB HL in trial 10 (–), or at 30 dB HL in trial 11 (–), but he does hear the tone at 35 dB in trial 12 (+). We have again approached a response from below in 5 dB steps.

The "down 10" rule now calls for us to present trial 13 at 25 dB HL, where we find no response (−). Trial 14 is thus presented at 30 dB HL according to the "up 5" rule. Because the tone is still not heard (−) at 30 dB HL, it is raised again by 5 dB, to be presented at 35 dB HL in trial 15. The patient hears the 35 dB HL tone in trial 15 (+). We have now completed a third ascending run ending in a + outcome at 35 dB HL. This completes the threshold search for this stimulus, and establishes the threshold to be 35 dB HL.

This is a good time to look at Figure 5–5 as a whole. Notice that there are −s at the hearing levels below the +s. Further, it is very sound reasoning to assume that the patient would have heard the tone almost all the time at HLs above the +s. In other words, each + represents one estimate of the lowest level at which the tone was audible, that is, one estimate of threshold. We have been using a clinical definition of threshold as the lowest HL where we find three responses out of six theoretical presentations. In this example, there was one + at 30 dB HL and three +s at 35 dB HL. The single + at 30 dB HL is below the 50% criterion, so that the threshold must be above 30 dB HL. Similarly, the three +s at 35 dB HL means that we have already reached the "three out of six" criterion for 50%. Thus, 35 dB HL is the patient's threshold for this tone because it is the lowest level at which he responded to the tone at least 50% of the time (conceptually based on six presentations).

Test Sequence for Pure-Tone Thresholds

The testing sequence described in this section is recommended for routine situations. However, one often encounters special circumstances that call for flexibility in one's testing approach, for example, pediatric assessments, and when evaluating difficult-to-test patients or those with poor reliability.

Air-conduction is tested for each ear, followed by bone-conduction. For air-conduction, the right ear is tested before the left ear unless there is reason to believe that one ear is better than the other. In the latter case, the apparently better ear is tested before the poorer one. Air-conduction is tested for the octave frequencies in the following order: 1000, 2000, 4000, 8000,

1000, 500, and 250 Hz. (It is also acceptable to routinely test the left ear before the right, or 500 to 250 Hz before 2000 to 8000 Hz. The point is that following the same sequence whenever possible results in the fewest tester errors.) The 1000-Hz retest is done as a reliability check, and is expected to be within +5 dB of the other 1000-Hz threshold in that ear. The semi-octaves (750, 1500, 3000, and 6000 Hz) are tested whenever there is a difference of >20 dB between two adjacent octave frequencies (e.g., 1500 Hz is tested if the thresholds at 1000 and 2000 Hz differ by 20 dB or more). The 125-Hz threshold should be obtained when there is an appreciable loss in the low frequencies. Bone-conduction is usually tested in the following order: 1000, 2000, 4000, 1000, 500, and 250 Hz. Many audiologists do not perform the 1000 Hz reliability check or test semi-octaves by bone-conduction unless there is reason to do so.

Many clinicians test certain semioctave frequencies on a regular basis. For example, 3000 Hz may be routinely tested because it is often needed to calculate the percentage of hearing impairment for legal purposes. However, it is not justifiable to test all of the frequencies on the dial just because they are there. The added information to be gained by an extra pure-tone threshold must be weighed against the cost of obtaining it. Patient fatigue and clinician time must be considered because other tests will follow, and pure-tone thresholds often have to be repeated with masking.

False Responses

A **false-positive** response means that the patient responds when he should not have responded. In contrast, a **false-negative** response means that he fails to respond when he should have responded. False-negative responses can occur for several reasons. Equipment problems or tester errors can prevent a signal from reaching the patient, or cause it to be presented in a manner that was not intended. Some patients are confused by tinnitus if their ear noises are similar to the test tones. The patient may not have fully understood the instructions or learned the proper mode of response. For example, some elderly patients have extremely strict criteria for when they will consider the tone present (i.e., they want to be very sure the tone is there) before they will respond. As we shall see in Chapter 14, there are also patients who do not respond because they are trying to make their hearing appear to be worse than it really is for conscious or unconscious reasons. False-negative responses can also occur for technical reasons, such as collapsed ear canals and standing waves, which are discussed later.

False-positive responses make thresholds difficult to obtain and unreliable from test to test. Some false-positives are caused by tactile stimulation and/or acoustical radiations (discussed later). Others are the result of confusion between test tones and tinnitus. Many false-positive responses are behavioral and are often due to misunderstood or improperly learned instructions, or to very lax response criteria. Behaviorally based false-positives can often be reduced by refamiliarizing the patient with the test tones and reinstructing him about exactly when and how to respond.

The tester can inadvertently encourage false-positives by presenting tones rhythmically. Remembering that most of the tones are hardly audible to begin with, learning the tester's rhythm makes the patient expect tones at certain times, and thus biases him to respond at those times.

A difficult situation can develop if a patient's *false* response coincidentally occurs at just the right moment after a *real* tone presentation. Because the false-response had every appearance of being a real one, the tester might even confirm its correctness for the patient. This problem can interact with rhythmic tone presentations. Not only does presenting the tones in a rhythmic pattern cause the patient to expect tones at certain intervals, but a rhythmic pattern also makes it more likely that the false responses will occur at the "right" times.

Avoiding Equipment Problems and Tester Errors

Several strategies can minimize equipment problems and tester errors. Daily equipment checks are the first line of defense. Errors due to incorrect equipment settings can be minimized by establishing a set of "start-up" positions that are always the same (e.g., frequency at 1000 Hz, HL dial at 0 dB, input selector to "tone," output selector to right earphone, etc.). By always resetting the audiometer to these initial setup positions after each patient, the clinician can avoid errors caused by a control inadvertently set at the wrong position. An added benefit of resetting the audiometer is never having a control in the wrong position. Simply returning everything to the start-up position, and then setting up the test from a "clean slate" is a lot easier and more effective than looking for the error. The ultimate version of this strategy is possible with digital audiometers that automatically return to their default positions when they are turned on. One should not be too eager to use the reset button or to turn the power off and (after waiting) on again. However, this can be the only solution when a digital audiometer "locks up" because of programming bugs or design flaws.

Recording Pure-Tone Thresholds on the Audiogram

The Audiogram Form   The patient's thresholds at each frequency are recorded on an **audiogram**, which is usually shown as a graph. Many audiologists record the information for both ears on the same audiogram form, whereas others use a separate graph for each ear. The audiogram form and symbols recommended by ASHA (1990) are shown in Figure 5–6. Frequency is shown on the abscissa, going from 125 Hz on the left to 8000 Hz on the right, and it is customary to label the frequency axis along the top. Notice that octaves are equally spaced. In other words, the distance covered by any doubling of frequency (e.g., 125 to 250 Hz, 1000 to 2000 Hz, 1500 to 3000 Hz, 4000 to 8000 Hz) is always the same. This means that the frequency scale on an audiogram is logarithmic. Hearing level is shown in dB HL (ANSI/ISO or ANSI S3.6-1996) along the y-axis, with intensity increasing from –10 dB HL at the top to the maximum level (120 dB HL in the figure) at the bottom.

An audiogram form can be of any convenient size but its *relative dimensions* are critical. Specifically, the distance covered by one octave must be equal to the distance covered by 20 dB. We could also say that it is made up of squares that are 1 octave wide by 20 dB high. The relative dimensions are important so that the configuration of a patient's audiogram will always have the same perspective. If the relative dimensions were not uniform, then the shape of the same hearing loss might have a steeply sloping appearance on one form and a shallow slope on another form.

Masking Noise Levels   The table below the audiogram in Figure 5–6 is used to record the amount of masking noise that has been used, if any. Masking is covered in Chapter 9. Here, "AC" means masking that is used during air-conduction testing, and "'BC" means masking that is used during bone-conduction testing. Notice that this table refers to the ear that receives the masking noise (the "nontest ear") as opposed to the ear being tested.

Audiogram Symbols   All audiogram forms should always include a key that explicitly describes the symbols used to plot information on the audiogram. Figure 5–6 shows the

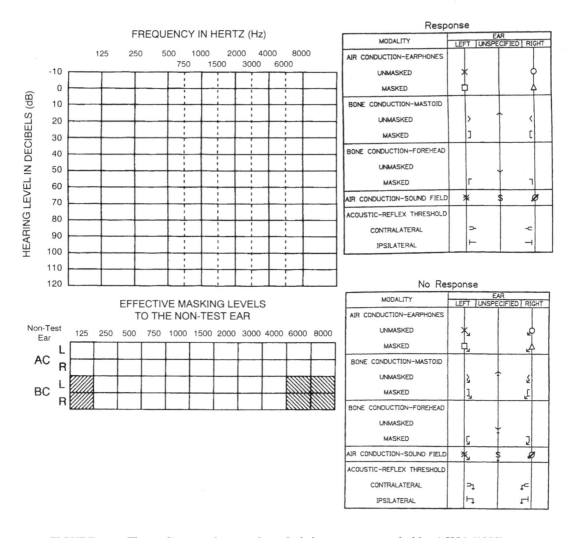

FIGURE 5–6   The audiogram form and symbols keys recommended by ASHA (1990).

symbols recommended by ASHA (1990). Do not be frustrated by the fact that many of the symbols refer to concepts that are unfamiliar at this point. It would be redundant to expand upon the symbol descriptions given in the key, except to highlight some key concepts and the most commonly used symbols. **"Unmasked"** means thresholds that were obtained in the way already described in this chapter, and **"masked"** means that the threshold was obtained with noise in the opposite ear. For air-conduction, the unmasked symbols are a circle for the right ear and an X for the left ear, and the masked symbols are respectively a triangle and a square.

The bone-conduction symbols refer to where the bone vibrator is located, which can be on the right or left mastoid or on the forehead. The right unmasked and masked mastoid bone-conduction symbols are < and [, and the equivalent left symbols are a > and], respectively. The student will soon learn that bone-conduction signals are picked up by the better cochlea no matter where the vibrator is placed. Hence, the unmasked "right" and "left" mastoid bone-conduction symbols (< and >) really refer to the position of the vibrator and not necessarily which ear heard the signal. In recognition of this point, some audiologists prefer to use the "unspecified" bone-conduction symbol unless masking has been used. Unlike air-conduction symbols, which are drawn on the grid line for the test frequency, the bone-conduction symbols are drawn near the frequency grid line. This is done to make the audiogram more readable.

The soundfield threshold is represented by an **S** and is described on the key as "unspecified" because either or both of the two ears could have heard the signal (discussed later in this chapter).

If there is no response to a signal at the maximum level provided by the audiometer, then a downward-pointing arrow is added to the symbol. No-response symbols should be located on the audiogram at the highest testable level. For example, if there is no response to a bone-conduction tone at a maximum testable level of 70 dB HL, then

the no-response symbol would be placed at 70 dB HL.

In order to make it easier to distinguish left ear and right ear symbols on the same audiogram, it has been traditional to plot right symbols in red and left symbols in blue or black. However, this convention is probably overemphasized because the red-blue distinction is lost whenever information must be shared: standard Xeroxing, carbon paper, and NCR paper all make single-color copies; printed material comes in black-and-white; and certain blues and reds do not photocopy well. Hence, although the use of red and blue is very convenient, it is no longer strictly required.

Numerical Audiograms   Instead of plotting symbols on a graph, many audiologists prefer to record the results numerically in tabular form. The disadvantages of numerical audiograms are largely related to the issue of whether one can visualize the audiometric pattern from the numbers. However, numerical audiograms have practical advantages when it comes to rapidly recording results and making calculations about masking (Chapter 9). Tabular arrangements of audiometric records are valuable when comparing audiograms over time, in which case the serial audiograms are recorded on separate lines of a table, one under the other. They also lend themselves to computerized record keeping. "No responses" should be indicated on numerical audiograms along with the maximum testable level. For example, a no response to a maximum bone-conduction signal of 70 dB HL could be written as "NR70," "70NR," "70+," or "70↓." However, just writing "NR" is ambiguous because one does not know what the highest level was, and the practice of writing the next-higher level (75 in this case) is very misleading.

Some audiologists (including the author) prefer to use the numerical format during the course of the evaluation and then plot the *final* threshold values onto a graphic audiogram. This approach takes advantage of the ease with which numbers can be written and used for calculations, and also results in a

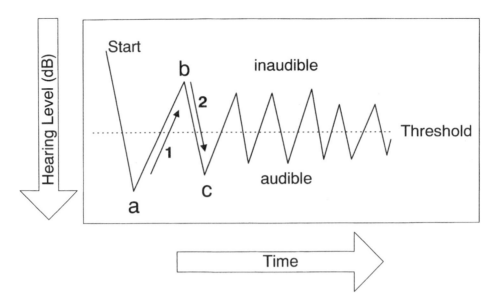

FIGURE 5–7   Bekesy (self-tracking) audiometry (see text).

very neat graph that represents the "bottom line," rather than being cluttered by numerous extra symbols.

Automatic Audiometry

Computerized Audiometry

Pure-tone audiometry does not always have to be done manually. It can also be done automatically with **microprocessor** or **computerized audiometers**. These instruments are programmed to test the patient (who responds by pressing a button) according to the same strategies that are used in manual audiometry, and can also be programmed for masking. Microprocessor audiometers can be useful for such large-scale testing applications as screening and industrial hearing conservation programs, providing the population being tested is able and willing to follow the test instructions. However, they are poorly suited for clinical use where patient variability and tester flexibility are the rule rather than the exception.

Another form of automatic audiometry involves the self-recording or tracking method, and is discussed in the next section.

Bekesy (Self-Tracking) Audiometry

Bekesy (1947) described an easy way in which a person is able to record her own thresholds by pressing and releasing a response button. The audiometer has a motor that continuously changes the attenuator setting at a fixed rate, so the hearing level is always changing (usually at 2.5 dB/second). The patient's response button controls the direction in which the attenuator moves. Specifically, the level increases as long as the button is not being pressed, and decreases as long as the button is being held down. The patient listens for the test tone, presses the button when the tone is audible, and releases it when the tone cannot be heard. Thus, pressing and releasing the button causes the intensity of the tone to rise and fall. The motor also controls a recorder, and the recorder pen moves up and down on a special audiogram form as the tone level rises and falls.

Figure 5–7 shows how self-recording audiometry works. The y-axis shows the level of the tone in dB HL, with intensity increasing downward just as it does on a regular audiogram. The x-axis shows the progression of time while the threshold is being tracked. The dashed horizontal line represents the patient's threshold. The zigzag shows the pattern tracked by the recorder pen, which represents the level of the tone on the paper. In this example, the test tone is initiated at a low level ("start" on the graph). The patient does not press the button because the tone is inaudible. Hence, the level increases steadily until the patient realizes that she can now hear the tone, and responds at point **a**. This causes the motor to reverse direction, so that the intensity starts decreasing, and the pen moves upward on the audiogram (arrow 1). The tone then falls below her threshold, and the patient releases the button in response to the tone's inaudibility at point **b**. Releasing the button causes the motor to reverse direction again, so that the intensity starts rising, represented by the line drawn downward on the audiogram (arrow 2). The patient responds to the reappearance of the tone at point **c**, at which point she presses the button, and the process continues as described until the test is discontinued. This process causes the intensity of the tone to rise and fall around the patient's threshold, and the midpoint of the resulting zigzag pattern is taken as her threshold. [The attentive student will have noticed that the reversal points overshoot the dashed line representing threshold. This reflects (1) how far above (or below) the "threshold" value the intensity must be before

the patient decides that it is present (or absent); and (2) her reaction time, which is how long it then takes her to press the button.]

In the example, we have been assuming that the frequency of the test tone stays the same during the procedure just described, so that the Bekesy audiogram is for one frequency. This type of testing is called **fixed frequency** (or discrete-frequency) Bekesy audiometry. In **sweep-frequency** Bekesy audiometry, the frequency changes slowly over time, so that the patient's thresholds are tracked across the audiometric frequency range. Bekesy audiometry is covered in further detail in Chapter 10.

Comparing Air- and Bone-Conduction Thresholds

Remember that the outer and middle ears collectively make up the conductive mechanism, and the cochlea and auditory nerve compose the sensorineural mechanism (Chapter 2). Comparing the air-conduction thresholds to the bone-conduction thresholds allows us to figure out whether a hearing loss is coming from a problem located in the conductive mechanism or in the sensorineural mechanism, or from a combination of the two. Figure 5–8 represents the whole peripheral hearing mechanism. It is divided into two halves, rep-

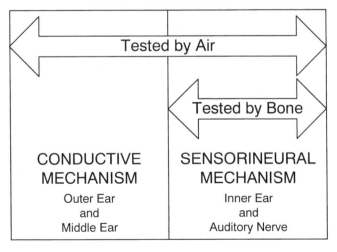

FIGURE 5–8 Air-conduction tests the entire system. Bone-conduction is said to "bypass" the conductive mechanism, so it tests only the inner ear (and auditory nerve).

TABLE 5-1   Air- and bone-conduction thresholds and air-bone-gaps, and the parts of a hearing loss represented by each

	Audiometric Measure	Represents
	Air-conduction threshold	Whole hearing loss
Minus	Bone-conduction threshold	Sensorineural part of the hearing loss
Equals	Air-bone-gap	Conductive part of the hearing loss

resenting the conductive mechanism (outer and middle ears) and the sensorineural mechanism (cochlea and auditory nerve). The entire ear is tested by air-conduction because the signal from an earphone must be processed through the outer, middle, and inner ear, and the auditory nerve. This notion is represented by the arrow labeled "tested by air" in the figure. All of these parts must be working properly for the air-conduction threshold to be normal, and a problem in any one (or more) of these locations would cause a hearing loss by air-conduction. Hence, the air-conduction threshold shows the total amount of hearing loss that is present. However, it cannot distinguish between a problem coming from one part of the ear versus the other. In contrast, the bone-conduction signal "bypasses" the outer and middle ears and directly stimulates the cochlea.[1] Hence, bone-conduction is considered to test just the sensorineural mechanism. This idea is represented by the arrow labeled "tested by bone" in the figure.

We can deduce the location of a problem from the following principles: (1) air-conduction tests the whole ear, and (2) bone-conduction tests the sensorineural part of the ear. Thus, a difference between the air- and bone-conduction thresholds implies that there is a problem with the conductive system. The difference between the air-conduction thresh-

old (AC) and the bone-conduction threshold (BC) at the same frequency is called an **air-bone-gap (ABG)**; that is, **AC − BC = ABG**. Table 5–1 summarizes the relationship between the air- and bone-conduction thresholds and the air-bone-gap, as well as the implications of each of these three audiometric measures.

Figure 5–9a represents an ear in which the thresholds are 55 dB HL by air-conduction thresholds and 55 dB HL by bone-conduction. It is assumed that the air- and bone-conduction thresholds are both obtained at the same frequency. The bone-conduction threshold tells us that 55 dB HL of the loss is coming from the sensorineural part of the ear, and the air-conduction threshold indicates that the whole loss is 55 dB HL. Consequently, the sensorineural part of the loss (55 dB HL) accounts for the total amount of the loss (55 dB HL). The air-bone-gap here is 55 − 55 = 0 dB. From this information we can easily figure out that the whole loss is coming from the sensorineural mechanism, and also that the conductive mechanism must be okay. This kind of impairment is called a sensorineural hearing loss. It is indicated by air- and bone-conduction thresholds that are equal, or at least very close to one another. Sensorineural losses can be caused by a disorder of the cochlea or auditory nerve, or both. The combined term *sensorineural* is used to highlight the fact that we cannot distinguish between cochlear (sensory) and eighth nerve (neural) disorders from the audiogram.

Figure 5–9b shows another case in which the air-conduction threshold is 55 dB HL. In this case, however, the bone-conduction threshold is normal at 0 dB HL. This means that none of the hearing loss is coming from the sensorineural mechanism, which leaves the conductive mechanism as the only possible

---

[1] It is useful to think in these terms even though it is not an altogether pristine concept. Bone-conduction also involves outer and middle ear components, and bone-conduction thresholds can be affected by conductive pathologies. This is why quotes are used when we say that the conductive mechanism is "bypassed." However, that bone-conduction thresholds principally represent hearing sensitivity at the cochlea is fundamentally correct and of great practical significance.

culprit. The size of the air-bone-gap in this case is 55 − 0 = 55 dB. Therefore, this 55 dB HL hearing loss is coming from the conductive mechanism, *i.e.*, the outer and/or middle ear. This kind of hearing loss is called a **conductive hearing loss**. It is revealed by a hearing loss by air-conduction but essentially no hearing loss by bone-conduction.

It is also possible to have a hearing loss that is partly due to a sensorineural problem and partly to a conductive problem, called a **mixed hearing loss**. The mixed loss concept is shown in Figure 5–9c. The 55 dB HL air-conduction threshold is the total amount of hearing loss coming from all sources, and the bone-conduction threshold of 30 dB HL represents the part of the loss that is due to problems in the sensorineural mechanism. If 30 dB of the 55 dB HL loss is coming from the sensorineural problem, then the remaining amount of 55 − 30 = 25 dB (which is the air-bone-gap) must be due to problems in the conductive system. In other words, the sensorineural part of a mixed loss is shown by the bone-conduction threshold, and its conductive component is represented by the air-bone-gap.

In principle, the air-bone-gap should be 0 dB unless there is a problem with the conductive mechanism. But this is not always the case, which is why it is suggested from the outset that the air-bone-gap should be at least 10 dB wide before it is considered significant. Let us see why this is so. One reason has to do with test-retest reliability. A given clinical threshold measurement is generally considered to be reliable within ±5 dB. Applying ±5 dB of variability to both the air- and bone-conduction measurements at the same frequency means that the spread between them (the air-bone-gap) can be as wide as 10 dB. Another reason has to do with the statistical relationship between air- and bone-conduction thresholds: it is the mean air-conduction threshold that equals the mean bone-conduction threshold. In other words, air- and bone-conduction thresholds are equal in normal ears *on average*, so that the normal air-bone-gap is 0 dB *on average*. Consequently there must also be normal ears with at least some amount of air-bone-gap, and even ears in which bone-conduction is poorer than air-conduction. This statistical distribution is such that most air- and bone-conduction thresholds are within ±10 dB of each other (Studebaker, 1967; Frank, Klobuka, & Sotir, 1983). These points also explain why it is possible and perfectly acceptable for a bone-conduction threshold to be a bit poorer

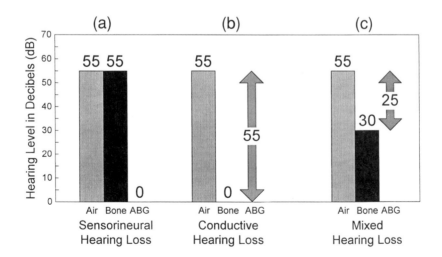

FIGURE 5–9 Air-conduction (Air) and bone-conduction (Bone) thresholds in cases of (a) sensorineural hearing loss, (b) conductive hearing loss, and (c) mixed hearing loss. The difference between the air- and bone-conduction thresholds is called the air-bone-gap (ABG), and represents the part of the loss coming from the conductive mechanism.

than the air-conduction thresholds at the same frequency (a so-called *"reverse air-bone-gap"* or *"bone-air-gap"*), even if everything is done correctly. Most certainly, a clinician should not "adjust" a bone-conduction threshold that is too high down to where it "should be." In addition, one should also be wary of the fact that bone-conduction may be worse than air-conduction because of an error. This often occurs if the bone vibrator slips or if it was improperly placed when it was applied.

Basic Audiogram Interpretation

A typical normal audiogram is shown in Figure 5–10. All of the air-conduction thresholds are in the vicinity of 0 dB HL for both ears. In addition, the air- and bone-conduction thresholds are very close to one another at each frequency, so that there are no significant air-bone-gaps. Why do we bother testing bone-conduction in a case such as this one, where the hearing is clearly normal? The reason for testing bone-conduction, even when the air-conduction thresholds are normal, is because 0 dB HL is the *average* threshold for normal people, so that thresholds

lower than 0 dB HL are expected to be found in many people, especially in children (Eagles, Wishik, & Doerfler, 1967). A middle ear problem in a person who normally has −15 dB HL thresholds can cause these thresholds to shift up to 0 or 5 dB HL. Here, the hearing sensitivity is within the normal range but there is also a conductive disorder. In cases such as this, testing bone-conduction would show a 15- to 20-dB air-bone-gap, thus revealing the problem. However, omitting bone-conduction testing would cause such a conductive impairment to be missed.

A **pure-tone average (PTA)** is usually calculated for each ear. The PTA, which is simply the mean of the air-conduction thresholds at 500, 1000, and 2000 Hz, is an attempt to summarize the degree of hearing loss. Table 5–2 shows the various categories of degrees of hearing loss. It indicates that pure-tone averages up to 15 dB HL are considered to be within the normal limits. The patient in Figure 5–10 has pure-tone averages of 0 dB HL for the right ear and 2 dB for the left ear, which are well within this normal range.

The pure-tone average was originally based on the 500-, 1000-, and 2000-Hz thresh-

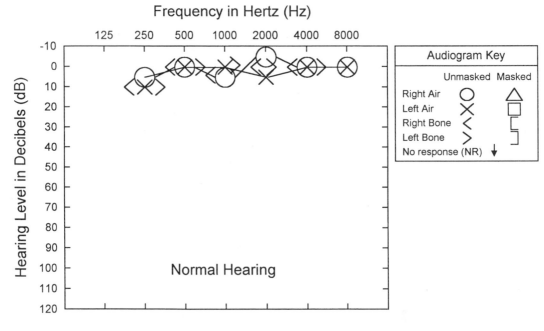

FIGURE 5–10   An example of a normal audiogram.

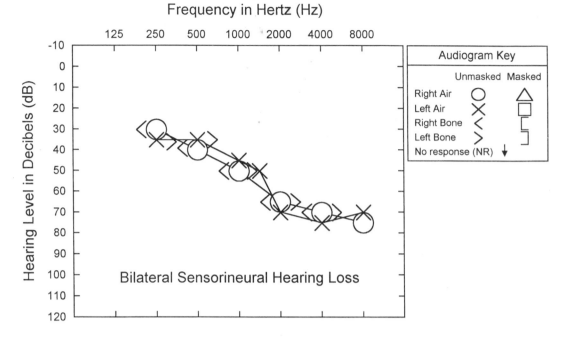

FIGURE 5–11   An example of a bilateral sensorineural hearing loss.

olds because it often agrees with hearing ability for speech (Fletcher, 1929). The PTA is usually compared to a measure of hearing for speech called the **speech reception threshold (SRT)**,[2] and significant differences between the PTA and SRT are of clinical significance (Chapters 8 and 14).

For this reason, 500, 1000, and 2000 Hz have come to be known as the *"speech frequencies."* However, this is a misnomer because adequate speech recognition actually depends on a much wider range of frequencies. Moreover, this three-frequency pure-tone average often fails to agree with the SRT, especially when the shape of the pure-tone audiogram slopes sharply. A **two-frequency pure-tone average** based on the best two of these three frequencies (usually 500 and 1000 Hz) is often used instead of the three-

frequency PTA under these circumstances (Fletcher, 1950). It is sometimes necessary to compare the SRT to the single frequency with the best threshold (often 500 Hz, and sometimes 250 Hz) to achieve agreement between the pure-tone and speech results (Gelfand & Silman, 1985, 1993).

The air-conduction thresholds in Figure 5–11 reveal that this patient has a hearing loss in both ears. A loss in both ears is said to be

TABLE 5-2   Typically used categories to describe the degree of hearing loss based on the pure-tone average

Pure-Tone Average in dB HL	Degree of Hearing Loss
≤15	Normal hearing
16–25	Slight hearing loss
26–40	Mild hearing loss
41–55	Moderate hearing loss
56–70	Moderately severe hearing loss
71–90	Severe hearing loss
>90	Profound hearing loss

[2] The SRT is the lowest level (in dB HL) at which a patient can correctly repeat spondee words 50% of the time. Spondee words have two syllables with equal emphasis on both syllables (e.g., "baseball" or "greyhound"). See Chapter 8.

bilateral. The left ear was tested at 1500 Hz because there was a spread of ≥20 dB between the thresholds at 1000 and 2000 Hz. The three-frequency pure-tone averages are 52 dB HL in the right ear and 50 dB HL in the left ear, so that the degree of hearing loss would be considered moderate according to Table 5–2. Because this audiogram has quite a slope, we would also calculate two-frequency PTAs based on 500 and 1000 Hz. These are 45 dB HL for the right ear and 40 dB for the left. The type of loss in this example is sensorineural because the air- and bone-conduction thresholds are essentially the same at each frequency, that is, there are no significant air-bone-gaps. This implies that the underlying disorders are located in the cochleae and/or eighth nerves. Finally, the configuration (shape) of the audiogram slopes downward with increasing frequency. It is easily understood why the interpretation of this audiogram would read as follows: "Moderate sloping sensorineural hearing loss, bilaterally."

Figure 5–12 is an example of a bilateral conductive hearing loss. It is the audiogram of a child who has middle-ear infections in both ears. The air-conduction thresholds are between 25 and 45 dB HL, but all of the bone-conduction thresholds are in the vicinity of 0 dB HL. According to the criteria shown in Table 5–2, the losses would be considered to be in the mild range because the pure-tone averages are 30 dB HL for the right ear and 38 dB for the left ear. Table 5–3 shows how to calculate each of the air-bone-gaps in this figure. Overall, we can see that the air-bone-gaps account for virtually the entire hearing losses of both ears. In broad terms, the configurations of these losses could be described as flat; however, notice that there is a slight tent-like shape for the right ear.

The patient whose audiogram is shown in Figure 5–13 has a **unilateral** hearing loss because it involves just one ear. The normal left ear has a pure-tone average of 2 dB. The impaired right ear has a mild hearing loss with a fairly flat configuration and a pure-

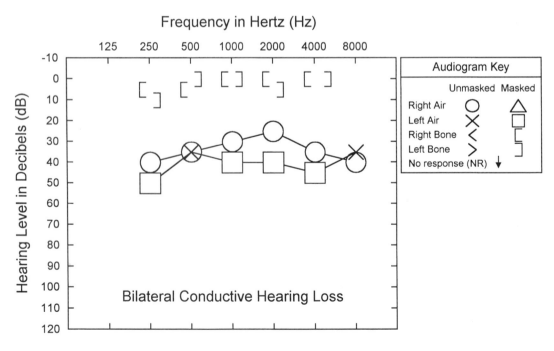

FIGURE 5–12 An example of a bilateral conductive hearing loss. Each of the air-bone-gaps is enumerated in Table 5–3. (Notice that both unmasked and masked symbols are used in this figure and subsequent ones.)

TABLE 5–3 How to calculate each of the air-bone-gaps in the audiogram shown in Figure 5–12

Frequency	Ear	AC Threshold (dB HL)	minus	BC Threshold (dB HL)	equals	Air-Bone-Gap (dB)
250 Hz	Right	40	–	5	=	35
	Left	45	–	10	=	35
500 Hz	Right	35	–	5	=	30
	Left	35	–	0	=	35
1000 Hz	Right	30	–	0	=	30
	Left	40	–	0	=	40
2000 Hz	Right	25	–	0	=	25
	Left	40	–	5	=	35
4000 Hz	Right	35	–	0	=	35
	Left	45	–	0	=	45

tone average of 32 dB HL. The hearing loss in the right ear is conductive because the bone-conduction thresholds approximate 0 dB HL in both ears. Let us calculate a couple of the air-bone-gaps for illustrative purposes. The air-bone-gap is 30 dB at 500 Hz because the air- and bone-conduction thresholds at this frequency are 35 dB HL and 5 dB HL, respectively. Similarly, the air-bone-gap at 4000 Hz is 25 – 0 = 25 dB.

Figure 5–14 shows the audiogram of a patient with normal hearing in his right ear and a sensorineural hearing loss in his left ear. The hearing loss is sensorineural because the air- and bone-conduction thresholds are essentially the same. The patient's thresholds were tested at 1500 Hz for the left ear because of the large drop-off between 1000 and 2000 Hz. Notice, however, that there was no response at the maximum testable bone-

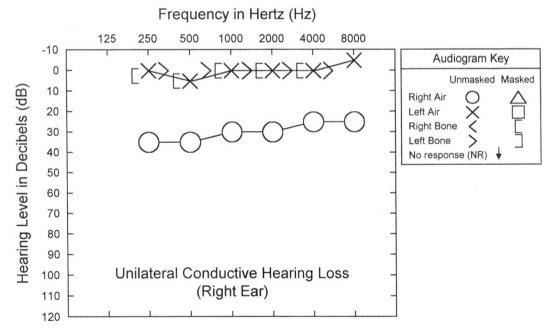

FIGURE 5–13 An example of a unilateral conductive hearing loss in the right ear (with normal hearing in the left ear).

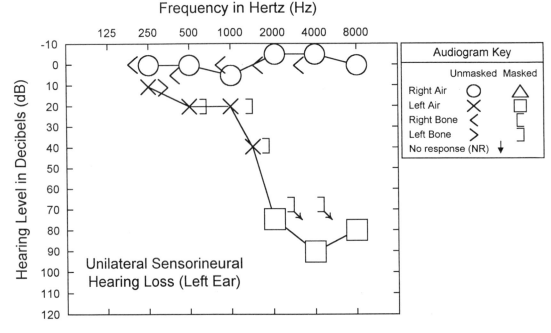

FIGURE 5–14   An example of a unilateral sensorineural hearing loss in the left ear (with normal hearing in the right ear).

conduction levels of 70 dB HL for both 2000 and 4000 Hz. This is no problem at 2000 Hz where the air-conduction threshold is only 75 dB HL, but we really *do not know for sure* whether or not there is an air-bone-gap at 4000 Hz where the air-conduction threshold is 90 dB HL. For the purpose of discussion, we accept the fact that other findings have confirmed this loss is completely sensorineural.

The normal right ear's pure-tone average is 0 dB HL. The impaired left ear has a three-frequency pure-tone average of 38 dB HL and a two-frequency PTA of 20 dB HL. Even if one of these averages agrees with the speech reception threshold, both of them clearly understate the amount of hearing loss in the higher frequencies. This shows how misleading it can be to describe a hearing loss solely on the basis of the pure-tone average. It is for this reason that the configuration of the hearing loss must not be overlooked. Hence, one might interpret this audiogram as indicating "a unilateral severe high frequency hearing loss in the left ear,

with normal hearing sensitivity in the right ear." The "severe" designation here is borrowed from the degrees of loss shown in Table 5–2. This is technically a misuse of the term because the degrees of loss shown in the table really apply only to the pure-tone average, and are intended to imply how much the hearing loss affects overall sensitivity for speech. Yet it has become common practice to describe other parts of the audiogram in these terms, as well. However, the author would consider it undesirable to say that this ear has "normal hearing in the low frequencies with a severe high-frequency sensorineural loss" even if all of the lower frequency thresholds would have been 0 dB HL. This objection is made because it is misleading to use the term *normal* to describe the thresholds at some of the frequencies in an *ear* that is not normal.

A mixed hearing loss occurs when both sensorineural and conductive impairments coexist in the same ear. In this case, the bone-conduction thresholds show the sensorineural portion of the loss, and the conductive component is represented by the air-bone-gap. The overall extent of the hearing loss is shown by the air-conduction thresholds. Figure 5–15 shows an example of a bilateral mixed hearing loss in which the pure-tone averages are 67 dB HL in the right ear and 75 dB HL in the left ear. The bone-conduction thresholds show the sensorineural components are similar for the two ears, sloping from about 10 to 15 dB HL at 250 Hz down to 55 to 60 dB HL at 4000 Hz. The air-bone-gaps are also similar for the two ears and also from one frequency to the other in this audiogram. However, it must be stressed that this is *not* always the case.

Sensation Level

Recall that *sound pressure level* expresses a sound's magnitude in dB compared to a physical reference (which is $2 \times 10^{-5} N/m^2$). In contrast, *hearing level* indicates the magnitude of a sound compared with the average threshold of that sound for the population of normal people. Hence, 0 dB HL will corre-spond to a different number of dB SPL at each frequency, as shown in Table 4-1 of Chapter 4. For example, 0 dB HL corre-sponds to 13.5 dB HL at 500 Hz. Similarly, 0 dB HL corresponds to 7.5 dB at 1000 Hz, and 0 dB HL at 4000 Hz will have a sound pres-sure level of 10.5 dB. However, we often want to know the intensity of a sound above an *individual* person's own threshold. This is called **sensation level (SL)**. For example, 25 dB SL means that the sound in question is 25 dB above the patient's threshold.

Consider a patient whose 1000-Hz thresh-old is 30 dB HL, which means that she can just perceive the tone when it is 30 dB above 0 dB HL. In other words, 30 dB HL is *at her threshold*. Hence, 30 dB HL *for her* corre-sponds to a *sensation level* of 0 dB. This is so because one's own threshold is the refer-ence value for sensation level, and a reference value has a level of 0 dB. Consequently, a threshold corresponds to 0 dB *SL*. Now, suppose we present this patient with a 1000-Hz tone at 65 dB HL. This tone is 35 dB *above her threshold*; therefore, its *sensation level* is 35 dB SL.

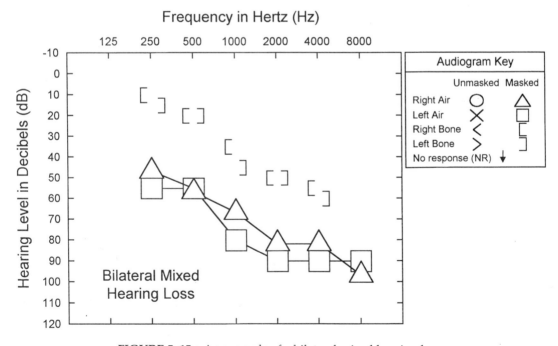

FIGURE 5–15 An example of a bilateral mixed hearing loss.

As an exercise, let us determine the sensation levels for various tones using the audiograms just described. A 500-Hz tone at 70 dB HL tone would have sensation levels of (a) 70 dB SL in each ear for Figure 5–10, (b) 30 dB SL for the right ear and 35 dB SL for the left ear in Figure 5–11, and (c) 15 dB SL for both ears in Figure 5–15. Now consider several tones with different frequencies, all of which are presented at 90 dB HL. For the left ear in Figure 5–14, 90 dB HL would correspond to 70 dB SL at 500 Hz, 50 dB SL at 1500 Hz, 15 dB SL at 2000 Hz, and 0 dB SL at 4000 Hz. Using the right ear in Figure 5–15, the sensation levels of these 90 dB HL tones would be 45 dB SL at 250 Hz, 25 dB SL at 1000 Hz, and 10 dB SL at 2000 Hz.

Factors That Affect Pure-Tone Results

Many factors can affect the validity and reliability of the audiogram. The implications of calibration, regular instrumentation checks, and an appropriate test environment were covered in Chapter 4. We have also covered such issues as patient seating, instructions, false responses, etc. In this section we will address several very real phenomena that nonetheless produce incorrect outcomes on the audiogram. We will also briefly look at a couple of audiometric configurations that sometimes reveal possible errors. These points are introduced after covering basic audiometric interpretation because they require some basic understanding of audiograms and hearing losses. However, it will be apparent that these issues need to be in your mind while you are testing the patient.

Standing Waves

The distance between the eardrum and the diaphragm of the earphone can be very close to the wavelength of an 8000-Hz tone (which is about 4.25 cm or 1.68 inches). If they just match, then a standing wave can develop in the ear canal. Under these conditions the tone and its reflections within the ear canal will be 180° out-of-phase, which will *cancel* the tone. This will cause the patient's 8000-Hz

threshold to be higher than its real value. A standing wave artifact is generally suspected if the 8000-Hz threshold is appreciably below the threshold at 4000 Hz. It is confirmed if altering the fit or orientation of the earphone causes the 8000-Hz threshold to get better, in which case the improved threshold is more likely to be the correct one. Using insert receivers can be helpful in these cases. These points should be kept in mind with respect to 6000 Hz as well, because standing wave problems are occasionally found at this frequency.

Tactile Responses

Patients with very severe hearing losses who cannot hear the sounds being presented might still respond if they *feel* the vibrations produced by the bone vibrator or earphones (Nober, 1970). These tactile responses are most likely to occur at low frequencies (especially 125 and 250 Hz) where the skin is more sensitive to vibratory stimulation.

Tactile responses cause two kinds of problems. First, they can give the false impression that the patient's thresholds are better than they actually are, or that the patient has hearing where there is none. For example, the tactile threshold at 250 Hz might be 75 dB HL when the actual threshold would have been 90 dB HL or even no response. Second, a false bone-conduction threshold due to a tactile response can create an artificial air-bone-gap, so that a sensorineural hearing loss would appear to be mixed. For example, suppose a patient has an 85 dB HL sensorineural loss. A tactile response to bone-conduction at 45 dB HL would give the false impression that this is an 85 dB HL mixed loss that includes a 40-dB air-bone-gap.

Dealing with tactile responses often involves simply asking the patient if the stimulus was heard or felt. However, this is not always possible with young children, especially those with very severe hearing losses who have had little or no experience with sound.

Acoustical Radiations

The bone-conduction vibrator can cause a sound to be radiated into the air. The radiations then enter the ear canal, and may be heard via the air-conduction route. These acoustical radiations are sometimes heard at presentation levels that are below (better than) the patient's true bone-conduction threshold. This causes a false air-bone-gap above 2000 Hz, which is usually most prominent at 4000 Hz (Bell, Goodsell, & Thornton, 1980; Shipton, John, & Robinson, 1980; Frank & Crandell, 1986). The artificial high-frequency air-bone-gap can make a sensorineural loss appear to be mixed. For example, hearing the acoustical radiations produced by a 55-dB HL bone-conduction tone can cause a 75-dB HL sensorineural loss to appear to include a 20-dB air-bone-gap.

The problem of acoustical radiations is easily alleviated by inserting earplugs into the ears during bone-conduction testing, but this is certainly not needed on a routine basis. Frank and Crandell (1986) suggested that bone-conduction should be retested with earplugs when there is an air-bone-gap

of >10 dB above 2000 Hz and no other evidence of conductive impairments.

Collapsed Ear Canals

It is possible for the pressure from the earphones to cause the cartilaginous portion of the ear canal to collapse during air-conduction testing (Ventry, Chaiklin, & Boyle, 1961). Collapse of the ear canal obstructs the flow of sound while the earphone pressure is being applied, and results in (1) an apparent high-frequency conductive hearing loss and (2) poor test-retest reliability. An example is shown in Figure 5–16. The size of the air-bone-gap artifact can range from 10 to 50 dB HL (Coles, 1967). The problem is more common in elderly patients than in other groups because tissue elasticity often becomes reduced with age, but the incidence rate is unclear because of variability among samples. For example, Marshall, Martinez, and Schlaman (1983) found collapsed ear canals

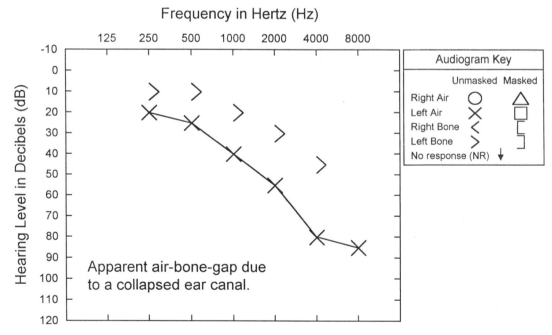

FIGURE 5–16 Audiogram of a patient with a sensorineural hearing loss who has a collapsed ear canal effect. Notice how the ear canal collapse makes the loss appear to be mixed, and how the size of the apparent air-bone-gap gets larger as frequency gets higher. Only one ear is represented for clarity.

in none of their elderly subjects, whereas Randolf and Schow (1983) reported a 36% incidence rate.

One must be alert to the possibility of a collapsed ear canal when there is an air-bone-gap that is greater in the higher frequencies because this artifact can lead to misdiagnosis. The traditional ways to confirm and overcome this artifact involve (1) inserting a tube into the ear canal to hold it open, or (2) removing the earphone from the headset and holding it loosely at the ear to do away with the pressure. Two other methods are now preferred. One is to retest with insert earphones, which by their very nature hold the canals open. The other method is to retest the air-conduction thresholds while the patient is holding his jaw open (Reiter & Silman, 1993). Before doing this, the patient should be asked whether he has any problems that would contraindicate the jaw opening technique (e.g., temporomandibular joint disorders). This technique alleviates the collapsed ear canal effect because the mandible contributes to the wall of the external auditory meatus, so that the movements involved in jaw opening can distort and therefore open the collapsed canal. Reiter and Silman (1993) found similar thresholds are obtained with insert earphones and the open jaw method. They suggested that patients with air-bone-gaps can be screened for ear canal collapse by retesting them with the jaw open at 4000 Hz, which is where the artifact is usually largest. A collapsed ear canal is suspected if the air-conduction threshold improves by ≥15 dB with the jaw open.

Configurations That Should Be Confirmed

Several audiometric configurations can indicate the presence of a possible error. Hearing losses that are unilateral or identical for both ears are audiometric configurations that should be confirmed because they could also be due to artifacts, errors, and/or false responses.

Unilateral hearing losses can be caused by equipment problems affecting one ear-phone, especially when there is no response at all for one ear. The most likely culprits are damaged earphone wires or jacks that have been dislodged from their sockets. A typical tester error that can cause a false unilateral loss is setting the output selector to the wrong transducer. Under these conditions, the clinician should (1) listen to the sounds produced by both earphones, and (2) retest the patient with the earphones reversed (i.e., right phone on left ear, left phone on right ear). It is often wise to do a Stenger test to rule out a functional component when faced with a unilateral loss (Chapter 14).

Identical thresholds in both ears usually means a symmetrical hearing loss, but it sometimes indicates that the clinician tested the same ear twice. It is wise to double check if there is any question that this error may have occurred.

Supplemental Pure-Tone Tests

Occlusion Effect and Audiometric Bing Test

Recall that the occlusion effect (1) causes a low-frequency bone-conduction threshold to be lower (better) than it would be with the ear uncovered, and (2) occurs when the conductive mechanism is normal but not when there is a conductive disorder. The Bing test was originally a tuning fork technique used to determine whether the occlusion effect is present (see below). The audiometric Bing test uses a bone-conduction vibrator in place of a tuning fork. Because the audiometric Bing test also reveals the *size* of the occlusion effect, it is used to help determine how much noise is required when bone-conduction is tested with masking (Chapter 9), and this is the major use of the test.

The **audiometric Bing test** is administered as follows: Bone-conduction thresholds are obtained in the regular way, with the ears uncovered. The low-frequency (<1000 Hz) thresholds are then retested while the test ear is occluded by one of the earphones. The opposite earphone is located on the opposite side of the head (usually between the opposite ear and eye, or high on the opposite cheek) but *not* covering the other ear. The audiometric Bing test is positive if the occluded thresholds are significantly better (lower) than the unoccluded thresholds. A positive result means that the occlusion effect is present, and suggests that a conductive disorder is not present. This would occur when the ear is normal or when the hearing loss is sensorineural. The size of the occlusion effect is simply the difference between the occluded and unoccluded thresholds at any given frequency. The test is negative if the occluded and unoccluded thresholds are essentially the same, indicating that the occlusion effect is absent. This result suggests that there is a problem with the conductive mechanism and implies that the hearing loss is either conductive or mixed.

Sensorineural Acuity Level (SAL) Method

An indirect technique for estimating the sensorineural component of a hearing loss was originated by Rainville (1959) and modified for more efficient clinical use as the **Sensorineural Acuity Level (SAL)** test by Jerger and Tillman (1960). The SAL test is no longer used routinely, but it is occasionally helpful when one needs to know about a patient's hearing sensitivity at the cochlea, even though the standard bone-conduction thresholds are equivocal. Even if the test is not used, an understanding of how the SAL works will help the student bring together a number of important audiological concepts.

In the SAL test the patient's air-conduction thresholds are tested while a noise is being presented from a bone vibrator at the forehead. This noise is thus transmitted by bone-conduction to the cochlea, where it will interfere with the ability to hear the air-conduction test tone. This is an example of **masking** (Chapters 3 and 9). Raising the level of the air-conduction tone will enable the patient to hear it over the noise. The SAL test involves measuring the size of this threshold shift for a given patient. Before using the SAL test on patients, we must find out how much masking is produced by the noise being used. This is done by testing a

group of normal persons. Suppose we find that our noise causes the air-conduction thresholds of normal people to *shift* from 0 dB HL to 40 dB HL. Clinically, we would expect the same amount of threshold shift if the patient's hearing is normal *at the cochlea* and less of a threshold shift (or none at all) if there is a hearing loss *at the cochlea*.

Because the cochlea is normal when there is a conductive loss, all of the masking noise from the bone vibrator will be just as effective as it is in a person with normal hearing. Therefore, the bone-conduction noise will cause the threshold for the test tone to *shift* by the same amount (40 dB with our noise) in a conductive loss as it does in normal people. For example, a 30 dB HL threshold would shift by 40 dB to 70 dB HL. On the other hand, the masking noise will cause a smaller amount of threshold *shift* in cases of sensorineural loss because less (or even none) of the masking noise will be heard by the disordered cochlea. For example, the masking noise in our example would be barely (if at all) audible at the cochlea of somebody with a 40 dB HL sensorineural loss. Hence, the original 40 dB HL threshold would remain *unshifted* at 40 dB HL while the noise is present.

Tuning Fork Tests

Tuning forks were used to test hearing long before the development of the audiometer. A set of tuning forks used for this purpose is shown in Figure 5–17. Four of the more well known of these tests are the Schwabach, Weber, Bing, and Rinne tests. Even though the Schwabach test is rarely if ever used anymore, it is still worthy of some discussion because it uses interesting principles and highlights the limitations of methods that compare the patient to the tester. The Weber, Bing, and Rinne tests are still used, and can also be done audiometrically. Table 5–4 summarizes the outcomes and clinical implications associated with these three tests.

Schwabach Test The Schwabach test is a technique for estimating a patient's hearing

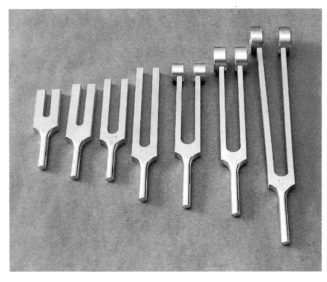

FIGURE 5–17   A complete set of tuning forks used for hearing assessment.

sensitivity by bone-conduction. The test has two principal characteristics: (1) it makes use of the fact that the tone produced by a tuning fork becomes softer with time after it has been struck due to damping, and (2) the patient's hearing is expressed in relative terms compared with the examiner's hearing ability. This comparison is done by timing how long the tuning fork is heard by the patient and how long it is heard by the examiner. The basic procedure involves placing the base of the vibrating fork on the patient's mastoid process until the tone fades away. The clinician then moves the fork to his own mastoid and times how long he can hear it. Compared to how long the examiner can hear the tone, it is expected that the patient will hear the tone (1) for a shorter period of time if she has a sensorineural loss, (2) for a longer period of time (or perhaps the same length of time) if she has a conductive loss, and (3) for the same amount of time if she has normal hearing. Schwabach outcomes are problematic when dealing with mixed losses. The Schwabach test provides a relative estimate of hearing at best, and its validity is completely dependent on the tenuous assumption that the examiner really has normal hearing. It is not surprising this test is rarely if ever used.

TABLE 5–4   Outcomes and diagnostic implications of the most commonly used tuning fork tests

Test	Outcome	Diagnostic Implications
Weber	Sound lateralized to	
	Midline or both ears equally	Normal (or sensorineural loss)
	Better ear	Sensorineural loss
	Poorer ear	Conductive loss
Bing	Positive (occluded louder)	Normal or sensorineural loss
	Negative (no difference)	Conductive loss
Rinne	Positive (air > bone)	Normal or sensorineural loss
	Negative (bone > air)	Conductive loss

Weber Test The Weber test is used to help determine whether a unilateral hearing loss is sensorineural or conductive. It is a **lateralization** test because the patient is asked to indicate the direction from which a sound appears to be coming. Before starting this test, the patient should be advised that it *is* possible for the tone to be heard from the good side *or* the poorer side, or any other location for that matter. The procedure involves putting the base of the vibrating tuning fork somewhere on the midline of the skull, most commonly on the center of the forehead or the top of the head. The audiometric Weber test uses the bone-conduction vibrator instead of tuning forks. The patient is asked to indicate *where* the tone is heard. Hearing the tone in the *better* ear implies that there is a *sensorineural loss* in the poorer ear, whereas hearing the tone in the *poorer ear* suggests a *conductive loss* in that ear. The tone is heard in the middle of the head, "all over," or equally in both ears when the patient has normal hearing, although some patients with sensorineural losses also report such midline lateralizations. If there is a mixed loss, the tone will be lateralized to the better ear if its level is below the poorer ear's bone-conduction threshold. The Weber test will fail to detect the conductive component of a mixed loss in such cases.

The Weber test works for several reasons, all of which are related to the idea that the bone-conduction tone from the tuning fork reaches both cochleae at the same intensity. The tone lateralizes to the better ear with sensorineural losses for either of two reasons: (1) The tone will only be heard in the better ear if its level is lower than the bone-conduction threshold of the poorer ear. (2) The second mechanism is due to the **Stenger effect**, which means that a sound presented to both ears is perceived only in the ear where it is louder. The intensity of the tone from the tuning fork will have a higher sensation level in the better ear than in the impaired ear. Hence, it will be louder in the better ear and will be perceived there. Several explanations can explain why a bone-conduction tone would be louder in (and thus lateralized to) the poorer ear. These mechanisms are just briefly mentioned because they are beyond the scope of an introductory text: (1) outer ear obstructions (e.g., impacted cerumen) may cause an occlusion effect, (2) mass loading of the middle ear system caused by effusions or ossicular chain interruptions may lower its resonance, and (3) phase advances may be caused by fixations or interruptions of the ossicular chain.

Bing Test The Bing test is used to determine if closing off the patient's ear canal results in an occlusion effect. The audiometric version of the test has already been discussed. In the traditional Bing test the patient is asked to report whether a tuning fork sounds louder with the ear canal open or closed. The base of a vibrating tuning fork is held against the patient's mastoid process. The tester then presses the tragus down over the entrance of the ear canal to occlude it. The usual technique is to alternately occlude and unocclude the ear canal to help the patient make a reliable louder-softer judgment. It is desirable to make sure that the tuning fork sounds louder when the ear is closed and softer when the ear is open, instead of just asking whether the tone pulses between louder and softer. Unlike the audiometric version that involves thresholds and thus quantifies the amount of the occlusion effect, the outcome of the tuning fork Bing test is based completely on a subjective judgment of louder versus not louder.

If the occlusion effect is present, covering the ear canal should cause the tuning fork to sound louder. This is called a positive result and implies that the ear is either normal or has a sensorineural hearing loss. A negative result occurs if closing off the ear canal fails to make the tuning fork sound louder, and implies that there is either a conductive or mixed hearing loss.

Rinne Test The Rinne test is a tuning fork procedure that compares hearing by air-conduction and bone-conduction; however, the approach used is different from the one used in pure-tone audiometry. The Rinne test is based on the idea that the hearing mechanism is normally more efficient by air-conduction than it is by bone-conduction. For this reason, a tuning fork will sound louder by air-conduction than by bone-conduction. However, this air-conduction advantage is lost when there is a conductive hearing loss, in which case the tuning fork sounds louder by bone-conduction than by air-conduction.

Administering the Rinne test involves asking the patient to indicate whether a vibrating tuning fork sounds louder when its base is held against the mastoid process (bone-conduction) or when its prongs are held near the pinna, facing the opening of the ear canal (air-conduction). After striking the fork, the clinician alternates it between these two positions so that the patient can make a judgment about which one is louder. The bone-conduction vibrator is used instead of the tuning fork in the audiometric version of the Rinne test, and the patient indicates whether the vibrator sounds louder on the mastoid or in front of the ear canal. Masking noise must be put into the opposite ear to make sure that the Rinne results are really coming from the test ear.

The outcome of the Rinne test is traditionally called "positive" if the fork is louder by air-conduction, and this finding implies that the ear is normal or has a sensorineural hearing loss. The results are called "negative" if bone-conduction is louder than air-conduction, which is interpreted as revealing the presence of a conductive abnormality. This terminology is confusing because the examiner is often concerned with identifying a conductive loss with this test. Consequently, many clinicians prefer to describe Rinne results as "air better than bone" (AC > BC) versus "bone better than air" (BC > AC). In these terms, AC > BC implies normal hearing or sensorineural impairment, and BC > AC implies a conductive disorder.

Sometimes, the air- and bone-conduction signals sound equally loud to the patient (AC = BC). This equivocal outcome can usually be overcome by using the timed Rinne test

(Gelfand, 1977). This more accurate way to administer the Rinne test involves *timing* how long the patient can hear the tuning fork at the two locations. In this case, the results are (1) positive (AC > BC) when the tone is heard longer by air-conduction, and (2) negative (BC > AC) when it is heard longer by bone-conduction. Another variation of the timed Rinne test involves holding the tuning fork at the mastoid until the tone has faded away, and then moving it to the ear canal (and vice versa). Here, the result is (1) AC > BC if the tone can still be heard by air-conduction after it faded away by bone-conduction, and (2) BC > AC if the tone can still be heard by bone-conduction after it faded away by air-conduction. These timed versions of the Rinne test are well established (Johnson, 1970; Sheehy, Gardner, & Hambley, 1971). They are more accurate than the loudness comparison method, but are also more cumbersome and time consuming. For this reason, they are not used unless the quicker and easier technique yields equivocal results.

Comments on Tuning Fork Tests Tuning fork tests are quick and easy to administer and do not require special instrumentation, so they can provide general, on-the-spot clinical insights, and they provide important (albeit limited) diagnostic information, especially when an audiogram is not available. However, tuning fork tests fall short of audiological measures in their ability to assess the patient's hearing status. This is due to the greater precision of audiometric tests made possible by calibrated electronic equipment and systematic testing strategies. Moreover, tuning fork tests are subject to considerable variability in administration and subjectivity in interpretation. Several limitations have already been mentioned with respect to individual tests, and others are worthy of mention. Which frequencies are tested varies among clinicians; some test only at 512 Hz and others use various combinations of frequencies. The intensity of the tone produced by the tuning fork depends on how hard it is struck each time, which causes stimulus levels to be inconsistent. Subjective patient responses can be a confounding variable, especially when dealing with younger children, and when the perception is "not logical" (e.g., when a tone is heard in the bad ear or gets louder when the ear is closed off). Also, tuning fork tests are usually done in examination rooms and clinics that are not sound isolated. Hence, noises that can mask the test signal and/or distract the patient are often a real issue.

It is therefore not surprising that carefully done studies have shown that tuning forks are less accurate than audiometric methods. Wilson and Woods (1975) found that both the Bing and Rinne tests failed to achieve a high level of accuracy in properly identifying conductive versus nonconductive losses. Gelfand (1977) studied the diagnostic accuracy of the Rinne test. All of the tuning fork tests were done with masking of the opposite ear. He found that the Rinne test cannot identify a conductive loss with reasonable accuracy until the size of the air-bone-gap becomes at least 25 to 40 dB wide (Table 5–5). Thus, mild conductive hearing losses that are easily revealed audiometrically are frequently missed by tuning fork tests like the Rinne.

Some tuning fork test problems are exacerbated by how and where the test is done. For example, the need for masking with certain tuning fork tests, particularly the Rinne, is well established in the otological literature (Shambaugh, 1967; Johnson, 1970; Sheehy et al, 1971). However, few physicians actually perform the Rinne test this way.

TABLE 5–5 Minimum air-bone-gaps needed for Rinne test to identify conductive losses with 75% accuracy (Gelfand, 1977)

Frequency (Hz)	Air-Bone-Gaps (dB)
128	25–30
256	5–40
512	55–60
1024	45–0
2048	None[a]

[a]Correct identification of conductive losses failed to reach chance at 2048 Hz, no matter how large the size of the air-bone-gap.

Soundfield Testing

A **soundfield** is an environment where sound is present. Testing from *loudspeakers* is called **soundfield testing** because the sound is delivered into the air in the test room (the soundfield), which then transmits it to the patient's ears. This means that the sound reaching the patient's ears will be affected by the acoustical characteristics of the room and any objects in the room, including the patient himself. Due to the acoustical differences between sounds from earphones and loudspeakers, it is necessary for the earphone and soundfield testing systems to be calibrated separately. In addition, because of the nature of standing waves (Chapter 1), (1) pure tones and other very narrow band signals are not appropriate for soundfield testing, and (2) the sound levels produced by the loudspeaker may not be the same throughout the test room. In addition, recall from Chapter 4 that different reference levels are used depending on the direction of the loudspeaker relative to the patient's head (ANSI S3.6-1996). The beginning audiology student and those planning to be speech-language pathologists should be aware of these acoustical factors even though they are actually advanced issues.

Once the sound reaches the ear, it follows the air-conduction route that was described for earphones. But here, too, there are at least two major differences between earphone and loudspeaker testing. The first difference is that the ears are uncovered during soundfield testing but are covered by the earphones and their cushions during headphone testing. Covering the ears blocks out room noises that can reach the eardrum when the ears are uncovered. This noise can mask, or interfere with the ability to hear, soft sounds. This quieter environment at the eardrum during earphone testing can make it possible to get lower (better) thresholds than could be obtained in the soundfield. We encountered this issue when considering the maximum allowable noise levels for audiometric test rooms in Chapter 4.

The second difference between earphone and soundfield testing has to do with the ability to test the two ears separately. Earphones allow us to test each ear separately because each ear has its own receiver. In contrast, the sound from a loudspeaker is picked up by both ears, so that they are not being tested separately. This means that a given soundfield threshold must be coming from the *better ear* if the ears are different, or from both ears if they are the same. Consider the case of 2-year-old Johnny who will not put on earphones but responds to sounds as low as 10 dB HL from loudspeakers. Here are the possible choices:

1. The response at 10 dB HL is really from both ears, which are the same. In this case, he is normal in both ears.
2. He really heard the 10 dB HL sound in his right ear. In this case, the right ear is fine, but the left ear could be *anything* from just a bit poorer than the right all the way to completely deaf.
3. He really heard the 10 dB HL sound in his left ear. Here, the left ear is okay, but the right ear could be just a bit worse, completely deaf, or anywhere in between.

The disturbing problem is that we simply do not know which of these alternatives is the right answer. This is why the soundfield threshold symbol (S) is described as "ear unspecified" on the audiogram key.

One way to help distinguish between the right and left ears during soundfield testing is to "block" one ear at a time. This can be done by (1) putting the earphone headset on the patient's head so that only one ear is covered by one of the earphones and its cushion and/or (2) inserting an earplug into the ear, or (3) covering one ear with an earphone that also directs a masking noise into that ear. These techniques are used to test one ear at a time in soundfield for special purposes, but they would not be much help for cases like little Johnny, who will not put on a headset to begin with.

REFERENCES

American National Standards Institute (ANSI). 1997. *Methods for Manual Pure-Tone Threshold Audiometry.* ANSI S3.21-1978 (R1997). New York: ANSI.

American National Standards Institute (ANSI). 1996. *American National Standard Specifications for Audiometers.* ANSI S3.6-1996. New York: ANSI.

American Speech and Hearing Association, Committee on Audiometric Evaluation (ASHA). 1978. Guidelines for manual pure-tone threshold audiometry. *ASHA* 20, 297–301.

American Speech and Hearing Association, Committee on Audiometric Evaluation (ASHA). 1990. Guidelines for audiometric symbols. *ASHA* 32 (suppl), 25–30.

Bekesy G. 1947. A new audiometer. *Arch Otolaryngol* 35, 411–422.

Bell J, Goodsell S, Thornton ARD. 1980. A brief communication on bone conduction artifacts. *Br J Audiol* 14, 73–75.

Carhart R, Jerger J. 1959. Preferred method for clinical determination of pure-tone thresholds. *J Speech Hear Dis* 24, 330–345.

Coles P. 1967. External meatus closure by audiometer earphones. *J Speech Hear Dis* 32, 296–297.

Dirks, D. 1964. Factors related to bone conduction reliability. *Arch Otolaryngol* 79, 551–558.

Dirks D, Malmquist C. 1969. Comparison of frontal and mastoid bone conduction thresholds in various conduction lesions. *J Speech Hear Res* 12, 725–746.

Dirks D, Swindeman JG. 1967. The variability of occluded and unoccluded bone-conduction thresholds. *J Speech Hear Res* 10, 232–249.

Eagles EL, Wishik SM, Doerfler LG. 1967. Hearing sensitivity and ear disease in children: A prospective study. *Laryngoscope Monogr* Suppl, 1–274.

Elpern B, Naunton RF. 1963. The stability of the occlusion effect. *Arch Otolaryngol* 77, 376–384.

Fletcher H. 1929. *Speech and Hearing in Communication.* Princeton: Van Nostrand Reinhold.

Fletcher H. 1950. A method for calculating hearing loss for speech from an audiogram. *J Acoust Soc Am* 22, 1–5.

Frank T, Crandell C. 1986. Acoustic radiation produced by B-71, B-72, and KH-70 bone vibrators. *Ear Hear* 7, 344–347.

Frank T, Klobuka CS, Sotir PJ. 1983. Air-bone-gap distributions in normal-hearing subjects. *J Aud Res* 23, 261–269.

Gelfand SA. 1977. Clinical precision of the Rinne test. *Acta Otolaryngol* 83, 480–487.

Gelfand SA, Silman S. 1985. Functional hearing loss and its relationship to resolved hearing levels. *Ear Hear* 6, 151–158.

Gelfand SA, Silman S. 1993. Relationship of exaggerated and resolved hearing levels in unilateral functional hearing loss. *Br J Audiol* 27, 29–34.

Goldstein DP, Hayes CS. 1965. The occlusion effect in bone-conduction. *J Speech Hear Res* 8, 137–148.

Harris JD. 1979. Optimum threshold crossings and time window validation in threshold pure-tone audiometry. *J Acoust Soc Am* 66, 1545–1547.

Hughson W, Westlake H. 1944. Manual for program outline for rehabilitation of aural casualties both military and civilian. *Trans Am Acad Ophthalmol Otolaryngol* 48 (suppl), 1–15.

Huizing EH. 1960. Bone conduction: The influence of the middle ear. *Acta Otolaryngol* 155 (suppl), 1–99.

Jerger J, Tillman T. 1960. A new method for clinical determination of sensorineural acuity level (SAL). *Arch Otolaryngol* 71, 948–953.

Johnson E. 1970. Tuning forks to audiometers and back again. *Laryngoscope* 80, 49–68.

Link R, Zwislocki J. 1951. Audiometrische knochen-leitungsuntersuchungen. *Arch Klin Exp Ohr Nas Kehkopfheik* 160, 347–357.

Marshall L, Martinez S, Schlaman M. 1983. Reassessment of high-frequency air-bone-gaps in older adults. *Arch Otolaryngol* 109, 601–606.

Nober EH. 1970. Cutile air and bone conduction thresholds in the deaf. *Except Child* 36, 571–579.

Rainville MJ. 1959. New method of masking for determination of bone conduction curves. *Trans Beltone Instrum Res*, No. 11.

Randolf L, Schow R. 1983. Threshold inaccuracies in an elderly clinical population: Ear canal collapse as a possible cause. *J Speech Hear Res* 26, 54–58.

Reiter LA, Silman S. 1993. Detecting and remediating external meatal collapse during audiologic assessment. *J Am Acad Audiol* 4, 264–268.

Shambaugh G. 1967. *Surgery of the Ear*. Philadelphia: WB Saunders.

Sheehy J, Gardner G, Hambley W. 1971. Tuning forks in modern otology. *Arch Otolaryngol* 94, 132–138.

Shipton MS, John AJ, Robinson DW. 1980. Air radiated sounds from bone vibrator transducers and its implications for bone conduction audiometry. *Br J Audiol* 14, 86–99.

Studebaker GR. 1962. Placement of vibrator in bone conduction testing. *J Speech Hear Res* 5, 321–331.

Studebaker GR. 1967. Intertest variability and the air-bone-gap. *J Speech Hear Dis* 32, 82–86.

Tyler ES, Wood EJ. 1980. A comparison of manual methods for measuring hearing thresholds. *Audiology* 19, 316–329.

Ventry TM, Chaiklin JB, Boyle WF. 1961. Collapse of the ear canal during audiometry. *Arch Otolaryngol* 73, 727–731.

Wilson WR, Woods LA. 1975. Accuracy of the Bing and Rinne tuning fork tests. *Arch Otolaryngol* 101, 81–85.

6

Auditory System and Related Disorders

This chapter gives an overview of the disorders of the auditory system. We will address the nature of various pathologies, where and when they occur, their major signs and symptoms, how hearing is affected, and the ways they are treated. Further coverage of auditory disorders, their diagnosis and treatment, may be found in many fine otolaryngology texts (e.g., Hughes, 1985; Buckingham, 1989; Bluestone & Stool, 1996; Paparella, Shumrick, Gluckman, & Meyerhoff, 1991; Tos, 1993, 1995; Hughes & Pensak, 1997; Lalwani & Grundfast, 1998; Wetmore, Muntz, & McGill, 2000).[1]

Hearing impairments are caused by abnormalities of structure and/or function in the auditory system, which are often called **lesions**. Using this terminology, a hearing loss may be viewed as one of the manifestations of a lesion somewhere in the ear, as are other symptoms such as pain, ringing in the ears, and dizziness. We are interested in the nature of the lesion, as well as its severity, etiology (cause), location, and time course (including when it began and how it has progressed). Disorders are often called **idiopathic** if a specific underlying cause cannot be identified. The interactions among these various factors can often be important. Consider, for example, the distinction between "congenital" and "hereditary." A disorder is **congenital** if it is present at birth—a matter of timing. On the other hand, a disorder is **hereditary** or **genetic** if it is transmitted by the genetic code that the

child inherits from her parents; otherwise it is **acquired**, which is a matter of causation. A congenital disorder may be caused by a genetic problem or other factors that interfere with normal embryological development or occur during the birth process. Similarly, genetic disorders are often present at birth, but others are delayed, manifesting themselves long after birth. Moreover, some degree of hereditary predisposition is involved in many acquired disorders.

We are equally interested in the nature, severity, and time course of the hearing impairment itself. Although the nature of a hearing loss goes hand in hand with that of the lesion, the same cannot always be said about severity and time course. For example, middle ear infections cause conductive losses, but the magnitude of the hearing loss is not clearly related to the severity of the infection. Similarly, hair cell damage due to noise exposure and/or aging is typically under way long before the patient notices (or at least admits to) a hearing problem. A more dramatic issue has to do with when a severe hearing loss develops in a child and when it is identified and addressed. **Prelingual** impairments occur before the development of speech and language, and have a catastrophic effect on this process, precipitating serious communicative impairments and interference with academic development. **Postlingual losses** develop after speech and language have been established, and have a *relatively* smaller effect. The earlier the onset, and the longer the child is deprived of auditory stimulation, the more the loss will interfere with speech and language development, and

---

[1] These texts served as references for material used throughout this chapter.

hence the more devastating its effect. Conversely, the earlier that a significant hearing impairment is identified, the sooner its effects can be mitigated by appropriate intervention techniques.

The Case History

The case history includes information about the patient that provides insight into his auditory status and related factors, and that contributes to the development of a diagnostic impression, a plan for audiological remediation, and appropriate referrals to other professionals. Thus, the clinical case history involves obtaining a complete picture of the patient's auditory and communicative status, historical information about factors known to influence or to be related to auditory functioning, and his pertinent medical and family history. These points should be kept in mind while reading this chapter, and necessitate addressing the issue of case histories at this point.

Exactly how the case history is obtained is often a matter of personal style and interviewing skills. At one extreme is the use of a formal "case history form" that the patient completes in advance, which is then reviewed and discussed with the patient. The other extreme involves conducting an open-ended interview, in effect asking, "What's a nice person like you doing in a place like this?" This method is quite effective in the hands of a "master clinician," but it is easy for those with less experience to lose control of an open-ended interview, or to omit information that would have been obtained with a more structured approach. For this reason, those who prefer the open-ended approach are often well served by completing items on a prepared form during the interview rather than starting with a blank sheet of paper. Many audiologists prefer to use a structured interview in which they ask the patient a predetermined set of questions, and then probe further depending on the answers.

A "case history form" is not included here because what is covered in a clinical case history should stem from an integrated knowledge and understanding of the nature, signs, and symptoms of auditory and related disorders. The case history can only be meaningful if one has an integrated knowledge and understanding of normal auditory functioning and the characteristics of auditory and related disorders. Otherwise, one is filling out the form for the sake of filling out the form. The serious student will find that an instructive and useful exercise is to derive a case history questionnaire on the basis of the material in this chapter and elsewhere in the text, particularly Chapters 12 and 13.

Conductive, Sensorineural, and Mixed Impairments

Sensorineural lesions involve the cochlea and/or auditory nerve, and may affect sensory receptor (hair) cells, auditory neurons, and/or any of the many structures and processes that enable them to be activated and function properly. The resulting impairment of auditory functioning is called a **sensorineural hearing loss**. *Nerve deafness* and *perceptive loss* are obsolete terms for sensorineural hearing loss, but are occasionally encountered. Using the term *sensorineural* (sometimes *sensori-neural* or *neurosensory*) highlights the anatomical and physiological interdependence of the cochlea and the eighth nerve. In addition, cochlear and auditory nerve lesions cannot be distinguished on the audiogram because both result in threshold shifts that are the same for air- and bone-conduction (i.e., no air-bone-gaps). Moreover, sensory and neural lesions can coexist because, for example, the absence of cochlear hair cells can result in degeneration of the auditory neurons associated with them, and an eighth nerve tumor can indirectly damage the cochlea by putting pressure on its blood supply. In spite of these points, it is not uncommon to find that *sensorineural loss* is being used to mean or imply "sensorineural loss of cochlear origin," in which case the intended meaning is usually understood from the context. Disorders of the eighth nerve are often described as being **retrocochlear**, meaning beyond the cochlea. Let us review some of the more common characteristics of sensorineural losses, which are due to cochlear lesions in the preponderance of cases. We will then go over conductive impairments, so that the student can appreciate the major differences between these two broad categories. The characteristics associated with neural lesions, per se, will be covered later in the section on retrocochlear disorders.

Cochlear disorders result in a loss of hearing sensitivity that is essentially the same for air- and bone-conduction. There is a rather systematic relationship between *where a lesion occurs* along the cochlear spiral and *which frequencies* have elevated thresholds on the audiogram: High-frequency hearing losses are associated with damage toward the *base* of the cochlea, and the hearing loss includes successively lower frequencies as the damage to the cochlea extends upward toward the apex. Similarly, lesions affecting the *apical* regions of the cochlea are associated with low-frequency sensorineural hearing losses, and the loss widens to include successively higher frequencies as the cochlear abnormality spreads downward toward the base. The outer hair cells are generally more susceptible to damage than the inner hair cells, and lesions involving the outer hair cells alone are typically associated with mild to moderate degrees of hearing loss. Damage to both the outer and inner hair cells usually produces more severe losses. However, it is difficult to establish a clear relationship between the *severity of cochlear damage* and the *amount of hearing loss* it causes.

Unlike the situation for many conductive disorders, medicine and surgery cannot correct sensorineural hearing losses because they are due to cochlear and/or neural damage that is permanent. In effect, missing hair cells and neurons do not regenerate. The student should be aware that hair cell regeneration can occur in birds (Corwin & Cotanche, 1988; Ryals & Rubel, 1988; Cotanche, Lee, Stone, & Picard, 1994; Tsue, Oesterle, & Rubel, 1994). This is an avenue of critically

important research that might provide hope for the future. However, counseling skill is often needed to help patients be aware (and accept) that while research on hair cell regeneration and related issues is critically important, it is also unrealistic to expect practical benefits for hearing improvement within the foreseeable future.

Sensorineural hearing losses can be of *any* shape and degree, but the most common configurations have thresholds that get worse as frequency increases. In other words, sensorineural impairments often involve a greater loss of hearing sensitivity at higher frequencies than at lower frequencies, so that the audiometric configuration may be described as sloping. This creates a burdensome problem for the hearing impaired patient because many of the acoustical cues that distinguish speech sounds involve the higher frequencies, and because, on average, the intensity of the speech signal gets weaker as frequency increases.

Most patients with sensorineural hearing losses complain that they can *hear* speech, but that it is *unclear or hard to understand*, and that this problem becomes worse when noise or competing sounds are present. These ubiquitous complaints occur for several reasons. Many high-frequency speech cues are rendered inaudible or barely audible by the frequency dependence of many sensorineural losses described previously. In addition, speech cues are distorted because inner ear lesions cause a variety of auditory impairments above and beyond elevated thresholds, such as the dulling of fine frequency and temporal distinctions. As a result, the auditory representation of speech cues is less faithfully encoded and noisy. In other words, cochlear lesions impair the clarity of speech due to both attenuation and distortion.

Patients with cochlear disorders often experience aberrations of pitch and loudness perception, such as diplacusis and loudness recruitment. **Diplacusis** means that more than one pitch (a perception) is heard in response to the same pure tone (i.e., frequency). This phenomenon is called monaural diplacusis when the same tone elicits different pitch sensations within the same ear, and binaural diplacusis when there is a pitch difference for the same tone between the two ears. **Loudness recruitment** means that the loudness of a sound (a perception) grows abnormally rapidly as the intensity of the sound (its physical level) is raised above the patient's threshold. For example, suppose a patient has a 50 dB HL cochlear loss in one ear and normal hearing (0 dB HL) in the other ear. A 100 dB HL sound would be 100 dB above the threshold in the normal ear but only 50 dB above threshold in the abnormal ear; yet 100 dB would sound equally loud in both ears. In other words, a 50-dB increment in the impaired ear sounds as loud as the 100-dB increment in the normal ear. As a result, many sounds are either too soft to hear adequately or too loud to hear comfortably. This is why a hearing impaired patient might ask you to "speak up" and then ask you to "stop shouting" after you comply with the first request. It also creates a dilemma for hearing aid use because the same amount of amplification that makes softer sounds audible also makes more intense sounds too loud.

Patients with severe-to-profound degrees of sensorineural hearing loss will not be able to hear speech without amplification. The inability of these patients to monitor their own speech can lead to aberrations in vocal pitch and loudness, as well as articulation errors. Along with language disorders, speech production problems are a major issue for patients with prelingual hearing losses, but are less common than once thought among adults with adventitious impairments.

Conductive lesions impair the *transmission* of sound from the environment to the cochlea, so that the signal reaching the sensorineural system is weaker than it should be. A **conductive hearing loss** is the amount by which the signal is attenuated (weakened) due to the disorder, and is expressed by the size of the air-bone-gap (Chapter 5). For example, a 30-dB conductive hearing loss means that the signal reaching the cochlea is 30 dB weaker than it would have been if the

conductive mechanism had been normal, resulting in a 30 dB HL hearing loss. Assuming that the patient has a normal sensorineural system (with a bone-conduction threshold of 0 dB HL), this 30-dB conductive loss would cause (1) a 40 dB HL signal to sound softer than normal because the signal reaches the cochlea at $40 - 30 = 10$ dB HL, and (2) a 25 dB HL signal to be inaudible because it reaches the cochlea below threshold at $25 - 30 = -5$ dB HL.

The size of the conductive hearing loss is not necessarily related to the severity of the underlying disease (e.g., an ear infection), but rather depends on how the lesion impedes the transmission of energy to the cochlea (e.g., by interfering with the middle ear transformer function). In contrast to the sloping configuration of the "typical" sensorineural impairment, conductive losses as a group tend to have *relatively* little variation in the amount of hearing loss from frequency to frequency. Notice that the emphasis is on the word *relatively*, and that conductive audiograms do not have to be "flat" any more than sensorineural audiograms have to be sloping; there are many exceptions to both generalities.

Because conductive disorders affect energy transmission to the cochlea but not the sensory processes within the cochlea, we expect the patient's complaints to reveal that she is experiencing a loss of intensity but not distortions or a loss of clarity; for example, "Speech is too soft but it does sound clear once it's loud enough." However, patients do not necessarily characterize their perceptual experiences using our concepts. Thus, when the patient says something like "Speech sounds *muffled*," we need to find out what she means by "muffled." Does it mean that speech is *too low* unless people speak loudly (a typical conductive loss complaint) or that speech is *lacking in clarity* even though it is loud enough (often associated with sensorineural loss)?

Relatively intense sounds are generally less bothersome to patients with conductive hearing losses because these sounds are reduced in level before entering the cochlea.

In one sense, the conductive loss is like an "ear plug" that lowers sounds by the amount of the air-bone-gap. For example, a 100 dB HL sound will reach the cochlea of a patient with a 40-dB conductive loss (air-bone-gap) at only 60 dB HL (i.e., 100 − 40 = 60). In contrast, the same 100 dB HL sound would reach a normal person's cochlea at 100 dB HL, and thus be very loud. This phenomenon is advantageous when these patients use hearing aids because it permits many sounds to be amplified without becoming too loud. However, this apparent "benefit" of a conductive hearing loss is no larger than the size of the air-bone-gap, and certainly does *not* shield the ear from sounds that are intense enough to cause a tactile sensation or pain.

Patients with conductive losses may report that speech is heard better in a noisy environment than in a quiet one. This phenomenon is the opposite of the normal experience and is called **paracusis willisii**. It occurs for the following reasons: Normal people have no trouble hearing conversational speech in a quiet room, but this speech is too low for the patient with a conductive loss. People talk louder in the presence of a background noise because of the Lombard voice reflex (see Chapter 14). However, the background noise level is still high enough to interfere with the ability to hear the talker's voice for normal hearing people. In contrast, the background noise is effectively lowered (or even made inaudible) by the conductive hearing loss, while at the same time the talker's increased vocal effort makes his speech intense enough to become audible above the noise for people with conductive losses. In other words, the noise makes the talker speak louder, and the conductive loss makes the noise sound lower. It is also common (but certainly not universal) to find that patients with conductive losses speak relatively softly. This occurs because the patient hears her own speech loud-and-clear via bone-conduction (which is normal), while at the same time fails to adjust her vocal level to account for environmental noises that are rendered inaudible or very low due to the hearing loss.

A **mixed hearing loss** is the combination of a sensorineural loss and a conductive loss in the same ear. Mixed losses may be caused by the presence of two separate disorders in the same ear (e.g., noise-induced hearing loss plus otitis media) or by a single disorder that affects the conductive and sensorineural systems (e.g., head trauma or advanced otosclerosis).

Tinnitus

Tinnitus is the abnormal perception of sounds for which there is no external stimulus. It is frequently associated with both sensorineural and conductive hearing losses, but it can also occur when hearing is within normal limits. The sensations are often described as "ringing in the ears," "head noises," or "ear noises," and are characterized by a host of terms such as "tonal," "ringing," "buzzing," "roaring," "hissing," "chirping," "pulsing," "humming," etc. Some sensations tend to be more commonly associated with sensorineural losses and others with conductive disorders. Certain kinds of tinnitus are particularly important, for example, pulsating tinnitus, which is timed to the patient's pulse, leads one to suspect the possibility of a glomus tumor. However, tinnitus per se is too common and too variable in how it is described to be used as a distinguishing diagnostic attribute.

Bothersome tinnitus may be the most common health-related complaint, occurring in anywhere from about 6% to 20% of the population, and it is severe enough to interfere with day-to-day activities in about 1%. Hence, although we are concentrating on tinnitus as a concomitant of hearing loss at this introductory level, the student should realize that it is a clinically relevant problem in and of itself, so that the nature, evaluation, and management of tinnitus is an area of audiological interest (Hazell, 1987; Tyler, Aran, & Dauman, 1992; Henry & Meikle, 2000; Jacobson, Henderson, & McCaslin, 2000; Sandlin & Olsson, 2000).

Fundamentally, several kinds of approaches have been used to assess tinnitus, such as (1) psychoacoustic measurements of the pitch, loudness, quality, and duration of the tinnitus (e.g., matching the loudness of the tinnitus to that of real sounds); (2) electrophysiological measurements such as auditory brainstem responses and otoacoustic emissions; and (3) determining the impact of the tinnitus on the patient in terms of annoyance, sleep interference, emotional stress, and handicap.

Unfortunately, the direct management of tinnitus has been largely disappointing. Medicines and surgery have been unsuccessful in alleviating tinnitus. Some patients have been helped by devices called **tinnitus maskers**, which mask the disturbing tinnitus with a more acceptable masking noise. Psychological techniques such as counseling, biofeedback, behavior modification, relaxation training, cognitive therapy, and reassurance have been used with various degrees of success. A meta-analysis[2] by Andersson and Lyttkens (1999) showed that psychological techniques reduce the annoyance caused by tinnitus, but do not produce lasting benefits in terms of reducing its loudness.

Congenital and Hereditary Disorders

Genetic Influences

The information needed to make a particular person (the genetic code) exists in the form of deoxyribonucleic acid (DNA) molecules packaged as chromosomes in every cell. Genes are segments of DNA that occur at fixed locations on the chromosomes, and operate as the biological units of inheritance. In other words, hereditary characteristics (traits) are carried by genes, which are arranged along the chromosomes. Humans have 46 chromosomes arranged in 23 pairs. One pair is different for females (XX) and males (XY), and the other 22 pairs are autosomes, or the same for both sexes. Each parent contributes half of each pair.

A **genetic** or **hereditary disorder** is an abnormal trait that is transmitted by an abnormal gene. Disorders may be the result of single- or multiple-gene abnormalities, or multifactorial inheritance, which is the combined effect of genetic and environmental factors. Hereditary hearing losses can occur alone or in combination with other genetic abnormalities, and may be transmitted by autosomal-dominant, autosomal-recessive, and X-linked inheritance, and by mitochondrial mutations (Jacobson, 1995; Smith, 1995; Tomaski & Grundfast, 1999; Keats, 2000; Post, 2000). Syndromes involving hearing loss are discussed later in this chapter. In addition, nonsyndromic genetic hearing losses have been associated with many loci (chromosome locations of the genes) in the human genome.[3]

Autosomal-dominant inheritance means that only one abnormal gene is needed in order for the trait to appear (hence, it is dominant). Suppose one parent is hearing impaired due to an autosomal-dominant gene and the other parent is normal. It does not make a difference which parent is affected because both the sperm and egg contribute half of each chromosome pair. If the mother is affected, then there will be a 50% chance that a given egg will contain the abnormal gene. If the father is affected, then half of his sperm will carry the abnormal gene and half will not. In either case, the chances are 50-50 for any pregnancy to result in a hearing impaired child, as illustrated by the pedigree diagram in Figure 6–1a. Approximately 15 to 20% of hereditary hearing losses are caused by autosomal-dominant transmission.

---

[2] Meta-analysis is a sophisticated statistical approach for combining results across studies.

[3] Research in this area is progressing very actively. As of this writing, 26 loci were identified for nonsyndromic autosomal-recessive hearing loss, 28 for autosomal dominant, 5 for X-linked, and 2 for mitochondrial defects. For up-to-date information, see the Hereditary Hearing Loss (VanCamp & Smith) site on the Internet, available at: http://dnalab-www.uia.ac.be/dnalab/ hhh. For information on the Human Genome Project, see http://www.ornl.gov/TechResources/Human_Genome/ home/html and http://www.nhgri.nih. gov/.

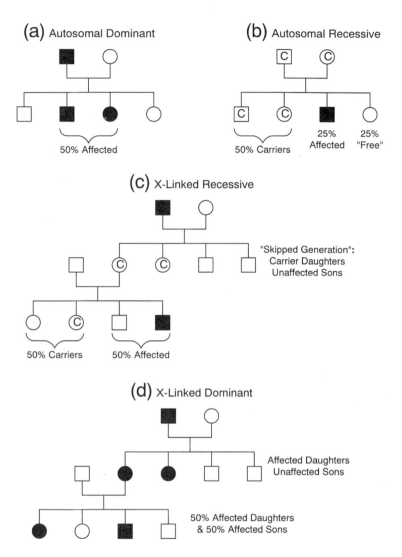

FIGURE 6–1 Pedigree diagrams for disorders based on (a) autosomal dominant, (b) autosomal recessive, (c) X-linked recessive, and (d) X-linked dominant inheritance. Circles, females; squares, males; open symbols, individuals free of the abnormal gene; filled symbols, affected individuals with the abnormal gene; "C," unaffected carriers of the abnormal gene.

The situation is different with **autosomal-recessive** inheritance because both genes in the pair must be present for the trait to manifest itself. There are three possibilities with respect to the abnormal recessive gene: (1) One may be altogether free of the abnormal gene. (2) A person with both abnormal genes will have the disorder and will be able to transmit the disorder to an offspring. Such

an individual is a **homozygote** because the same (*homo*) kind of abnormal gene was contributed by both parents when the fertilized egg (*zygote*) was produced. (3) An individual may have only one abnormal recessive gene, while the other one in the pair is normal. This is a **heterozygote** because the two genes in the pair are different (*hetero*). He will not have a hearing loss because he has only one abnormal gene and it is recessive, but he is a **carrier** because he can transmit the abnormal gene to his offspring.

Let's see what happens when both parents are normal hearing carriers of a certain recessive gene for hearing loss, that is, heterozygotes with one abnormal gene and one normal gene (Fig. 6–1b). The probability of getting the mother's abnormal gene is 0.5 and the probability of getting the father's abnormal gene is also 0.5. Therefore, the probability of getting *both abnormal genes* is $0.5 \times 0.5 = 0.25$. In other words, a given pregnancy has a 25% chance of producing a child who has both abnormal genes and is hearing impaired. On the other hand, the probability of getting *both normal genes* is also $0.5 \times 0.5 = 0.25$, which means a 25% chance that a given pregnancy will result in a child who is altogether free of the abnormal gene. What about the other 50%? These are the two remaining combinations (normal gene from the mother with abnormal from the father, and abnormal from the mother with normal from the father), both of which produce an unaffected carrier of the abnormal gene. Approximately 75 to 80% of inherited hearing losses are transmitted by autosomal-recessive inheritance. Autosomal-recessive hearing losses can be very hard to trace because a particular kind of abnormal gene can be transmitted across a number of generations before two unaffected (and unaware) carriers coincidentally find each other and fail to beat the odds.

X-linked (or **sex-linked**) inheritance occurs when the gene is associated with the X chromosome instead of being autosomal, and accounts for roughly 2% of hereditary hearing impairments. With an **X-linked recessive** disorder (Fig. 6–1c), an affected male transmits the abnormal gene to all of his daughters, who become unaffected carriers of the trait, but not to his sons. In turn, a female carrier has a 50% chance of having sons who are affected and a 50% chance of having daughters who are unaffected carriers. In **X-linked dominant** inheritance (Fig. 6–1d), an affected male will have all affected daughters and no affected sons. An affected female has a 50%

chance of having affected children, whether they are males or females.

Mitochondrial defects account for less than 1% of hereditary hearing losses, and appear to be related to aminoglycoside ototoxicity (Prezant et al, 1993; Fischel-Ghodsian, 1998). Ototoxicity is discussed later in this chapter.

Maternal Infections

Fetuses and newborns are adversely affected in various ways by at least 16 viruses and 6 bacteria. The major offenders are called the **TORCH complex**, of toxoplasmosis, other (including syphilis), rubella, cytomegalovirus, and herpes simplex. Many authorities have replaced TORCH with **STORCH** or **(S)TORCH** to recognize the importance of congenital syphilis in this group.

Syphilis (lues) is a sexually transmitted bacterial infection caused by the spirochete *Treponema pallidum*, which can be passed to the fetus from an infected mother. The number of reported cases of congenital syphilis increased dramatically from only 160 in 1981 to 2,867 in 1990 (Shimizu, 1992). Congenital syphilis is associated with notched incisor teeth, interstitial keratitis (a chronic inflammation of the cornea with the appearance of ground glass), and sensorineural hearing loss. The hearing loss can develop at any time during childhood or adulthood, even as late as about 60 years old. The sensorineural hearing loss is usually bilateral, symmetrical, and progressive, typically becoming severe- to-profound in degree. It is not uncommon for the loss to have a sudden onset or to fluctuate over time. Vertigo and/or tinnitus can also occur. **Vertigo** is a specific kind of dizziness in which the patient experiences a sensation of *whirling* or *rotation*. It is associated with nystagmus (Chapter 11) and is often accompanied by nausea. The shape of the audiogram is often flat or rising, but any configuration is possible. It is sometimes possible to arrest (and possibly even reverse) the progression of early-onset luetic hearing loss with high doses of penicillin and steroids.

Toxoplasmosis is a parasitic infection caused by the protozoan *Toxoplasma gondii*, and is often contracted from contaminated raw meats and eggs, as well as from contact with cat feces. The disease is transmitted to the developing fetus via the placenta, often from a mother who does not have any symptoms herself. The risk of adverse effects in the infant is great for infections incurred during the first trimester but small during late pregnancy. The incidence of toxoplasmosis is roughly 1.1 in 1000 births. Congenital toxoplasmosis causes a variety of disorders, including central nervous system disorders (e.g., microcephaly, hydrocephaly, intracranial calcifications, mental retardation), chorioretinitis (inflammation of the choroid and retina) and other eye disorders, and bilateral sensorineural hearing loss that may be moderate to severe and progressive. Hearing losses have been reported in 14 to 26% of children with congenital toxoplasmosis. Optimistically, Stein and Boyer (1994) found no hearing losses in 58 children treated with antiparasitic and sulfonamide drugs for 12 months beginning when they were less than 2.5 months old, although long-term follow-up studies of these children are still needed.

Rubella (German measles) is a viral disease transmitted from the mother to the fetus via the placenta. Epidemics in the United States during the 1960s have probably made it the most infamous viral cause of congenital hearing impairment, but the rubella vaccine has reduced the number of congenital rubella cases to about 50 per year (Strasnick & Jacobson, 1995). Babies affected by congenital rubella may have heart disorders, kidney disorders, mental retardation, visual defects, and hearing loss. The risk for congenital rubella is greatest if the fetus is exposed during the first trimester (roughly 50% in the first month, 20% in the second month, and 10% in the third), but the possibility of significant risks extends out to the 16th week. Sensorineural hearing loss is the most frequent sequela, with an incidence of about 50% when rubella is contracted during the first trimester and about 20% in the

second and third trimesters. Congenital rubella is typically associated with bilateral sensorineural hearing losses that are severe-to-profound in degree, and either flat, bowl-shaped, or sloping in configuration.

Cytomegalovirus (CMV) affects 2 to 3% of live births, and is the most common viral cause of congenital hearing loss. It is a herpes-type virus often contracted by sexual contact, and is also known to be transmitted by close associations with infected children. Pregnant women can be infected by a new exposure or by the reactivation of latent viruses already present in their bodies, and are usually asymptomatic when they do have the infection. The major consequences of CMV are associated with transmissions to the developing fetus, whereas postnatal CMV infections do not seem to present any major risks for an otherwise healthy child.

The severe outcomes of congenital CMV may include death, microcephaly, pneumonia, mental retardation, liver disease, dental defects, visual lesions, and sensorineural hearing loss (Stagno, 1990; Schildroth, 1994; Strasnick & Jacobson, 1995). About 10% of CMV-infected newborns are *symptomatic*, with one or more manifestations such as a purple rash, jaundice, "blueberry muffin" skin discolorations, and various signs of infection. About 90% are *asymptomatic*, having "silent" CMV infections. Stagno (1990) reported that 92% of symptomatic newborns have one or more serious sequela (including a 30% death rate) compared to only 6% for asymptomatic infants. Some examples are shown in Figure 6–2. About 10 to 15% of the cases eventually have one or more serious complications of congenital cytomegalovirus.

Cytomegalovirus causes a wide variety of sensorineural hearing losses ranging from mild to profound, which may be bilateral or unilateral, progressive or stable. A recent survey of children with hearing losses due to CMV revealed that approximately 88% have severe-to-profound impairments, and 50% have at least one additional disability (Schildroth, 1994).

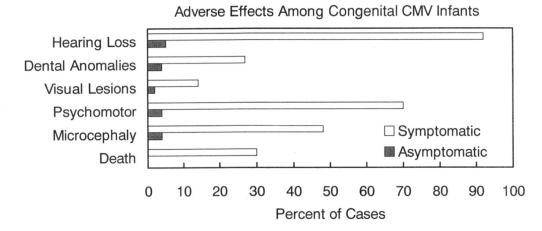

FIGURE 6–2 Percentage of cases with various adverse effects among 97 symptomatic and 267 asymptomatic infants with congenital cytomegalovirus (CMV) infections. "Psychomotor" refers to psychomotor retardation and neuromuscular disorders. Based on Stagno (1990).

Herpes simplex is a sexually transmitted viral disease that can be passed from an infected mother to the developing fetus either during pregnancy or during delivery (perinatally). Infected infants are affected by central nervous system problems (e.g., microcephaly and psychomotor disorders), growth deficiencies, retinal dysplasia, and moderate-to-severe sensorineural hearing loss in one or both ears.

Other Influences in the Maternal Environment

Maternal infections are not the only adverse influences that can cause or contribute to hearing impairments in the developing fetus. Another group of causes includes drugs, chemicals, and other agents in the maternal environment (Strasnick & Jacobson, 1995). For example, congenital hearing loss can be caused by the maternal use of certain medications that may be passed to the fetus via the placenta. The most prominent group of drugs are the **aminoglycoside antibiotics**, such as kanamycin and gentamicin, and streptomycin, which are sometimes essential in the treatment of severe infections. Other aspects of the maternal environment that can contribute to congenital hearing impairments and related anomalies include maternal diseases

such as toxemia and diabetes, nutritional deficiencies and disturbances, Rh-factor incompatibility between the mother and fetus, exposure to physical agents such as heat and radiation, and use of nonmedicinal drugs and chemicals such as alcohol.

Adverse factors that occur just before, during, and immediately after birth include compromises of the oxygen supply (asphyxia, anoxia, hypoxia), trauma during labor and/or delivery, hyperbilirubinemia (jaundice) leading to kernicterus, and infections. Borg (1997) reviewed 20 years of research to clarify the relationship between hearing loss and prenatal hypoxia (oxygen deficiency), ischemia (blood supply deficiency), and asphyxia (indicated by a low Apgar score). He found that the risk of permanent sensorineural hearing loss is greater for ischemia than for hypoxia; the central nervous system (CNS) is more susceptible to these kinds of insults than is the inner ear; and preterm infants are more susceptible than full-term babies. Interestingly, hearing losses were rarely caused by birth asphyxia alone, and hypoxia all by itself appeared to be associated with temporary hearing losses as opposed to permanent ones.

Some elucidation about **hyperbilirubinemia** is desirable because not every newborn with jaundice is at risk. The normal breakdown of spent red blood cells produces bilirubin, which is detoxified by the liver and excreted. Hyperbilirubinemia is a buildup of bilirubin in the blood and is observed as jaundice. Some degree of jaundice is common among newborns and is successfully treated by exposing the baby to ultraviolet light (phototherapy). However, **Rh-factor incompatibilities** between the mother (who is Rh-negative) and the fetus (who is Rh-positive) can result in the production of antibodies in the mother's blood, which can attack and break down red blood cells in the fetus. This disorder is called **erythroblastosis fetalis** or **hemolytic disease** of the neonate, and usually occurs in subsequent pregnancies where the fetus is Rh-positive. The concentration of bilirubin in the blood of the fetus can become high enough to cross the blood–brain barrier, causing **kernicterus**, or the deposit of bilirubin in the brain. Kernicterus causes brain damage because bilirubin is toxic to neural tissue. It can be widespread, but particularly affects the basal ganglia. Typical sequelae include athetoid cerebral palsy, mental retardation, and hearing impairment. Blood transfusions (exchange transfusions) are used to avert or minimize these effects in newborns with high bilirubin levels. A variety of sensorineural losses are found in about 4% of babies with hemolytic disease or hyperbilirubinemia (Hyman, Keaster, Hanson, Harris, Sedgwick, Wursten, & Wright, 1969). However, there is an unresolved controversy about whether hearing losses in kernicterus patients come from damage to the brainstem centers (such as the cochlear nuclei) or to coincidental peripheral impairments.

Congenital Anomalies of the Ear

Outer and Middle Ear

Dysplasia means an abnormality in the development of an anatomical structure. These congenital anomalies can affect the outer, middle, and/or inner ear, and can occur alone or as part of syndromes. The conductive system anomalies span a range of severity from barely noticeable cosmetic aberrations to a complete lack of development (**aplasia**). Outer and middle ear anomalies may occur alone or together, as well as in combination with inner ear dysplasia, especially in more severe cases.

The major external ear anomalies are microtia and atresia, which often occur together. **Microtia** means an abnormally small pinna, but it actually refers to a wide range of auricle deformities. *Type I microtias* have recognizable parts, and can be more or less well-formed except for their size. Pinnas that are only partially formed, generally resembling a curved or straight ridge, are *type II microtias*. A *type III microtia* is a tissue mass that does not resemble a pinna. Finally, the auricle may be completely absent, which is called **agenesis** (or **aplasia**) of the pinna, or **anotia**. Microtias are a major cosmetic problem, but do not cause substantial hearing losses in and of themselves. (This is not to undervalue the important auditory role of the pinna in such processes as directional hearing.) In contrast, considerable degrees of hearing loss can be produced by **aural atresia**, which is the absence of an external auditory meatus. If the canal opening is abnormally narrow, then the condition is called **aural stenosis**.

There are many kinds of congenital middle ear anomalies, such as the following:

1. The middle ear cavity and antrum may be grossly malformed, slit-like, or altogether absent.
2. The tympanic membrane may be rudimentary or absent.
3. Ossicles may be abnormally formed, e.g., the malleus and incus are often conglomerated into a unit.
4. Ossicles may be missing.
5. Ossicles may be attached to the abnormally formed middle ear cavity either directly or via bony bridges.
6. Facial nerve abnormalities are also frequently encountered.

Outer and middle ear anomalies produce a conductive hearing loss, provided the inner ear is not also affected. The degree of the conductive loss depends on the nature and extent of the abnormalities and is often about 60 dB. Surgical reconstruction of the conductive mechanism is generally possible, provided there is a serviceable cochlea behind the abnormal conductive mechanism. Depending on the nature of the abnormal anatomy, it is often possible to reduce the conductive loss to the 30-dB range, which is a considerable degree of improvement. Surgical reconstruction for the microtia provides the child with cosmetic improvements, the importance of which should not be underestimated.

Inner Ear

The congenital anomalies of the inner ear also exist along a continuum of severity from slight to complete. The worst case is the total absence of any inner ear structures, known as **Michel's aplasia**. It is possible for this to occur even with a normal conductive mechanism. Incomplete anomalies and developmental failures of the bony and membranous ducts of the inner ear are known as **Mondini's dysplasia** and vary widely in severity. The most common abnormality is dysplasia of the membranous ducts of the cochlea and saccule, and is called

Scheibe's aplasia. It is generally believed that the Michel and Mondini anomalies are caused by autosomal-dominant traits, and that Scheibe's aplasia is transmitted by the autosomal-recessive route. **Alexander's aplasia** refers to congenital abnormalities of the cochlear duct, especially affecting the basal turn (high-frequency region) of the cochlea.

Syndromes Involving the Ear and Hearing

A **syndrome** is a pattern of abnormalities and/or symptoms that results from the same cause. Auditory disorders can be found in a great many syndromes, and extensive listings are readily available in the audiological literature (e.g., Northern & Downs, 1991; Hall, Prentice, Smiley, & Werkhaven, 1995; Jacobson, 1995; Smith, 1995). Several representative syndromes known to cause hearing impairments are outlined in Table 6–1. Notice that different syndromes are associated with different kinds of hearing losses, some of which appear to be present at birth (congenital), whereas others are delayed in onset. Several other syndromes are discussed elsewhere in this chapter.

TABLE 6–1   Examples of syndromes that affect hearing

Syndrome	Inheritance	Hearing Loss	Characteristics
Alpert syndrome	Autosomal dominant	Conductive (congenital)	Craniofacial anomalies affecting the ears, stapes fixation, fused fingers and toes, and spina bifida; associated with conductive hearing loss
Alport syndrome	Autosomal dominant (types I, V, VI) X-linked (types II, III, IV)	Sensorineural (delayed onset, progressive)	Varies by type: renal disease, ocular disorders, blood plate defect, hearing loss
Alström syndrome	Autosomal recessive	Sensorineural (delayed onset progressive)	Retinitis pigmentosa, cataract, diabetes mellitus, obesity, hearing loss
Branchio-oto-renal syndrome	Autosomal dominant	Sensorineural conductive mixed, (congenital or delayed onset)	Outer, middle, inner ear deformities, branchial fistulas/cysts, renal disorders, hearing loss
Crouzon syndrome	Autosomal dominant	Conductive mixed (congenital)	Prematurely fused cranial sutures, beak-shaped nose, exophthalmos, variable outer/middle ear anomalies, hearing loss

Syndrome	Inheritance	Hearing Loss	Characteristics
Down (trisomy 21) syndrome	Chromosome abnormality	Conductive mixed	Multisystem disorder; mental retardation; characteristic facial features (tilted palpebral fissures, epicanthal folds, broad nasal bridge, flattened profile, open mouth with protruding tongue); outer/middle/inner ear hypoplasia have been reported; muscular hypotonia; short hands with simian line, congenital heart disease; frequent upper respiratory infections; recurrent otitis media, hearing loss
Friedreich's ataxia	Autosomal recessive	Sensorineural (delayed onset, progressive)	Ataxia, nystagmus, optic atrophy, hearing loss
Goldenhar syndrome (oculoauriculo-vertebral dysplasia)	Autosomal recessive	Conductive (congenital)	Facial asymmetry, microtia, atresia, preauricular tags, eye anomalies, oral defects, clubfoot, hemivertebrae, congenital heart disease, abnormal semicircular canals, hearing loss
Klippel-Feil sequence [a]	Autosomal dominant	Sensorineural conductive (congenital)	Fused cervical vertebrae, short neck, decreased head mobility, low occipital hairline, ossicle abnormalities, hearing loss
Hunter syndrome	X-linked	Sensorineural, conductive, mixed (progressive)	Skeletal deformities, dwarfism, coarse facial features, corneal clouding, cardiovascular disorders, mental retardation, mucopolysaccharide accumulations in tissues result in progressive characteristics, hearing loss, males affected only (cf. Hurler syndrome)
Hurler syndrome	Autosomal recessive	Sensorineural, conductive, mixed (progressive)	Same features as Hunter syndrome, but may be more severe, affects both sexes
Osteogenesis imperfecta	Autosomal dominant	Sensorineural, conductive, mixed (progressive)	Fragile bones, large skull, triangular facies, hemorrhage tendency, stapes fixation, hearing loss
Pendred syndrome	Autosomal dominant	Sensorineural (variable, congenital, progressive)	Hearing loss and thyroid enlargement (goiter), both variable, hearing loss
Treacher Collins syndrome (mandibulofacial dysostosis)	Autosomal dominant	Conductive, mixed (congenital)	Facial anomalies (depressed zygomatics, eyes slant downward laterally, receding mandible, mouth large and fish-like, dental anomalies, cleft palate); outer and middle ear deformities, hearing loss
Usher syndrome (Vestibulocerbellar ataxia)	Autosomal recessive	Sensorineural (congenital)	Usher I: retinitis pigmentosa, vestibular dysfunction, profound hearing loss Usher II: retinitis pigmentosa, sloping hearing loss (variable degree) (A third type may exist)

[a] A sequence is a group or pattern of abnormalities that result from a primary anomaly.

(continued)

Syndrome	Inheritance	Hearing Loss	Characteristics
Waardenburg syndrome	Autosomal dominant	Sensorineural (congenital)	White forelock in hair, prominent root of nose, differently colored eyes, hyperplasia of medial third of eyebrows, medial canthi displaced laterally; inner ear dysplasia, hearing loss

CHARGE Association   An **association** is a group of abnormalities that occur together too often to be due to chance. One such heterogeneous grouping that includes hearing impairment is called **CHARGE association** (Pagon, Graham, Zonana, & Yong, 1981), which stands for its major characteristics: (1) coloboma, which is a malformation of the iris (giving the pupil a "keyhole" appearance), disk, or retina; (2) congenital **h**eart defects; (3) **a**tresia of the choanae, so that the posterior nasal airway is obstructed; (4) retarded development and/or **g**rowth; and (5) **e**ar anomalies and/or hearing loss. The hearing loss is typically mixed and may be progressive. It is rare for one person to have all of the characteristics that can occur in CHARGE association, and the presence of any of these aberrations is reason enough to investigate for the presence of the others (Toriello, 1995).

Acquired Disorders

Head Trauma

Traumatic head injuries can cause conductive, sensorineural, and mixed hearing losses, depending on the nature and extent of the injuries. Head trauma causes a conductive hearing loss by such mechanisms as injuries to the eardrum and/or ossicles, accumulations of blood and debris in the ear canal and middle ear, and temporal bone fractures. Traumatic sensorineural losses are typically caused by concussion to the inner ear and fractures of the temporal bone directly injuring the inner ear structures.

Temporal bone fractures are classified according to whether the fracture line is in the same direction as the axis of the petrous pyramid (longitudinal) or across it (transverse). The relationships of these fractures to the structures of the ear are shown in Figure 6–3.

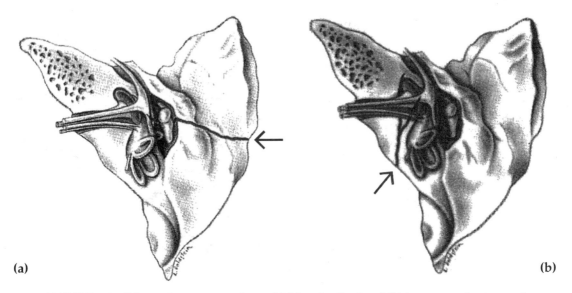

(a)   **(b)**

FIGURE 6–3   Schematic representations of (a) longitudinal and (b) transverse fractures of the temporal bone and how they relate to ear structures. Adapted from Swartz and Harnsberger (1998), with permission.

Longitudinal fractures go through the ear canal and middle ear and usually bypass the inner ear structures, so that they are most likely to produce conductive losses. About 80% of temporal bone fractures are longitudinal. In addition, concussion to the cochlea can result in a sensorineural loss (generally high-frequency) even though the inner ear structures are not directly involved in the longitudinal fracture. In contrast, **transverse fractures** cut through the inner ear, often resulting in profound sensorineural hearing loss and vertigo. Facial nerve paralysis occurs in about 50% of patients with transverse fractures. Mixed fractures are also common.

Outer Ear Disorders

Impacted Cerumen

Cerumen is a waxy substance that is supposed to be in the ear canal, where it serves lubricating and cleansing functions and also helps to protect the ear from bacteria, fungi, and insects. The cerumen is produced by glands in the cartilaginous portion of the ear canal and migrates out over time. Small amounts of cerumen often accumulate in normal ears, typically seen as yellow to brown globs that do not obstruct the ear canal. **Impacted cerumen** is an accumulation of wax in the ear canal that interferes with the flow of sound to the eardrum. Impacted cerumen occurs naturally in many patients who produce excessive amounts of cerumen, which builds up over time. It is also the fate of many Q-tip–wielding patients who inadvertently pack cerumen further back into the canal (and frequently against the eardrum) in an ironic attempt to clean their ears.

Impacted cerumen commonly produces conductive hearing loss, itching, tinnitus, vertigo, and external otitis. The hearing loss gradually worsens as the cerumen builds up, and can reach about 45 dB when the canal is completely occluded. Some patients may experience a "sudden" hearing loss in the shower or swimming pool if they have a small opening in the cerumen plug that is abruptly closed by the water.

The treatment for excessive cerumen is to remove it. **Cerumen management** procedures (e.g., Ballachanda & Peers, 1992; Roeser & Wilson, 2000) are undertaken only after an otoscopic examination and a complete history is taken. Cerumen removal may be preceded by the use of a wax softening product, and is accomplished by one technique or a combination of techniques including irrigation of the ear with water, removal with a blunt curette designed for this purpose, and by suction. Although cerumen management has traditionally been a medical function, it is now within the scope of audiological practice (e.g., ASHA, 1992, 1997).

Foreign Bodies

A seemingly endless assortment of **foreign bodies** can get into the ear. Some of these may get pushed into the ear where they can produce traumatic injuries to the canal wall, tympanic membrane, and middle ear structures. Others get stuck in the canal. Others do both. Foreign bodies that get stuck in the canal may be inorganic or organic, including live insects, and can produce the same effects as impacted cerumen *plus* traumatic injuries and/or infection depending on the nature of the object. Foreign objects in the ear should be removed by an otologist.

Growths and Tumors

The outer ear can be the site of cysts as well as benign and malignant tumors that should be addressed medically. Hearing becomes a factor if the ear canal is obstructed. **Exostoses** are the most common tumors of the ear canals, and are regularly encountered audiologically. These are benign, skin-covered bony growths from the canal walls that are smooth and rounded. They are usually found bilaterally. The development of exostoses is encouraged by repeated encounters with cold water and are common among swimmers. It is uncommon to find exostoses that will fully occlude the external auditory meatus by themselves, but their presence makes it easier for the canal to be blocked by cerumen or debris in the canal.

Infections

External otitis (otitis externa) is a diffuse infection of the external auditory meatus usually caused by pseudomonas (and less often by staphylococcus) bacteria. It is occasionally known as "swimmer's ear" because of its association with swimming in inadequately maintained pools. External otitis produces a considerable amount of pain, as well as edema (swelling), discharge, itching, and a conductive hearing loss if the canal is occluded by the swelling and debris. It is treated with antibiotic drops or creams that are frequently mixed with hydrocortisone to help reduce the edema. When there is considerable edema a gauze wick may be impregnated with the antibiotic/cortisone cream and gently pushed into the swollen ear canal to act as a medication applicator.

Otitis externa can develop into an aggressive and life-threatening form of the infection called **necrotizing (malignant) external otitis** in diabetics and other susceptible patients, and requires extensive antibiotic and other medical treatment.

The **furuncle** is an example of a more circumscribed outer ear infection. It is a staphylococcus infection of a hair follicle in the cartilaginous portion of the ear canal. Furuncles are treated with oral antibiotics, the placement of an alcohol-soaked wick in the ear canal until it spontaneously opens and drains, and/or incision and drainage of the furuncle under local anesthesia.

Middle Ear Disorders

Bullus myringitis is a very painful viral infection seen as inflamed, fluid-filled blebs or blister like sacs on the tympanic membrane and nearby ear canal walls. It often occurs in association with upper respiratory infections as well as with otitis media. Very little hearing loss is associated with this condition even though it does impair the mobility of the tympanic membrane to some extent. Bullus myringitis is usually self-limiting, and a thin fluid (perhaps with blood) is discharged when the blebs rupture. Antibiotics are often used to avoid secondary infections.

Tympanosclerosis refers to a variety of tissue changes that occur as the result of repeated middle ear infections. It is often seen as chalky white calcium plaques and scar tissue on the pars tense of the eardrum, which has little if any effect on hearing sensitivity. Tympanosclerosis also affects the other structures of the middle ear, and can affect hearing if the calcification or other changes impair the mobility of the ossicular chain.

Perforations of the tympanic membrane can be caused by ear infections and various kinds of traumatic insults. Typical traumatic causes include (1) punctures; (2) chemical injuries; and (3) forceful pressure changes due to an explosion, a slap to the ear, intense sound (**acoustic trauma**), and sudden changes in air pressure while flying or water pressure while diving (**barotrauma**). As illustrated in Figure 6–4, the opening is described as a central, marginal, or attic perforation, according to its location on the eardrum. Attic perforations involve the pars flaccida and are often associated with cholesteatoma, as discussed below. Eardrum perforations produce conductive hearing losses because they (1) reduce the size of the drum's vibrating

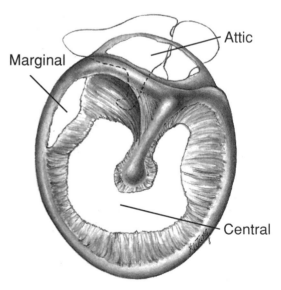

FIGURE 6–4 Examples of central, marginal, and attic perforations of the tympanic membrane. Adapted from Hughes (1985), with permission.

surface area, which reduces the eardrum-to-oval window area advantage; (2) impair the coupling of the eardrum to the ossicular chain so that signal transmission is reduced; and (3) interfere with the proper phase relationship at the oval and round windows by allowing sound to impact upon the round window. In general, the magnitude of the conductive hearing loss gets worse as the size of the perforation increases.

Many tympanic membrane perforations heal spontaneously. Healed perforations are associated with the development of *scar tissue* and thin areas that do not have a fibrous middle layer, which are sometimes called *monomeric membranes*. Larger perforations and those associated with chronic middle ear infections generally do not heal on their own, and require a surgical repair of the eardrum called a **myringoplasty**.

Otitis Media and Associated Pathologies

Inflammations of the middle ear are called **otitis media**, and constitute the most common cause of conductive hearing losses. Otitis media affects people of all ages, but the incidence among children is particularly high. For example, most children have at least one case of otitis media by age 3, and at least three episodes occur by age 3 in about 33% of children overall and in about 80% of those in day-care centers (Denny, 1984; Teele, Klein, & Rosner, 1984; Preliner, Kalm, & Harsten, 1992).

The implications of otitis media in children go beyond the medical ramifications of the pathology and the direct interference with communication caused by the conductive hearing loss. Young children with recurrent otitis media are subjected to frequent and sustained periods of conductive hearing impairment during critical learning periods. For this reason, recurrent otitis media in young children has been associated with deficits affecting auditory processing, language development, cognitive and academic skills (e.g., Jerger, Jerger, Alford, & Abrams, 1983; Friel-Patti & Finitzo, 1990; Menjuk, 1992;

Gravel & Wallace, 1992; Brown, 1994; Downs, 1995; Schwartz, Mody, & Petinou, 1997; Mody, Schwartz, Gravel, & Ruben, 1999).

Otitis media can take on several forms depending on such factors as the development and time course of the disease, whether a bacterial infection is present, the nature of the fluid in the middle ear space, and the kinds of complications that exist. The easiest way to address these issues is to trace the development of the disease.

A properly functioning Eustachian tube provides the middle ear with ventilation and drainage, and maintains the same amount of pressure on both sides of the tympanic membrane. **Eustachian tube dysfunction** exists when the tube does not open properly, is not patent, or is blocked in one way or another. The tube might be blocked by edema (swelling) and/or fluid caused by an upper respiratory infection, sinusitis, inflamed adenoids, or allergies; obstruction by hypertrophic (enlarged) adenoids; or obstruction or encroachment by a nasopharyngeal tumor or other growth. The Eustachian tube may fail to open appropriately (e.g., upon swallowing or yawning) due to structural or functional abnormalities affecting the tensor palatini muscle. This problem is common among cleft palate patients.

Unlike the adult Eustachian tube, which tilts downward by about 45°, infants and young children have almost horizontal Eustachian tubes (Fig. 6–5), which are also

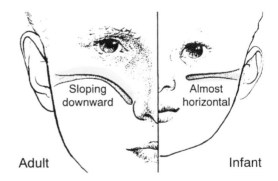

FIGURE 6–5 The Eustachian tube slopes downward in adults but is closer to being horizontal in infants and young children. Adapted from Pulec and Horwitz (1973), with permission.

relatively shorter and wider; in addition to which their tensor palatini muscles operate less efficiently. These factors, which improve with growth and development, increase the chances of Eustachian tube dysfunction and middle ear disease among infants and young children.

Eustachian tube dysfunction prevents the middle ear from being ventilated, causing the air within the middle ear cavity to become stagnant. Part of the stagnant air is then absorbed by the tissues of the middle ear. As a result, the air pressure will be lower inside the middle ear than it is outside in the surrounding atmosphere. This situation is called **negative pressure** in the middle ear.[4] This pressure difference on the two sides of the tympanic membrane (higher outside, lower inside) causes it to be drawn inward, or **retracted**. The same nonpatency of the Eustachian tube that caused the air to be trapped within the middle ear cavity also prevents ventilation of the middle ear that would reequalize the pressure and "unclog" the ears. If this problem is caused by an abrupt pressure change, it is called **aerotitis** or **barotrauma**. Aerotitis is usually caused by the abrupt air pressure increase of an airplane descent, which causes the tympanic membrane to retract and prevents the Eustachian tube from opening.

The next step in the development of otitis media is **effusion**, or the accumulation of fluid. The presence of fluid in the middle ear is described as **otitis media with effusion**. In their clinical practice guideline pertaining to young children, Stool, Berg, Berman, Carney, Cooley, Culpepper, Eavey, Feagans, Finitzo, Friedman, et al (1994) defined otitis media with effusion as the presence of middle ear fluid in the absence of infection, although this restriction on the definition is not universal. Different kinds of effusions may accumulate in the middle ear. **Serous fluid** is a watery and clear transudate that is free of cells and other materials, whereas **mucoid fluid** is an

exudate that is thicker, cloudy, and more viscous, containing white blood cells and other cellular material. The effusion may also contain blood from broken vessels. Blood in the middle ear is called **hemotympanum**. Effusions initially contain serous fluid that is drawn from the middle ear tissues by the negative pressure. This is **serous otitis media**. Continuation of the process may involve mucoid fluid from secretory (goblet) cells in the middle ear mucosa. At this stage the condition would be described as **secretory otitis media**. The term **mucoid otitis media** would eventually be applied with the continued thickening of the effusion. Because serous fluid is absorbed by the middle ear mucosa with time, the effusion can become progressively thicker and more viscous, eventually leading to **adhesive otitis media** or "**glue ear**," which causes a conductive loss by preventing the motion of the ossicles.

Middle ear fluid can sometimes be detected otoscopically by seeing a fluid line or **meniscus** if the middle ear is not completely filled with liquid, or by the presence of bubbles. It is often not possible to distinguish between the presence or absence of effusion if the tympanum is completely filled with serous fluid. The ability to accurately diagnose a fluid-filled middle ear effusion involves the use of a **pneumatic** or **Siegel otoscope** (Stool et al, 1994), which has a rubber bulb and tube that allows the examiner to change the air pressure against the eardrum (by squeezing the bulb). Middle ear fluid is indicated if the air pressure fails to cause observable eardrum movement. However, it is difficult at best to differentiate between serous and secretory otitis, and many otologists consider the distinction to be academic.

So far we have been assuming that the patient has a middle ear effusion that is **nonsuppurative** or **nonpurulent**, which means that it is free of bacterial infection. However, middle ear fluid is a wonderful place for bacteria to live, so that infections can readily develop once the microbes gain access to the middle ear. The usual route to the middle ear is from the nasopharynx via the Eustachian tube. Otitis media becomes **suppurative** or **purulent** when bacteria invade the middle

---

[4] The nonpatent Eustachian tube explanation appears to account for negative pressures up to only about −100 dekapascal (daPa) (Cantekin et al, 1980; Yee & Cantekin, 1986), so that other mechanisms may also be involved in creating abnormally negative middle ear pressures.

ear system. The most common bacteria responsible for **acute suppurative otitis media** are *Streptococcus pneumoniae, Haemophilus influenzae,* and *Branhamella catarrhalis.*

Acute purulent (suppurative) otitis media typically occurs during or soon after an upper respiratory infection. The typical course of events begins with **hyperemia** (engorgement of the tissues with blood), often seen as reddening on the tympanic membrane, accompanied by **otalgia** (ear pain) and possibly fever. After a couple of days this is followed by **exudation**, in which the middle ear space is filled with fluid containing white blood cells, red blood cells, mucus, and other materials. The eardrum is red and thickened so that landmarks cannot be seen, and it bulges due to pressure from the exudate in the middle ear. This comes with increased pain, fever, and a conductive hearing loss. The **suppuration** stage occurs when the building pressure causes the eardrum to rupture, resulting in the drainage of pus and other materials from the infected middle ear. Such a purulent discharge from the ear is called **otorrhea**. It is preferable for the drainage to be effected by a small surgical incision of the eardrum, called a myringotomy. (The indications for a myringotomy are discussed below.) Drainage relieves the pressure and pain, and there is often spontaneous healing of the tympanic membrane.

Ongoing or repeated episodes of acute otitis media are called **chronic otitis media**, which is often associated with a perforated tympanic membrane. However, ongoing ear pathology can occur even without a perforation. Hence, the distinction between acute and chronic otitis media may also be made on the basis of how long the disease lasts. For example, a case of otitis media might be **acute** if it lasts up to 3 weeks, **chronic** if it lasts more than 12 weeks, and **subacute** for intermediate durations. One often encounters the term **recurrent otitis media** for the same reason. Some cases of chronic otitis media with intact eardrums are not detected clinically or may even be undetectable, and have been termed **silent otitis media** (Paparella, Goycoolea, Bassiouni, & Koutroupas, 1986).

Complications and Sequelae of Otitis Media

Otitis media can result in quite a few sequelae and complications of major medical significance, some of which can have life-threatening consequences. Cholesteatoma is a common problem, and is discussed below. Facial paralysis can result if the infection erodes the fallopian canal and affects the seventh cranial nerve. Spread of the infection to the inner ear results in labyrinthitis. Recall that the tympanum communicates with the mastoid antrum and air cell system, so that otitis media can spread to infect the mastoid, producing **mastoiditis**. Mastoiditis can lead to the further spread of the infection to the central nervous system, as well as to other sites.

Conductive hearing loss is certainly the effect with which we are most directly concerned. Any amount of conductive loss can occur with otitis media, and fluctuation is common. These audiograms tend to be reasonably flat, but it is not uncommon to find losses that are poorer in the low frequencies, and others that are somewhat tent-shaped (Fig. 6–6). Otitis media can also cause a sensorineural loss, particularly in the high frequencies. The sensorineural component may be caused by the transmission of toxins to the perilymph via the round window. However, conductive lesions can affect bone-conduction thresholds, which might account for some of the sensorineural components seen in these patients, at least in part (see Chapter 5, and the section on otosclerosis in this chapter).

Otitis media can lead to a continuing conductive hearing loss by causing such conditions as (1) perforated eardrums; (2) adhesions, tympanosclerosis, and glue ear, which restrict or prevent motion of the ossicles; and (3) ossicular chain discontinuities that occur when the infective process causes part of the chain to be eroded away.

A **cholesteatoma** is a cyst made of layers of keratin producing squamous epithelium filled with an accumulation of keratin and cellular debris. It is also known as a **keratoma** or an **epidermoid inclusion cyst**. Even though *keratoma* is the less popular term, it is actually

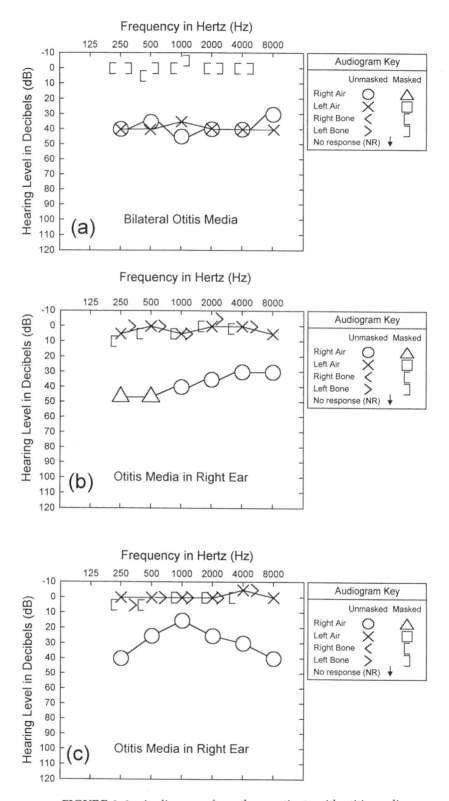

FIGURE 6–6   Audiograms from three patients with otitis media.

more appropriate because cholesteatomas contain considerable amounts of keratin but little if any cholesterol.

Cholesteatomas are usually associated with chronic otitis media, and with perforated and retracted tympanic membranes. They also occur spontaneously in a small percentage of patients and can develop in the middle ear, eardrum, or petrous portion, and even intracranially. The most common sites for cholesteatoma formation are pars flaccida and marginal perforations. Let us consider the development of an attic cholesteatoma, which is a very common type. The cholesteatoma might begin as a small retracted pouch (retraction pocket) in the pars flaccida, often encouraged by ongoing negative pressure in the middle ear. The sac retains keratin and debris. Inflammation of the sac causes it to swell and expand. The cholesteatoma may lie dormant for some time, or it may grow slowly or quickly. The invasion route begins in the epitympanic recess, or attic, as shown in Figure 6–7. Notice in the figure that a cholesteatoma that appears tiny when viewed from the outside can actually be quite large. The expanding cholesteatoma destructively encroaches upon the middle ear space and

structures. As it continues to grow, the cholesteatoma has the potential to invade other locations, such as the mastoid, labyrinth, and cranium. This aggressive capability makes the cholesteatoma a potentially life-threatening lesion that must be removed surgically.

Infections (as well as traumatic injuries) can also result in various kinds of middle ear defects, such as **ossicular discontinuities**, which are interruptions in the ossicular chain, and other disorders that prevent the ossicular chain from vibrating effectively or at all, such as extensive tympanosclerosis or adhesions. Figure 6–8 compares a normal conductive system to a simple perforation, a perforation with an ossicular chain interruption involving the malleus, and an ossicular discontinuity with an intact eardrum.

Treatment of Otitis Media and Related Pathologies

Acute otitis media is generally treated with oral antibiotics. Typical choices are amoxicillin, ampicillin, erythromycin, trimethoprim-sulfa preparations, and cephalosporins, depending on the microbe and the patient's drug sensitivities. The effectiveness of anti-

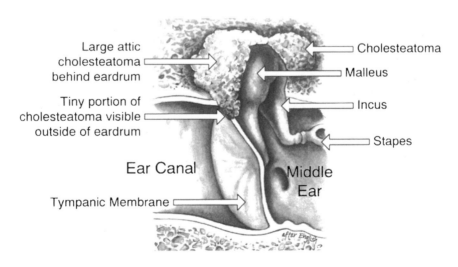

FIGURE 6–7 Example of a large attic cholesteatoma. Notice that only a tiny portion of the cholesteatoma is visible outside the tympanic membrane. Adapted from Hughes (1985), with permission.

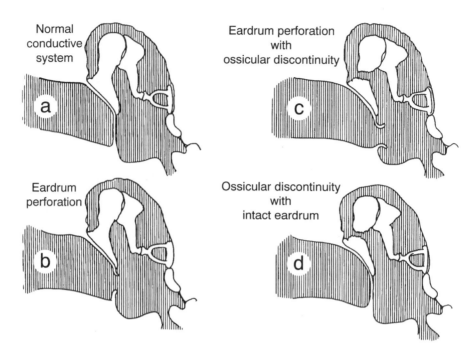

FIGURE 6–8 (a) Normal tympanic membrane and ossicular chain; (b) perforated eardrum with intact ossicles; (c) perforated eardrum with interrupted ossicular chain due to eroded malleus; (d) intact eardrum with interrupted ossicular chain due to eroded malleus. Adapted from Hughes and Pensak (1997), with permission.

histamines and decongestants is questionable, unless the underlying problem is allergic.

Several mechanical methods can also be used to ventilate clogged ears by opening the patient's nonpatent Eustachian tubes. Patients can use the **Valsalva maneuver**, provided they do not have an upper respiratory infection that could be spread to the middle ear. This method involves forcing the Eustachian tube open by blowing forcefully with the mouth closed tightly and the nose pinched closed. The middle ear can also be ventilated by **politzerization**. This procedure uses a rubber tube with a compressible rubber bulb. The physician places the free end of the tube into one nostril (with the other one pinched closed) and air is forced in by squeezing the bulb. Other air pressure sources can also be used. An effective but thoroughly unpleasant method for ventilating the middle ear involves forcing air directly into the Eustachian tube orifice in the nasopharynx through a catheter inserted into the nose.

Adenoidectomy (removal of the adenoids) is considered a treatment for recurrent otitis media with effusion in children when the problem can be attributed to a blockage of the Eustachian tube by hypertrophic adenoids. Some otolaryngologists may also perform a **tonsillectomy** (removal of the tonsils) in combination with the adenoidectomy. It appears that children with middle ear effusion may be helped by adenoidectomy, but adding a tonsillectomy does not provide any additional benefit (e.g., Mau, 1984; Stool et al, 1994).

A **myringotomy** or **paracentesis** is a surgical incision in the tympanic membrane usually performed for the purpose of draining the middle ear. Myringotomies are commonly done in children who have persistent or recurrent middle ear effusions to remove the fluid, thereby alleviating the conductive hearing loss, and helping prevent recurrences by keeping the middle ear ventilated. In cases of acute otitis media, myringotomies may be performed to prevent the rupturing of a markedly distended eardrum, and when there is severe pain, high fever, toxicity, evidence of medical complications, or poor responsiveness to antibiotics.

The myringotomy procedure is straightforward (Fig. 6–9): A small incision is made in the eardrum, which is commonly placed in the anteroinferior quadrant. The fluid is then aspirated (removed with suction) from the middle ear. Finally, a **pressure equalization (PE)** or **ventilation tube** (or **grommet**) is usually inserted into the incision to keep it open. These tubes are made of many different kinds of materials and come in a wide variety of designs. The purpose of the PE tube becomes apparent when we realize that removing the fluid does not fix the Eustachian tube problem, which is usually the underlying culprit. Pressure equalization tubes help prevent the recurrence of effusions by keeping the middle ear ventilated and preventing the development of negative pressure, and also provide a route for any continued drainage. In effect, ventilation tubes replace the functions of a dysfunctional Eustachian tube. Ventilation tubes are usually left in place for several months or until they are naturally extruded by the eardrum. The major concerns are (1) clogging or premature extrusion of the tubes, (2) water getting into the middle ear through the tubes, (3) persistence of the Eustachian tube blockage leading to recurrence of the disease once the tubes are out, and (4) medical complications such as otorrhea, tympanosclerosis, and cholesteatoma.

At least three kinds of audiological services are important for patients with ventilation tubes: (1) Custom-made earplugs often called "swimming earmolds" are needed to prevent water from entering the middle ear via the PE tubes when the patient swims, showers, and engages in similar activities. (2) Periodic monitoring with acoustic immittance tests (Chapter 7) is needed to determine if the PE tube is still in place and patent, or if it has become clogged or dislodged. (3) Audiological assessments are necessary so that residual hearing impairments or changes in hearing over time can be identified and addressed. Notice that the first two activities address

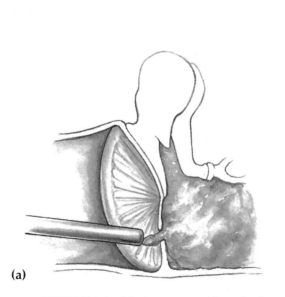

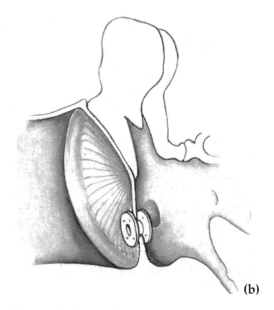

(a)

(b)

FIGURE 6–9 Myringotomy with aspiration of middle ear fluid (a) and placement of a pressure equalization tube in the eardrum (b). Adapted from Hughes (1985), with permission.

medical concerns and the status of the PE tube. The third directly addresses the patient's auditory status.

Surgery for more severe cases of otitis media and mastoiditis is less common than in the past when antibiotics were unavailable. However, surgery is still necessary for chronic conditions, when antibiotics are not fully effective, and when the infection becomes sufficiently severe, such as when it invades bone tissue. Cholesteatomas must always be removed unless the patient has general medical/surgical contraindications for surgery. Usage varies, but the term **mastoidectomy** generally describes the surgical removal of disease, and **tympanoplasty** often refers to the surgical reconstruction of the eardrum and middle ear structures. The two may be done in one combined procedure, or surgical reconstruction may be attempted at a later time, after the disease has been alleviated. A **radical mastoidectomy** is done when the disease is so widespread, severe, or aggressive that the surgeon must remove much or all of the mastoid along with the entire contents of the middle ear. As expected from the description of what is removed, a radical mastoidectomy leaves the patient with a structural defect called a mastoidectomy cavity and a very large conductive hearing loss. Thus, it is important for the patient to understand that the purpose of this kind of surgery is to preserve life rather than to address a hearing loss.

A **modified radical mastoidectomy** involves the surgical removal of the pathological tissue and alleviation of the disease process without sacrificing the eardrum and ossicles. An optimal result does not necessarily worsen the hearing loss, and might even improve hearing to some extent by removing a lesion that interferes with sound transmission or by being done in combination with a tympanoplasty. This approach is often used when there is a cholesteatoma in locations such as the attic or antrum. A **simple mastoidectomy** removes diseased tissue in the mastoid without "breaking through" the posterior canal wall (which would constitute

a modified radical mastoidectomy). Surgery to reconstruct the sound transmission system and restore hearing is covered later in this chapter.

Otosclerosis

Otosclerosis is a disease of the temporal bone in which normal bone is progressively resorbed and replaced with *spongy* bone that may harden to become sclerotic. Many authorities prefer to call the disorder **otospongiosis** because of the spongy nature of the otosclerotic deposits. Otosclerosis develops at isolated locations and usually affects the oval window and stapedial footplate (**stapedial otosclerosis**). Otoscerlosis is usually bilateral, but often progresses at different rates for the two ears. **Clinical otosclerosis** exists when the patient begins to experience a hearing problem due to the disorder. This occurs because the otosclerotic material interferes with the normal motion of the stapedial footplate at the oval window, eventually resulting in complete **ankylosis** or **fixation** (Fig. 6–10). The progressive and eventually complete impediment of the ossicular chain's ability to effectively transmit signals to the cochlea produces a progressive conductive hearing loss. **Cochlear otosclerosis** may occur in advanced cases, in which case the disease process encroaches upon the inner ear, adding a sensorineural component to the hearing loss. Stapedial fixation that occurs in association with fragile, easily fractured bones (**osteogenesis imperfecta tarda**) and a bluish tint to the whites of the eyes (**blue sclerae**) is known as **van der Hoeve's syndrome**, and may be related to otosclerosis.

Patients with otosclerosis usually complain about a slowly progressive *hearing loss* that is frequently accompanied by *tinnitus*, and they often typify the characteristics of conductive losses that were outlined earlier in the chapter. Assuming that otosclerosis is the only problem, these patients generally have no other otologic or related complaints and are otoscopically normal. However, it is

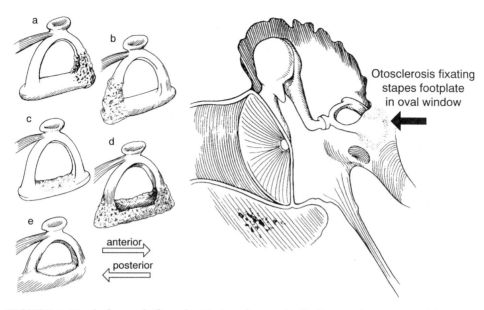

FIGURE 6–10   Left panel: Otosclerotic involvement affecting various parts of the stape-dial footplate [(a) to (d)] as well as complete obliteration of the oval window (e). Right panel: Otosclerosis fixating the stapes in the oval window. Adapted from Hughes (1985), with permission.

sometimes possible to see a reddish/pinkish coloration of the cochlear promontory through the eardrum called **Schwartze's sign**, which is due to vascularization associated with active otosclerosis. The following generalities about otosclerosis can be helpful when assessing a patient's case history, and also reveal that it is a multifactorial disorder with both hereditary and nonhereditary components: (1) otosclerosis tends to run in families; (2) it typically begins to show up clinically during the second to fourth decades of life; (3) it is about twice as common in women than in men; and (4) progression is often noticed in association with hormonally active periods like pregnancy and menopause.

The audiological picture of otosclerosis involves a conductive hearing loss in the affected ear(s). The size of the loss depends on the degree of progression of the disease at the time of testing and can be anywhere from mild to as severe as 65 to 70 dB HL. The loss tends to be somewhat worse in the lower frequencies, at least initially (Fig. 6–11a), and

flatter as the loss progresses. In addition, there is often an elevation of the bone-conduction threshold at 2000 Hz, called **Carhart's notch** (Carhart, 1950). However, this does not reflect a true sensorineural component of the disorder. Instead, Carhart's notch is thought to occur because the mechanical advantage provided by the 2000-Hz resonance of the ossicular chain is altered by the ankylosis, which prevents the ossicles from vibrating normally. Moreover, it can be alleviated by surgery that restores normal ossicular chain vibration. This should not be altogether surprising. Recall from Chapter 5 that it is not unusual for conductive impairments to affect bone-conduction thresholds. In more advanced cases the presence of cochlear otosclerosis will add a sensorineural component to the conductive loss produced by stapedial otosclerosis, resulting in a mixed loss (Fig. 6–11b). The typical acoustic immittance characteristics of otosclerosis include essentially normal tympanometric peak pressure, abnormally low static acoustic admittance, and absent acoustic reflexes.

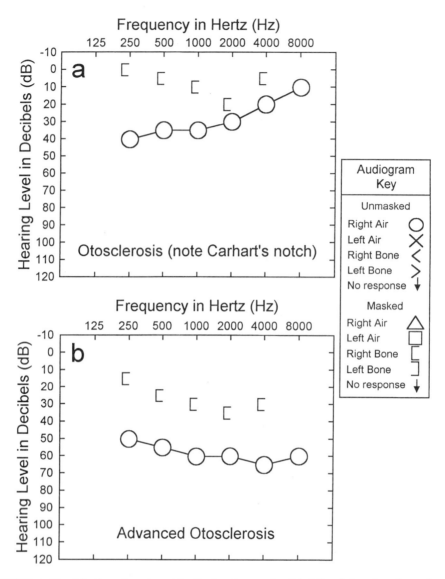

FIGURE 6–11 (a) Otosclerosis with Carhart's notch. (b) Mixed hearing loss due to advanced cochlear and stapedial otosclerosis. (Opposite ears not shown for clarity.)

Surgery is often considered the treatment of choice for otosclerosis that produces a clinically significant hearing impairment because it is the only available means to ameliorate the conductive loss. Hearing aids are a viable alternative, particularly when surgery is not indicated, but of course cannot reverse the loss or arrest its progression. Shambaugh and Causse (1974) found that medical treatment with sodium fluoride was successful in arresting the progression of oto-

sclerosis in 80% of 4000 patients, but yielded some degree of improvement in only 3%. A "good candidate" for otosclerosis surgery should be medically appropriate for elective surgery and the risks it entails, and should have a substantial conductive hearing loss (air-bone-gap), normal or near-normal bone-conduction thresholds, and a relatively good speech recognition score for the ear in question. The latter two criteria are sometimes referred to as good "cochlear reserve."

Surgery to Improve/Restore Hearing

Otosclerosis Surgery

The three general types of operations that have been used to improve hearing in cases of otosclerosis are the fenestration (Lempert, 1938), stapes mobilization (Rosen, 1953), and stapedectomy (Shea, 1958) procedures.[5] The **fenestration** procedure (Lempert, 1938) completely bypasses the fixated stapes and was a popular operation for otosclerosis for quite some time. The incus and most of the malleus are excised. The unusable oval window is replaced by a new window (*fenestra*) that is drilled into the lateral semicircular canal and covered with a soft tissue flap derived from the tympanic membrane. The new fenestra enables sound to be transmitted to the cochlea by taking advantage of the shared perilymph system of the hearing and balance parts of the inner ear, provided that the round window is still compliant. Fenestrations successfully reduce the size of large conductive losses to about 25 to 30 dB, but do not completely eliminate air-bone-gaps because they do not restore the middle ear transformer mechanism.

Stapes mobilization directly addresses the fixated stapes by palpating the incus, incudostapedial joint, and/or stapes until the footplate essentially breaks free of its fixation by the otosclerotic growth and is again mobilized in the oval window. Compared to fenestration, the surgery involved in stapes mobilization is far less extensive and invasive, and has fewer complications. It also effectively reestablishes the normal physiologic activity of the ossicular chain. However, refixation of the stapes often occurs over time, which of course comes with recurrence of the hearing loss.

Stapes mobilizations and fenestrations have been almost completely replaced by the **stapedectomy** operation and its variations. A total stapedectomy involves removing the ankylosed stapes and footplate, and sealing the oval window with a connective tissue or

vein graft, or some other suitable material. The stapes is then replaced with a **prosthesis** that connects the incus to the oval window, and thus reestablishes the ability of the ossicular chain to transmit signals to the cochlea via the normal route. The prosthesis itself may be a wire, strut, or piston made of a synthetic material, metal, cartilage, etc. The procedure is illustrated in Figures 6–12a,b. A **partial stapedectomy** may be done if only the anterior aspect of the stapes is fixated (the most common site). It involves removing only the anterior footplate and anterior crus, leaving the posterior crus to transmit signals to the cochlea. **Stapedotomy** (Fisch, 1980; Lesinski, 1989) is a modification of the stapedectomy in which the fixated stapedial footplate is left in the oval window. A hole (fenestra) is then bored through the footplate using either a drill or a laser. One end of a piston prosthesis is then inserted into the fenestra and the other end is attached to the incus, completing the connection between the oval window and the ossicular chain (Figs. 6-12c,d). Assuming a normal cochlea, stapedectomies tend to result in normal or near-normal hearing in about 80 to 90% of cases, with a 1 to 3% risk of deafness. Stapedotomy outcomes appear to be at least comparable to those obtained by stapedectomy (McGee, 1981; Levy, Shvero, & Hadar, 1990). Success rates are low and complication rates are higher for revision stapedectomies, that is, when an ear is operated on again due to progression of the otosclerosis or complications. When surgery is planned for both ears it is desirable to operate on one ear first (the poorer one if there is a difference) and to defer the second procedure for at least several months to ensure that the initial result has been successful and that no delayed complications have arisen.

Tympanoplasty

Structural defects of the conductive system may be the result of a congenital anomaly, injury, or disease. The surgical repair and reconstruction of the tympanic membrane and/or middle ear is known as a **tym-**

---

[5] The origins of these procedures actually date back to the latter part of the 19th century (Jahn, 1981).

Stapedectomy

Stapedotomy

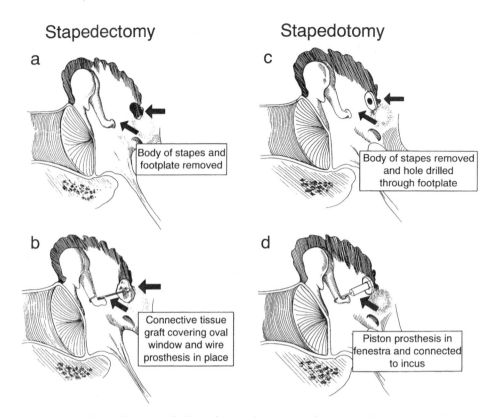

a

Body of stapes and footplate removed

b

Connective tissue graft covering oval window and wire prosthesis in place

c

Body of stapes removed and hole drilled through footplate

d

Piston prosthesis in fenestra and connected to incus

FIGURE 6–12   Stapedectomy (left) and stapedotomy (right) procedures for otosclerosis. Adapted from Hughes (1985), with permission.

panoplasty, and is intended to resolve (or at least minimize) the conductive hearing loss due to structural deficits. These procedures may be done along with operations used to eradicate the ear disease (e.g., mastoidectomy), or at a later time, depending on what is medically and surgically appropriate.

Traditional tympanoplasty procedures are classified by type from I to V. We will outline the traditional classifications, but one should be aware that quite a few classification systems have been proposed (e.g., Farrior, 1968; Bellucci, 1973; Kley, 1982; Wullstein & Wullstein, 1990; Tos, 1993). According to the classical approach, a simple perforated eardrum is repaired with a *type I tympanoplasty* or **myringoplasty**, and typically results in normal or near-normal hearing. It involves patching the eardrum defect with a graft made of various materials, such as muscle facie, perichondrium, and homografts (transplanted

material). Types II to IV are used when there is an ossicular discontinuity, providing that the remaining segments of the ossicular chain leading to the oval window are mobile so that they can transmit vibrations to the cochlea. Depending on what is missing, the eardrum graft may be attached to the incus (*type II*, head of the stapes (*type III*), or even to the stapes footplate (*type IV*). The *type V* tympanoplasty is used when the stapes footplate is fixated rather than mobile. In the traditional procedure (*type Va*) the fixated footplate is ignored, and a new window (fenestra) is drilled into the horizontal semicircular canal, to which the eardrum graft is connected. Sizable air-bone-gaps can remain after these procedures because they do not fully restore the middle ear transformer mechanism (especially in types IV and V). The traditional approaches have largely been superseded by ossicular reconstruction methods that bridge the gap in the ossicular chain with a bone or cartilage graft, or by substituting the missing structures with a homograft or a prosthesis. The traditional type Va tympanoplasty has largely been replaced by the *type Vb* procedure, which uses a prosthesis to bridge the missing ossicles and to transmit signals to the oval window, as in the stapedectomy operation for otosclerosis.

Growths and Tumors

Benign and malignant tumors can occur anywhere in the temporal bone, including the tympanum, although middle ear tumors are relatively rare. **Glomus tumors** (paragangliomas or chemodectomas) are particularly relevant audiologically (Woods, Strasnick, & Jackson, 1993; Baguley, Irving, Hardy, Harada, & Moffat, 1994). Glomus tumors are highly vascular tumors that arise from glomus bodies (which serve as chemoreceptors) that are associated with branches of the glossopharyngeal and vagus (ninth and tenth cranial) nerves that course through the temporal bone, as well as elsewhere in the body. They are called **glomus tympanicum tumors** when they develop within the middle ear cavity and **glomus jugulare tumors** when they develop from the crest of the jugular bulb under the floor of the middle ear. Glomus tumors invade the middle ear and other parts of the temporal bone, and can also extend intracranially. They are usually unilateral and are more common in women than in men by a ratio of roughly three-to-one. The most common characteristics of patients with glomus tumors are pulsing tinnitus that is synchronized to the patient's vascular pulse and a conductive or mixed hearing loss, which is unilateral in a wide majority of cases. Bleeding from the ear occurs in some cases, and patients may also experience a feeling of pressure in the ear. Other complaints may also occur but are highly variable. Glomus tumors are usually seen as a reddish mass behind the tympanic membrane, often with a "rising sun" appearance; one might also see it pulsating, and possibly causing the eardrum to bulge. Glomus tumors are treated surgically.

Cochlear Disorders

Noise-Induced Hearing Loss

High sound levels can produce both temporary and permanent hearing losses due to over stimulation and/or mechanical trauma (Miller, 1974; Schmiedt, 1984; Henderson & Hamernik, 1986; Saunders, Dear, & Schneider, 1985; Boettcher, Henderson, Gratton, Danielson, & Byrne, 1987; Clark, 1991; Hamernik and Hsueh, 1991; Hamernik, Ahroon, & Hsueh, 1991; Melnick, 1991; Saunders, Cohen, & Szymko, 1991; Ward, 1991). A sensorineural hearing loss produced by the damaging effects of overstimulation by high sound levels, usually over a long period of time, is called a **noise-induced hearing loss**. In contrast, the term *acoustic trauma* usually refers to the hearing loss produced by extremely intense and impulsive sounds like explosions or gun shots. They can mechanically traumatize the eardrum, middle ear, and/or cochlear structures in addition to producing damage by overstimulation, and often from a single insult.

Almost everybody has experienced temporary hearing difficulty (often with tinnitus) after being exposed to high sound levels of one kind or another, such as loud music, construction noise, lawn mowers, subways, etc. This short-term decrease in hearing sensitivity is sensorineural in nature and is called a **temporary threshold shift (TTS)**. In general, a TTS can be produced by sound levels greater than about 80 dB sound pressure level (SPL). As the intensity and/or duration of the offending sound increases, the size of the TTS gets bigger and the time it takes for recovery gets longer. A **permanent threshold shift (PTS)** exists when the TTS does not recover completely, that is, when hearing sensitivity does not return to normal. Because PTS could refer to just about any permanent hearing loss, we generally lengthen the term to **noise-induced permanent threshold shift (NIPTS)** for clarity. The nature and severity of a NIPTS is determined by the intensity, spectrum, duration, and time course of the offending sounds; the overall duration of the exposures over the years; and the patient's individual susceptibility to the effects of noise. In addition, the amount of hearing loss produced by noise exposure is exacerbated if vibration is also present and by the use of potentially ototoxic drugs.

The kinds of anatomical and physiological abnormalities caused by noise exposure range from the most subtle disruptions of hair cell metabolic activities and losses of stereocilia rigidity (leading to "floppy cilia") to the complete degeneration of the organ of Corti and the auditory nerve supply. Some of the abnormalities include metabolic exhaustion of the hair cells, structural changes and degeneration of structures within the hair cells, morphological changes of the cilia (so that they become fused and otherwise distorted), ruptures of cell membranes, and complete degeneration and loss of hair cells, neural cells, and supporting cells. Mild metabolic disruptions and floppy cilia can be reversible, and are thought to be related to TTS. Greater amounts of interference and damage are associated with permanent hearing losses. Both outer and inner hair cells are damaged by noise, but outer hair cells are more susceptible.

Noise-induced impairments are usually associated with a notch-shaped high-frequency sensorineural loss that is worst at 4000 Hz (Fig. 6–13), although the notch often occurs at 3000 or 6000 Hz, as well. The reason for the notch in this region is not definitively established. One explanation is that this region is most susceptible to damage due to the biology and mechanics of the cochlea. Another rationale is that commonly encountered noises have broad spectra that reach the cochlea with a boost in the 2000- to 4000-Hz region because of the resonance characteristics of the outer and middle ear. Noise-induced losses tend to be bilateral and more or less symmetrical; however, there are many exceptions, especially when one ear has been subjected to more noise than the other.

Not all "noise-induced" audiograms conform to the idealized picture in Figure 6–13. Analyses of the progression of noise-induced hearing losses across many studies have revealed that the general audiometric pattern of noise-induced hearing loss evolves as noise exposure continues over the course of many years (Passchier-Vermeer, 1974; Rösler, 1994). The hearing loss typically begins as a notch at 4000 Hz. As noise exposure continues, the notch widens to include a wider range of frequencies, but continues to progress most

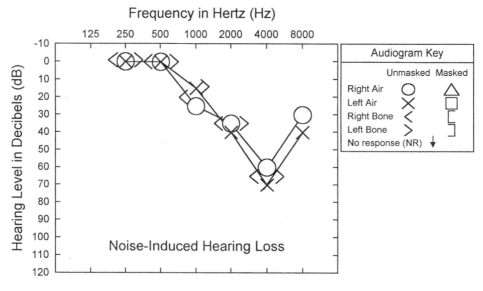

FIGURE 6–13   The audiogram of a patient with a bilateral sensorineural hearing loss due to noise exposure.

noticeably at 4000 Hz. After perhaps 10 to 15 years of exposure, the progression of the loss at 4000 Hz often slows down, and progression now becomes more apparent at other frequencies, such as 2000 Hz.

Meniere's Disease

Meniere's disease or syndrome (endolymphatic hydrops) is an inner ear disease attributed to excessive endolymphatic fluid pressure in the membranous labyrinth, causing Reissner's membrane to become distended. It is characterized by episodic attacks of (1) vertigo, (2) hearing loss, (3) tinnitus, and (4) a feeling of fullness or pressure in the ear. Attacks last for as little as 20 minutes or as long as several hours. The tinnitus is usually described as roaring or as a low pitch noise, but this can vary. The vertigo can be extremely severe and debilitating and is the principal problem for most patients. Endolymphatic hydrops commonly produces a low-frequency (rising) sensorineural hearing loss (Fig. 6–14), but the loss often extends to include the higher frequencies so that there is often a flat configuration as the disease progresses. It is possible for the loss

to eventually become profound. The impairment fluctuates because the hearing loss and tinnitus often improve between attacks, and may even resolve between attacks in the early stages of the disease. However, the long-term trend is in the direction of constant hearing loss and tinnitus that worsens during attacks. Two variants of the classical disorder are also recognized. These are identified as cochlear Meniere's disease when the symptoms do not include vertigo, and as vestibular Meniere's disease when there is no hearing loss. Meniere's disease is unilateral in roughly 70 to 85% of the cases, but the incidence of bilateral cases increases with the duration of the disease, reaching about 40% after 15 years (Morrison, 1976).

Meniere's disease has been attributed to may different causes, such as food allergies, hypothyroidism, adrenal and pituitary gland insufficiencies, vascular diseases, stenosis of the internal auditory meatus, trauma, syphilis, viral infections, and genetic origins. However, it is generally viewed as an idiopathic disorder because the precise etiology is difficult to establish.

Medical treatment for Meniere's disease generally consists of a low-salt diet, diuretics,

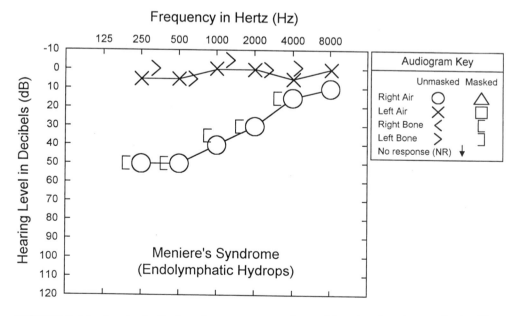

FIGURE 6–14 A principally low-frequency sensorineural hearing loss in a patient with Meniere's disease.

and the use of vestibular suppressants and sedatives to control the vertigo. Surgical treatment is used when medical treatment is ineffective in controlling the vertigo. Endolymphatic sac surgery is used to control debilitating vertigo while preserving the patient's hearing. These operations attempt to relieve the hydrops by removing bone to alleviate pressure on the endolymphatic sac (*endolymphatic sac decompression*), or by decompressing the sac and then providing a route for the endolymph to drain into the subarachnoid space or mastoid (*endolymphatic subarachnoid shunt*). Destructive approaches can also be used to control intractable vertigo. However, destructive procedures are reserved for cases where there is no serviceable hearing in the affected ear because they result in deafness. For example, the diseased labyrinth might be surgically removed (*labyrinthectomy*) or destroyed, and/or the vestibular nerve may be cut (*vestibular neurectomy*). Ototoxic drugs that principally destroy the vestibular end-organs have also been used to control debilitating vertigo with less invasive surgery or nonsurgically, for example, by applying gentamicin locally at the round window, or giving a series of streptomycin injections in cases of bilateral disease.

Ototoxicity

Ototoxicity means damage to the ear due to the toxic effects of various chemical agents, especially drugs. The most ototoxic medications belong to a class of antibiotics called **aminoglycosides**, such as amikacin, dihydrostreptomycin (no longer used), gentamicin (typically as Garamycin), kanamycin, neomycin, netilmicin, streptomycin, and tobramycin. Aminoglycosides are generally administered in cases of very severe or life-threatening infections, and to newborns who are in a state of sepsis. Other kinds of antibiotics can also be ototoxic, such as capreomycin, vancomycin, and even erythromycin. However, the suffix "mycin" does not necessarily mean a drug is ototoxic; for example, clindamycin, Terramycin, and Vibramycin are not ototoxic (although they do have other

adverse reactions). Among the other kinds of ototoxic drugs are cisplatinum, an antineoplastic, and quinine, which was popular in the treatment of malaria. Salicylates (aspirin) are ototoxic in large doses, but the hearing loss is usually reversible.

Loop diuretics such as bumetanide (Bumex), ethacrynic acid (Edecrin), and furosemide (Lasix) are also ototoxic, although the effect can be reversible. Diuretics are commonly used in the treatment of congestive heart disease and other edematous disorders.

Typical ototoxic chemicals include heavy metals, tetrachlorocarbon and sulfur compounds, benzol, nitrobenzol, aniline, organic phosphates, and carbon monoxide. Occupational exposures to one or more of these toxins are possible in a number of industries.

Most ototoxic drugs affect both the cochlear and vestibular parts of the inner ear. However, some are relatively more cochleotoxic (e.g., neomycin) and others are more vestubulotoxic (e.g., streptomycin). Ototoxic drugs cause hearing losses by affecting the cochlear hair cells and the strict vascularis. The outer hair cells are usually affected before the inner hair cells, and damage usually begins in the basal part of the cochlea. As a result, the hearing loss usually begins in the high frequencies and then proceeds to include successively lower frequencies. The hearing loss is usually bilateral, but can be unilateral as well. Tinnitus usually accompanies or precedes the hearing loss, but not always. Vestibulotoxicity can produce symptoms such as vertigo, general unsteadiness or disequilibrium, and/or ataxia. Most ototoxic effects occur during or soon after administration, but hearing losses due to aminoglycoside ototoxicity can develop or continue for many months after treatment has ended, depending on the drug.

The major factors affecting the risk of ototoxicity are dosage, duration of treatment, the adequacy of the patient's renal (kidney) functioning, and whether other potentially ototoxic agents are also being used. The ototoxic effects of aminoglycosides are substantially greater when the patient is also receiving diuretics. Ototoxic drugs also interact with noise to produce greater amounts of hearing loss (Boettcher et al, 1987). A further complication is that many ototoxic drugs are also toxic to the kidneys.

To minimize the risk of hearing loss, it is important to closely monitor those patients receiving ototoxic drugs for renal functioning, drug levels in their blood, and hearing status throughout the treatment period. A baseline audiological evaluation should be obtained as soon as possible, although the degree of illness often makes a preadministration baseline unrealistic. It is important to keep in mind that the decision to use ototoxic medications depends on the nature and severity of the patient's illness, and that it is sometimes necessary to continue their use even if a hearing loss develops. Because of the risk of delayed onset and/or progression of hearing loss, periodic audiological monitoring should continue for quite some time after treatment is over.

Infections

Herpes zoster oticus, also known as **Ramsay-Hunt syndrome**, is observed as a painful chicken pox or shingles-like rash involving the pinna and ear canal, and often appears over portions of the face and neck. This viral infection typically occurs in adults and can cause sensorineural hearing loss, vertigo, and facial palsy.

Syphilis is an infection that was discussed earlier in the context of congenital infections. Acquired syphilis can also cause sensorineural hearing impairments and is known for its ability to mimic other disorders, such as Meniere's disease.

Several kinds of infections commonly cause hearing losses even though they are not ear diseases per se. Many of these diseases are typically associated with infancy and childhood, but are not limited to those years. Sensorineural hearing loss can be a complication of the common viral illnesses of childhood— measles, chicken pox, and mumps— as well as influenza. Measles and mumps are particularly noteworthy. **Measles** has been known to produce sudden-onset bilateral sensorineural hearing losses that are severe in degree and

sloping in configuration in ≥5% of cases. **Mumps** is probably the most common cause of acquired unilateral sensorineural hearing loss in children. Mumps has been known to cause various degrees of sensorineural hearing loss ranging from a mild high-frequency impairment to deafness on the side of the infection, and profound losses are the most common. The hearing loss usually has a sudden onset and has been known to occur even in cases where there was no apparent swelling of the parotid gland. It is reasonable to expect that the use of vaccines for these common illnesses should reduce the incidence of acquired sensorineural hearing losses among children.

Bacterial meningitis is an acute central nervous system infection that can result in brain damage and hearing loss among those who survive the disease. Historically, about 70% of the cases were caused by the *Haemophilus influenzae* type b (Hib) bacteria, and the rest were meningococcal, pneumococcal, and streptococcal infections. However, there has been a substantial decrease in the incidence of Hib infections since the introduction of anti-Hib vaccines in the late 1980s.

A severe-to-profound sensorineural hearing loss is the most common permanent sequela of bacterial meningitis, and occurs when the cochlea is invaded by the infection. Transitory conductive losses have also been reported. The prevalence of sensorineural hearing loss due to bacterial meningitis is variable due to differences in the underlying pathogens and in how the disease was treated. For example, the incidence of hearing loss is between 3 and 16% for Hib meningitis, compared to 10.5% for meningococcal, and between 31 and 50% for pneumococcal infections (Dodge, Davis, Feigin, et al, 1984; Stein & Boyer, 1994). There appears to be a reduction in hearing losses suffered by those who do contract the disease when they are treated with several newer cephalosporin antibiotics and corticosteroids.

Perilymphatic Fistulas

A perilymphatic fistula is a leak of perilymph from a rupture of the oval and/or round windows, and is a common cause of sudden hearing loss. The fistula itself can be quite small and even microscopic. Oval and round window fistulas can result from explosions, barotrauma, and increased intracranial pressure due to straining or physical exertion, sneezing, coughing, Valsalva maneuvers, and other precipitating events. Fistulas may also be the result of bone erosion due to a cholesteatoma or infection, and of untoward outcomes of stapes surgery.

The **fistula test** is usually administered to a patient who is suspected of having a perilymphatic fistula. Air is pumped into the ear canal by squeezing the bulb of a Siegel (pneumatic) otoscope or using the pressure pump of an acoustic immittance device (Chapter 7). The positive pressure is expected to cause a considerable amount of vertigo and nystagmus if the patient has a perilymphatic fistula. Here is why: The air pressure causes an inward displacement of the tympanic membrane that is transmitted to the stapes footplate, which in turn presses in on the perilymph. There will be an abnormally large amount of fluid displacement because the fistula acts like an open valve. The excessive fluid displacement overstimulates the receptors in the semicircular canals, resulting in vertigo and nystagmus. Positive outcomes are highly suggestive of a fistula. However, false-negative outcomes occur in about half the cases (e.g., Goodhill, 1981), so that a negative test result does not rule out a fistula.

Once a perilymphatic fistula is diagnosed, the otologist might choose to treat it conservatively, or to perform a surgical exploration of the middle ear (tympanotomy) to find and repair the fistula. The conservative approach might include bed rest with the head elevated and avoidance of straining. The surgical repair of a fistula involves patching it with materials such as perichondrium, a vein graft, or fat. Successful surgery can arrest the progression of hearing loss or even improve hearing to some extent if performed soon enough.

Retrocochlear Disorders

Retrocochlear disorders involve the structures that are medial to the cochlea. In the broadest sense, this includes any problem that involves the statoacoustic (eighth cranial) nerve or any part of the central auditory nervous system. In practice, however, **retrocochlear** usually refers to a disorder involving the eighth cranial nerve or the cerebellopontine angle (CPA). Disorders are generally classified as **central** when the abnormality is in the central nervous system. Particularly when dealing with brainstem disorders, the term **extraaxial** is often used to describe a lesion that is located *outside* the brainstem (e.g., a CPA tumor that is pressing on the brainstem from without), and the term **intra-axial** is used when the lesion is actually *inside* the brainstem itself.

Eighth Cranial Nerve and Cerebellopontine Angle Tumors

The great majority of eighth nerve tumors are unilateral. Approximately 5% are bilateral and are associated with a genetic syndrome called neurofibromatosis type 2. Eighth nerve tumors are most commonly referred to as **acoustic neuromas**, **acoustic neurilemomas**, **acoustic neurinomas**, and **acoustic tumors**. These are misnomers because most eighth nerve tumors are actually composed of *Schwann* cells and affect the *vestibular* division of the nerve rather than its auditory branch. Thus, the technically preferred term is **vestibular schwannoma** (NIH, 1991). Yet the misnomers are so firmly entrenched in clinical usage that the NIH Consensus Statement stresses that the term *vestibular schwannoma* is itself called *Acoustic Tumor*, probably to maximize recognition of its content. Almost everybody uses these terms interchangeably, but it is important to remember that the primary site is usually the vestibular branch of the nerve. In addition to schwannomas, other kinds of space-occupying lesions of the CPA are also encountered, such as neurilemomas, meningiomas, and cholesteatomas. Tumors located in (or expanding into) the CPA are also called cerebello-pontine angle or posterior fossa tumors.

Vestibular schwannomas can occur anywhere along the eighth nerve, either within the internal auditory meatus or medial to it in the cerebello-pontine angle. Tumors inside the internal auditory meatus erode the bony walls of the canal as they grow, and often expand medially into the CPA because this is the road of least resistance. The eighth nerve is compressed, deformed, and displaced by the growing tumor. Pressure from the tumor can also interfere with the blood supply to the cochlea, which is probably why many "retrocochlear patients" have "cochlear findings" such as loudness recruitment. As tumor size increases, pressure can also be exerted on other cranial nerves, especially the facial (seventh) and trigeminal (fifth), and can even displace the brainstem. As a result, vestibular schwannomas can produce extensive and even life-threatening consequences even though they are benign and usually slow growing.

The presenting complaints of patients with eighth nerve tumors vary widely, depending largely on the size and location of the lesion. Even though impressive neurological complaints are mentioned in the traditional literature, these are no longer as common because retrocochlear lesions now tend to be identified before tumors grow large enough for many of these symptoms to occur. The most common complaint is a hearing disturbance in one ear. It is usually slowly progressive but can be sudden. Other complaints include tinnitus, dizziness and/or imbalance, facial numbness, gait disturbances, and headaches. It might seem odd that hearing disturbances are the preponderant complaint when most eighth nerve tumors originate on the vestibular branch. The most likely reason is that the slowly developing vestibular problem is offset by central compensation.

The majority of these patients have at least some degree of high-frequency loss, but *any* audiometric configuration is possible, varying from normal thresholds to a profound sensorineural hearing losses. The retrocochlear indications of audiological tests are covered in Chapters 8, 10, and 11, but the importance of physiological tests such as the auditory brainstem response and acoustic reflexes should be highlighted. The diagnosis of acoustic tumors and related lesions depends on the use of radiological techniques, and magnetic resonance imaging (MRI) with gadolinium enhancement is currently the "definitive" test.

The treatment of choice for acoustic tumors is surgical removal. The tumor may be approached by three general routes, as shown by the arrows in Figure 6–15. Craniotomy via the *suboccipital (retrosigmoid)* route can be used for both large and small lesions and is the major neurosurgical approach for acoustic tumor surgery. The *middle fossa* approach is usable for small tumors. These approaches make it possible for the patient's hearing to be preserved (at least for many small tumors) because they do not involve dissecting the inner ear structures. The *translabyrinthine* route is the otologic approach to the acoustic tumor by dissecting through the temporal bone. By approaching the tumor laterally via the temporal bone, the translabyrinthine approach avoids manipulating brain tissue and also allows the surgeon to identify and protect the integrity of the seventh cranial (facial) nerve. On the other hand, it results in deafness on the operated side because the route to the tumor involves drilling through the labyrinth. Combined

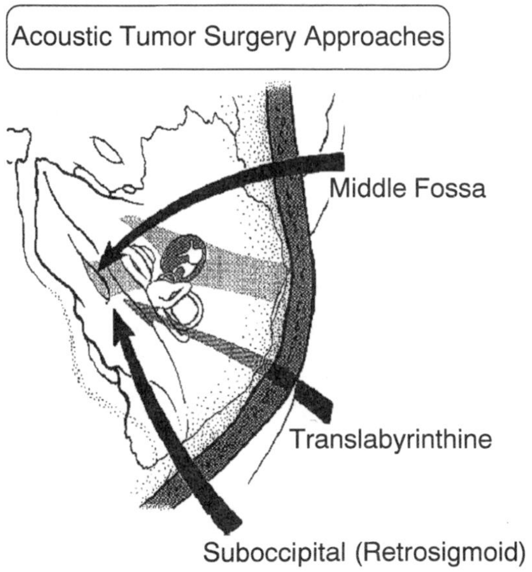

FIGURE 6–15 The three arrows show the major approaches used in acoustic tumor surgery. Adapted from Buckingham et al (1989), with permission.

neurologic-otologic approaches are also used. A radiological technique called *radiosurgery* is an option for patients who cannot (or are not willing to) have traditional surgery, although more information is needed about the long-term outcomes and complications of this approach.

The choice of surgical approach must consider whether the patient has usable preoperative hearing in the pathological ear, as well as the size and location of the tumor, and general medical/surgical issues. The hearing ability of the opposite ear must also be considered in eighth nerve tumor management. For example, using a technique that is more likely to preserve hearing becomes a major consideration when the patient already has a significant hearing impairment in the opposite ear.

Neurofibromatosis Acoustic tumors are commonly associated with a hereditary disease known as neurofibromatosis. However, neurofibromatosis actually refers to two different disorders that have different characteristics and genetic origins (NIH, 1991; Pikus, 1995). **Neurofibromatosis type 1 (NF1)**, or **von Recklinghausen's disease**, is an autosomal-dominant syndrome associ-

ated with chromosome 17. Individuals with NF1 typically have neurofibromas involving the skin, CNS tumors, skeletal deformities including macrocephaly, visual system disorders, and characteristic *café-au-lait spots* (coffee-with-milk colored blotches). These stigmata are observed in early childhood and increase with age.

Neurofibromatosis type 2 (NF2) is an autosomal-dominant syndrome associated with chromosome 22. It is characterized by bilateral eighth nerve tumors, and the possibility of other tumors of the brain and/or spinal cord, but not the dramatic outward characteristics of NF1. Thus, bilateral eighth nerve tumors are virtually the hallmark of neurofibromatosis type 2, but are rare in type 1. This important distinction is missed by the older notion that von Recklinghausen's disease was a singular, unified syndrome, which permeates the traditional literature. Diagnostic criteria for NF1 and NF2 (NIH, 1991) are enumerated in Table 6–2 for ready reference.

Other Retrocochlear Disorders

Although the issue of retrocochlear pathology usually focuses on eighth nerve and cerebello-pontine angle tumors of one type or the other, these are certainly not the only

---

TABLE 6–2   Diagnostic criteria for Neurofibromatosis Type 1 (NF1) and Neurofibromatosis Type 2 (NF2) based on NIH (1991)

NF1 is revealed by the presence of ≥2 of the following characteristics:
   ≥6 café-au-lait spots that are
      ≥5 mm in diameter before puberty
      ≥15 mm in diameter after puberty
   ≥2 neurofibromas of any type even 1 plexiform fibroma
   Freckling in the axillary (armpit) region or inguinal (groin) region
   Optic glioma
   ≥2 Lisch nodules (pigmented iris hamartomas)
   Having a parent/sibling/child with NF1 (based on the above criteria)
NF2 is revealed by the presence of any of the following characteristics:
   Bilateral eighth nerve tumors
   Having a parent/sibling/child with NF2 *and either* a unilateral eighth nerve tumor
      or any one of the following:
      Neurofibroma
      Meningioma
      Glioma
      Schwannoma
      Posterior capsular cataract or opacity at an early age

kind of retrocochlear disorders. For example, as mentioned earlier, hair cell destruction (a cochlear lesion) leads to the retrograde degeneration of auditory nerve fibers (a retrocochlear lesion), and this effect can be quite extensive when the cochlear impairment is severe or profound. Neural presbycusis is a form of age-associated hearing impairment characterized by a loss of auditory neurons. Bone pathologies such as Paget's disease and temporal bone tumors can interfere with the eighth nerve. The eighth nerve can also be compressed by a vascular loop of the anterior inferior cerebellar artery. Neural degeneration or viral infection of the vestibular branch of the eighth nerve can produce acute or chronic vertigo, nausea, and vomiting, known as **vestibular neuronitis**. The eighth nerve can also be affected by such diverse diseases as multiple sclerosis and syphilis.

Auditory Neuropathy

The term **auditory neuropathy** refers to hearing disorders in which physiological tests show that the eighth cranial nerve or the lower auditory brainstem is functioning abnormally even though the outer hair cells are operating normally.[6] Radiological tests do not show retrocochlear lesions of the types just described, such as tumors or multiple sclerosis. Auditory neuropathy occurs among all ages from infancy throughout adulthood. Rance, Beer, Cone-Wesson, Shephert, Dowell, King, Rickards, and Clark (1999) reported an incidence rate of 1 per 433 cases in a large sample of infants and young children who were at risk for hearing impairment, although the overall prevalence of auditory neuropathy is unclear.

The nature of auditory neuropathy has been described in some detail (Sininger,

Hood, Starr, Berlin, & Picton, 1995; Starr, Picton, Sininger, Hood, & Berlin, 1996): The hallmark of auditory neuropathy is (1) a *neural abnormality* demonstrated by an absent or very abnormal *auditory brainstem response (ABR)* in spite of (2) *normally functioning outer hair cells*, which may be shown by normal results for *otoacoustic emissions or cochlear microphonics* (see Chapter 11). Other tests of auditory neural integrity also show abnormalities, such as absent *acoustic reflexes* (see Chapter 7) and absent *masking level differences* (see Chapter 10). Patients with auditory neuropathy can have sensorineural hearing losses of any degree from mild to severe, and their speech recognition performance is usually poorer than what would be expected on the basis of the pure-tone audiogram. In contrast to sensorineural hearing losses of cochlear origin, those with auditory neuropathy derive little if any benefits from the use of conventional hearing aids, and effective treatment approaches are still being sought for these patients.

Central Disorders

Disorders of the auditory central nervous system can be caused by many factors, including age-related deterioration, congenital and/or hereditary disorders, degenerative and demyelinating diseases, developmental disorders, chemical- or drug-induced problems, head trauma, infections (e.g., encephalitis, meningitis), tumors, kernicterus, metabolic disturbances, vascular diseases, and even surgically induced lesions (e.g., sectioning of the corpus callosum). Disturbances of central auditory functioning have also been associated with chronic middle ear effusion, as discussed earlier, and auditory deprivation.

Central auditory lesions generally do not produce a hearing loss per se because information from each ear is represented in both the right and left auditory pathways. Recall from Figure 2–47 of Chapter 2 that this redundant, bilateral representation exists as low as the superior olivary complex, and that there is communication between the two sides at all levels except the medial geniculates. On the

---

[6] Notice that the *outer* hair cells are working normally—not necessarily the cochlea as a whole. Auditory neuropathy probably can have more than just one cause, including problems affecting the inner hair cells and how they operate as a functional unit with the auditory nerve. This is why auditory neuropathy is being listed separately from the other retrocochlear disorders.

other hand, central disorders adversely affect the processing of auditory information in myriad ways, so that the patient might experience one or several of the following problems (ASHA, 1996): Disturbances of speech perception are often experienced when there is noise or a competing signal, as well as when the signal is degraded in some way. Dichotic speech processing, which involves dealing with different messages that are presented to the two ears, is frequently impaired. There may be impairments of various binaural processes, such as directional hearing (localization and lateralization) and spatial orientation, masking level differences, and the ability to put together signals that have been presented to the two ears (often described as binaural fusion or resynthesis). Further, there may be problems with various temporal aspects of hearing (temporal integration, resolution, masking, ordering), as well as with auditory pattern recognition. Auditory tests that address these and other aberrations are discussed in Chapters 10 and 11.

Aphasia is the general term used to describe a variety of central speech and language disorders resulting from lesions affecting the language dominant hemisphere of the brain. **Auditory agnosia** is the inability to recognize sound that has been heard, and **verbal agnosia** is the inability to recognize linguistic material, often called **word deafness.** However, pure word deafness in the absence of aphasia is extremely rare. Cases of central deafness resulting from bilateral temporal lobe damage have been reported from time to time (e.g., Landau, Goldstein, & Kleffner, 1957; Jerger, Weikers, Sharbrough, & Jerger, 1969; Trumo, Bharucha, & Musiek, 1990). The most exhaustive coverage of this rare disorder is a 20-year longitudinal case study by Hood, Berlin, and Allen (1994).

Sudden Hearing Loss

Sudden hearing loss means the rapid onset of a hearing loss, which might develop instantaneously, overnight, or over the course of a few days. The hearing loss is usually unilateral, but it can be bilateral, and any degree of severity is possible. It is almost always accompanied by tinnitus, and a feeling of pressure or fullness in the affected ear(s) is also very common; vertigo may or may not be present.

The possible etiologies that must be considered as the cause of sudden hearing loss include a variety of viral infections; perilymphatic fistula; interference with the cochlear blood supply due to, for example, vascular disease, blood disorders (e.g., sickle cell), embolisms, and vascular spasms; perilymph hypertension; rupturing of Reissner's membrane; Meniere's disease; and acoustic tumor. Recent head trauma, acoustic trauma, and exposure to ototoxic drugs are often omitted from the list, but the author has come across cases of sudden hearing loss attributable to each of these. Finally, we cannot forget that impacted cerumen as well as acute Eustachian tube occlusion can also lead to sudden hearing losses. It is true that these conductive disorders are not what we have in mind here, but we do not know the cause until after the patient has been seen. No matter what the etiology eventually turns out to be, *a current complaint of sudden hearing loss constitutes a medical emergency.*

The expected course of sudden hearing loss is difficult to project because it depends on the underlying cause of the symptoms. Some of these losses resolve spontaneously. Some cases are responsive to medical or surgical treatment, which may have to be initiated quickly to avert a permanent hearing loss. Others are permanent, and others still may be progressive. The treatment for sudden hearing loss is usually medical, and might consist of corticosteriods, vasodilators, anticoagulants, rebreathing of 95% oxygen/5% carbon dioxide, diuretics, and/or a low-sodium diet, depending on the diagnosis. Outcomes run the gamut from no effect to dramatic improvement. Unfortunately, controlled studies of treatment effectiveness for sudden hearing loss are distinguished by their absence. Byle (1984) found no better results for any treatment than what would have been expected from spontaneous recovery. When specific underlying causes are identified (e.g.,

Meniere's disease, underlying systemic diseases, acoustic tumor), they are treated appropriately. Surgery may be indicated if there is evidence of a perilymphatic fistula.

Presbycusis

The aging process comes with some degree of deterioration at most and probably all levels of the auditory system, resulting in age-related auditory impairments that are collectively known as **presbycusis** (Marshall, 1981; Roush, 1985; CHABA, 1988). There is a general consensus that presbycusis is the result of various kinds of physiological degeneration due to the normal aging process (theoretically "pure presbycusis")

plus the accumulated effects of noise exposure, ototoxicity, medical disorders and their treatment, as well as the possibility of hereditary susceptibilities (CHABA, 1988).

Presbycusis is usually described in terms of how hearing thresholds change with increasing age (Corso, 1963; Spoor, 1967; Robinson & Sutton, 1979; Kryter, 1983; Moscicki, Elkins, Baum, & McNamara, 1985; Robinson, 1988; Gates, Cooper, Kannel, & Miller, 1990; Brant & Fozard, 1990; Weinstein, 2000). Differences exist among presbycusis curves, reflecting differences between the populations sampled, degrees of exposure to social and/or occupational noises, and the extent to which people with otological disorders were excluded from the samples. Represen-

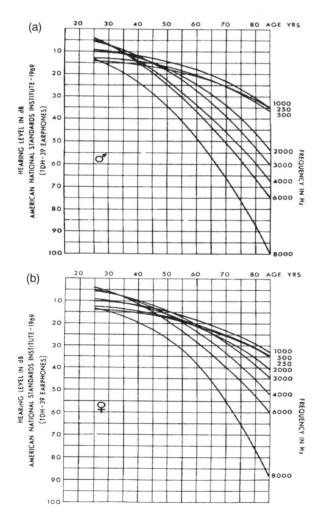

FIGURE 6–16 Hearing level as a function of age (presbycusis curves) for (a) males and (b) females (Data by Spoor, 1967. Adapted from Lebo CP, Reddell RC. 1972. The presbycusis component in occupational hearing loss. *Laryngoscope* 82, 1399–1409, with permission).

tative curves are shown in Figure 6–16. Notice that (1) age-related threshold shifts are greater and begin sooner for the higher frequencies, suggesting greater involvement toward the base of the cochlea; and (2) males are affected more than females, presumably reflecting more exposure to occupational and recreational noises. Figure 6–17 shows the audiogram of a typical patient with presbycusis, showing a sloping sensorineural hearing loss that is essentially symmetrical in both ears.

Difficulty with speech recognition is the most common complaint of presbycusics. There is a general trend for speech recognition scores in quiet to decrease with age, but there is also considerable variability, and it has been suggested that the performance of the elderly is comparable to that of young persons with similar audiograms when they are tested at adequate intensity levels (Marshall, 1981). Gates et al (1990) found that only 3 out of 1026 elderly subjects (0.3%) had disproportionately low speech recognition scores with respect to their audiograms. In contrast, it is clear that speech intelligibility decreases with aging for speech that is presented under *difficult listening conditions* (noise, time compression, rever-

beration, interruptions, competition, etc). The presbycusic effect for degraded speech becomes evident as early as the fifth decade of life (years 40–49) (Bergman, 1980).

Various histological types of presbycusis have been described, as illustrated in Figure 6-18. However, the student should be aware that many patients have more than one kind of histological deterioration, and that not all of the idealized types of presbycusis have been observed by all investigators. The four classical types of presbycusis were based on a combination of clinical and histological findings by Schuknecht (1955, 1964, 1974): **Sensory presbycusis** is due to the degeneration of the sensory hair cells and supporting cells mainly toward the basal turn of the cochlea, and can also include atrophy of the associated neurons as a secondary effect. It is associated with a sloping (often steeply) high-frequency sensorineural hearing loss and speech recognition scores that are consistent with the nature of the audiogram. **Neural presbycusis** is related to primary degeneration of the auditory neurons. The reduced neuronal population is characterized clinically by speech recognition scores that are lower than what would be expected

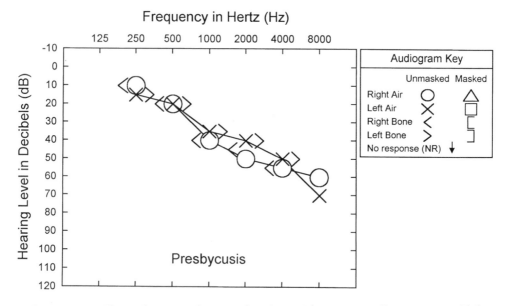

FIGURE 6–17   The audiogram of a typical patient with an essentially symmetrical bilateral sloping sensorineural hearing loss associated with presbycusis.

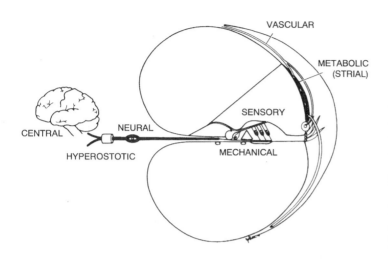

FIGURE 6–18 Schematic representation of the various kinds of presbycusis described in the text. Adapted from Johnsson & Hawkins (1979). Age-related degeneration of the inner ear. In Han SS, Coons DH (Eds.): *Special Senses in Aging.* Ann Arbor: Institute of Gerontology, University of Michigan, 119–135, with permission.

from the audiogram. Atypically poor speech recognition in presbycusis is sometimes called phonemic regression (Gaeth, 1948), but this phenomenon appears to be rare (Gates et al, 1990).

Metabolic or **strial presbycusis** is caused by degeneration of the strict vascularis, causing a relatively flat sensorineural hearing loss with speech recognition scores that are in line with the audiogram. **Mechanical** or **cochlear conductive presbycusis** is attributed to structural changes in the basilar membrane, affecting its mass and stiffness, which would in turn affect the mechanics of the cochlea and produce a sloping sensorineural hearing loss. This kind of presbycusis may be hypothetical.

Two additional forms of presbycusis have also been identified (Johnsson & Hawkins, 1979; Hawkins & Johnsson, 1985): **Vascular presbycusis** is associated with deterioration of the blood supply to the lateral wall of the cochlear duct and the spiral lamina, and may play a part in the deterioration of the strict vascularis and spiral ligament (Johnsson & Hawkins, 1972; Johnsson, 1973). **Hyperostotic presbycusis** occurs when abnormal bone growth (hyperostosis) in the modiolus or internal auditory meatus compresses auditory nerve cells so that they degenerate (Krmpotić-Nemanić, 1969; Krmpotić-Nemanić, Nemanić, & Kostović, 1972; Hawkins & Johnsson, 1985).

Central presbycusis is due to deterioration at various levels of the auditory system up to and including the auditory cortex (CHABA, 1988), although the amount of anatomical evidence in this area has been disappointing. The central component of presbycusis is generally revealed by performance deficits on auditory tests associated with central auditory processing disorders (Chapter 10). Central presbycusis does not appear to be based on cognitive deficits (e.g., Jerger et al, 1989; Jerger, Mahurin, & Pirozzolo, 1990), and increases in prevalence with advancing age (Stach, Spretnjak, & Jerger, 1990).

Paget's Disease

Paget's disease (osteitis deformans) is a chronic and progressive skeletal disease in which bone is resorbed and replaced with dystrophic bone tissue that is often enlarged and prone to fracture and other complications. Typical sites of the disease include the pelvis, spine, legs, and skull. Paget's disease is generally not diagnosed before the fifth decade, often as an incidental finding. Involvement of the temporal bone affects all parts of the ear.

Paget's disease is often thought of in the context of conductive disorders, but it usually produces hearing losses that are mixed or sensorineural, probably including a sizable presbycusic component. Harner, Rose, and Facer

(1978) reviewed a large sample of Paget's disease patients with known audiograms. About 4% of their sample also had otosclerosis. Figure 6–19 shows that most of the hearing losses were sensorineural or mixed, and that less than 2% of the losses were purely conductive regardless of whether the disease affected the skull. However, the percentage of mixed losses was greater when the disease also affected the skull.

Calcitonin has been used to treat hearing loss in Paget's disease with disappointing or inconclusive results. For example, even though Soloman, Evanson, Canty, & Gill (1977) found that hearing improved in calcitonin-treated patients and deteriorated in untreated control subjects, Walker, Evanson, Canty, & Gill (1979) found no differences between subjects from the two groups when they were retested after 3 years.

Obscure Auditory Dysfunction

Many patients have essentially normal hearing on routine tests but still complain of hearing problems, particularly in noisy and other relatively difficult listening situations. Saunders and Haggard (1989) use the term **obscure auditory dysfunction (OAD)** to describe the situation in which a patient has convincing complaints about hearing difficulty in spite of essentially normal hearing thresholds and no disorders that could explain the problem. It is tempting to discount these complaints because they are unjustified by the patient's thresholds and to send her

off with little more than comforting words of reassurance, which has generally been the common practice of many clinicians. However, these complaints can be quite real and may reflect any of several kinds of disorders that do not show up as elevated pure-tone thresholds (Saunders & Haggard, 1989, 1992a,b; Baran & Musiek, 1994; Higson, Haggard, & Field, 1994). These may include one or a combination of disorders of the peripheral ear or central auditory system, cognitive dysfunctions, psychosocial factors, changing acoustical environments or communicative demands, linguistic factors, and age-related effects (although Saunders and Haggard apply the term OAD to those who are <55 years old).

It is desirable to confirm and if possible explain a patient's OAD-like complaints. The most compelling argument is that these complaints can signal the presence of a significant pathology, but this is not the only reason. We also need to know what kinds of referrals and counseling are appropriate for a particular patient, as well as who can be reassured on the basis of normal test results. Of course, patients with normal results are encouraged to return if their subjective problems worsen.

A test battery for OAD has been developed and standardized by Saunders and Haggard (1989, 1992a,b). It includes several tests and interview methods for auditory dysfunctions, central or cognitive deficits, and personality-related factors including the underestimation of hearing ability on the

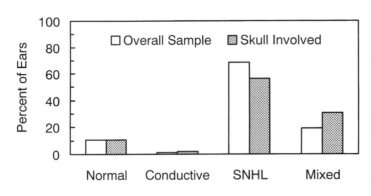

FIGURE 6–19 Percentages of ears with normal hearing and with conductive, sensorineural (SNHL), and mixed hearing losses for a large sample of patients with Paget's disease and a subgroup with Paget's disease of the skull (recalculated from data by Harner, Rose, & Facer, 1978).

part of the patient. Higson, Haggard, and Field (1994) found that the protocol revealed performance deficits in 81% of OAD patients and were able to categorize 73% of them on the basis of one or more auditory, cognitive, and/or personality factors.

Baran and Musiek (1994) recommended that patients should be evaluated when they have auditory complaints that are disproportionately severe compared to their hearing losses, and/or when their auditory complaints are persistent. Formal testing is needed when the complaints cannot be explained by the clinical interview and case history. Noting that many of these problems have a central origin, Baran and Musiek suggested a top-down search, beginning with tests of the higher auditory pathways, then moving to the brainstem level, and finally looking for evidence of subclinical problems involving the cochlea.

Nonorganic Hearing Loss

It is possible for a patient to have a hearing disturbance that is not attributable to a structural abnormality, or which manifests itself in one or more ways that do not occur with organically based hearing losses. These kinds of apparent hearing problems are variously described as nonorganic, functional, psychogenic, feigned, or exaggerated hearing losses, or as malingering or pseudohypacusis. The topic of nonorganic hearing loss is covered in Chapter 14.

References

American Speech-Language-Hearing Association (ASHA). 1992. External auditory canal examination and cerumen management. *ASHA* 34 (suppl), 22–24.

American Speech-Language-Hearing Association Task Force on Central Auditory Processing Consensus Development (ASHA). 1996. Central auditory processing: Current status of research and implications for clinical practice. *Am J Audiol* 5, 41–54.

American Speech-Language-Hearing Association (ASHA). 1997. *Preferred Practice Patterns for the Profession of Audiology*. Rockville Pike, MD: ASHA.

Andersson G, Lyttkens L. 1999. A meta-analysis review of psychological techniques for tinnitus. *Br J Audiol* 33, 201–210.

Baguley DM, Irving RM, Hardy DG, Harada T, Moffat A. 1994. Audiological findings in glomus tumours. *Br J Audiol* 28, 291–297.

Ballachanda BB, Peers CJ. 1992. Cerumen management. *ASHA* 34, 43–46.

Baran DJ, Musiek FE. 1994. Evaluation of the adults with hearing complaints and normal audiograms. *Hearing Today* 6, 9–11.

Bellucci R. 1973. Dual classification of tympanoplasty. *Laryngoscope* 83, 1954–1958.

Bergman M. 1980. *Aging and the Perception of Speech*. Baltimore: University Park Press.

Bluestone CD, Stool SE, Kenna MA (Eds.). 1996. *Pediatric Otolaryngology*, 3rd ed. Philadelphia: WB Saunders.

Boettcher FA, Henderson D, Gratton MA, Danielson RW, Byrne CD. 1987. Synergistic interactions of noise and other ototraumatic agents. *Ear Hear* 8, 192–212.

Borg, E. 1997. Prenatal asphyxia, hypoxia, ischemia and hearing loss: An overview. *Scand Audiol* 26, 77–91.

Brant LJ, Fozard JL. 1990. Age changes in pure-tone hearing thresholds in a longitudinal study of normal human aging. *J Acoust Soc Am* 88, 813–820.

Brown DP. 1994. Speech recognition in recurrent otitis media: Results in a set of identical twins. *J Am Acad Audiol* 5, 1–6.

Buckingham RA (Ed.), Becker W, Naumann HH, Pfaltz CR. 1989. *Ear, Nose and Throat Diseases*. New York: Thieme.

Byle FM Jr. 1984. Sudden hearing loss: Eight years experience and suggested prognostic table. *Laryngoscope* 94, 647–661.

Cantekin EI, Doyle WJ, Phillips DC, Bluestone CD. 1980. Gas absorption in the middle ear. *Ann Otol Rhinol Laryngol* 89 (suppl 68), 71–75.

Carhart R. 1950. Clinical application of bone conduction. *Arch Otolaryngol* 51, 798–807.

Clark WW. 1991. Recent studies of temporary threshold shift (TTS) and permanent threshold shift (PTS) in animals. *J Acoust Soc Am* 90, 155–163.

Committee on Hearing, Bioacoustics and Biomechanics Working Group on Speech Understanding & Aging, National Research Council (CHABA). 1988. Speech understanding and aging. *J Acoust Soc Am* 83, 859–895.

Corso JF. 1963. Age and sex differences in pure-tone thresholds. *Arch Otolaryngol* 77, 385–405.

Corwin JT, Cotanche DA. 1988. Regeneration of sensory hair cells after acoustic trauma. *Science* 240, 1772–1774.

Cotanche DA, Lee KH, Stone JS, Picard DA. 1994. Hair cell regeneration in the bird cochlea following noise damage or ototoxic drug damage. *Anat Embryol* 189, 1–18.

Denny F. 1984. Otitis media. *Pediatr News* 18, 38.

Dodge PR, Davis H, Feigin RD, et al. 1984. Prospective evaluation of hearing impairment as a sequela of acute bacterial meningitis. *N Engl J Med* 311, 869–874.

Downs MP. 1995. Contribution of mild hearing loss to auditory language learning problems. In Roeser R, (Ed.), *Auditory Disorders in School Children*, 3rd ed. New York: Thieme, 188–200.

Farrior B. 1968. *Tympanoplasty in 3-D*. Tampa: American Academy of Ophthamology and Otolaryngology.

Fisch U. 1980. *Tympanoplasty and Stapedotomy: A Manual of Techniques*. New York: Thieme-Stratton.

Fischel-Ghodsian N. 1998. Mitochondrial mutations and hearing loss: Paradigm for mitochondrial genetics. *Am J Hum Genet* 62, 15–19.

Friel-Patti S, Finitzo T. 1990. Language learning in a prospective study of otitis media with effusion in the first two years of life. *J Speech Hear Res* 33, 188–194.

Gaeth JH. 1948. Study of phonemic regression in relation to hearing loss. Unpublished dissertation. Evanston: Northwestern University.

Gates GA, Cooper JC, Kannel, WB, Miller NJ. 1990. Hearing in the elderly: The Framingham cohort. Part 1: Basic audiometric test results. *Ear Hear* 11, 247–256.

Goodhill V. 1981. Leaking labyrinthine lesions, deafness, tinnitus and dizziness. *Ann Otol Rhinol Laryngol* 90, 96–106.

Gravel JS, Wallace IF. 1992. Listening and language at 4 years of age: Effects of early otitis media. *J Speech Hear Res* 35, 588–595.

Hall JW, Prentice CH, Smiley G, Werkhaven J. 1995. Auditory dysfunction in selected syndromes and patterns of malformations. *J Am Acad Audiol* 6, 80–92.

Hamernik RP, Ahroon WA, Hsueh KD. 1991. The energy spectrum of an impulse: Its relation to hearing loss. *J Acoust Soc Am* 90, 197–208.

Hamernik RP, Hsueh KD. 1991. Impulse noise: Some definitions, physical acoustics and other considerations. *J Acoust Soc Am* 90, 189–196.

Harner SG, Rose DE, Facer GW. 1978. Paget's disease and hearing loss. *Otolaryngol* 86, 869–874.

Hawkins JE, Johnsson L-G. 1985. Otopathological changes associated with presbycusis. *Sem Hear* 6, 115–133.

Hazell J. 1987. *Tinnitus*. London: Churchill-Livingstone.

Henderson D, Hamernik RP. 1986. Impulse noise: Critical review. *J Acoust Soc Am* 80, 569–584.

Henry JA, Meikle MB. 2000. Psychoacoustic measures of tinnitus. *J Am Acad Audiol* 11, 138–155.

Higson JM, Haggard MP, Field DL. 1994. Validation of parameters for obscure auditory disfunction (OAD)—robustness of determinants of OAD status across samples and test methods. *Br J Audiol* 28, 27–39.

Hood LJ, Berlin CI, Allen P. 1994. Cortical deafness: A longitudinal study. *J Am Acad Audiol* 5, 330–342.

Hughes GB (Ed.). 1985. *Textbook of Otology*. New York: Thieme-Stratton.

Hughes GB, Pensak ML. (Eds.) 1997. *Clinical Otology*, 2nd ed. New York: Thieme.

Hyman C, Keaster V, Hanson V, Harris I, Sedgwick R, Wursten H., Wright A. 1969. CNS abnormalities after hymolyte disease or hyperbilirubinemia. *Am J Dis Child* 117, 395–405.

ISO-1999. 1990. *Acoustics—Determination of Occupational Noise Exposure and Estimation of Noise-Induced Hearing Impairment*. Geneva: International Standards Organization.

Jacobson GP, Henderson JA, McCaslin DL. 2000. A re-evaluation of tinnitus reliability testing. *J Am Acad Audiol* 11, 156–161.

Jacobson JT. 1995. Nosology of deafness. *J Am Acad Audiol* 6, 15–27.

Jahn A. 1981. Stapes surgery in the 19th century. *Am J Otol* 3, 74–78.

Jerger J, Jerger S, Oliver T, Pirozzolo F. 1989. Speech understanding in the elderly. *Ear Hear* 10, 79–89.

Jerger J, Mahurin R, Pirozzolo F. 1990. The separability of central auditory and cognitive deficits: Implications for the elderly. *J Am Acad Audiol* 1, 116–119.

Jerger J, Weikers N, Sharbrough F, Jerger S. 1969. Bilateral lesions of the temporal lobe. *Acta Otolaryngol* 258 (suppl), 5–51.

Jerger S, Jerger, J, Alford BR, Abrams S. 1983. Development of speech intelligibility in children with recurrent otitis media. *Ear Hear* 4, 138–145.

Johnsson L-G. 1973. Vascular changes in the human inner ear. *Adv Otorhinolaryngol* 20, 197–220.

Johnsson L-G, Hawkins JE. 1972. Vascular changes in the human inner ear associated with aging. *Ann Otol Rhinol Laryngol* 81, 364–376.

Johnsson L-G, Hawkins JH. 1979. Age-related degeneration of the inner ear. In Han, SS, Coons DH (Eds.): *Special Senses in Aging*. Ann Arbor: Institute of Gerontology, University of Michigan, 119–135.

Keats BJB. 2000. Genetic intervention and hearing loss. In Roeser RJ, Valente M, Hosford-Dunn H (Eds.): *Audiology Diagnosis*. New York: Thieme, 593–614.

Kley W. 1982. Surgical treatment of chronic otitis media. In Naumann, HH (Ed.): *Head and Neck Surgery, Vol. 3: Ear*. Stuttgart: Thieme.

Krmpotić-Nemanić J. 1969. Presbycusis and retrocochlear structures. *Int Audiol* 8, 210–220.

Krmpotić-Nemanić J, Nemanić D, Kostović I. 1972. Macroscopical and microscopical changes in the bottom of the internal auditory meatus. *Acta Otolaryngol* 73, 254–258.

Kryter KD. 1983. Presbycusis, sociocusis and nosocusis. *J Acoust Soc Am* 73, 1897–1917 [and addendum/erratum, *J Acoust Soc Am* 74, 1907–1909].

Lalwani AK, Grundfast KM. 1998. *Pediatric Otology and Neurotology*. Philadelphia: Lippincott-Raven.

Landau W, Goldstein R, Kleffner F. 1957. Congenital aphasia: A clinicopathologic study. *Neurology* 7, 915–921.

Lebo CP, Reddell RC. 1972. The presbycusis component in occupational hearing loss. *Laryngoscope* 82, 1399–1409.

Lempert J. 1938. Improvement of hearing in cases of otosclerosis. *Arch Otolaryngol* 28, 42–97.

Lesinski S. 1989. CO_2 laser stapedotomy. *Laryngoscope* 99 (suppl 46), 20–24.

Levy R, Shvero J, Hadar T. 1990. Stapedotomy technique results: Ten years' experience and comparative study with stapedotomy. *Laryngoscope* 100, 1.

Marshall L. 1981. Auditory processing in aging listeners. *J Speech Hear Dis* 46, 226–240.

Mau A. 1984. Chronic otitis media with effusion and adenotonsilectomy: A prospective randomized controlled study. In Lim DJ, et al (Eds.). *Recent Advances in Otitis Media with Effusion*. Philadelphia: Decker, 299–302.

McGee T. 1981. Comparison of small fenestra and total stapedectomy. *Ann Otol Rhinol Laryngol* 90, 633–636.

Melnick W. 1991. Human temporary threshold shift (TTS) and damage risk. *J Acoust Soc Am* 90, 147–154.

Menjuk P. 1992. Relationship of otitis media to speech and language development. In Katz J, Stecker N, Henderson D (Eds.): *Central Auditory Processing: A Transdisciplinary Approach*. St. Louis: Mosby, 187–197.

Miller JD. 1974. Effects of noise on people. *J Acoust Soc Am* 56, 729–764.

Mody M, Schwartz RG, Gravel JS, Ruben RJ. 1999. Speech perception and verbal memory in children with and without histories of otitis media. *J Speech Lang Hear Res* 42, 1069–1079.

Morrison AW. 1976. The surgery of vertigo: Saccus drainage for idiopathic endolymphatic hydrops. *J Laryngol Otol* 90, 87–93.

Moscicki EK, Elkins EF, Baum HM, McNamara PM. 1985. Hearing loss in the elderly: An epidemiological study of the Framingham heart study cohort. *Ear Hear* 6, 184–190.

National Institutes of Health (NIH). 1991. *Consensus Statement on Acoustic Neuroma.* 9, 1–24.

Northern JL, Downs MP. 1991. *Hearing in Children,* 4th ed. Baltimore: Williams & Wilkins.

Pagon RA, Graham JM, Zonana J, Yong S. 1981. Coloboma, congenital heart disease, and choanal atresia with multiple anomalies: CHARGE association. *J Pediatr* 99, 223–227.

Paparella MM, Goycoolea M, Bassiouni M, Koutroupas S. 1986. Silent otitis media: Clinical applications. *Laryngoscope* 96, 978–985.

Paparella MM, Shumrick DA, Gluckman JL, Meyerhoff WL (Eds.). 1991. *Otolaryngology.* Philadelphia: WB Saunders.

Passchier-Vermeer W. 1974. Hearing loss due to continuous exposure to steady-state broad-band noise. *J Acoust Soc Am* 56, 1585–1593.

Pikus AT. 1995. Pediatric audiologic profile in type I and type II neurofibromatosis. *J Am Acad Audiol* 6, 54–62.

Post JC. 2000. Genetics principles. In Wetmore RF, Muntz JR, McGill TJ (Eds.): *Pediatric Otolaryngology: Principles and Practice Pathways.* New York: Thieme, 65–86.

Preliner K, Kalm O, Harsten G. 1992. Middle ear problems in childhood. *Acta Otolaryngol Suppl* 493, 93–98.

Prezant TR, Agapian JV, Bohlman MC, et al. 1993. Mitochondrial ribosome RNA mutation associated with both antibiotic and non-syndromic deafness. *Nature Genet* 4, 289–294.

Pulec JL, Horwitz MJ. 1973. Diseases of the eustachian tube. In Paparella MM, Shumrick A (Eds.): *Otolaryngology Vol. 2: Ear.* Philadelphia: WB Saunders, 75–92.

Rance G, Beer DE, Cone-Wesson B, Shephert RK, Dowell RC, King AM, Rickards FW, Clark GM. 1999. Clinical findings for a group of infants and young children with auditory neuropathy. *Ear Hear* 20, 238–252.

Robinson DW. 1988. Threshold of hearing as a function of age and sex for the typical unscreened population. *Br J Audiol* 22, 5–20.

Robinson DW, Sutton GJ. 1979. Age effect in hearing—a comparative analysis of published threshold data. *Audiology* 18, 320–334.

Roeser RJ, Wilson PL. 2000. Cerumen management. In Hosford-Dunn H, Roeser RJ, Valente M (Eds.): *Audiology Practice Management.* New York: Thieme, 273–290.

Rosen S. 1953. Mobilization of the stapes to restore hearing in otosclerosis. *NY State J Med* 53, 2650–2653.

Rösler G. 1994. Progression of hearing loss caused by occupational noise. *Scand Audiol* 23, 13–37.

Roush J (Ed.). 1985. Aging and hearing impairment. *Semin Hear* 6, 99–219.

Ryals BM, Rubel EW. 1988. Hair cell regeneration after acoustic trauma in adult *Coturnix* quail. *Science* 240, 1774–1776.

Sandlin RE, Olsson RT. 2000. Subjective tinnitus: Its mechanisms and treatment. In Valente M, Hosford-Dunn H, Roeser RJ (Eds.): *Audiology Treatment.* New York: Thieme, 691–714.

Saunders GH, Haggard MP. 1989. The clinical assessment of obscure auditory disfunction—1. Auditory and psychological factors. *Ear Hear* 10, 200–208.

Saunders GH, Haggard MP. 1992a. A clinical test battery for obscure auditory disfunction (OAD): Development, selection and use of tests. *Br J Audiol* 26, 33–42.

Saunders GH, Haggard MP. 1992b. The clinical assessment of "obscure auditory disfunction" (OAD) 2: Case controls analysis of determining factors. *Ear Hear* 13, 241–254.

Saunders JC, Cohen YE, Szymko YM. 1991. The structural and functional consequences of acoustic injury in the cochlea and peripheral auditory system: A five year update. *J Acoust Soc Am* 90, 136–146.

Saunders JC, Dear SP, Schneider ME. 1985. The anatomical consequences of acoustic injury: A review and tutorial. *J Acoust Soc Am* 78, 833–860.

Schildroth AN. 1994. Congenital cytomegalovirus and deafness. *Am J Audiol* 3, 27–38.

Schmiedt RA. 1984 Acoustic injury and the physiology of hearing. *J Acoust Soc Am* 76, 1293–1317.

Schuknecht F. 1955. Presbycusis. *Laryngoscope* 65, 402–419.

Schuknecht F. 1964. Further observations on the pathology of presbycusis. *Arch Otolaryngol* 80, 369–382.

Schuknecht F. 1974. *Pathology of the Ear.* Cambridge: Harvard University Press.

Schwartz RG, Mody M, Petinou K. 1997. Phonological acquisition and otitis media: Speech perception and speech production. In Roberts J, Wallace I, Henderson F (Eds.): *Otitis Media in Young Children: Medical, Developmental and Educational Considerations.* Baltimore: Brookes.

Shambaugh G, Causse J. 1974. Ten years experience with fluoride in otosclerotic (otospongiotic) patients. *Ann Otol Rhinol Laryngol* 635.

Shea JJ. 1958. Fenestration of the oval window. *Ann Otol Rhinol Laryngol* 67, 932–951.

Shimizu H. 1992. Childhood hearing impairment. *AAS Bull* 17, 15–37.

Sininger YS, Hood LJ, Starr A, Berlin CI, Picton TW. 1995. Hearing loss due to auditory neuropathy. *Audiology Today* 7, 10–13.

Smith SD. 1995. Overview of genetic auditory syndromes. *J Am Acad Audiol* 6, 1–14.

Soloman L, Evanson J, Canty D, Gill N. 1977. Effect of calcitonin treatment on deafness due to Paget's disease of bone. *Br Med J* 2, 485–487.

Spoor A. 1967. Presbycusis values in relation to noise induced hearing loss. *Int Audiol* 6, 48–57.

Stach BA, Spretnjak ML, Jerger J. 1990. The prevalence of central presbycusis in a clinical population. *J Am Acad Audiol* 1, 109–115.

Stagno S. 1990. Cytomegalovirus. In Remington J, Klein J (Eds.): *Infectious Diseases of the Fetus and Newborn Infant,* 3rd ed. Philadelphia: WB Saunders, 240–281.

Starr A, Picton TW, Sininger YS, Hood LJ, Berlin CI. 1996. Auditory neuropathy. *Brain* 119, 741–753.

Stein LK, Boyer KM. 1994. Progress in the prevention of hearing loss in infants. *Ear Hear* 15, 116–125.

Stool SE, Berg AO, Berman S, Carney CJ, Cooley JR, Culpepper L, Eavey RD, Feagans LV, Finitzo T, Friedman EM, et al. 1994. *Otitis Media with Effusion in Young Children: Clinical Practice Guideline.* AHCPR publ. no. 94–0622. Rockville, MD: Agency for Health Care Policy and Research, Public Health Service, US Department of Health & Human Services.

Strasnick B, Jacobson JT. 1995. Teratogenic hearing loss. *J Am Acad Audiol* 6, 28–38.

Swartz JD, Harnsberger HR (Eds.). 1998. *Imaging of the Temporal Bone*, 3rd ed. New York: Thieme.

Teele DW, Klein JL, Rosner BA, et al. 1984. Otitis media with effusion during the first three years of life and development of speech and language. *Pediatrics* 74, 282–287.

Tomaski SM, Grundfast KM. 1999. A stepwise approach to the diagnosis and treatment of hereditary hearing loss. In Roizen NJ, Diefendorf AO (Eds.): *Hearing Loss in Children. Pediatr Clin North Am* 46, 35–48.

Toriello HV. 1995. CHARGE association. *J Am Acad Audiol* 6, 47–53.

Tos M. 1993. *Manual of Middle Ear Surgery: Vol. 1. Approaches, Myringoplasty, Ossiculoplasty, and Tympanoplasty.* Stuttgart: Thieme.

Tos M. 1995. *Manual of Middle Ear Surgery: Vol. 2. Mastoid Surgery and Reconstructive Procedures.* Stuttgart: Thieme.

Trumo M, Bharucha J, Musiek FE. 1990. Music perception and cognition following bilateral lesions of the auditory cortex. *J Cognit Neurosci* 2, 195–212.

Tsue TT, Oesterle EC, Rubel EW. 1994. Hair cell regeneration in the inner ear. *Otolaryngol Head Neck Surg* 111, 281–301.

Tyler RS, Aran J, Dauman R. 1992. Recent advances in tinnitus. *Am J Audiol* 1, 36–44.

Walker G, Evanson J, Canty D, Gill N. 1979. Effect of calcitonin on deafness due to Paget's disease. *Br Med J* 4, 364–365.

Ward WD. 1991. The role of intermittence in PTS. *J Acoust Soc Am* 90, 164–169.

Weinstein B. 2000. *Geriatric Audiology.* New York: Thieme.

Wetmore RF, Muntz HR, McGill TJ (Eds.). 2000. *Pediatric Otolaryngology: Principles and Practice Pathways.* New York: Thieme.

Woods CI, Strasnick B, Jackson CG. 1993. Surgery for glomus tumours: The otology group experience. *Laryngoscope* 103 (suppl), 93–99.

Wullstein HL, Wullstein S. 1990. *Tympanoplasty: Osteoplastic Epitympanoplasty.* Stuttgart: Thieme.

Yee AL, Cantekin EI. 1986. Effect of changes in systemic oxygen tension on middle ear gap exchange. *Ann Otol Rhinol Laryngol* 95, 369–372.

Acoustic Immittance Assessment

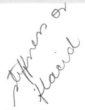

*tiffness or
flaccid*

Immittance Instrumentation

We learned in Chapter 1 that **acoustic immittance** is the general term used to describe the various aspects of acoustic impedance and admittance. Let us quickly review the major terms. **Acoustic impedance** (Z_a) is the opposition to the flow of sound energy, measured in ohms. Acoustic impedance is the ratio of sound pressure (P) to sound flow, or volume velocity (U); or $Z_a = P/U$. The reciprocal of acoustic impedance is **acoustic admittance** (Y_a), expressed in acoustic *millimhos (mmhos)*. Acoustic admittance is the ease of sound flow, or $Y_a = U/P$. Acoustic impedance is composed of (1) a frictional component called **acoustic resistance** (R_a), (2) a stiffness component called **negative (stiffness) acoustic reactance** ($-X_a$), and (3) a mass component called **positive (mass) acoustic reactance** ($+X_a$). Their reciprocals are respectively the components of acoustic admittance: (1) **acoustic conductance** (G_a); (2) **positive (compliant or stiffness) acoustic susceptance** ($+B_a$), and (3) **negative (mass) acoustic susceptance** ($-B_a$).

The immittance of the ear is derived from its various sources of mechanical and acoustical springiness, mass, and resistance (Van Camp, Margolis, Wilson, Creten, & Shanks, 1986): (1) The *stiffness (springiness) components* come from the volumes of air in the outer ear and middle ear spaces, the tympanic membrane, and the tendons and ligaments of the ossicles. (2) The *mass components* are due to the ossicles, the pars flaccida of the eardrum, and the perilymph. (3) *Resistance (friction)* is introduced by the perilymph, the mucous membrane linings of the middle ear spaces, the narrow passages between the middle ear and mastoid air cavities, and also by the tympanic membrane and the various middle ear tendons and ligaments. Contractions of the middle ear muscles also change the immittance of the ear, usually by increasing the stiffness component. Various pathologies cause changes in the admittance characteristics of the ear that can help us to detect their presence and to distinguish among them. This is why we use acoustic immittance testing in clinical audiology. Admittance measurements are employed clinically because they are more straightforward than those using impedance. The acoustic admittance characteristics of the ear can be assessed using a device such as the one described in Figure 7–1.

The acoustic immittance of the ear is measured by inserting an ear piece called a **probe tip** into the ear canal. The probe tip is encased in a flexible plastic cuff to create an airtight connection between the ear canal and the probe tip, called a **hermetic seal**. The probe tip includes four tubes. One tube is connected to a **receiver** (loudspeaker), which is used to deliver a tone into the ear canal. This sound is called the **probe tone**. The second tube is connected to a measuring **microphone** and is used to monitor the probe sound within the ear canal. The third tube is connected to an air **pressure pump** and **manometer** (pressure meter), and the fourth tube connects to another receiver used to present stimuli for testing the acoustic reflex. In addition to the probe tip in one ear, a second earphone goes to the opposite ear and is

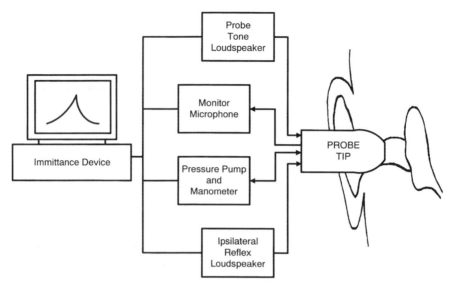

FIGURE 7–1 Block diagram of the major components of a clinical acoustic immittance device.

used for acoustic reflex tests. The latter earphone may be a standard audiometric earphone or an insert receiver, depending on the device being used. The acoustic admittance (in mmhos or mL) measured with such a device is displayed on a meter or video display and is usually plotted on paper. Figure 7–2 shows a photograph of a typical clinical acoustic immittance instrument.

The process of measuring the ear's admittance employs the first two tubes just described, that is, those connected to the receiver that produces the probe tone, and to the measuring microphone. The basic approach is to introduce an 85 dB sound pressure level (SPL) probe tone into the ear canal, where it will be affected by the admittance properties of the ear. This will be

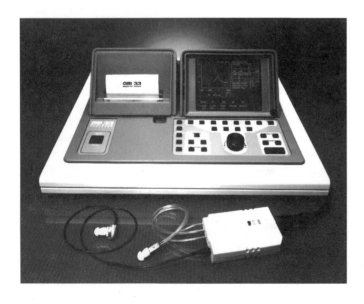

FIGURE 7–2 A clinical acoustic immittance device. Photograph courtesy of Grason-Stadler, Inc.

revealed as an increase or decrease in the level of the probe tone as it is monitored by the measuring microphone. The details of immittance device technology are beyond the current scope of this book, but the beginning student should be aware that instruments called **bridges** involve a manual intensity adjustment to bring the probe level in the ear to 85 dB SPL, whereas those referred to as **meters** use an automatic volume control to keep the probe level at 85 dB SPL. In addition to measuring overall admittance (Y), most admittance meters also provide separate measurements of susceptance (B) and conductance (G). This is done by analyzing the monitored signal in terms of in-phase (for G) and out-of-phase (for B) components. The characteristics and calibration of acoustic immittance devices are given in the ANSI S3.39-1987 (R1996) standard.

Most routine immittance tests use a 226-Hz (or a 220-Hz) probe tone. Low-frequency probe tones such as these were originally chosen because they are sensitive to changes in stiffness reactance, comprising a major part of the normal ear's impedance. In addition, admittance devices are calibrated in terms of the admittance of an **equivalent volume** of air. In other words, when the meter indicates that the admittance of an ear is 1.8 mmhos at 226 Hz, it means that the admittance of the ear corresponds to that of a 1.8-milliliter (mL) volume of air. Let us see why. Suppose we have several stainless steel containers (i.e., hard-walled cavities) with various volumes, ranging from perhaps 0.2 to 2.5 mL or cc. The air volume in such a cavity constitutes an acoustical spring, so that its admittance is essentially a compliant susceptance (and its impedance a stiffness reactance). Inserting our probe tip into each of these containers would show that admittance increases (or the impedance decreases) as the volume of the cavity becomes larger. Repeating this experiment with different probe tone frequencies in the same cavity would result in different amounts of admittance at each frequency. This reflects the fact that admittance depends on frequency. We

would also find that admittance (in mmhos) is equal to the volume (in mL) when the probe tone is 226 Hz. For example, the acoustic admittance (Y_a) at 226 Hz will be 2.0 mmhos for a 2-mL (cc) container, 1.2 mmhos for a 1.2 mL container, 0.3 mmhos for a 0.3-mL volume, etc. This is why 226 Hz has become the preferred low-frequency probe tone frequency. Higher frequency probe tones provide other kinds of information and are often used as well.

Immittance at the Plane of the Eardrum

For diagnostic purposes we are mainly concerned with the immittance of the middle ear because it provides information about (1) middle ear pathologies, and (2) middle ear muscle contractions due to the acoustic reflex. However, the probe tip monitors the immittance of the ear from the perspective of its location, which is in the general vicinity of the ear canal entrance. Thus, the probe tip measures the *total immittance* of the ear, which includes the combined effects of the outer ear and the middle ear. This is a problem because ear canal volume (size) is usually not clinically relevant, yet its influence on the total immittance value (at the probe tip) is often big enough to cloud the effects of the clinically significant middle ear immittance value. For example, a patient with abnormally low middle ear admittance due to a conductive disorder may have a normal total admittance value due to a large ear canal volume. Another individual whose middle ear is normal might seem to have unusually low total admittance because her ear canal volume is quite small. A third patient might have low total admittance due to otitis media when first evaluated. The middle ear problem might be completely resolved (i.e., the middle ear immittance has returned to normal) when she returns for reassessment, but the total Y_a might still be abnormally low simply because her outer ear volume was made to appear smaller by a very deeply inserted probe tip. This can happen because the volume under the probe tip will be different depending on how deeply it has been inserted.

We must remove the outer ear component from the total admittance value at the probe tip to get an undistorted representation of the middle ear's admittance at the eardrum. In other words, removing the effect of the ear canal moves the measurement location from the end of the probe tip to the *plane of the tympanic membrane*. We can achieve this goal by taking advantage of the fact that total admittance (Y_{TOTAL}) is simply the sum of the admittances of the outer ear (Y_{OE}) and the middle ear (Y_{ME})[1]:

$$Y_{TOTAL} = Y_{OE} + Y_{ME}.$$

Consequently, subtracting the admittance of the outer ear from the total admittance leaves the middle ear admittance, which is the value that we need:

$$Y_{ME} = Y_{TOTAL} - Y_{OE}. \quad outer ear$$

This simple, additive relationship is one of the main reasons why we use measurements based on admittance rather than impedance.[2]

The procedure for determining the admittance of the middle ear (i.e., at the plane of the ear drum) is simple and straightforward: The first step is to measure the total admittance (Y_{TOTAL}) of the ear (Fig. 7–3a). The second step is to measure the ear's admittance again while pressure is being exerted on the tympanic membrane. This measurement reflects the admittance of the outer ear (or ear canal) alone, and is depicted in Figure 7–3b. The pressure change is accomplished using the pressure pump connected to one of the tubes in the probe tip. The rationale for this tactic is that the heightened air pressure puts the

eardrum under so much tension that it acts like a hard wall, so that essentially no sound energy can be transmitted into the middle ear. This strategy prevents the probe tip from measuring the admittance of the middle ear. In this case, we say that the middle ear has been excluded from the measurement. Hence, the admittance obtained under these conditions comes from the outer ear alone.

We now know the total admittance (of the outer and middle ear combined) from the first measurement and the admittance of the outer ear from the second measurement.

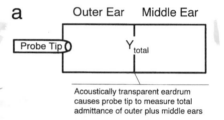

a   Outer Ear   Middle Ear

Probe Tip Y_{total}

Acoustically transparent eardrum causes probe tip to measure total admittance of outer plus middle ears

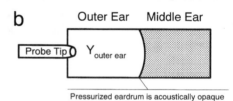

b   Outer Ear   Middle Ear

Probe Tip $Y_{outer ear}$

Pressurized eardrum is acoustically opaque to middle ear, causing probe tip to measure admittance of outer ear only.

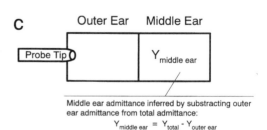

c   Outer Ear   Middle Ear

Probe Tip $Y_{middle ear}$

Middle ear admittance inferred by substracting outer ear admittance from total admittance:

$$Y_{middle\ ear} = Y_{total} - Y_{outer\ ear}$$

---

[1] Y_{ME} can also be called Y_{TM}, which stands for the admittance at the plane of the tympanic membrane.

[2] The equivalent impedance formula is more complicated:

$$Z_{ME} = \frac{(Z_{OE} \times Z_{TOTAL})}{(Z_{OE} - Z_{TOTAL})}$$

where Z_{TOTAL} is the total impedance, Z_{OE} is outer ear impedance, and Z_{ME} is middle ear impedance.

FIGURE 7–3   (a) Total admittance (Y_{TOTAL}) at the probe tip includes the combined admittances of the outer and middle ears. (b) The middle ear is excluded from the admittance measurement by using air pressure to tense the eardrum. The probe tip now registers the admittance of just the outer ear (Y_{OE}). (c) Admittance at the plane of the drum, or middle ear admittance (Y_{ME}) is inferred by subtracting Y_{OE} from Y_{TOTAL}.

The third step (Figure 7–3c) is to figure out the previously unknown middle ear admittance (Y_{ME}) by simply subtracting the outer ear admittance (Y_{OE}) from the total admittance (Y_{TOTAL}).

Tympanometry

Tympanometry involves measuring the acoustic admittance of the ear with various amounts of air pressure in the ear canal. We can control the amount of air pressure in the ear canal because the probe tip makes a hermetic seal with the ear canal, and one of its tubes is connected to an air pump and manometer. The amount of air pressure is expressed in terms of **dekapascals (daPa)** or of millimeters of water pressure (mm H_2O),[3] relative to the atmospheric pressure in the room where the test is being done. Hence, 0 daPa implies that the pressure in the ear canal is equal to the atmospheric pressure, positive pressure (e.g., +100 daPa) means that the ear canal pressure is greater than atmospheric pressure, and negative pressure (e.g., –100 daPa) means it is less than atmospheric pressure. This information is shown on a diagram called a **tympanogram** (Fig. 7–4a), with admittance in mmhos (or equivalent volume in mL) on the y-axis, and pressure in daPa (or mm H_2O) on the x-axis. Notice in the figure that atmospheric pressure (0 daPa) is in the middle, with positive pressure increasing to the right and negative pressure increasing to the left.

Because most instruments generate tympanograms automatically, we can concentrate on what is happening and why. (Here, as elsewhere, it is assumed that the ear and related structures have already been inspected.) The first step in tympanometry is to properly insert the probe so that it makes a hermetic seal with the external auditory

meatus. The probe tip should face the drum and not the ear canal wall, and the path to the tympanic membrane should not be blocked. Cerumen will be problematic if it gets into the probe tip tubes or completely obstructs the path to the tympanic membrane, but the simple presence of some wax is usually not a problem. The next step is to select the probe frequency and the admittance parameter(s) to be measured. We will measure overall acoustic admittance (Y) with a 226-Hz probe tone. The appropriate button(s) on the immittance device are then pushed to initiate the following tympanometry procedure:

The 226-Hz probe tone is turned on and the pressure in the ear canal is then raised to +200 daPa. This amount of positive pressure is usually assumed to tense the eardrum sufficiently to prevent the admittance of the middle ear from being measured, as described in the previous section and illustrated in Figure 7–3b. A useful analogy is to imagine that the +200 daPa pressure causes the tympanic membrane to become "opaque" to sound, so that the probe cannot "see" the middle ear through it. Thus, the admittance obtained at +200 daPa is assumed to represent just the outer ear. In Figure 7–4a, the admittance at +200 daPa is 1.0 mmhos (point 1). This means that the acoustic admittance of the outer ear is 1.0 mmhos, and that the ear canal volume is 1.0 mL because mmhos equals volume at 226 Hz. The air pressure is then decreased at a steady rate while we continue to measure the admittance. Notice that the tympanogram curve slowly rises as the pressure decreases below +200 daPa. The total admittance rises by about 0.1 mmhos, to reach 1.1 mmhos, when the pressure is +100 daPa (point 2). It then increases more rapidly as the pressure drops further, and achieves 1.75 mmhos at 0 daPa, or at atmospheric pressure (point 3).

Why is this happening and what does it mean? As the pressure in the ear canal is steadily reduced, the tension on the tympanic membrane also diminishes. The middle ear is no longer being completely blocked from the view of the probe tip. Instead, the

How to apply a tympanogram →

[3] The relationship between these two units of pressure is so close (1 daPa = 1.02 mm H_2O, and 1 mm H_2O = 0.98 daPa) that we can think of them interchangeably for most purposes.

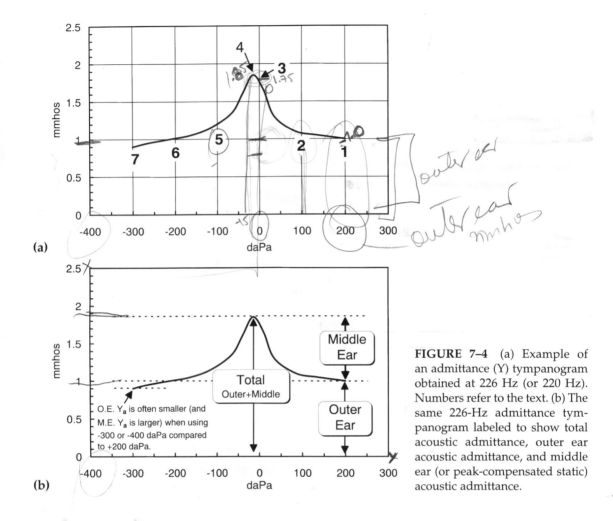

FIGURE 7–4 (a) Example of an admittance (Y) tympanogram obtained at 226 Hz (or 220 Hz). Numbers refer to the text. (b) The same 226-Hz admittance tympanogram labeled to show total acoustic admittance, outer ear acoustic admittance, and middle ear (or peak-compensated static) acoustic admittance.

probe tip is now picking up more and more of the middle ear's admittance. The less the pressure, the less the tension on the eardrum, and the more the middle ear contributes. It is as though the eardrum has changed from being completely "opaque" to being progressively more "translucent." Because we know that 1.0 mmho is coming from the ear canal, we can deduce that the additional amounts of admittance (above 1.0 mmho) must be coming from the middle ear. Hence, the 1.75 mmhos of total admittance at 0 daPa represents 1.0 mmho from the ear canal and 0.75 mmho from the middle ear.

Returning to the tympanometry procedure, the pressure continues to be reduced below 0 daPa. Air is now being pumped out

of the ear canal instead of into it, so that the pressure is becoming increasingly negative. We see that the admittance continues rising until it reaches a maximum of 1.85 mmhos when the pressure in the outer ear is –15 daPa (*point 4*). The total admittance then begins to fall again as the negative pressure increases. The maximum point is called the peak of the tympanogram. Using our visual analogy, this is where there is no longer any tension being imposed on the tympanic membrane, so that it becomes "transparent," allowing the probe tip to "see" all of the middle ear admittance. Because we know that the maximum (or peak) *total* admittance is 1.35 mmhos and that the *outer ear* admittance is 1.0 mmho, we can deduce that the *middle ear* admittance is

0.85 mmho. (The middle ear admittance is often referred to as the *static* admittance, or more accurately as *peak-compensated static admittance*, discussed below.)

By reducing the pressure below 0 daPa we are actually increasing the negative pressure. This causes the admittance to fall to 1.2 mmhos at −100 daPa (*point 5*), and to 1.0 mmho at −200 daPa (*point 6*). The falling admittance values indicate that the negative pressure is tensing the tympanic membrane, so that it again becomes progressively more opaque to sound. Continuing to increase the negative pressure causes the admittance to fall to only 0.9 mmho at −300 daPa (*point 7*), which is the lowest pressure used here. Thus, the admittance at −300 daPa is actually smaller than it was at +200 daPa. This means that the middle ear can be excluded from the measurement by applying either positive or negative pressure (i.e., at *points 1 or 7*, which are often called the positive and negative "tails").

Even though many audiologists use +200 daPa to estimate outer ear volume, the lowest point on the tympanogram is often obtained at −300 to −400 daPa. Compared to +200 daPa, it has been shown that −400 daPa more effectively removes the middle ear admittance and thus provides a more accurate measure of the outer ear volume (Shanks & Lilly, 1981). It is suggested that (1) tympanograms should be obtained over a pressure range from +200 daPa down to −400 daPa (or at least −300 daPa); and that (2) the admittance of the middle ear should be based on (a) the tympanogram peak as the total admittance value and (b) the lower of the two "tails" as the outer ear admittance value.

Figure 7–4a is redrawn in Figure 7–4b to summarize the major components of the typical 226-Hz (or 220-Hz) tympanogram. Because the y-axis shows admittance in mmhos (or equivalent volume in mL), the overall height of the peak relative to 0 mmhos gives total admittance, and the overall height of the "tail" (at +200 daPa or −300 daPa) gives the outer ear volume. The height of the tympanogram's peak above its own baseline (i.e., one of the two tails) gives the middle ear admittance.

The peak of the tympanogram also provides us with an estimate of the pressure within the middle ear, which is −15 daPa in this example. Here is why: Recall that we exclude the middle ear by using air pressure to stress the eardrum. This stress occurs because there is more pressure on one side of the tympanic membrane than on the other (higher pressure in the outer ear than in the middle ear, or vice versa). The admittance will be highest (the peak) when the eardrum is not experiencing any stress due to a pressure difference. Thus, the positive or negative pressure used to obtain the peak pressure should be the same as the pressure that exists on the other side of the eardrum, that is, within the middle ear. This is so because having the same pressure on both sides of the eardrum will result in the least tension on the drum, and hence the highest total admittance value, so that the tympanogram peak provides us with an estimate of the pressure inside the middle ear.

Interpreting 226-Hz (Low-Frequency) Tympanograms

The major considerations that come into play when interpreting 226-Hz (or 220-Hz) tympanograms include static acoustic admittance, tympanometric gradient or width, ear volume, the pressure at which the tympanometric peak occurs, and the shape of the tympanogram. It is also possible to categorize tympanograms into a reasonably small number of types that summarize the majority of configurations found clinically. Several systems have been proposed for classifying 220-Hz (226-Hz) tympanograms (Liden, 1969; Jerger, 1970; Liden, Peterson, & Bjorkman, 1970; Jerger, Anthony, Jerger, & Mauldin, 1974; Liden, Harford, & Hallen, 1974; Feldman, 1975; Paradise, Smith & Bluestone, 1976; Silman & Silverman, 1991). The most widely utilized tympanogram classification systems was originated by Jerger (1970). Figure 7–5 shows most of the tympanogram types in this system. These types were based

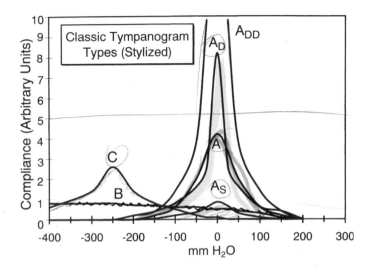

FIGURE 7–5 Stylized examples of the Jerger's (1970) classical 220-Hz (226-Hz) tympanogram types (shown in terms of the arbitrary compliance units used by relative immittance devices).

on relative tympanograms obtained with an immittance bridge, and this format is retained in the figure. Notice that these tympanograms are expressed in arbitrary compliance units instead of absolute admittance in mmhos (static acoustic admittance and ear canal volume were measured separately). Type A tympanograms had a distinctive peak in the vicinity of atmospheric pressure and were typical of normal patients, as well as those with otosclerosis. If the type A tympanogram had a very shallow peak it was classified as type A$_S$, which was generally associated with otosclerosis but could also occur with otitis media. In contrast, very high (deep) type A tympanograms were designated as type A$_D$. These were found in otherwise normal ears that had scarred or flaccid eardrums, or in cases of ossicular interruptions. The type A$_{DD}$ tympanogram was so deep that the peak was off-scale, and was found in ears with ossicular discontinuities. Type B tympanograms were essentially flat across the pressure range, and were characteristic of patients with middle ear fluid and cholesteatoma. However, type B tympanograms can also be caused by entities such as eardrum perforations or impacted cerumen (or other obstructions) in the ear canal. Type C tympanograms had negative pressure peaks beyond –100 daPa (mm H$_2$O) indicating negative middle ear pressure.

They were associated with Eustachian tube disorders, and were also found in cases of middle ear fluid.

Not shown in the figure are tympanograms with notched peaks, which were classified as **type D** if the notch was narrow and **type E** if it was wide. These are rare occurrences when using 226-Hz (220-Hz) probe tones. Type D was associated with hypermobile or scarred (but otherwise normal) eardrums, whereas type E was found in cases of ossicular disruption.

STATIC ACOUSTIC IMMITTANCE

Static acoustic immittance is the immittance of the middle ear at some "representative" air pressure. It was originally considered to be the middle ear impedance or admittance obtained under conditions of atmospheric pressure (Zwislocki & Feldman, 1970; Feldman, 1975, 1976). This point might seem confusing because we pressurized the ear to figure out the middle ear admittance. However, remember that the *total* admittance can be measured *without* applying any pressure, that is, at atmospheric pressure of 0 daPa. Pressure is used to stiffen the eardrum to obtain the outer ear component. This "pressurized" outer ear value is then *removed* from the total admittance at atmospheric pressure, leaving the middle ear admittance at the eardrum, which is also at atmospheric pressure. In any case, this is the situation that presumably exists in the patient's ear "under regular conditions" when the probe tip is not there. On the tympanogram, it is the value of Y_{ME} obtained at 0 daPa, which is 0.75 mmho in Figure 7–4a (*point 3*). We will call this measurement "atmospheric static." The alternative approach is to measure static admittance at whatever pressure corresponds to the peak of the tympanogram (Brooks, 1969; Jerger 1970; Jerger, Jerger & Maudlin, 1972; Jerger et al, 1974a; Margolis & Popelka, 1975). We will call this value "peak static." (More accurately, it is the *peak-compensated static* admittance.) It occurs at –15 daPa in Figure 7–4a, where Y_{ME} is 0.85 mmho (*point 4*). The peak static method is preferred because it provides a more stable picture of middle ear admittance (Wiley, Oviatt, & Block, 1987).

The static acoustic admittance measurements obtained from a patient are compared to the applicable normative admittance values. These norms are usually expressed as 90% normal ranges, which means that they include the admittance values that fall between the 5th and 95th percentiles for a large group of subjects with normal middle ears. Table 7–1 shows some representative normal ranges for the static acoustic admittance of adults, children, and infants. The student should be aware that different normal ranges have been reported by other studies. These differences are largely due to disparities in methodology and the criteria

used for normalcy. This point also applies to the normal ranges used for the other tympanometric variables discussed below.

Two procedural variables warrant special mention. One of these is the effect of which "tail" is used for the ear canal value, as already discussed. The other major procedural variable is pump speed, or how fast the pressure is changed while obtaining the tympanogram. As illustrated in Table 7–2, different pump speeds result in different normal ranges. This is an important variable to consider when interpreting tympanograms, especially when fast pump speeds are used, as is often the case during screening tests.

A given static admittance measurement is considered to be (1) within normal limits if it falls within the normal range, (2) abnormally low if it falls below the lower limit of the normal range, and (3) abnormally high if it is above the upper limit of the normal range. The seven tympanograms in Figure 7–6 show static admittance values ranging from 2.6 mmhos for the tympanogram with the highest peak down to only 0.1 mmho for the lowest one, which is close to being flat. Let us compare these to the normal range for adults in Table 7–1. The tallest tympanogram is abnormally high because its static admittance (2.6 mmhos) is well above the upper limit of 1.66 mmhos. The static value for the second tympanogram from the top is 1.7 mmhos, which is right on the upper limit (rounded to the nearest tenth of mmho). We would probably consider it to be just within normal limits, especially if there is no air-

TABLE 7–1 Representative 90% normal ranges for peak static acoustic admittance (mmhos) for adults, children, and infants

Group	90% Normal Range
Adults[a]	0.37–1.66
Children[b]	0.35–1.25
Infants[c]	0.26–0.92

[a]Wiley (1989).

[b]Silman, Silverman, and Arick (1992).

[c]Margolis & Popelka (1975).

TABLE 7–2 Differences in 90% normal ranges for peak static acoustic admittance (mmhos) at slow and fast pump speeds[a]

Pump Speed	Adults[b]	Children (3–5 years)[c]
Slow (≤ 50 daPa/sec)	0.50–1.75	0.35–0.90
Fast (200 daPa/sec)	0.57–2.0	0.40–1.03

[a]Modified from Van Camp et al (1986).

[b]Based on data from Wilson, Shanks, and Kaplan (1984).

[c]Based on data from Koebsell and Margolis (1986).

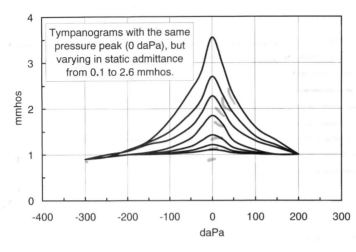

FIGURE 7–6 Examples of tympanograms with static admittance values ranging from (top to bottom) 2.6, 1.7, 1.3, 0.9, 0.4, 0.2, and 0.1 mmho. These values are the distances in mmhos between the height of the peaks and the ear canal value of 1.0 mmho at +200 daPa.

bone-gap. (It is also within the upper limit of 1.75 mmhos in Table 7–2.) The third and fourth curves have static values of 1.3 and 0.9 mmhos and are clearly within normal limits. The next tympanogram (third from the bottom) shows a static admittance value of 0.4 mmhos, which is just above the lower limit of 0.37. (Even though 0.4 mmhos is below the 0.5 mmho lower limit in Table 7–2, most clinicians use lower limits closer to those in Table 7–1, and some use even lower criteria taken from other studies.)

The second tympanogram from the bottom in Figure 7–6 reveals static admittance of 0.2 mmho, and the static admittance shown on the lowest one is 0.1 mmho. Both of these are abnormally low compared to the normal range shown in Table 7–1.

Abnormally low static acoustic admittance corresponds to abnormally high impedance and is generally associated with disorders such as otitis media, cholesteatoma, and otosclerosis. On the other hand, abnormally high static admittance (and thus abnormally low impedance) is often associated with disorders such as ossicular discontinuity. Unfortunately, the range of static admittance values found with the various types of disorders overlaps the normal range (Jerger, 1970; Jerger, Anthony, et al, 1974; Feldman, 1976; Shahnaz & Polka, 1997). There is even some degree of overlap between the ranges of static admittance values obtained from ears

with otosclerosis and ossicular discontinuity (Silman & Silverman, 1991).

If we apply the classical tympanogram types to the examples in Figure 7–6 we would categorize those having static admittance within the normal range as type A. The tympanogram with abnormally high admittance would be classified as either type A_D or A_{DD}. The two tympanograms with abnormally low admittance would be classified as A_S, although the lowest one might be considered "flat" enough to be categorized as type B. Notice that the tympanograms in this group have peaks at 0 daPa, so that the type A categories are straightforward. If these tympanograms had peak pressures of perhaps −165 daPa, then they would all have been classified as type C, and the differences in static admittance would have been obscured. (A possible exception is the lowest one, which might have been classified as type B.) This issue emphasizes the idea that details can be lost if one makes the mistake of considering tympanograms only by their letter designations.

TYMPANOMETRIC GRADIENT AND WIDTH

We see in Figure 7–6 that the tympanogram peak becomes smaller as the static admittance becomes lower. If the admittance becomes low enough, then there will be no discernible peak, so that the tympanogram is described as *flat*. This is a common finding in ears with otitis media and cholesteatoma, where the static admittance may be as low as 0.06 or less (Jerger, Anthony, et al, 1974). The flatness (versus peakedness) of a tympanogram can also be quantified by its **gradient**, which describes the relationship of its height and width. The gradient was originally calculated in terms of arbitrary units of compliance (Brooks, 1969), as shown in Figure 7–7a, and is determined as follows: (1) Draw a horizontal line where the width of the tympanogram is 100 mm H_2O (or daPa). (2) Measure the height of the peak above this line (hp), as well as the total height (ht) of the tympanogram from its peak to its baseline. In the figure hp is 3.6 compliance units and ht is 8 units. (3) Find the gradient by dividing hp/ht, which is 3.6/8 = 0.45 in the figure. The same procedure can be used to calculate

the gradient of absolute tympanograms, except that the heights are measured in terms of mmhos or mL.

Tympanometric gradients less than 0.2 are considered to be abnormally low (Nozza, Bluestone, Kardatzke, & Bachman, 1992) and are associated with the presence of middle ear fluid (Brooks, 1969; Paradise, Smith, & Bluestone, 1976; Fiellau-Nikolajsen, 1983; Nozza et al, 1992).

Another way to quantify the flatness of a tympanogram is to determine the **tympanometric width** (Koebsell & Margolis, 1986; ASHA 1997), which is simply the width of the tympanogram in daPa measured at 50% of its static acoustic admittance value. The method for determining tympanometric width is illustrated by the example in Figure 7–7b. The static admittance value is measured at the tympanogram peak and is found

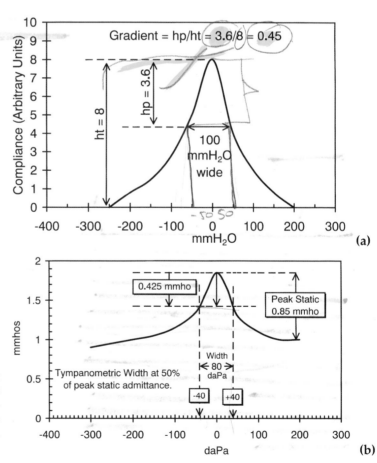

FIGURE 7–7 Examples illustrating how to measure (a) tympanometric gradient (shown in terms of the arbitrary compliance units that were used by relative immittance bridges), and (b) tympanometric width.

Type B [handwritten annotation]

to be 0.85 mmho in this example. We measure down 0.425 mmho from the peak because this distance is half the static value, and draw a horizontal line intersecting both sides of the tympanogram. Next, we draw vertical lines from these intersection points down to the x-axis. The tympanogram width is the distance between these two lines. In the example the tympanogram width is 80 daPa because the vertical lines cross the x-axis at −40 daPa and +40 daPa (which are 80 daPa apart).

Tympanometric widths that are too wide are associated with middle ear effusion, and normative data may be used to help determine when this is the case (e.g., Koebsell & Margolis, 1986; Margolis & Heller, 1987; Nozza, Bluestone, Kardatzke, & Bachman, 1992, 1994; Silman, Silverman, & Arick, 1992; Roush, Bryant, Mundy, Zeisel, & Roberts, 1995; AAA, 1997; ASHA, 1997; Shahnaz & Polka, 1997; DeChicchis, Todd, & Nozza, 2000). Representative upper cutoff values for tympanometric width are 235 daPa for infants and 200 daPa for 1-year-olds through school-age children (ASHA, 1997). Typical 90% normal ranges for adults are 51 to 114 daPa (Margolis & Heller, 1987) and 48 to 134 daPa (Shahnaz & Polka, 1997).

EAR VOLUME

Tympanograms with extremely small or absent peaks are often referred to as essentially flat. These findings are usually attributed to extremely low middle ear admittance, and are typically associated with middle ear pathologies such as otitis media and cholesteatoma. However, we can reach this conclusion only if the volume (admittance at 226 Hz) measured at +200 daPa (or at −300 or −400 daPa) is attributable to the ear canal. If the volume is too large, then the flat tympanogram may be due to such causes as (1) a perforated tympanic membrane; (2) a patent myringotomy tube, if one is present; or (3) the absence of a hermetic seal. It is reasonable to consider the volume to be larger than normal when it exceeds 2.0 mL (mmhos) in children and 2.5 mL (mmhos) in adults (Van Camp et

al, 1986; Silman & Silverman, 1991). On the other hand, the following causes are associated with volumes that are too small: (1) a clogged probe tip; (2) a probe tip that is pushed against the canal wall; (3) impacted cerumen or another obstruction in the ear canal; and (4) a clogged myringotomy tube, if one is present. These cases are usually identified by volumes at or close to 0 mL (mmhos). Figure 7–8 demonstrates how the flat tympanograms associated with tympanic membrane perforation, otitis media with effusion, and a clogged probe tip are differentiated on the basis of their ear canal volumes. It is very important to keep this issue in mind when tympanograms are classified by type because the letter designation does not account for the ear volume. For example, we could not attribute the type B tympanogram in Figure 7–5 to middle ear effusion unless we also know the ear volume.

TYMPANOMETRIC PEAK PRESSURE

We know the pressure on the outer ear side of the eardrum because it is generated and measured using the air pump and manometer connected to the probe tip. In addition, we have learned that the tympanogram peak occurs when the same pressure exists on both sides of the tympanic membrane. Consequently, the ear canal pressure corresponding to the tympanogram peak is also an estimate of the pressure within the middle ear. Figure 7–9 shows otherwise identical tympanograms with peak pressures of 0, −50, −150, and −250 daPa. Notice how increasingly negative tympanometric peak pressures are shown moving to the left of 0 daPa. Even though "tympanometric peak pressure" and "middle ear pressure" are often used interchangeably, we distinguish between the two terms here to point out that they are not always the same, especially when the patient has a flaccid tympanic membrane (Elner, Ingelstedt, & Ivarsson, 1971; Renvall & Liden, 1978; Margolis & Shanks, 1985).

Abnormally negative tympanometric peak pressures are associated with Eustachian tube disorders, which can occur either with

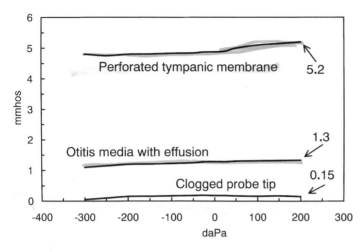

FIGURE 7–8 Flat tympanograms from cases with tympanic membrane perforation (top), otitis media with effusion (middle), and a clogged probe tip (bottom). Ear canal volumes at +200 daPa are indicated for each.

or without the presence of middle ear fluid. The amount of negative pressure needed to consider the tympanometric peak pressure *abnormally negative* is not clearly identifiable in the literature. Suggested cutoff values vary widely, including values such as –25 daPa (Holmquist & Miller, 1972), –30 daPa (Feldman, 1975), –50 daPa (Porter, 1972), –100 daPa (Jerger, 1970; Jerger, Jerger, Mauldin, 1972; G. Jerger, Jerger, Mauldin, & Segal, 1974; Fiellau-Nikolajsen, 1983; Silman, Silverman & Arick, 1992), –150 daPa (Renvall & Liden, 1978; Davies, John, Jones, & Stephens, 1988), and –170 daPa (Brooks, 1969). In practice, –100 daPa appears to be a reasonable low cutoff value for tympanometric peak pressure. Lower pressures suggest the possibility of Eustachian tube dysfunction. Unfortunately, there does not seem to be a particular tympanometric peak pressure cutoff value that successfully distinguishes between the presence and absence of middle ear effusion.

One can sometimes follow the course of recovery from a case of otitis media as tympanometric peak pressures that become progressively less negative over time (Feldman, 1976). This course of events can be seen in stylized form by imagining that the series of tympanograms in Figure 7–9 follows a sequence going from –250 daPa toward 0 daPa over a period of several days.

Unlike the situation for negative middle ear pressure, the significance of abnormally

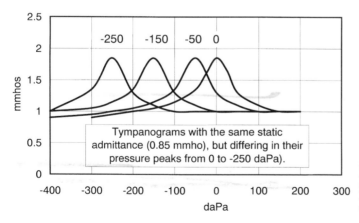

FIGURE 7–9 Examples of tympanograms with tympanometric peak pressures of 0 daPa, –50 daPa, –150 daPa, and –250 daPa.

high *positive* peak pressures (e.g., >50 daPa) is not clear. In spite of the extensive literature on tympanometry and middle ear pathology, only a few papers have reported positive pressures in some cases of otitis media (Paradise, Smith, & Bluestone, 1976; Feldman, 1976; Ostergard & Carter, 1981). In addition, positive peak pressure has also been associated with nonpathologic causes such as rapid elevator rides, crying, or nose blowing (Harford, 1980).

TYMPANOGRAM SHAPE

Low-frequency probe tones like 226 Hz are mainly sensitive to changes in stiffness (or compliance). The shapes of most 226-Hz (220-Hz) tympanograms do not provide much information because they are usually single-peaked or flat. The infrequent exception is the presence of a notch in the tympanogram peak. Notched tympanograms are produced when mass becomes a significant component of the ear's immittance, which occurs near and above its resonant frequency. For this reason notching is common with high-frequency probe tones, (e.g., 660 or 678 Hz) (Vanhuyse, Creten, & Van Camp, 1975; Van Camp, Creten, Van de Heyning, Decraemer, & Vanpeperstraete 1983; Van Camp et al, 1986; Wiley, Oviatt, & Block, 1987). Notching of the 226-Hz tympanogram is abnormal because it means that something is causing mass to play a greater than normal role in the ear. These changes can be produced by a scarred or flaccid tympanic membrane (even in an otherwise normal ear), as well as abnormalities such as ossicular discontinuities (which produce substantial hearing losses). Recall that these are the aberrations associated with type D and E tympanograms.

VASCULAR PULSING

Although most tympanograms are smooth, they sometimes have regular ripples or undulations that are synchronized with the patient's pulse, which is their origin. Medical referral is indicated when vascular pulsing is present on the tympanogram because it tends to occur in patients with glomus jugulare tumors (Feldman, 1976).

678-Hz (660-Hz) Tympanograms

"High-frequency" tympanograms are obtained with probe tones higher than the traditional "low-frequency" 226-Hz (or 220-Hz) probe tone. The "high-frequency" probe tone is usually 678 Hz (or 660 Hz). The combined use of 226-Hz and 678-Hz tympanograms is sometimes called **multiple frequency (or multifrequency) tympanometry**. However, this term is also used to describe various tympanometric methods that involve testing at many frequencies to arrive at the resonant frequency of the ear and other measures. Abnormally high resonant frequencies are associated with stiffening disorders, such as otosclerosis, whereas abnormally low resonant frequencies are associated with disorders that increase the mass component of the system, like ossicular discontinuity. The details of these and other advanced approaches are not covered here, but the interested student will find many readily available sources (e.g., Shanks, Lilly, Margolis, Wiley, & Wilson, 1988; Shanks & Sheldon, 1991; Hunter & Margolis, 1992; Margolis & Goycoolea, 1993; Shahnaz & Polka, 1997).

Separate tympanograms are obtained for susceptance (B) and conductance (G) when testing at 678 Hz (or 660 Hz) instead of a single admittance (Y) tympanogram. Depending on the instrumentation used, the B and G tympanograms may be obtained simultaneously (which is preferred), or they may be done one after the other. In either case, the interpretation is easier when they are plotted on the same tympanogram form.

NORMAL 678(660)-HZ TYMPANOGRAMS

In contrast to 226-Hz tympanograms, 678-Hz (660-Hz) B-G tympanograms are interpreted on the basis of their shapes and configurations (or morphology). There are four types of normal 678-Hz B-G tympanograms (Vanhuyse, Creten, & Van Camp, 1975; Van Camp et al, 1983, 1986; Wiley et al, 1987). They are named on the basis of the number of positive and negative peaks and must also meet a criterion for tympanogram width.

The first normal type of 678-Hz tympanogram is called **1B1G** because there is one peak for the B tympanogram and one peak for the G tympanogram (Fig. 7–10a). The other three normal variations involve notches on one or both of the tympanograms. The second normal type has a notched peak on the B tympanogram and a single peak on the G tympanogram. Notice that the notch on the B tympanogram can be viewed as two positive peaks with a negative peak between them. The convention is to count these "peaks" or "extrema." Thus, this normal variation is called **3B1G** because B has three peaks and G has one peak (Fig. 7–10b). The third normal variation is called **3B3G** because there are three peaks on both tympanograms (Fig. 7–10c). The last type of normal 678-Hz (or 660-Hz) configuration is called **5B3G** because it has five peaks on the B tympanogram and three peaks on the G tympanogram (Fig. 7–10d). In addition to having a maximum of five peaks for B and three peaks for G, the distance between the outermost peaks of normal 678-Hz B-G tympanograms should be (1) ≤75 daPa wide for 3B3G tympanograms and ≤100 daPa for 5B3G tympanograms, and (2) narrower for the G tympanogram than for the B tympanogram. Table 7–3 shows the percentages of normal adults with each of the 678-Hz B-G tympanogram types.

As a general rule, normal tympanograms are single-peaked at 220 or 226 Hz and often multiple-peaked at 660 or 678 Hz. However, an important exception to the typical relationship was pointed out by Sprague, Wiley,

TABLE 7–4 Percentages of ears with single-peaked (1B1G), multiple-peaked (3B1G, 3B3G, 5B3G) and flat tympanograms in normal neonates

	Single-Peaked	Multiple-Peaked	Flat
220 Hz	17	83	0
660 Hz	99	0	1

Based on Sprague, Wiley, and Goldstein, 1985.

and Goldstein (1985) in a study of normal neonates less than 1 week old. Their data are summarized in Table 7–4, where we see that neonates usually have single-peaked tympanograms at 660 Hz and a large proportion of multiple-peaked tympanograms at 220 Hz, which is the reverse of the typical arrangement.

ABNORMAL 678(660)-Hz TYMPANOGRAMS

A 678-Hz (660-Hz) B-G tympanogram is considered abnormal if it fails to meet the criteria just outlined, that is, if it (1) has too many peaks, and/or (2) is too wide. Abnormal 678(660)-Hz B-G tympanograms are principally associated with ossicular discontinuities, but they can also occur with tympanic membrane abnormalities. We can often distinguish between them because ossicular discontinuities usually cause significant amounts of hearing loss and appreciably alter the acoustic reflex, which is generally not the case with eardrum abnormalities per se. In addition, many tympanic membrane abnormalities can be visualized otoscopically.

The 678-Hz (660-Hz) B-G tympanograms often help us to distinguish between ossicu-

TABLE 7–3 Percentages of normal 678-Hz (or 660-Hz) B-G tympanograms

	1B1G	3B1G	3B3G	5B3G
Van Camp et al (1983)	56.8	28.1	6.0	9.1
Wiley, Oviatt, and Block (1987)	75.8	17.4	5.5	1.2
Weighted average	69.4	21.0	5.7	3.9

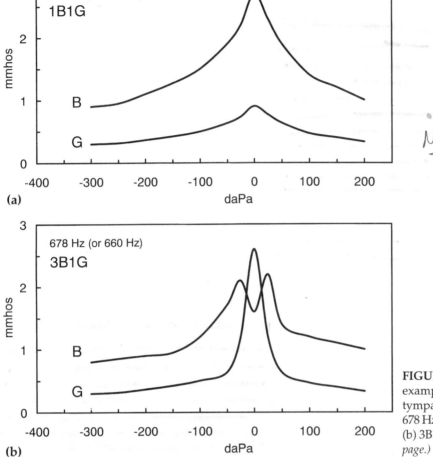

FIGURE 7–10 Illustrative examples of normal B-G tympanograms obtained at 678 Hz (or 660 Hz): (a) 1B1G, (b) 3B1G. *(Continued on next page.)*

lar discontinuities and other disorders, even when they are indistinguishable on the 226 Hz (220-Hz) tympanograms. Figure 7–11 shows 660-Hz B-G tympanograms from a case of ossicular discontinuity. This highly abnormal example is extremely wide and has an excessive number of peaks. In addition to being very abnormal this tympanogram is from a case that highlights the value of using 678(660)-Hz tympanometry. It is from a patient who previously had stapedectomy surgery in both ears for bilateral otosclerosis. He complained that the hearing in both ears worsened several years after the surgery, although he was not sure about the timing of the progression. His complaints were confirmed by much larger air-bone-gaps on his

new audiogram. On the surface, this seemed to be a case of otosclerosis that progressed bilaterally after the surgery. No insights could be gleaned from the 220-Hz tympanograms. The 660-Hz tympanogram had not appreciably changed in his left ear, where the ossicular chain was again fixated by progression of the otosclerosis. However, the 660-Hz B-G tympanogram shown in the figure was a new finding in his right ear, revealing an ossicular discontinuity that occurred when the surgically installed prosthesis (Chapter 6) became dislodged.

It is possible for there to be a "stiffening" disorder like otosclerosis *medially* and a "loosening" anomaly such as a scarred or flaccid eardrum *laterally* in the same ear.

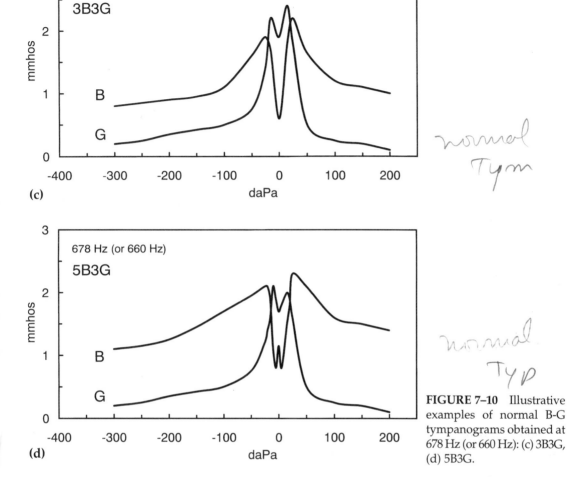

normal Tym

normal Typ

(c)

(d)

FIGURE 7–10 Illustrative examples of normal B-G tympanograms obtained at 678 Hz (or 660 Hz): (c) 3B3G, (d) 5B3G.

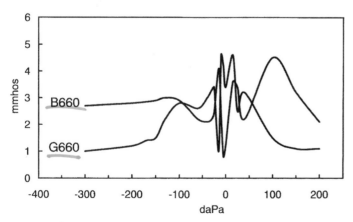

Abnormal Tympanogram

FIGURE 7–11 The abnormal 660-Hz B-G tympanogram of a patient with ossicular discontinuity (see text for discussion).

Under these conditions the tympanogram will reflect characteristics of the more lateral eardrum problem (Feldman, 1976).

Eustachian Tube Function Tests

We have already seen that Eustachian tube dysfunctions are inferred from the peak pressure of the tympanogram as a matter of routine. Further testing is occasionally desirable when it is important to determine the adequacy of Eustachian tube functioning in a given patient. For example, adequate Eustachian tube functioning is often a factor when dealing with matters such as inserting or removing a myringotomy tube, repairing a perforated tympanic membrane, adenoidectomy, and cleft palate surgery (e.g., Holmquist, 1968; Bluestone, Paradise, Berry, & Wittel, 1972; Hughes, 1985; Hughes & Pensak, 1997).

Eustachian tube functioning is usually assessed with an inflation test when the eardrum has a perforation or when a myringotomy tube is present (Bluestone, 1975, 1980). This method involves using the immittance device to pump air into the ear through the probe tip while monitoring the increasing pressure on the manometer. A properly functioning Eustachian tube should be forced open by the increasing air pressure. Opening of the Eustachian tube releases the built-up air pressure, which is seen as a reasonably abrupt drop of the air pressure back down toward 0 daPa on the manometer. A second step is needed if the built-up air pressure does not open the tube. In this case the patient is instructed to swallow several times, which should cause the Eustachian tube to open, causing the pressure to fall back to 0 daPa on the manometer. A Eustachian tube dysfunction is considered to be present if the pressure cannot be completely vented by swallowing.

Several Eustachian tube function tests are used when the tympanic membrane is intact, including the Valsalva, Toynbee, and inflation/deflation tests (Bluestone, 1975, 1980; Seifert, Seidemann, & Givens, 1979; Riedel, Wiley, & Block, 1987). Each of them involves

determining (1) whether the pressure within the middle ear can be changed by a given activity, and (2) if swallowing will successfully ventilate the middle ear so that the pressure can return to its original value. The procedures outlined here are the ones proposed by Riedel, Wiley, and Block (1987).

VALSALVA TEST

To perform the Valsalva maneuver the patient is instructed to close her mouth and nose (by pinching her nostrils) and then to blow hard so that her cheeks puff up and air is forced into her ears, creating a sensation of fullness. The first step in the Valsalva test is to do a pretest tympanogram, which provides a baseline value for peak pressure. The patient is then instructed to perform the Valsalva maneuver. She is told not to swallow, and a second tympanogram is then obtained. It is expected that the peak pressure will increase in the positive direction compared to the baseline value, indicating that the maneuver successfully increased the middle ear pressure. The patient is then asked to swallow several times. This may be done while drinking water ("wet") or without drinking water ("dry"). These swallows are expected to open the Eustachian tube, so that the middle ear is ventilated and its pressure can return to normal (i.e., to the pretest baseline value). A third tympanogram is then done to determine whether the peak pressure returned to the baseline value as a result of the swallowing.

TOYNBEE TEST

In the Toynbee maneuver the patient is instructed to swallow (dry) while holding his nose closed (by pinching his nostrils). The Toynbee maneuver is typically expected to make the middle ear pressure more negative, but it actually causes *either* a positive *or* negative shift in middle ear pressure (Riedel et al, 1987). The Toynbee test follows the same procedures used for the Valsalva test, except that the Toynbee maneuver is used. (Although it is not an audiological technique, one should be aware that the **Politzer test** involves supplementing this maneuver by forcing air into one of the nostrils from a rubber bulb or other air pressure source.)

INFLATION AND DEFLATION TESTS

The inflation and deflation tests are based on the notion that fairly large amounts of pressure in the outer ear will cause a slight change in middle ear pressure. The mechanism will become apparent as the test procedure is described. The first step in the inflation test is to measure the baseline peak pressure with a pretest tympanogram. Positive pressure of +400 daPa is then pumped into the ear canal. This is expected to push in on the tympanic membrane, making the middle ear volume slightly smaller. The patient is told to swallow (wet) several times while the positive pressure is being applied. This is expected to cause a small amount of negative pressure in the middle ear. A second tympanogram is now done, which is expected to show that the peak pressure is slightly more negative than the baseline. The pressure is then returned to 0 daPa and the patient is asked to swallow several times (wet or dry) in an attempt to ventilate the middle ear. A third tympanogram is then done, which is expected to show that the peak pressure has moved back to its baseline value. The inflation method appears to be the least useful of the various Eustachian tube tests because it produces the smallest amounts of pressure change.

The deflation test is procedurally identical to the inflation test, except that −400 daPa is used. The negative pressure in the outer ear is expected to pull back on the eardrum, so that the middle ear volume becomes slightly larger. The expected results are a slight increase in peak pressure during the second tympanogram, which returns to the baseline value on the third tympanogram.

There is no question that Eustachian tube tests should be performed when there is a specific need for the general information that they provide. However, it is noteworthy that Eustachian tube tests have not enjoyed general acceptance in spite of their longevity and the medical implications of Eustachian tube dysfunctions. This is at least partly due to the scarcity of criteria for normality and abnormality on these tests. Norms are not available for children. There are some adult norms for the sizes of the pressure shifts produced by each of the methods (Riedel et al, 1987), but how well they can discriminate between normal and abnormal patients is not known. These points suggest that Eustachian tube function testing should be used and interpreted conservatively.

The Acoustic Reflex

Presenting a sufficiently intense sound to either ear results in the contraction of the stapedius muscle in both ears, which is called the **acoustic** (or **stapedius**) **reflex**. This reflexive muscle contraction stiffens the conductive mechanism via the stapedius tendon, and therefore changes the ear's immittance. The acoustic reflex is easily measured because the immittance change is picked up by the probe tip and displayed on the immittance device meter.

Acoustic Reflex Arc

The acoustic reflex arc was described by Borg (1973), and its basic features are shown in Figure 7–12. Let us follow this pathway assuming that the right ear was stimulated (highlighted by the shaded arrows in the figure). The afferent (sensory) part of the arc involves the auditory (eighth) nerve from the right ear, which goes to the right (ipsilateral) ventral cochlear nucleus. Neurons then go to the superior olivary complexes on both sides of the brainstem. The right and left superior olivary complexes send signals to the facial (seventh) nerve nuclei on their respective sides. Finally, the efferent (motor) legs of the acoustic reflex arc involve the right and left facial nerves, which direct the stapedius muscles to contract in both ears. Notice that the acoustic reflex involves the stapedius muscles. While the tensor tympani muscles do respond to extremely intense sounds, this is actually part of a startle reaction, and the

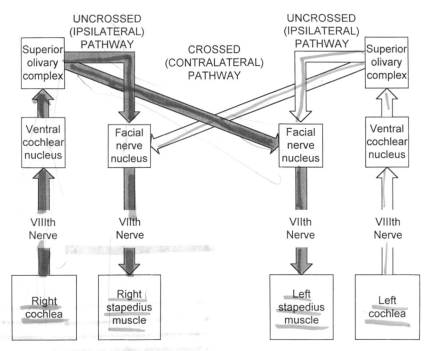

FIGURE 7–12   Schematic diagram of the acoustic reflex arc. The shaded arrows highlight the ipsilateral (uncrossed) and contralateral (crossed) reflex arcs resulting from stimulation of the right cochlea.

accumulated evidence reveals that the acoustic reflex in humans is a stapedius reflex (Gelfand, 1998). Certain kinds of non-acoustic stimulation also elicit contractions of the stapedius muscles (e.g., tactile stimulation of the external ear), or of both middle ear muscles (e.g., an air puff to the eye). These reflexes can be used in advanced diagnostic methods (Wiley & Block, 1984).

Acoustic Reflex Tests

The basic acoustic reflex testing procedure involves presenting a sufficiently intense tone or noise to activate the reflex, and observing any resulting immittance change, which is usually seen as a decrease in the ear's admittance (i.e., an increase in its impedance). The immittance change caused by the contraction of the stapedius muscle is measured in the ear containing the probe tip, which is called the **probe ear**. The ear receiving the stimulus used to activate the reflex is called the **stimulus ear**. Either ear can be the stimulus ear because the stimulus can be delivered from the receiver in the probe tip (the fourth tube described earlier) or the earphone on the opposite ear. The **ipsilateral** or **uncrossed** acoustic reflex is being measured when the stimulus is presented to the probe ear, which is the same ear in which the immittance change is being monitored. In contrast, the **contralateral** or **crossed** acoustic reflex is being measured when the probe tip is in one ear and the stimulus goes to the opposite ear.

It is easy to identify whether the right or left ear is being tested for the ipsilateral reflex because the reflex is activated and monitored in the same (probe) ear. However, there can be confusion about which ear is the "test ear" with contralateral reflexes because the stimulus and probe are in opposite ears. In fact, both ears (and the reflex pathway between them) are really being tested with the contralateral reflex. The convention is to identify a contralateral acoustic reflex according to the simulated ear. Hence, a "right contralateral acoustic reflex" means that the stimulus is in the right ear (with the probe in the left ear), and a "left contralateral acoustic reflex" means that the stimulus is in the left ear (with the probe in the right ear). Another way to avoid confusion is to describe the test results as, for example, "stimulus right" or "probe left." The testing arrangements are shown schematically Figure 7–13. The usual reflex testing order is to do the left contralateral and right ipsilateral reflexes while the probe is in the right ear (Fig. 7–13, upper frame), and then to reverse the headset and do the right contralateral and left ipsilateral reflex test while the probe is in the left ear (Fig. 7–13, lower frame). To help the student sort out what goes where, Figure 7–14 summarizes the various reflex

test arrangements in terms of both (a) the stimulus and the probe and (b) the right and left ears.

A variety of acoustic reflex tests are regularly used in clinical assessment. The two basic measurements are discussed here: the **acoustic reflex threshold**, which is the lowest stimulus level that produces a reflex response; and **acoustic reflex decay**, which is a measure of how long the response lasts if the stimulus is kept on for a period of time. Some more advanced techniques include (1) **acoustic reflex magnitude and growth functions** (how the size of the response depends on stimulus level); (2) acoustic reflex latency (the time delay between the stimulus and the reflex response); and (3) **nonacoustic reflexes** (middle ear muscle reflexes that are stimulated tactually, electrically, or with air puffs instead of sound). The interested stu-

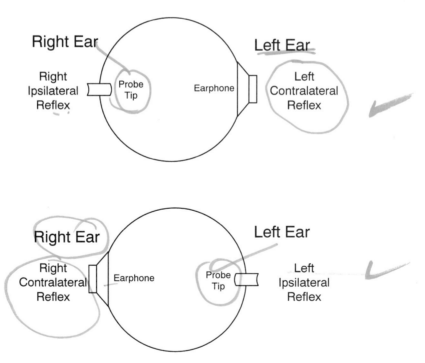

FIGURE 7–13   The stimulus and probe are in opposite ears for the contralateral (crossed) acoustic reflex and in the same ear for the ipsilateral (uncrossed) acoustic reflex. Expressing the reflex according to the ear being stimulated, we measure the right ipsilateral and left contralateral reflexes when the probe is in the right ear (upper frame), and the left ipsilateral and right contralateral reflexes when the probe tip is in the left ear (lower frame).

Arrangement in Terms of Stimulus and Probe		
TEST CONDITION	STIMULUS	PROBE
Right Contralateral (Crossed)	Right Ear	Left Ear
Left Contralateral (Crossed)	Left Ear	Right Ear
Right Ipsilateral (Uncrossed)	Right Ear	Right Ear
Left Ipsilateral (Uncrossed)	Left Ear	Left Ear

Arrangement in Terms of Right Ear and Left Ear		
TEST CONDITION	RIGHT EAR	LEFT EAR
Right Contralateral (Crossed)	Stimulus	Probe
Left Contralateral (Crossed)	Probe	Stimulus
Right Ipsilateral (Uncrossed)	Stimulus & Probe	
Left Ipsilateral (Uncrossed)		Stimulus & Probe

FIGURE 7–14   Summary of acoustic reflex testing arrangements and terminology in terms of the stimulus and probe (above) and the right ear and left ear (below).

dent will find these and related topics covered in many sources (Silman & Gelfand, 1982; Bosatra, Russolo, & Silverman, 1984; Silman, 1984; Wiley & Block, 1984; Silman & Silverman, 1991; Wilson & Margolis, 1991; Northern & Gabbard, 1994; Gelfand, 2000).

ACOUSTIC REFLEX THRESHOLD

Acoustic reflex threshold (ART) testing involves finding the lowest level of a stimulus that causes a measurable change in acoustic immittance. Figure 7–15 shows the measurement of an ART under laboratory conditions and illustrates several characteristics of the reflex response. Notice that the immittance changes attributed to the reflex are associated in time with the stimulus presentations, and that the magnitude of the

reflex response increases as the stimulus level is raised above the ART. Hence, we may also say that the ART is the smallest discernible immittance change that is associated in time with the presentation of a stimulus, and that responses should also be present (and generally larger) at higher stimulus levels. Clinical ARTs are usually obtained using pure-tone stimuli at 500, 1000, and 2000 Hz. Even though some clinicians also use 4000 Hz, it is not recommended because even young, normal hearing persons experience elevated ARTs at this frequency due to rapid adaptation (Gelfand, 1984). Clinically, pure-tone ARTs are obtained by changing the intensity of the stimulus in 5-dB steps while watching for admittance changes caused by the stimuli. These admittance changes are observed by watching for deflections on the admittance

Stimulus Presentation (Event) Markers and Sound Pressure Levels:

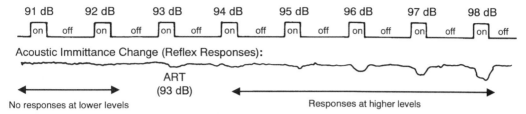

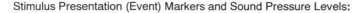

FIGURE 7–15 The acoustic reflex threshold is the lowest stimulus level resulting in an observable immittance change that is "time-locked" to a stimulus presentation. These data were obtained under laboratory conditions, using 1-dB stimulus steps and simultaneous recording of the stimulus presentations ("event marker") and reflex responses.

device meter, and the ART is considered to be the lowest intensity causing a deflection that can be distinguished from the background activity on the meter. This approach is often called "visual monitoring with 5-dB steps." It is sometimes necessary to test reflex thresholds using **broadband noise (BBN)** stimuli. Unlike pure-tone ART testing, which can use visual monitoring with 5-dB steps, 1- or 2-dB steps and recorded responses are needed to accurately measure ARTs for *broadband noise* stimuli even for clinical purposes. This is due to the very small size of the reflex response at and just above the ART when broadband noise is used (Silman, Popelka, & Gelfand, 1978; Gelfand, 1984; Silman, 1984; Silman, Piper, Silverman, Gelfand, & VanFrank, 1984). These small reflex responses are often missed with visual monitoring, and the lowest level at which they occur is obscured with 5-dB steps. As a result, visual monitoring with

5-dB steps often causes the normal *BBN* ART to appear higher (poorer) than it really is, and also shrinks the size of the normal 20-dB noise-tone difference (Gelfand & Piper, 1981; Gelfand, 1984).

Normal ARTs occur between about 85 and 100 dB SPL for *pure tones* and approximately 20 dB lower when the stimulus is *broadband noise* (Gelfand, 1984). Most clinical measurements involve pure-tone ARTs. Table 7–5 shows a representative set of contralateral and ipsilateral ARTs (in dB HL) for normal hearing individuals. In addition, the difference between the ARTs for pure tones and broadband noise is the basis of many methods that attempt to identify or predict hearing loss from ARTs (Silman, Gelfand, Piper, Silverman, & VanFrank, 1984; Silman, Gelfand, & Emmer, 1987), as discussed below.

Acoustic reflex testing is usually done with a 220- or 226-Hz probe tone. An important

TABLE 7–5 Acoustic reflex thresholds in dB HL for normal hearing subjects

	Pure Tones (Hz)				Broadband Noise
	500	*1000*	*2000*	*4000*	
Contralateral ART					
Mean	84.6	85.9	84.4	89.8	66.3
Standard deviation	6.3	5.2	5.7	8.9	8.8
Ipsilateral ART					
Mean	79.9	82.0	86.2	87.5	64.6
Standard deviation	5.0	5.2	5.9	3.5	6.9

Based on Wiley, Oviatt, and Block, 1987.

TABLE 7–6   Pure-tone (1000 Hz) and broadband noise acoustic reflexes in normal neonates using 220-Hz versus 660-Hz probe tones

Probe Frequency (Hz)		Present (%)		Mean ART (dB HL)	
		220	660	220	660
1000 Hz	Ipsilateral	43	81	82.6	81.7
	Contralateral	34	60	92.2	89.1
Broadband noise	Ipsilateral	51	74	60.9	54.6
	Contralateral	49	83	70.0	70.1

Based on Sprague, Wiley, and Goldstein, 1985.

exception occurs when testing neonates because their acoustic reflexes are often elevated or absent with a 226-Hz probe tone but are more likely to be present with ARTs more or less similar to those found in adults when using higher-frequency probe tones (Bennett & Weatherby, 1982; Gelfand, 1984; Sprague, Wiley, & Goldstein, 1985). Table 7–6 compares the effects of 220-Hz versus 660-Hz probe tones on the percentages of normal newborns' present reflexes and ARTs. These data show that newborns are more likely to have measurable reflexes and better ARTs with the 660-Hz probe tone, especially when testing ipsilaterally with a broadband noise stimulus.

ACOUSTIC REFLEX DECAY

In addition to the ART, it is also common practice to test for acoustic reflex decay (or adaptation), which is a measure of whether a reflex contraction is maintained or dies out during continuous stimulation (Anderson, Barr, & Wedenberg, 1970; Jerger, Harford, Clemis, & Alford, 1974; Wilson, Shanks, & Lilly, 1984). Reflex decay is tested at both 500 and 1000 Hz. Higher frequencies are not tested because even normal people can have rapid reflex decay above 1000 Hz. The test involves presenting a stimulus tone continuously for 10 seconds at a level 10 dB above the reflex threshold. The magnitude of the reflex response will either stay the same or decrease over the course of the 10-second stimulus, as shown in Figure 7–16. The central issue is whether the response decays to half of its original magnitude. If the magnitude of the reflex response does not decrease to 50% of its original size during the 10-second test period (Fig. 7–16a,b), then the outcome is considered negative. The test is considered positive if the magnitude of the reflex response does decay by 50% or more within this time period (Fig. 7–16c).

CONDUCTIVE HEARING LOSS

Conductive hearing losses cause acoustic reflexes to be either "elevated" or "absent." By "elevated" we mean that the ART is higher than normal, that is, it takes more intensity to reach the reflex threshold than would have been needed if there was no conductive loss. An "absent" reflex means that a reflex response cannot be obtained, even with the most intense stimulus available (which is usually 125 dB HL on most modern immittance devices). The effects of conductive loss can be summarized by two basic rules:

1. **Probe-ear rule:** The presence of conductive pathology in the probe ear causes the acoustic reflex to be absent. Here, even though the stapedius muscle itself may actually be contracting, the presence of the pathology prevents us from being able to register any change in acoustic admittance that can be picked up by the probe tip. In fact, Jerger, Anthony, Jerger, and Mauldin (1974) found that the chances of

having a measurable acoustic reflex fell to 50% when the air-bone-gap in the probe ear (averaged across frequencies) was only 5 dB.

2. **Stimulus-ear rule:** A conductive loss in the stimulus ear causes the ART to be elevated by the amount of the conductive impairment. This occurs because the amount of the stimulus that actually reaches the cochlea will be reduced by the amount of the air-bone-gap. For example, suppose an otherwise normal patient develops otitis media with a 25-dB air-bone-gap. The 25-dB air-bone-gap causes the signal reaching her cochlea to be 25 dB weaker than the level presented from the earphone. If her ART would normally have been 85 dB HL (without the conductive loss), then the stimulus would now have to be raised by 25 dB to 110 dB HL to reach her cochlea at 85 dB HL. Hence, her ART would now be elevated to 110 dB HL. In addition, if the air-bone-gap is large enough, then the ART will be elevated so much that the reflex will be absent. This occurs because the highest available stimulus level cannot overcome the size of the air-bone-gap and still deliver a large enough signal to the cochlea. Jerger, Anthony, et al (1974) found that the chances of having an absent acoustic reflex reached 50% when the conductive loss (averaged across frequencies) was 27 dB in the stimulus ear. This occurred because the (otherwise normal) average ART of about 85 dB HL plus an average air-bone-gap of 27 dB is more than 110 dB HL, which was the highest stimulus level available at that time. Modern immittance instruments allow testing up to 125 dB HL, so that the 50% point for absent reflexes is not reached until there is a 42-dB air-bone-gap in the stimulus ear (Gelfand, 1984).

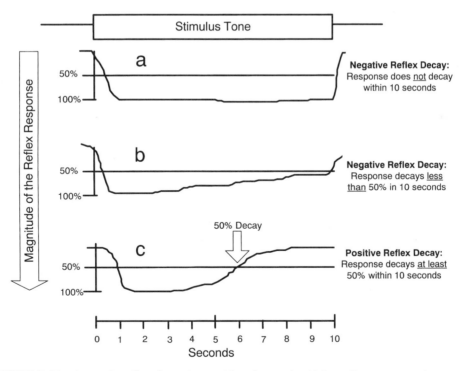

FIGURE 7–16   Acoustic reflex decay is considered negative if the reflex response does not decrease (tracing a) or if it decreases by less than half of its original magnitude (tracing b). Reflex decay is positive if the magnitude falls by 50% or more (tracing c).

The following acoustic reflex configurations result from the two principles just described: For unilateral conductive losses, contralateral acoustic reflexes tend to be (1) absent when the probe is in the pathological ear, and (2) elevated or absent when the probe is in the normal ear. Contralateral acoustic reflexes tend to be absent in both ears when there is a bilateral conductive impairment. Ipsilateral acoustic reflexes are affected by both principles at the same time; that is, the air-bone-gap reduces the effective level of the stimulus that actually reaches the cochlea and the conductive pathology prevents an immittance change from being monitored even if the reflex is activated. Consequently, ipsilateral acoustic reflexes tend to be absent when testing an ear with a conductive disorder, regardless of the condition of the opposite ear. These findings are illustrated in Figure 7–17 for a unilateral conductive loss and in Figure 7–18 for a bilateral conductive disorder.

SENSORINEURAL HEARING LOSS

Acoustic reflex thresholds depend on hearing sensitivity in a rather peculiar way (Popelka, 1981; Silman & Gelfand, 1981; Gelfand, Piper, & Silman, 1983; Gelfand, 1984; Gelfand & Piper, 1984; Gelfand, Schwander, & Silman, 1990). In this context "hearing sensitivity" represents a continuum going from normal hearing through various magnitudes of sensorineural hearing loss due to cochlear disorders. Figures 7–19 through 7–21 show the 10th, 50th, and 90th percentiles of the ARTs at 500, 1000, and 2000 Hz for patients who have normal hearing or sensorineural

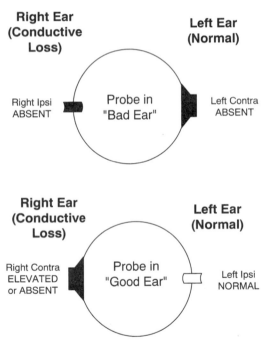

FIGURE 7–17   Configuration of contralateral and ipsilateral acoustic reflexes in unilateral conductive hearing loss. The conductive loss affects the right ear in this example. Contralateral reflexes are absent with the probe in the abnormal ear ("probe-ear rule," upper frame), and are elevated (or absent) with probe in the good ear and the contralateral stimulus going to the bad ear ("stimulus ear rule," lower frame). The ipsilateral reflexes are absent when the probe is in the abnormal right (upper frame) ear, and normal when the probe is in the normal left ear (lower frame).

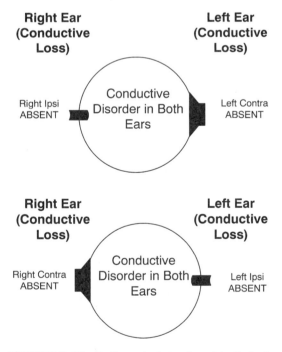

FIGURE 7–18   Both contralateral and both ipsilateral reflexes tend to be absent when there is a bilateral conductive disorder.

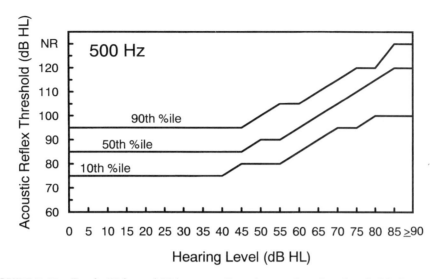

FIGURE 7–19 Tenth, 50th, and 90th percentiles of acoustic reflex thresholds for a 500-Hz stimulus as a function of the hearing level at 500 Hz for people with normal hearing and sensorineural hearing losses of cochlear origin. Adapted from Gelfand, Schwander, & Silman (1990), with permission of American Speech-Language-Hearing Association.

losses associated with cochlear disorders. For example, Figure 7–19 provides the following information about patients who have thresholds of 5 dB HL at 500 Hz: 10% of them have ARTs up to 75 dB HL, 50% have ARTs up to 85 dB HL, and 90% have ARTs up to 95 dB HL. Similarly, Figure 7-20 shows that among patients who have thresholds of 60 dB HL at 1000 Hz: 10% have ARTs up to 85 dB HL, 50% have ARTs up to 95 dB HL, and 90% have ARTs up to 110 dB HL. Using the median (50th percentile) curves as a guide,

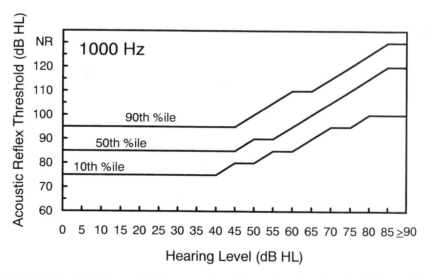

FIGURE 7–20 Tenth, 50th, and 90th percentiles of acoustic reflex thresholds for a 1000-Hz stimulus as a function of the hearing level at 1000 Hz for people with normal hearing and sensorineural hearing losses of cochlear origin. Adapted from Gelfand, Schwander, & Silman (1990), with permission of American Speech-Language-Hearing Association.

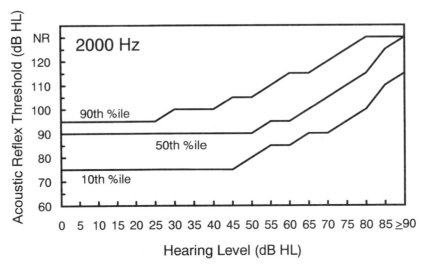

FIGURE 7–21   Tenth, 50th, and 90th percentiles of acoustic reflex thresholds for a 2000-Hz stimulus as a function of the hearing level at 2000 Hz for people with normal hearing and sensorineural hearing losses of cochlear origin. Adapted from Gelfand, Schwander, & Silman (1990), with permission of American Speech-Language-Hearing Association.

we see that pure-tone acoustic reflex thresholds (1) are about the same for people with normal hearing and sensorineural hearing losses of cochlear origin *up to roughly* 50 dB HL, and (2) become progressively higher as the amount of cochlear hearing loss increases *above about* 50 dB HL.

It is well established that patients with retrocochlear pathologies have acoustic reflexes that are elevated, often to the extent that the reflex is absent (Gelfand, 1984). However, the decision about when an ART is "elevated" must account for the fact that the ARTs depend on the magnitude of the hearing loss in patients who do not have retrocochlear involvement. The 90th percentiles provide us with upper cutoff values for ARTs that meet this need. In fact, many prior inconsistencies about the diagnostic usefulness of the reflex were resolved by the introduction of 90th percentiles that account for the degree of hearing loss (Silman & Gelfand, 1981; Gelfand, 1984).

Two sets of 90th percentile values are shown in Table 7–7 (Silman & Gelfand, 1981; Gelfand, Schwander, & Silman, 1990) because both are in common use and distinguish

between cochlear and retrocochlear ears with considerable success (Olsen, Bauch, & Harner, 1983; Gelfand, 1984; Sanders, 1984; Gelfand et al, 1990; Silman & Silverman, 1991; Gelfand, 2000).

In practice, the patient's ARTs are compared to the respective 90th percentiles that apply to his hearing thresholds for the frequencies tested. If an ART falls on or below the relevant 90th percentile, then it is considered to be essentially within the normal and/or cochlear distribution. However, ARTs that fall above the applicable 90th percentiles are considered elevated because only a small proportion of normal and/or cochlear-impaired ears have ARTs that are so high. If the abnormally elevated or absent reflexes are not attributable to a conductive disorder, then the patient is considered to be at risk for eighth nerve pathology in the ear that receives the stimulus. In contrast, many patients with functional impairments (Chapter 14) have ARTs that are below the 10th percentiles (Gelfand, 1994).

Abnormal reflex decay means that the response decreases rapidly, and is associated with retrocochlear disorders (Anderson,

TABLE 7–7   Acoustic reflex threshold 90th percentile cutoff values as a function of hearing level at 500, 1000, and 2000 Hz

	90th Percentile Acoustic Reflex Threshold Norms (dB HL)					
	Silman & Gelfand (1981)			Gelfand, Schwander, & Silman (1990)		
Hearing Threshold (dB HL)	500 Hz	1000 Hz	2000 Hz	500 Hz	1000 Hz	2000 Hz
0	95	100	95	95	95	95
5	95	100	95	95	95	95
10	95	100	100	95	95	95
15	95	100	100	95	95	95
20	95	100	100	95	95	95
25	95	100	100	95	95	95
30	100	100	105	95	95	100
35	100	100	105	95	95	100
40	100	105	105	95	95	100
45	100	105	105	95	95	105
50	105	105	110	100	100	105
55	105	105	110	105	105	110
60	105	110	115	105	110	115
65	105	110	115	110	110	115
70	115	115	125	115	115	120
75	115	115	125	120	120	125
80	125	125	125	120	125	NR
85	125	125	125	NR	NR	NR
≥90	125	125	125	NR	NR	NR

NR, no response at 125 dB HL.

Barr, & Wedenberg, 1970; Jerger, Harford, Clemis, & Alford, 1974; Wilson, Shanks, & Lilly, 1984). It is prudent to be suspicious of retrocochlear pathology in the stimulated ear if the reflex response decays by 50% or more within 10 seconds (as in Figure 7–16c) at either 500 Hz and/or 1000 Hz. However, the student should be aware that there are differences in approach regarding whether abnormal decay should occur during the first 5 seconds versus any time during the 10 second test, as well as how to interpret reflex decay that occurs at one frequency and/or the other (Anderson, Barr, & Wedenberg, 1970; Jerger, Harford, Clemis, & Alford, 1974; Hirsch & Anderson, 1980; Olsen, Stach, & Kurdziel, 1981; Wilson et al, 1984).

We have seen that acoustic reflex abnormalities such as elevated/absent reflexes and/or positive reflex decay are associated with retrocochlear pathologies in the ear receiving the stimulus tone. Testing both ARTs and reflex decay and considering a positive result on *either or both* tests as the criterion for suspecting retrocochlear pathology has been referred to as *acoustic reflexes combined* (ARC) (Turner, Frazer, & Shepard, 1984; Turner, Shepard, & Frazer, 1984). Acoustic reflex thresholds *and* decay should be routinely tested *because ARC with 90th percentiles* has a hit rate of about 85% for retrocochlear pathology and a false-positive rate of only 11% (Silman & Silverman, 1991).

ACOUSTIC REFLEX CONFIGURATIONS

We have already seen that patients with conductive disorders typically have certain configurations of acoustic reflex findings (Figs. 7–17 and 7–18). It has also been pointed out that eighth nerve pathology (e.g., acoustic neuroma) is associated with reflex abnormalities affecting the stimulated ear, which is expected because the eighth nerve is the sensory leg of the acoustic reflex arc. A typical example is depicted in Figure 7–22. Notice

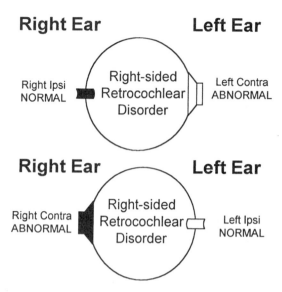

FIGURE 7–22 Typical configuration of acoustic reflex findings for an eighth nerve (extraaxial retrocochlear) disorder in the right ear.

that the right ear's ipsilateral (uncrossed) and contralateral (crossed) reflexes are both abnormal because they both stimulate the pathological auditory nerve, whereas both of the left ear reflexes are unaffected because they involve stimulating the normal eighth nerve.

In addition to retrocochlear lesions affecting the eighth nerve, acoustic reflex abnormalities are also associated with brainstem pathologies and facial nerve disorders, as well as demyelinating (e.g., multiple sclerosis) and neuromuscular (e.g., myasthenia gravis) diseases (Bosatra et al, 1984; Gelfand, 1984; Mangham, 1984; Wiley & Block, 1984; Wilson, Shanks, & Lilly, 1984). Acoustic reflexes are typically absent in patients with auditory neuropathy (Starr, Picton, Sininger, Hood, & Berlin, 1996). Cortically involved patients have the same ARTs as normal and cochlear-impaired patients with similar hearing sensitivity (Gelfand & Silman, 1982). Acoustic reflex configurations can help us distinguish among at least some of these categories of disorders, such as brainstem pathologies affecting the crossed reflex pathway and disorders of the facial nerve.

Pathologies *within* the brain stem are often called **intraaxial** to distinguish them from disorders such as acoustic tumors that are located outside the brainstem proper (which might be called **extraaxial**). Intra axial brainstem pathologies often affect the reflex pathways going from one side to the other, while not impacting on the ipsilateral pathways (Jerger & Jerger, 1977, 1983). This situation is shown in Figure 7–23. Notice how the contralateral (crossed) reflexes are abnormal because they are affected by the intraaxial lesion, whereas the unaffected ipsilateral (uncrossed) reflexes are normal.

In contrast to eighth nerve disorders that are associated with acoustic reflex abnormalities when the abnormal side is stimulated, *facial (seventh) nerve disorders* (e.g., Bell's palsy) are associated with abnormal reflexes when the probe tip is on the pathological side (Alford, Jerger, Coats, Peterson, & Weber, 1973; Citron & Adour, 1978; Wiley & Block, 1984). This occurs because the facial nerve is the motor leg of the acoustic reflex arc that innervates the stapedius muscle. Hence, the abnormality is seen in the probe ear because this is where the effects of the muscle contraction are being monitored (Fig. 7–24). Facial nerve disorders are generally

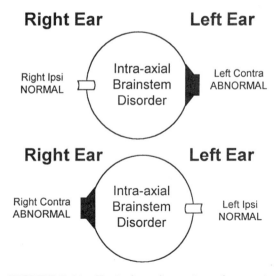

FIGURE 7–23 Typical configuration of acoustic reflex findings for intraaxial brainstem disorders.

**Right Ear
(Facial Nerve
Disorder)**

**Left Ear
(Normal)**

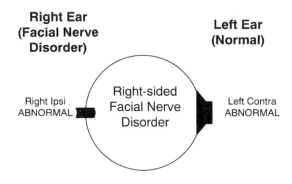

Right Ipsi
ABNORMAL

Right-sided
Facial Nerve
Disorder

Left Contra
ABNORMAL

**Right Ear
(Facial Nerve
Disorder)**

**Left Ear
(Normal)**

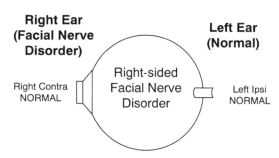

Right Contra
NORMAL

Right-sided
Facial Nerve
Disorder

Left Ipsi
NORMAL

FIGURE 7–24 Abnormal acoustic reflex findings occur when the probe tip is located on the side of the facial nerve disorder. Thus, a right-sided facial nerve disorder will affect the right ipsilateral and left contralateral acoustic reflexes.

discovered by observable signs of facial involvement and other neurological indicators besides stapedius reflex abnormalities. Thus, one of the major uses of acoustic reflexes has been to monitor the course of Bell's palsy through its recovery. However, it has been shown that seventh nerve disorders can cause ipsilateral and contralateral acoustic reflex decay (with the probe tip on the abnormal side) even when there are no signs of facial palsy (Silman, Silverman, Gelfand, Lutolf, & Lynn, 1988). Consequently, the possibility of seventh nerve involvement should be kept in mind whenever acoustic reflexes are being interpreted.

Hearing Loss Identification and Prediction

Several approaches have been devised that attempt to identify the presence of hearing loss or to predict its extent from ARTs

(Popelka, 1981; Silman & Gelfand, 1982; Silman, Gelfand, et al, 1984; Silman, Gelfand, & Emmer, 1987). As with other physiological methods, these acoustic reflex techniques were developed because we often have to evaluate the hearing of patients who cannot or will not respond reliably on routine behavioral tests. This might occur because the patient is too young for behavioral testing, or because the patient has one or more physical, cognitive, and/or emotional impairments that make behavioral testing difficult or impossible. Acoustic reflex-based methods for identifying or predicting hearing loss rely in various ways on the relationships of pure-tone and broadband noise ARTs, and how these are affected by hearing loss. Recall that there is a 20-dB difference between the normal pure-tone and broadband noise ARTs, and that tonal ARTs are independent of hearing thresholds for sensorineural losses up to roughly 50 to 60 dB HL, above which ARTs get higher as the amount of hearing loss increases. The opposite relationship exists for broadband noise ARTs, which become higher as hearing loss increases up to about 50 to 60 dB HL, and then remain more or less constant for greater amounts of hearing loss (Popelka, 1981). These relationships are illustrated in Figure 7–25.

The earliest hearing loss prediction methods attempted to predict the degree of hearing loss in decibels (Niemeyer & Sesterhenn, 1974) or in categories (Jerger, Burney, Mauldin, & Crump, 1974). The latter method, called **sensitivity prediction from the acoustic reflex (SPAR)**, was revised several times (Jerger, Hayes, Anthony, & Mauldin, 1978). Unfortunately, these types of procedures were found to have large error rates in terms of false-positive and false-negative rates and the accuracy with which the severity of hearing loss was predicted (Silman, Gelfand, et al, 1984). Another kind of approach tried to predict hearing loss from ARTs using formulas derived from statistical procedures called regression analyses (e.g., Baker & Lilly, 1976; Rizzo & Greenberg, 1979), although the predictive accuracy of these approaches was not very high (Hall & Koval, 1982; Silman, Gel-

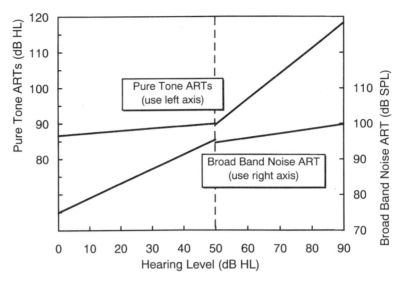

FIGURE 7–25 Acoustic reflex thresholds are related to the degree of hearing loss in different ways for pure-tone (left axis, dB HL) and broadband noise (right axis, dB SPL) stimuli. The relationships are shown as separate straight line functions for hearing losses below and above 50 dB HL to highlight the general concepts. Based on data from Gelfand, Schwander, & Silman (1990) for pure tones and Popelka (1981) for broadband noise.

fand, et al, 1984). The problems faced by methods that try to predict the degree of loss were due to several factors, such as: (1) the peculiarities of the relationships shown in Figure 7–25 (e.g., the noise-tone difference gets smaller and then widens again as hearing loss increases); (2) regression formulas use the ART as the independent variable and hearing loss as the dependent variable, which is the opposite of the actual relationship; and (3) the range of ARTs is roughly 20 dB wide for any given amount of hearing loss (Popelka, 1981; Gelfand, 1984; Silman, Gelfand, et al, 1984; Silman, Gelfand, & Emmer, 1987).

A more successful approach involves the more conservative goal of simply identifying whether a significant hearing loss is present rather than trying to predict its magnitude. One approach of this type uses just the broadband noise ART because it is sensitive to even small amounts of hearing loss. Keith (1977) found that BBN ARTs were ≤85 dB SPL in 86.5% of normal hearing individuals, and >85 dB SPL in 96.9% of hearing impaired patients. He therefore suggested using a broadband

noise ART of 85 dB SPL as a cutoff value for distinguishing between normal and impaired hearing. However, Keith's sample did not include losses between 20 and 33 dB HL, and the age range of the subjects was unspecified. Silman, Gelfand, et al (1984) and Silman, Silverman, Showers, and Gelfand (1984) found that adults with mild and high-frequency hearing losses had BBN reflex thresholds on both sides of the 85 dB SPL cutoff value. Although these factors limit the direct application of the 85 dB SPL cutoff value, especially with adults, they certainly do not detract from the value of the basic approach.

Another approach that has been widely used is the bivariate method, which uses both tonal and BBN ARTs (Popelka & Trumph, 1976; Popelka, 1981). It is called the **bivariate method** because the ART data are plotted on an x-y graph (Fig. 7–26). The x-axis shows the ratio of patient's BBN ARTs to tonal ARTs, and the y-axis shows the pure-tone ARTs. A sample of reflex data from people with known hearing thresholds is then used to draw vertical and diagonal cutoff lines on the graph. In the original bivariate

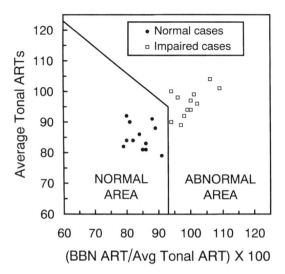

(BBN ART/Avg Tonal ART) X 100

FIGURE 7–26 Example of the bivariate plotting method. The original bivariate method places the cutoff lines where ≥90% of normal ears are in the normal area. The modified bivariate method places the cutoff lines where normal and impaired ears are maximally separated and ≥90% of ears with mild and sloping losses are outside of the normal area. Examples of typical normal and hearing loss cases are plotted.

method (Popelka & Trumph, 1976; Popelka, 1981), these lines were placed so that at least 90% of normal hearing subjects had reflex data falling in a "normal area" to the left of the vertical line and under the diagonal. Young patients with significant hearing losses, defined as a pure-tone average of 32 dB HL or more, were successfully identified by reflex data falling outside this normal area.[4]

Correct identification rates with the bivariate method can be disappointing when trying to identify hearing losses in adults who

may have mild and/or high-frequency as well as significant losses, especially when patients are ≥45 years old (Silman & Gelfand, 1979; Silman, Gelfand, et al, 1984; Silman, Silverman, Showers, & Gelfand, 1984; Silverman, Silman, & Miller, 1983). These problems are addressed by the **modified bivariate method** (Silman, Gelfand, et al, 1984; Silman, Silverman, et al, 1984), which differs from the original approach in terms of how the cutoff values are determined, and is used for patients who are under 45 years old. Using a reasonably large sample of patients with known thresholds, the cutoff lines of the modified bivariate plot are drawn to produce the best possible separation between normal and impaired ears, including the requirement that at least 90% of mild and sloping losses fall outside the normal area. Using the same group of 20- to 44-year-olds, the original bivariate correctly identified 97% of normals but only 69% of hearing impaired subjects, whereas the modified bivariate correctly identified 86% of normals and 96% with hearing losses (Silman, Gelfand, et al, 1984; Silman, Silverman, et al, 1984). Identifying hearing losses in adults who are ≥45 years old remains problematic; however, it was recommended that a hearing loss should be suspected for a patient in this population when the ART is >95 dB SPL for broadband noise, or ≥105 dB SPL for 1000 or 2000 Hz (Silman, Gelfand, et al, 1984; Silman, Silverman, et al, 1984). Applying these critera under clinical conditions correctly identified 93% of the patients whose hearing was within normal limits and 77% of those with hearing losses (Wallin, Mendez-Kurtz, & Silman, 1986).

Some Comments on High Stimulus Levels and the Acoustic Reflex

Before leaving this topic, the student should be aware that the high stimulus levels involved in acoustic reflex testing do have rare but possible untoward effects. Several cases of threshold shifts attributable to the high stimulus levels used during acoustic reflex testing have been reported over the

---

[4] Using the bivariate method involves plotting a patient's ART results at their x-y coordinates. The y coordinate is obtained by converting the 500-, 1000-, and 2000-Hz ARTs into dB SPL, and then averaging them. The x-coordinate is obtained by dividing the patient's ART for broadband noise (in dB SPL) by the same tonal ART average that was used for the y-coordinate, and then multiplying the result by 100.

years (Portmann, 1980; Tanka, Ohhashi, & Tsuda, 1981; Lenarz & Gulzow, 1983; Miller, Hoffman, & Smallberg, 1984; Arriaga & Luxford, 1993; Hunter, Ries, Schlauch, Levine, & Ward, 1999). Yet, these instances are at least very uncommon, and the full diagnostic potential of reflex testing often depends on the complete range of available testing levels (125 dB HL on contemporary instruments). Purely scientific and clinical considerations do not provide a resolution for this issue, let alone a neat one. One very defendable approach is to raise the stimulus level until a reflex response is obtained or the maximum level of 125 dB HL is reached. The opposite strategy is to limit testing to some presumably safe limit. Various limits have been suggested, such as 110 dB *SPL* (Wilson & Margolis, 1999), 115 dB *SPL* (Hunter et al, 1999), and 110 dB *HL* except when there is an air-bone-gap (Stach & Jerger, 1991). Another possibility is to test up to an appropriately selected upper cutoff value, such as the 90th percentile (above which the reflex would be considered elevated), but no higher. The situation is more complicated for reflex decay testing because it is typically done 10 dB above the acoustic reflex threshold. Regardless of which philosophy the clinician adopts, it is clear that one should be alert to complaints of hearing changes, tinnitus, etc., after acoustic reflex testing.

REFERENCES

Alford B, Jerger J, Coats A, Peterson C, Weber S. 1973. Neurophysiology of facial nerve testing. *Arch Otolaryngol* 97, 214.

American Academy of Audiology Position Statement (AAA). 1997. Identification of hearing loss and middle-ear dysfunction in preschool and school-age children. *Audiol Today* 9, 21–23.

American National Standards Institute (ANSI). 1996. *American National Standard Specifications for Instruments to Measure Aural Acoustic Impedance and Admittance (Aural Acoustic Immittance).* ANSI S3.39-1987 (R 1996). New York: ANSI.

American Speech-Language-Hearing Association (ASHA). 1997. *Guidelines for Audiologic Screening.* Rockville Pike, MD: ASHA.

Anderson H, Barr B, Wedenberg E. 1970. The early detection of acoustic tumors by the stapedial reflex test. In Wolstenholme GEW, Knight J (Eds.): *Sensorineural Hearing Loss.* London: Churchill, 275–289.

Arriaga MA, Luxford WM. 1993. Impedance audiometry and iatrogenic hearing loss. *Otolaryngol Head Neck Surg* 108, 70–72.

Baker S, Lilly DJ. 1976. Prediction of hearing level from acoustic reflex data. Paper presented at Convention of American Speech-Language-Hearing Association, Houston.

Bennett MJ, Weatherby LA. 1982. Newborn acoustic reflexes to noise and pure-tone signals. *J Speech Hear Res* 25, 383–387.

Bluestone CD. 1975. Assessment of Eustachian tube function. In Jerger J (Ed.): *Handbook of Impedance Audiometry.* Acton, MA: American Electromedics, 127–148.

Bluestone CD. 1980. Assessment of Eustachian tube function. In Jerger J, Northern J (Eds.): *Clinical Impedance Audiometry.* Acton, MA: American Electromedics, 83–108.

Bluestone CD, Paradise J, Berry Q, Wittel R. 1972. Certain effects of cleft palate repair on Eustachian tube function. *Cleft Palate J* 9, 183–193.

Borg E. 1973. On the neuronal organization of the acoustic middle ear reflex: A physiological and anatomical study. *Brain Res* 49, 101–123.

Bosatra A, Russolo M, Silverman CA. 1984. Acoustic-reflex latency: State of the art. In Silman S (Ed.): *The Acoustic Reflex: Basic Principles and Clinical Applications.* Orlando, FL: Academic Press, 301–328.

Brooks DN. 1969. The use of the electro-acoustic impedance bridge in the assessment of middle ear function. *Int Audiol* 8, 563–569.

Citron D, Adour K. 1978. Acoustic reflex and loudness discomfort in acute facial paralysis. *Arch Otolaryngol* 104, 303–308.

Davies JE, John DG, Jones AH, Stephens SDG. 1988. Tympanometry as a screening test for treatable hearing loss in the elderly. *Br J Audiol* 22, 119–121.

DeChicchis AR, Todd, NW, Nozza RJ. 2000. Developmental changes in aural acoustic admittance measurements. *J Am Acad Audiol* 11, 97–102.

Elner A, Ingelstedt S, Ivarsson A. 1971. The elastic properties of the tympanic membrane. *Acta Otolaryngol* 72, 397–403.

Feldman AS. 1975. Acoustic impedance-admittance measurements. In Bradford LJ (Ed.): *Physiological Measures of the Audio-Vestibular System.* NY: Academic Press, 87–145.

Feldman AS. 1976. Tympanometry—procedures, interpretation and variables. In Feldman AS, Wilber LA (Eds.): *Acoustic Impedance and Admittance: The Measurement of Middle Ear Function.* Baltimore: Williams & Wilkins, 103–155.

Fiellau-Nikolajsen M. 1983. Tympanometry and secretory otitis media. *Acta Otolaryngol* 394 (suppl), 1–73.

Gelfand SA. 1984. The contralateral acoustic reflex threshold. In Silman S (Ed.): *The Acoustic Reflex: Basic Principles and Clinical Applications.* Orlando, FL: Academic Press, 137–186.

Gelfand SA. 1994. Acoustic reflex threshold tenth percentiles and functional hearing impairment. *J Am Acad Audiol* 5, 10–16.

Gelfand SA. 1998. *Hearing: An Introduction to Psychological and Physiological Acoustics,* 3rd ed. New York: Marcel Dekker.

Gelfand SA. 2000. The acoustic reflex. In Katz J (Ed.): *Handbook of Clinical Audiology, 5th ed.* Baltimore: Lippincott Williams & Willkins, in press.

Gelfand SA, Piper N. 1981. Acoustic reflex thresholds in young and elderly subjects with normal hearing. *J Acoust Soc Am* 69, 295–297.

Gelfand SA, Piper N. 1984. Acoustic reflex thresholds: Variability and distribution effects. *Ear Hear* 5, 228–234.

Gelfand SA, Piper N, Silman S. 1983. Effects of hearing levels at the activator and other frequencies upon the expected levels of the acoustic reflex threshold. *J Speech Hear Dis* 48, 11–17.

Gelfand SA, Schwander T, Silman S. 1990. Acoustic reflex thresholds in normal and cochlear-impaired ears: Effects of no-response rates on 90th percentiles in a large sample. *J Speech Hear Dis* 55, 198–205.

Gelfand SA, Silman S. 1982. Acoustic reflex thresholds in brain damaged patients. *Ear Hear* 3, 93–95.

Givens GD, Seidemann MF. 1984. Acoustic immittance testing of the Eustachian tube. *Ear Hear* 5, 297–299.

Hall JW, Koval CB. 1982. Accuracy of hearing prediction by the acoustic reflex. *Laryngoscope* 92, 140–149.

Harford ER. 1980. Assessment of Eustachian tube function. In Jerger J, Northern J (Eds.): *Clinical Impedance Audiometry*. Acton, MA: American Electromedics, 40–64.

Hirsch A, Anderson H. 1980. Audiologic test results in 96 patients with tumors affecting the eighth nerve. *Acta Otolaryngol* 369 (suppl), 1–26.

Holmquist J. 1968. The role of the Eustachian tube in myringoplasty. *Acta Otolaryngol* 66, 289–295.

Holmquist J, Miller J. 1972. Eustachian tube evaluation using the impedance bridge. In Rose D, Keating LW. (Eds.): *Mayo Foundation Impedance Symposium*. Rochester, MN: Mayo Foundation, 297–307.

Hughes GB (Ed.). 1985. *Textbook of Clinical Otology*. New York: Thieme-Stratton.

Hughes GB, Pensak ML (Eds.). 1997. *Clinical Otology*, 2nd ed. New York: Thieme.

Hunter LL, Margolis RH 1992. Multifrequency tympanometry: Current clinical application. *Am J Audiol* 1, 33–43.

Hunter LL, Ries DT, Schlauch RS, Levine SC, Ward WD. 1999. Safety and clinical performance of acoustic reflex tests. *Ear Hear* 20, 506–514.

Jerger J. 1970. Clinical experience with impedance audiometry. *Arch Otolaryngol* 92, 311–324.

Jerger J, Anthony L, Jerger S, Mauldin L. 1974. Studies in impedance audiometry: III. Middle ear disorders. *Arch Otolaryngol* 99, 165–171.

Jerger J, Burney P, Mauldin L, Crump B. 1974. Predicting hearing loss from the acoustic reflex. *J Speech Hear Dis* 39, 11–22.

Jerger J, Harford E, Clemis J, Alford B. 1974. The acoustic reflex in eighth nerve disorders. *Arch Otolaryngol* 99, 409–413.

Jerger J, Hayes D, Anthony L, Mauldin L. 1978. Factors influencing prediction of hearing level from the acoustic reflex. *Maico Mongrs Contemp Audiol* 1, 1–20.

Jerger J, Jerger S, Mauldin L. 1972. Studies in impedance audiometry: I. Normal and sensorineural ears. *Arch Otolaryngol* 96, 513–523.

Jerger J, Jerger J. 1977. Diagnostic value of crossed vs. uncrossed acoustic reflexes: Eighth nerve and brain stem disorders. *Arch Otolaryngol* 103, 445–453.

Jerger S, Jerger J. 1983. Neuroaudiologic findings in patients with central auditory disorders. *Semin Hear* 4, 133–159.

Jerger S, Jerger J, Mauldin L, Segal P. 1974. Studies in impedance audiometry: II. Children less than six years old. *Arch Otolaryngol* 99, 1–9.

Keith RW. 1977. An evaluation of predicting hearing loss from the acoustic reflex. *Arch Otolaryngol* 103, 419–424.

Koebsell C, Margolis RH. 1986. Tympanometric gradient measured from normal preschool children. *Audiology* 25, 149–157.

Lenarz T, Gulzow J. 1983. Acoustic inner ear trauma by impedance measurement: Acute acoustic trauma? *Laryngol Rhinol Otol* 62, 58–61.

Liden G. 1969. The scope and application of current audiometric tests. *J Laryngol Otol* 83, 507–520.

Liden G, Harford E, Hallen O. 1974. Tympanometry for the diagnosis of ossicular disruption. *Arch Otolaryngol* 99, 23–29.

Liden G, Peterson JL, Bjorkman G. 1970. Tympanometry. *Arch Otolaryngol* 92, 248–257.

Mangham CA. 1984. The effect of drugs and systemic disease on the acoustic reflex. In Silman S (Ed.): *The Acoustic Reflex: Basic Principles and Clinical Applications*. Orlando: Academic Press, 441–468.

Margolis RH, Goycoolea HG. 1993. Multifrequency tympanometry in normal adults. *Ear Hear* 14, 408–413.

Margolis RH, Heller J. 1987. Screening tympanometry: Criteria for medial referral. *Audiology*, 26, 197–288.

Margolis RH, Popelka GR. 1975. Static and dynamic acoustic impedance measurements in infant ears. *J Speech Hear Res* 18, 435–443.

Margolis RH, Shanks JE. 1985. Tympanometry. In Katz J (Ed.): *Handbook of Clinical Audiology*, 3rd ed. Baltimore: Williams & Wilkins, 438–475.

Miller MH, Hoffman RA, Smallberg G. 1984. Stapedial reflex testing and partially reversible acoustic trauma. *Hear Instr* 35, 15, 49.

Niemeyer W, Sesterhenn G. 1974. Calculating the hearing threshold from the stapedius reflex threshold for different sound stimuli. *Audiology*, 13, 421–427.

Northern JL, Gabbard SA. 1994. The acoustic reflex. In Katz J (Ed.): *Handbook of Clinical Audiology*, 4th ed. Baltimore: Williams & Wilkins, 300–316.

Nozza RJ, Bluestone CD, Kardatzke D, Bachman R. 1992. Towards the validation of aural acoustic immittance measures for diagnosis of middle ear effusion in children. *Ear Hear* 13, 442–453.

Nozza RJ, Bluestone CD, Kardatzke D, Bachman R. 1994. Identification of middle ear effusion by aural acoustic admittance and otoscopy. *Ear Hear* 15, 310–323.

Olsen WO, Bauch CA, Harner SG. 1983. Application of the Silman and Gelfand (1981) 90th percentile levels for acoustic reflex thresholds. *J Speech Hear Dis* 48, 330–332.

Olsen WO, Stach BA, Kurdziel SA. 1981. Acoustic reflex decay in 10 seconds and in 5 seconds for Meniere's disease patients and for VIIIth nerve tumor patients. *Ear Hear* 2, 180–181.

Ostergard CA, Carter DR. 1981. Positive middle ear pressure shown by tympanometry. *Arch Otolaryngol* 107, 353–356.

Paradise JL, Smith CG, Bluestone CD. 1976. Tympanometric detection of middle ear effusion in infants and young children. *Pediatrics* 58, 198–210.

Popelka GR. 1981. The acoustic reflex in normal and pathological ears. In Popelka GR (Ed.): *Hearing Assessment with the Acoustic Reflex*. New York: Grune & Stratton, 5–21.

Popelka GR, Trumph A. 1976. Stapedial reflex thresholds for tonal and noise activating signals in relation to magnitude of hearing loss in multiple-handicapped children. Paper presented at Convention of American Speech-Language-Hearing Association, Houston.

Porter T. 1972. Normal otoadmittance values for three populations. *J Audiol Res* 12, 53–58.

Portmann M. 1980. Impedance audiometry is not always without risk. *Rev Laryngol* 101, 181–182.

Renvall U, Liden G. 1978. Clinical significance of reduced middle ear pressure in school children. In Harford ER, Bess FH, Bluestone CD, Klein JO (Eds.): *Impedance Screening for Middle Ear Disease in Children.* NY: Grune & Stratton, 189–196.

Riedel CL, Wiley TL, Block MG. 1987. Tympanometric measures of Eustachian tube function. *J Speech Hear Res* 30, 207–214.

Rizzo S Jr, Greenberg HJ. 1979. Predicting hearing loss from the acoustic reflex data. Paper presented at Convention of American Speech-Language-Hearing Association, Boston.

Roush J, Bryant K, Mundy M, Zeisel S, Roberts J. 1995. Developmental changes in static admittance and tympanometric width in infants and toddlers. *J Am Acad Audiol* 6, 334–338.

Sanders JW. 1984. Evaluation of the 90th percentile levels for acoustic reflex thresholds. Paper presented at Convention of American Speech-Language-Hearing Association, San Francisco.

Seifert M, Seidemann MF, Givens GD. 1979. An examination of the variables involved in tympanometric assessment of Eustachian tube functioning adults. *J Speech Hear Dis* 44, 388–396.

Shahnaz N, Polka L. 1997. Standard and multifrequency tympanometry in normal and otosclerotic ears. *Ear Hear* 18, 326–341.

Shanks JE, Lilly DJ. 1981. An evaluation of tympanometric estimates of ear canal volume. *J Speech Hear Res* 24, 557–566.

Shanks JE, Lilly DJ, Margolis RH, Wiley TL, Wilson RH. 1988. Tympanometry. *J Speech Hear Dis* 53, 354–377.

Shanks JE, Sheldon C. 1991. Basic principles and clinical applications of tympanometry. *Otolaryngol Clin North Am* 24, 299–328.

Silman S. 1984. Magnitude and growth of the acoustic-reflex. In Silman S (Ed.): *The Acoustic Reflex: Basic Principles and Clinical Applications.* Orlando, FL: Academic Press, 225–274.

Silman S, Gelfand SA. 1979. Prediction of hearing levels from acoustic reflex thresholds in persons with high-frequency hearing losses. *J Speech Hear Res* 22, 697–707.

Silman S, Gelfand SA. 1981. The relationship between magnitude of hearing loss and acoustic reflex threshold levels. *J Speech Hear Dis* 46, 312–316.

Silman S, Gelfand SA. 1982. The acoustic reflex in diagnostic audiology—part 2. *Audiology (J Continuing Educ)* 7, 125–138.

Silman S, Gelfand SA, Emmer M. 1987. Acoustic reflex in hearing loss identification and prediction. *Semin Hear* 8, 379–390.

Silman S, Gelfand SA, Piper N, Silverman CA, VanFrank L. 1984. Prediction of hearing loss from the acoustic-reflex threshold. In Silman S (Ed.): *The Acoustic Reflex: Basic Principles and Clinical Applications.* Orlando, FL: Academic Press, 187–223.

Silman S, Popelka GR, Gelfand SA. 1978. The effect of sensorineural hearing loss on acoustic stapedius reflex growth functions. *J Acoust Soc Am* 64, 1406–1411.

Silman S, Silverman CA. 1991. *Auditory Diagnosis: Principles and Applications.* San Diego: Academic Press.

Silman S, Silverman CA, Arick DS. 1992. Acoustic-immittance screening for detection of middle-ear effusion. *J Am Acad Audiol* 3, 262–268.

Silman S, Silverman CA, Gelfand SA, Lutolf J, Lynn DJ. 1988. Ipsilateral acoustic-reflex adaptation testing for detection of facial-nerve pathology: Three case studies. *J Speech Hear Dis* 53, 378–382.

Silman S, Silverman CA, Showers T, Gelfand SA. 1984. The effect of age on prediction of hearing loss with the bivariate plotting procedure. *J Speech Hear Res* 27, 12–19.

Silverman CA, Silman S, Miller MH. 1983. The acoustic reflex threshold in aging ears. *J Acoust Soc Am* 73, 248–255.

Sprague BH, Wiley TL, Goldstein R. 1985. Tympanometric and acoustic-reflex studies in neonates. *J Speech Hear Res* 28, 265–272.

Stach BA, Jerger JF. 1991. Immittance measures in auditory disorders. In Jacobson JT, Northern JL (Eds.): *Diagnostic Audiology.* Austin: Pro-Ed, 113–139.

Starr A, Picton TW, Sininger YS, Hood LJ, Berlin CI. 1996. Auditory neuropathy. *Brain* 119, 741–753.

Tanka K, Ohhashi K, Tsuda M. 1981. A case of unilateral acute sensorineural deafness after impedance audiometry. *Clin Otol Jpn* 8, 204–205.

Turner RG, Frazer GJ, Shepard NT. 1984. Formulating and evaluating audiological test protocols. *Ear Hear* 5, 321–330.

Turner RG, Shepard NT, Frazer GJ. 1984. Clinical performance of audiological and related diagnostic tests. *Ear Hear* 5, 187–194.

Van Camp KJ, Creten WL, Van de Heyning PH, Decraemer WF, Vanpeperstraete PM. 1983. A search for the most suitable immittance components and probe-tone frequency in tympanometry. *Scand Audiol* 12, 27–34.

Van Camp KJ, Margolis RH, Wilson RH, Creten WL, Shanks JE. 1986. Principles of tympanometry. *ASHA* monographs no. 24.

Vanhuyse VJ, Creten WL, Van Camp KJ. 1975. On the W-notching of tympanograms. *Scand Audiol* 4, 45–50.

Wallin A, Mendez-Kurtz L, Silman S. 1986. Prediction of hearing loss from acoustic-reflex thresholds in the older adults population. *Ear Hear*, 7, 400–404.

Wiley TL. 1989. Static acoustic-admittance measures in normal ears: A combined analysis for ears with and without notched tympanograms. *J Speech Hear Res* 32, 688.

Wiley TL, Block MG. 1984. Acoustic and nonacoustic reflex patterns in audiologic diagnosis. In Silman S (Ed.): *The Acoustic Reflex: Basic Principles and Clinical Applications.* New York: Academic Press, 387–411.

Wiley TL, Oviatt DL, Block MG. 1987. Acoustic-immittance measures in normal ears. *J Speech Hear Res* 330, 161–170.

Wilson RH, Margolis RH. 1999. Acoustic reflex measurements. In Musiek FE, Rintlemann WF (Eds.): *Contemporary Perspectives in Hearing Assessment.* Boston: Allyn & Bacon, 131–165.

Wilson RH, Margolis RH. 1991. Acoustic-reflex measurements. In Rintelmann WF (Ed.): *Hearing Assessment, 2nd ed.* Austin: Pro-Ed, 247–319.

Wilson RH, Shanks JE, Kaplan SK. 1984. Tympanometric changes at 226 Hz and 678 Hz across ten trials and for two directions of ear-canal pressure change. *J Speech Hear Res* 27, 257–266.

Wilson RH, Shanks JE, Lilly DJ. 1984. Acoustic-reflex adaptation. In Silman S (Ed.): *The Acoustic Reflex: Basic Principles and Clinical Applications.* Orlando, FL: Academic Press, 329–386.

Zwislocki J, Feldman AS. 1970. Acoustic impedance of pathological ears. *ASHA* monographs, no. 15.

Speech Audiometry

As the principal avenue of human communication and interaction, it is clear that speech is the most important signal we hear. Consequently, the pure-tone audiogram provides only a partial picture of the patient's auditory status because it does not give any direct information about his ability to hear and understand speech. To find out how a patient hears speech involves testing him with speech stimuli, and this process is called **speech audiometry**.

The instrument used for speech audiometry is the **speech audiometer**. Although devices designed specifically for speech audiometry were used in the past, this function is now incorporated into general-purpose clinical audiometers. The characteristics of audiometers, including those used for speech audiometry, are given in the *American National Standard Specifications for Audiometers* (ANSI S3.6-1996), and are described in Chapter 4. The **speech mode** (or the **speech channel**) of the clinical audiometer includes the following components: (1) various sources of recorded speech material, such as a tape deck, compact disk (CD) player, or even a computer; (2) a microphone for live-voice testing; (3) an input selector to choose the desired source of the speech material; (4) an input level control, which is used with a VU meter to ensure that the speech signals are at the levels necessary for them to be properly calibrated (Chapter 4); (5) an attenuator to control the level of speech being presented to the patient; (6) an output selector to direct the speech stimuli to the desired output transducer; and (7) output transducers (earphones, loudspeakers, bone vibrator). These compo-

nents are illustrated in Figure 8–1. In addition, there is a monitor earphone and/or loudspeaker (and level adjustment) to enable the audiologist to hear the speech signals that are being presented to the patient. Because speech audiometry is generally done in a two-room testing environment, there is also a patient (response) microphone that leads to an earphone and/or loudspeaker in the control room so that the audiologist can hear the patient's responses.

Recall that clinical audiometers have two channels because we sometimes need to present a signal to one ear and a masking noise to the opposite ear, or we might need to present different signals to the two ears on certain kinds of tests. The same thing applies to speech audiometry. Thus, a separate speech mode is provided for both channels of the audiometer. This allows us to send speech signals (not necessarily the same ones) to the two ears. Similarly, we might use one channel to present a speech test to one ear and use the second channel to present a masking noise to the opposite ear. Clinical masking is discussed in Chapter 9, and its appropriate use will be assumed throughout this chapter.

Calibrating the Test Signal(s) Calibration of the test materials is a necessary technical step in speech audiometry. Recorded materials always have a calibration signal, which is usually a 1000-Hz tone. The first steps are to select the appropriate input device (e.g., the tape deck) and set the interrupter switch to the constantly "on" position. The recorded calibration tone is then played while watching the level indicated on the VU meter. The

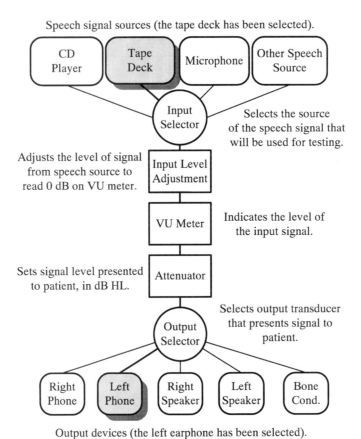

Speech signal sources (the tape deck has been selected).

Output devices (the left earphone has been selected).

FIGURE 8–1   Block diagram of the speech mode (channel) of a clinical audiometer. In this example the audiologist is using recorded speech from the tape deck and is presenting that signal to the patient via the left earphone.

input level dial is then turned up or down until the level of the calibration tone is at 0 dB on the VU meter. That's all there is to it. The input level control is kept in this position as long as this recording is being used. Now stop the calibration recording and proceed to administer the test materials on that recording. It will be necessary to recalibrate whenever you change recordings or move the input level dial. In practice it is desirable to calibrate the test material before each use. Throughout this chapter it will always be assumed that this simple calibration chore has already been completed for whatever tests are being used. Live-voice testing is trickier because the clinician must "balance" his vocal effort while talking into the microphone and

setting the input level control to keep his speech "peaking" at 0 dB on the VU meter.

Thresholds for Speech

The threshold of a nonspeech signal such as a tone has a clear meaning; it is the level at which the presence of the sound is just audible. However, the threshold for speech can mean the lowest level at which speech is either just audible or just intelligible. The lowest level at which the presence of a speech signal can be heard 50% of the time is called the **speech detection threshold (SDT)** or the **speech awareness threshold (SAT)**. In contrast, the lowest level at which a speech signal is intelligible enough to be recognized or identified 50% of the time is the **speech recognition threshold** or **speech reception threshold (SRT)**. The SRT is usually obtained by asking the patient to repeat **spondee (or spondaic) words**, which are two-syllable words that have equal emphasis on both syllables, such as "baseball" or "railroad." Spondaic words lend themselves well to this use because a very small intensity increase causes the recognition of spondees to rise very rapidly from 0% to 100%. The SRT has also been called the **spondee threshold (ST)** when measured with spondaic words (ASHA, 1979). All of these terms are readily understood in the field, but *speech detection threshold* and *speech recognition threshold* are the preferred usage (ASHA, 1988).

Speech detection and recognition thresholds should be different because the SDT depends on audibility alone, whereas the SRT requires the stimuli to be heard and identified. This expectation has been borne out repeatedly by the finding that the average SDT tends to be roughly 7 to 9 dB lower (better) than the mean SRT (Thurlow, Silverman, Davis, & Walsh, 1948; Chaiklin, 1959; Beattie, Edgerton, & Svihovec, 1975; Beattie, Svihovec, & Edgerton, 1975; Cambron, Wilson, and Shanks, 1991). Cambron et al (1991) found the mean SDT-SRT difference to be 8 dB for a male talker and 8.2 dB for a female talker.

The speech reception threshold has several clinical functions: (1) to serve as a measure for corroborating pure-tone thresholds, (2) to serve as a reference point for deciding on appropriate levels at which to administer suprathreshold speech recognition tests, (3) to determine hearing aid needs and performance, (4) to ascertain the need for aural (re)habilitation and progress in the management process, and (5) to determine hearing sensitivity for young children and others who are difficult to test. The speech detection threshold is generally used when an SRT is not obtainable.

RELATION TO THE PURE-TONE AUDIOGRAM

Recall from Chapter 5 that the pure-tone thresholds in the 500- to 2000-Hz range are associated with the SRT. We will see in Chapter 14 that a lack of reasonable consistency between the SRT and the pure-tone thresholds is associated with functional hearing losses. In fact, as already mentioned, it is commonly accepted that one of the principal applications of the SRT is to corroborate the pure-tone findings.

The SRT was originally compared to the pure-tone average (PTA) of 500, 1000, and 2000 Hz (Fletcher, 1929; Carhart, 1946a), but it soon became apparent that this three-frequency PTA is not necessarily the combination of pure-tone thresholds that comes closest to the SRT. This is especially true with sloping audiograms, where the pure-tone thresholds may be quite different from one frequency to the other. Agreement between the SRT and PTA is improved under these conditions by using other combinations. Fletcher (1950) recommended using the average of the best two of these three frequencies, usually 500 and 1000 Hz. Carhart (1971) suggested that PTA-SAT agreement is maximized by a simple formula that involves subtracting 2 dB from the average of the 500 Hz and 1000 Hz thresholds. Single-frequency comparisons to the SRT are also sometimes appropriate. Carhart and Porter (1971) found that the single frequency with the highest correlation to the SRT was 1000 Hz, unless there is a sharply sloping hearing loss. When the audiogram slopes precipitously, it is often useful to compare the SRT to the one frequency that has the best threshold, which is often 500 Hz, and can even sometimes be 250 Hz (Gelfand & Silman, 1985, 1993; Silman & Silverman, 1991).

Materials for SRT Testing

SPONDEE WORDS

As already indicated, most speech recognition thresholds are obtained using spondaic words, and we will concentrate on this method. Recorded 42-word spondee tests were originally developed at the Harvard Psychoacoustic Laboratory (PAL) by Hudgins, Hawkins, Karlin, and Stevens (1947). They tried to use phonetically dissimilar words from a familiar vocabulary that reasonably represented the sounds of English and were as homogeneous as possible with respect to their audibility. The PAL lists were provided in two recorded formats; all of the spondees were recorded at the same level in PAL Test No. 14, whereas they were attenuated by a fixed amount of 4-dB after every sixth word on PAL Test No. 9. Subsequently, Hirsh, Davis, Silverman, Reynolds, Eldert, and Benson (1952) of the Central Institute for the Deaf (CID) improved upon the original spondaic materials by reducing the list to the 36 most familiar spondees and by recording the words in a way that made them homogeneous with respect to difficulty. This was done by adjusting the recording level by −2 dB for the easiest spondees and by +2 dB for the hardest words. Six randomizations of the list were recorded with all of the spondees at the same level on the **CID W-1 Test**, and with an attenuation of 3-dB after every third word on the **CID W-2 Test**. In addition, each test word was preceded by the carrier phrase, "Say the word...," which was recorded at a level 10 dB higher than the test word itself. Contemporary studies using digital technology are addressing the issue of achieving homogeneous test materials in terms of the psychometric equivalence of recorded spondee words (e.g., Bilger, Matthies, Meyer, & Griffiths, 1998; Wilson & Strouse, 1999).

Numerous modifications and variations of the CID spondee materials have been introduced since the original lists and tests were distributed in the 1950s. A distinction is made between *lists* and *tests* because, for example, the CID W-1 Test refers to the specific recording just described. Presenting the same word list by live voice or from another recording actually constitutes a different test because of talker and recording differences. The spondaic word list recommended by ASHA (1979, 1988) is a revision of the CID W-1/W-2 list, emphasizing the criteria of dissimilarity among the words and homogeneous audibility. Recorded versions of the spondee tests (as well as many of the others discussed in this chapter) on cassette tapes and/or CDs are produced by Auditec of St. Louis, Virtual Corporation, and the Department of Veterans Affairs (VA). For example,

the psychometrically equivalent spondee tests using a female talker developed by Wilson and Strouse (1999) are included in a CD produced by the Department of Veterans Affairs (1998). In addition, ASHA (1988) has recommended a streamlined list of 15 highly homogeneous spondees based on research by Young, Dudley, and Gunter (1982), and a list of 20 spondees easily represented by pictures that are suitable for testing young children, based on findings by Frank (1980). Shortened lists like these are commonly used in clinical practice, but the student should be aware that shortening the word list lowers the SRT (Punch & Howard, 1985; Meyer & Bilger, 1997). Several examples of commonly used spondaic word lists may be found in the Appendices B through E.

SENTENCE TESTS

Although spondees are used in the overwhelming majority of routine clinical SRT measurements, the student should be aware that they are not the only materials available for this purpose. Sentences are the principal alternative materials used for SRT testing, especially in noise (Plomp & Mimpin, 1979; Hagerman, 1982; Gelfand, Ross, & Miller, 1988; Smoorenburg, 1992; Nilsson, Soli, & Sullivan, 1994; Versfeld, Daalder, Festen, & Houtgast, 2000). English-language sentence SRT materials have been developed by Gelfand, Ross, and Miller (1988) based on the PH-SPIN sentences (described later in this chapter) and by Nilsson, Soli, and Sullivan (1994) based on the BKB sentences (described in Chapter 12). The latter, known as the **Hearing in Noise Test (HINT)**, is more commonly encountered and includes 25 lists of 10 sentences each. Just as the spondee SRT is sometimes called the spondee threshold, sentence SRTs are often referred to as sentences reception thresholds.

Measuring the Speech Recognition Threshold

INSTRUCTIONS AND FAMILIARIZATION

The first part of the SRT testing process involves instructing the patient about the task and familiarizing him with the test words. As recommended by ASHA (1988), the instructions should indicate the nature of the task, that it involves speech material, how the patient is to respond, that he should continue responding even when the words are faint, and that guessing is encouraged. The following is an example of instructions that one might use:

> The next test is used to find the softest speech that you can hear and repeat back. I [*or, a recorded voice*] will say two-syllable words like "baseball" or "railroad," and your job is to repeat each word. The words will start out being loud so that you can familiarize yourself with them. They will then get softer and softer. Your job is to keep repeating the words back to me, no matter how soft they become, even if you have to guess. Do you have any questions? [*Address these questions as necessary.*]

Notice that these instructions also refer to the familiarization process that precedes the actual testing. The purpose of familiarization is to ensure that the patient knows the test vocabulary and is able to recognize each word auditorily, and that the clinician can accurately interpret the patient's responses (ASHA, 1988). The importance of the familiarization process is well established (Pollack, Rubenstein, & Decker, 1959; Tillman & Jerger, 1959; Conn, Dancer, & Ventry, 1975). For example, Tillman and Jerger (1959) found that the average SRT is about 4 to 5 dB lower with familiarization than without it.

Recorded versus Monitored Live-Voice Testing
Spondaic words may be presented to the patient using readily available recorded materials or by **monitored live voice**, which means the words are spoken into a microphone by the audiologist who monitors her voice level on the audiometer's VU meter. Recorded material is preferred for SRT testing, but presenting the stimuli by monitored live voice is also acceptable (ASHA, 1988). Compared to monitored live voice testing, recorded materials provide much better control over the level and quality of the speech signals being presented to the patient, as well as the obvious benefits of greater standardization. On

the other hand, the flexibility afforded by monitored live-voice testing is often desirable or essential when testing patients who require any kind of modification of the test procedure. Typical examples are elderly patients who might need more time to respond than is provided on the recording, children or others with restricted vocabularies, etc. The need for flexibility is not limited to patients who have special needs. For example, it is often desirable to test at a faster pace than is possible with recorded lists when testing some young, normal adults. In addition, the SRT is usually robust enough to withstand the limitations of live-voice testing, and has been found to be reliable under these conditions (Carhart, 1946b; Creston, Gillespie, & Krahn, 1966; Beattie, Forrester, & Ruby, 1976). In fact, modified live-voice is the most common way to present spondees for the SRT, and its use *for this purpose* is generally agreeable even to ardent proponents of recorded materials for most other kinds of speech recognition testing. However, the audiologic results should indicate that the SRT was obtained by monitored live voice when this is the case.

CARRIER PHRASE USE FOR SRT TESTING

Whether the test word is introduced by a carrier phrase (e.g., "Say the word . . .") does not appear to have any substantive effect upon the resulting SRT (Silman & Silverman, 1991). In fact, even though carrier phrases were included on the original Technisonics Studios phonograph recordings of W-1 and W-2, they are omitted from current commonly used spondee recordings such as those by Auditec of St. Louis and Virtual Corporation.

THE INITIAL (BALLPARK) SRT ESTIMATE

It would unnecessarily fatigue the patient and waste time and effort to present many test words at levels well above or below the actual SRT. For this reason, SRT testing usually has an initial phase in which the level of the spondee words is changed in relatively large steps to make a quick, rough estimate of where the SRT is probably located. This ballpark estimate provides an efficiently placed starting level for the actual threshold search. Most SRT protocols specify the starting hearing level and technique for making this ballpark estimate, and this initial testing phase will be mentioned for each of the four SRT methods described below. However, one should be aware that many audiologists select the level to present the first word based on the patient's behavior or pure-tone thresholds.

TESTING TECHNIQUES

It is generally accepted that the SRT is the lowest hearing level at which a patient can repeat 50% of spondee words, but there are many ways to find this point and no single technique is universally accepted. Most SRT testing methods share a number of common features even though their specific characteristics can vary widely. The most common characteristic is that a number of spondee words are presented to the patient one at a time at the same hearing level. The **descending methods** begin presenting these blocks of test words *above* the estimated SRT so that the patient is initially able to repeat them,

and then present subsequent blocks of spondee words at progressively lower hearing levels. This process is repeated until the patient misses a certain number of words, at which time the descending run is over. On the other hand, **ascending methods** start *below* the estimated threshold, where the patient cannot repeat the words, and then present subsequent blocks of test words at progressively higher hearing levels. This procedure is repeated until the patient correctly repeats a certain number of words, at which point the ascending run is terminated. What distinguishes among the methods are features such as how many words are in a block, what are the criteria for starting and stopping an ascending or descending run, and how one defines the "50% correct" level.

One general group of SRT methods considers the SRT to be the lowest hearing level where half (or at least half) of a block of the words is correct. Three examples are illustrated in Figure 8–2. The Chaiklin and Ventry (1964) method is a *descending technique* because it begins by presenting the spondee words at a level that is high enough for them to be

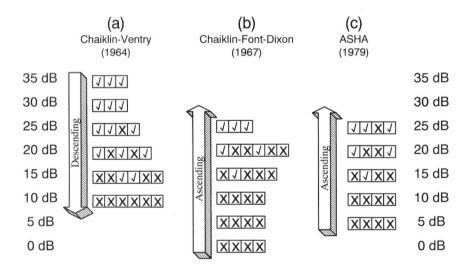

FIGURE 8–2 Examples of measuring the SRT with (a) descending Chaiklin & Ventry (1964), (b) ascending Chaiklin, Font, & Dixon (1967), and (c) ascending ASHA (1979) methods. The ASHA (1979) method includes a second ascending run beginning 10 dB below the first SRT measurement (not shown). The SRT is defined as the lowest hearing level where three out of a possible six spondee words are repeated correctly in (a) and (b), and as the lowest level where at least three of the spondees are repeated correctly in (c). (See text.)

heard and repeated easily, and then searches for the SRT by presenting words at progressively lower hearing levels. The method involves presenting the spondees one at a time in blocks of up to six words per level. The intensity is decreased in 5-dB steps to find the lowest level where three words are repeated correctly. Two-decibel steps may also be used, but Chaiklin and Ventry (1964) found that 2- and 5-dB step sizes yield comparable results for clinical purposes. The initial testing phase begins 25 dB above the patient's two-frequency pure-tone average, and involves presenting one word per level in decreasing 5-dB steps until one word is missed. The starting point for the main SRT search begins 10 dB above that level.

The Chaiklin-Ventry technique is illustrated in Figure 8–2a. Suppose the first word was missed at 25 dB HL during the initial phase of testing, so that the starting level for our SRT search is 10 dB higher, at 35 dB HL. It is not necessary to present more than three words at the 35-dB starting level because they are all correct. The rationale is that three correct words out of a possible six indicates the performance is already at least 50%, so that nothing would be gained by presenting any more words at this level. This is why many of the blocks in the figure have fewer than six words even though the method is theoretically based on six words per level. In any case, because the patient repeated three words at 35 dB HL, we now know that the SRT must be 35 dB HL *or lower*. The level is thus reduced to 30 dB HL, where the same thing occurs, so we know the SRT is 30 dB HL or lower. When the level is reduced to 25 dB HL, the first two words are right but the third one is wrong. We must now present another word because it is possible for the percentage of correct responses to be less than 50%. The fourth word is correct, bringing the tally to three right and one wrong at this level. Here, too, the score would be at least 50% if all six words were given, so there would be no benefit from presenting more words at this level. The SRT is now 25 dB HL or lower. Five words are needed at 20 dB HL. Let us see why. The first three words include

an error, so a fourth is needed. The fourth word brings the tally to two right and two wrong. Based on a possible six words, the score could still be 33% (2 of 6), 50% (3 of 6), or even 67% (4 of 6). A fifth word is therefore presented, which is correct. This brings the tally to three correct out of a possible six, again meeting the criterion. The SRT is now 20 dB HL or lower. The intensity is reduced to 15 dB HL, where the following is found: one right out of three, two correct out of four, and two right out of five. Here a sixth word is needed to determine whether the score is 50% (3 of 6) or 33% (2 of 6). Word six is wrong, indicating that 15 dB is *below* the SRT. Thus, the SRT is *20 dB HL* in this example, because this is the lowest level where half of the spondee words are repeated correctly (out of a possible 6). The figure shows that 10 dB HL was also tested because the Chaiklin-Ventry method requires that we continue testing until all six words in a block are wrong, which occurs here at the next lower level.

Chaiklin, Font, and Dixon (1967) described an *ascending* SRT method that is otherwise very similar to the Chaiklin-Ventry technique in that it uses the same number of words per level, step size, and definition of the SRT. This method is illustrated in Figure 8–2b. Because this is an ascending method, the starting level is now below the expected SRT. The initial testing phase with this approach begins at −10 dB HL, and involves presenting one word per level in ascending 10-dB steps until one word is repeated correctly. The main threshold search for SRT is then started 20 dB below that level. For example, if the first word was correctly repeated at 20 dB HL during the initial phase, then the starting level for the main test would be 20 dB lower, or 0 dB HL, which is shown in the figure. In the ascending method, we are working upward until the patient finally repeats correctly three out of a theoretical six words per level. The reasoning for how many words to use per level is analogous to the Chaiklin-Ventry method, except that we must be mindful of the direction. At least four words must be presented and missed before raising the test level because this is the smallest number of misses that can tell us that we are still *below* the SRT. In other words, the patient must miss four out of a possible six words before we really know that he cannot possibly repeat three out of them. This explains why four errors are shown at each ascending level from the starting level of 0 dB HL through 20 dB. Only four words are needed if the patient misses all of them (e.g., at 0, 5, and 10 dB HL), but five words must be used if one is correct (e.g., at 15 dB HL), and six words are needed if two are right (e.g., at 20 dB HL). The SRT in this example is *25 dB HL* because this is the first level where three words are repeated correctly. It is not necessary to go above this point because the SRT is defined as the lowest level where the patient correctly repeats three of a possible six spondees. Incidentally, just because the patient got all three words correct in a row in our example does not mean this is always the case. Any combination of three correct spondees in a block of up to six words at the same hearing level will do (e.g., "x✓x✓✓" or "x✓x✓x✓" or "xxx✓✓✓").

The *ascending* SRT method recommended by ASHA (1979) is illustrated in Figure 8-2c. Its initial testing phase is similar to the Chaiklin, Font, and Dixon (1967) approach, except that the starting level for the main test is 15 dB below the level where the first word is correctly repeated. This is why the two methods have different starting levels in the figure. The ASHA (1979) method has the following characteristics: Four spondee words are presented at each hearing level. The hearing level is increased by 5 dB until *at least three* of the words are correctly repeated at the same level (which is 25 dB HL in the figure). The intensity is then reduced by 10 dB, and a second ascending series of presentations is administered using the same technique (not shown in the figure). The SRT is defined as the lowest level at which at least three words are correctly repeated, based on at least two ascending runs.

The methods just described are similar in that the SRT is the hearing level of the block of words that meets some criterion (such as 3 of 6 or 3 of 4 words correct). Another general group of SRT methods involves interpolating the 50% correct level using the responses obtained from several blocks of words (Hudgins et al, 1947; Tillman & Olsen, 1973; Wilson, Morgan, & Dirks, 1973; ASHA, 1988), and is based on well-established statistical principles (Spearman, 1908). This approach is incorporated into the ASHA (1988) guidelines for SRT testing.

The initial phase of the ASHA (1988) method is a ballpark estimate. It begins by presenting one spondee word at 30 dB or 40 dB HL. If the original intensity is too low for the patient to repeat the first word, then it is increased in large, 20-dB steps (giving one word per step) to quickly find where she can repeat a word. Regardless of whether the first word is repeated at 30 dB HL or at 70 dB HL, then one word per level is presented in decreasing 10-dB steps until the patient misses a word, at which point a second word is presented. This descending strategy continues until she misses two consecutive words at the same level. The *starting level* for the main SRT determination will be 10 dB higher than the level where the two words were missed. Thus, if the patient misses two consecutive words at 40 dB HL, the starting level would be 50 dB HL.

Having arrived at a starting level, we are now ready to find the SRT using the ASHA (1988) procedure. The testing itself is similar to the other methods, except five words are given at every level and we keep track of whether each word is right or wrong on a tally sheet such as the one shown in Figure 8–3. First, five spondee words are presented one at a time at the starting level, where the patient usually repeats all of them correctly. We then decrease the hearing level by 5 dB and present another five words, tallying the results for each word. This *descending* procedure continues until the patient misses all five words at the same level. This "stopping level" is 35 dB HL in the example. Notice that the patient's performance goes from 100% correct at the starting level down to 0% correct at the stopping level. The SRT is interpolated from this range by, in effect, giving 1 dB of credit for each correctly repeated word.

Speech Level (dB HL)	Word Number				
	1	2	3	4	5
50	√	√	√	√	√
45	√	√	X	√	√
40	X	√	X	X	X
35	X	X	X	X	X

Starting Level

Stop: 5 missed on same level.

Count correct words from starting level to stopping level (10 in this example).

Calculation of the SRT (in dB HL):

Record the Starting Level:	50
Subtract number of correct words:	- 10
Sub-total:	40
Add the 2-dB Correction Factor:	+ 2
Speech Recognition Threshold (SRT) =	42

FIGURE 8–3 Tally sheet and calculation of the SRT with 5-dB steps according to the ASHA (1988) method.

The calculation is done by following these steps:

1. Record the starting level (50 dB in the example).
2. Count all the correct words, including the starting level (10 words in the example).
3. Subtract the number of correct words from the starting level (50 − 10 = 40).
4. Add a 2-dB correction factor to the difference found in step 3 (40 + 2 = 42).

The result in step 4 is the SRT, expressed in dB HL (SRT = 42 dB HL). The ASHA (1988) method can also be done with 2-dB steps (Fig. 8–4). Here, we present two words per level and stop testing when the patient misses five out of six words. The calculation is also the same, except that the correction factor is 1 dB.

In general, the differences between SRTs obtained with the various test methods tend to be either not statistically significant or too small to be of any major clinical relevance. For example, SRTs are about 2.7 to 3.7 dB better (lower) with the ASHA (1988) method compared with the ASHA (1979) procedure, but the 1979 method has a slight edge with respect to agreement between the SRT and pure-tone averages (Huff & Nerbonne, 1982; Wall, Davis, & Myers, 1984; Jahner, Schlauch, & Doyle, 1994). The 1988 method took less time to administer than the 1979 technique in two studies (Huff & Nerbonne, 1982; Wall,

Speech Level (dB HL)	Word No.	
	1	2
50	√	√
48	√	√
46	X	√
44	√	X
42	√	X
40	X	√
38	√	X
36	X	X
34	X	X

Starting Level

Stop: 5 of 6 words missed.

Count correct words from starting level to stopping level (9 in this example).

Calculation of the SRT (in dB HL):

Record the Starting Level:	50
Subtract number of correct words:	- 9
Sub-total:	41
Add the 1-dB Correction Factor:	+ 1
Speech Recognition Threshold (SRT) =	42

FIGURE 8–4 Tally sheet and calculation of the SRT with 2-dB steps according to the ASHA (1988) method.

Davis, & Myers, 1984), but Jahner, Schlauch, and Doyle (1994) found that the 1988 method took 4 seconds longer plus 11 seconds for the SRT calculation. It is hard to demonstrate a singularly "best" method, although the ASHA (1988) approach appears to be the most appealing one on conceptual grounds.

Testing by Bone-Conduction

Bone-conduction speech audiometry most often involves obtaining an SRT. This approach has been used to (1) help indicate whether a conductive loss is present (by comparison to the air-conduction SRT) in children and other patients when reliable pure-tone results are lacking, (2) provide insight about the status of the cochlea before and after middle ear surgery, and (3) corroborate bone-conduction pure-tone thresholds (Bess, 1983; Olsen & Matkin, 1991). Although reference values are provided for presenting speech stimuli by bone-conduction (see Chapter 4), it is a wise choice to calibrate on an empirical basis for the presentation of speech by bone-conduction.

Comfortable and Uncomfortable Listening Levels for Speech

The **most comfortable loudness level (MCL)** for speech is the hearing level at which the patient experiences speech material to be most comfortable, that is, where she prefers to listen to speech material. The basic method used in MCL testing involves adjusting the hearing level of speech until the patient indicates that it is comfortably loud. "Continuous discourse" speech material is often used for obtaining the MCL, although spondees and sentences are also usable. The "continuous discourse" is usually a recorded selection of some prose material. Relatively uninteresting selections are used so that the patient can concentrate on the perceived level of the material without being distracted by its content. Continuous discourse material is also known as "cold running speech" for this reason.

As they try to find *the* MCL, new clinicians learn rather quickly that many patients seem "unreliable" or even "uncooperative" because they report comfortable loudness at several hearing levels. This experience is not an example of patients trying to give the audiologist a hard time. On the contrary, it demonstrates the important concept that the MCL is really *a range of levels* instead of *a level* (Dirks & Morgan, 1983).

UNCOMFORTABLE LOUDNESS LEVEL

The **uncomfortable loudness level (UCL)** for speech is the hearing level at which the patient considers speech material to be uncomfortably loud. The same kinds of materials used for measuring the MCL for speech are also applicable to the UCL. When testing for the UCL, it is important for the patient to understand that he should indicate when the experience of loudness becomes uncomfortable (Dirks & Morgan, 1983). This is an important distinction because we are interested in when the sound becomes uncomfortably loud rather than the patient's capacity to endure pain. In other words, we are concerned with sound levels that begin to produce an uncomfortable *auditory* experience, as opposed to the *tactile* sensations (e.g., tickle, feeling, pain) associated with the highest tolerable sound intensities. For this reason, "uncomfortable loudness level" is preferred over other terms that include words like *discomfort* and *tolerance*, such as *loudness discomfort level, tolerance level,* or *threshold of discomfort.*

DYNAMIC RANGE FOR SPEECH

The range in decibels between the patient's SRT and UCL is called the **dynamic range**. It is, in effect, the patient's usable listening range. For example, if a patient has an SRT of 15 dB HL and a UCL of 100 dB HL, then her dynamic range would be 100 − 15 = 85 dB wide. This means that the patient's hearing can accommodate a range of sound intensities that is 85 dB wide. One of the major problems faced by many patients with sensorineural hearing losses is that their thresholds are elevated but their UCLs remain essentially unchanged, which results in a constricted dynamic range. For example, a patient's SRT might be elevated to 65 dB HL, but her UCL might still be 100 dB HL, so that her dynamic range would be 100 − 65 = 35 dB wide. Notice the difference between this situation and the prior example. There would be no problem "fitting" the wide range of intensities in the real world into a usable (dynamic) listening range that is 85 dB wide. However, the patient in the second example has a usable listening range that is only 35 dB wide, which is too narrow to accommodate the range of intensities found in the real world of sound. Imagine the implications of a restricted dynamic range for hearing aid use: Amplifying sound levels so they become audible (which is desirable) will also cause many sounds to exceed the patient's UCL (which is undesirable). Consequently, in addition to amplifying them, we must also try to "squeeze" the wide range of real-world sounds into the patient's narrower dynamic range.

Assessing Speech Recognition

There is a readily understandable distinction between the threshold for speech and the ability to understand the speech that is heard. Consider the following complaints expressed by a variety of hearing impaired patients: "I can hear speech but I can't understand it"; "words aren't clear"; "Speech sounds muffled [or distorted]"; or "I mistake one word for another." The common theme here is that the speech heard by the patient is lacking in intelligibility. This problem is experienced in terms of inaccurately received messages and/or reduced clarity. Speech recognition measures have been used in every phase of audiology, such as (1) to describe the extent of hearing impairment in terms of how it affects speech understanding, (2) in the differential diagnosis of auditory disorders, (3) for determining the needs for amplification and other forms of audiologic rehabilitation, (4) for making comparisons between various hearing aids and amplification approaches, (5) for verifying the benefits of hearing aid use and other forms of audiologic rehabilitation, and (6) for monitoring patient performance over time for either diagnostic or rehabilitative purposes.

Speech intelligibility can be tested clinically in a straightforward manner. The most common approach is to present the patient with a list of test words. The percentage of test words correctly repeated by the patient is called the **speech recognition score**, the **word recognition score**, or the **speech discrimination score**. *Speech recognition score* is the preferred term because it describes the task in terms of the patient's response, which involves recognizing or identifying the test items. It is often called the "suprathreshold speech recognition score" because these tests are typically performed at levels above the threshold for speech. *Word recognition score* is an equally acceptable term providing the test items are words, which is usually the case. Even though it is a popular term, *speech discrimination score* is less desirable because it refers to a different kind of test than that usually performed. Specifically, a speech *discrimination* test involves comparing two (or more) items and judging whether they are the same or different. Speech recognition scores are sometimes called "PB scores" for reasons that will become clear, although this term is technically correct only when "PB" materials are used. One sometimes sees references to "articulation testing" and "articulation scores," particularly in the older literature. Even though this term is rarely used anymore, it was actually quite appropriate because it alludes to the degree of correspondence between the stimulus and the response.

The student has probably noticed that *speech recognition score* looks and sounds a lot like *speech recognition threshold*. The possible confusion of these terms is one reason that many audiologists continue to use the terms *speech reception threshold* and *speech discrimination score* even though the preferred nomenclature is more descriptive and precise.

Traditional Test Materials

Speech recognition tests were originally devised to assess the effectiveness of telephone and radio communication systems, and various different kinds of speech material were used for this purpose. The most commonly used materials for clinical speech recognition testing are monosyllabic words that are presented in an open-set format. An **open-set** format means the patient must respond without any prior knowledge of what the possible alternatives might be, whereas a **closed-set** format means the patient is provided with a choice of several possible response alternatives. In other words, an open-set item is much like a fill-in question and a closed-set item is much the same as a multiple-choice question.

This section outlines the development of the W-22 and NU-6 lists, which are the most widely used speech recognition tests in general clinical practice. We can then discuss the fundamental aspects and implications of speech recognition testing without being overwhelmed by the details of alternative kinds of tests. Other speech recognition materials will be discussed later in the chapter.

The common features of the W-22 and NU-6 speech recognition tests include an open-set format; 50-word lists composed of reasonably familiar monosyllabic words, each of which is preceded by a carrier phrase (such as "You will say..." or "Say the word..."); and phonetic or phonemic balance within each list. Several recorded versions of these tests are commercially available. The CID W-22 and NU-6 test lists may be found in Appendices F and G.

The first monosyllabic word materials to enjoy wide clinical use were the Harvard **PAL PB-50 test** (Egan, 1948). The PB-50 test is the precursor of the W-22 and NU-6 materials, which have supplanted it in day-to-day speech recognition testing. Each of the 20 PB-50 lists included 50 words that were phonetically balanced (hence, the name "PB-50"). **Phonetic balance** means that the relative frequencies of the phonemes on the test list are as close as possible to the distribution of speech sounds used in English, which was in turn based on Dewey's (1923) analysis of 100,000 words in newsprint. To improve word familiarity and phonetic balance, Hirsh et al (1952) included 120 of the 1000 PB-50 words in the **CID W-22 test** lists. The W-22 test includes 200 words arranged in four 50-word lists (1–4), each of which was recorded using six randomizations. Phonetic balance on the W-22 lists is based on an analysis of

spoken English (business telephone conversations) by French, Carter, and Koenig (1930), as well as the Dewey word counts, where 95% of the words on the W-22 lists are among the 4000 most common words found by Thorndike (1932).

Northwestern University Auditory Test No. 6, or the **NU-6 test**, is composed of four lists of 50 phonemically balanced CNC words (Tillman & Carhart, 1966). Just as the W-22 test was derived from the PB-50 materials, the NU-6 lists were based on the earlier work of Lehiste and Peterson (1959, Peterson & Lehiste, 1962). Lehiste and Peterson (1959) modified the concept of phonetic balance to one of **phonemic balance** in recognition of the fact that speech recognition is accomplished on a phonemic rather than a phonetic basis. This is a real distinction because **phonemes** are actually groups of speech sounds (each of which is a **phonetic element**) that are classified as being the same by native speakers of the language. Thus, all phonetic differences are not phonemically relevant. For example, phonetically different variants of the phoneme /p/ (**allophones** of /p/) are identified as /p/ even though they vary in terms of their articulatory and acoustic (i.e., phonetic) characteristics in different speech sound contexts (e.g., /p/ as in /pat/ versus /pit/, or initially versus finally as in /pɛp/) and from production to production. To achieve a reasonable degree of phonemic balance, Lehiste and Peterson developed test lists from 1263 monosyllabic words. These were all consonant-vowel nucleus-consonant, or CNC words, drawn from the Thorndike and Lorge (1944) word counts. The original CNC lists were subsequently modified to replace the least familiar words (Peterson & Lehiste, 1962), so that all but 21 of the words on the final version of the CNC lists have a frequency of ≥5/million. Tillman, Carhart, and Wilber (1963) used 95 of Lehiste and Peterson's CNC words and five others to construct two 50-word lists known as the NU-4 test, which may be viewed as an intermediate step in the development of the NU-6 test. The 100 CNCs on the NU-4 lists were increased to 200 words (185 of which are from the Lehiste and Peterson materials) to develop the four 50-word lists that compose the NU-6 test (Tillman & Carhart, 1966).

Speech Recognition Testing

The speech recognition testing process is extremely simple. We will assume that the test is being done with either recorded W-22 or NU-6 materials, but the fundamentals are largely the same regardless of which test is used. The patient is instructed to listen to the test recording and to repeat each test word, guessing if necessary. The attenuator is then set to the desired presentation level, and the speech materials are presented to the patient through the desired output transducer (e.g., one of the earphones). The clinician keeps a tally of right and wrong responses during the test, and then calculates a percent correct score. Each word is worth 2% on a 50-word test. For example, the speech recognition score would be 92% if four words are missed or repeated incorrectly, 86% if seven words are wrong, etc. Foreign-language speakers and those who cannot give a verbal response can often be tested effectively by having them respond by pointing to the response word from a choice of alternative words or pictures (Spitzer, 1980; Wilson & Antablin, 1980; Comstock & Martin, 1984; Antablin McCullough, Cunningham, & Wilson, 1992; McCullough, Wilson, Birck, & Anderson, 1994; Aleksandrovsky, McCullough, & Wilson, 1998).

Speech recognition scores are generally expected to be approximately 90% to 100% in normal hearing individuals. The range of speech recognition scores is typically between 80% and 100% with most conductive losses (e.g., otitis media, otosclerosis), but has been found to be as low as 60% in cases of glomus tumor; and the range for sensorineural losses is anywhere from 0% to 100%, depending on etiology and degree of loss (Bess, 1983). In general, speech recognition scores that are "abnormally low" are associated with retrocochlear lesions; however, there is no clear cutoff value for this decision (e.g., Johnson, 1977; Olsen, Noffsinger, & Kurdziel, 1975; Bess, 1983). As we shall see in the next section, a lower than expected speech recognition score can also occur if the test level is not high

enough. Thus, an atypically low speech recognition score often means the clinician must retest at a higher hearing level.

When is a speech recognition score "too low" with respect to the patient's audiogram? There is a rough relationship in which speech recognition scores tend to become lower as sensorineural hearing loss worsens, but it is hardly predictive and is complicated because the notion of "better" and "worse" on an audiogram often involves considering both the amount and configuration of the loss. Some guidance was provided by 98% lower cutoff values for PB-50 test scores associated with various amounts of cochlear hearing loss among patients younger than 56 years of age (Yellin, Jerger, & Fifer, 1989). However, those cutoff values based on PB-50 test scores do not seem applicable to scores obtained with more commonly used tests such as CID W-22 (Gates, Cooper, Kannel, & Miller, 1990). Dubno, Lee, Klein, Matthews, and Lam (1995) reported 95% lower cutoff values for the NU-6 test (Auditec version) as a function of the patient's three-frequency PTA. These lower cutoff values are shown for both 50- and 25-word lists in Table 8–1.

PERFORMANCE-INTENSITY FUNCTIONS

The percentage of words that are repeated correctly depends on more than just the patient's speech recognition ability. It also depends on the conditions of the test, such as the intensity at which the words are presented. The graph in Figure 8–5 is called a **performance-intensity (PI) function** because it shows how the patient's speech recognition *performance* (in percent correct on the y-axis) depends on the *intensity* of the test materials (along the x-axis).[1] It is often called a **PI-PB function** when phonetically or phonemically balanced (PB) words are used. This PI function is from a normal-hearing individual. Notice how his

---

[1] A more correct term would be *performance-level function*, although it is rarely used. The student should also be aware that the PI function is a type of **psychometric function**, which shows performance (in this case speech recognition) as a function of some stimulus parameter (in this case the speech level).

TABLE 8–1 Lower 95% confidence limits for PB_{max} with the NU-6 test (Auditec), recommended by Dubno, Lee, Klein, Matthews, and Lam (1995)

500, 1000, 2000 Hz PTA (dB HL)	Lower 95% Confidence Limits in Percent for	
	25-Word Lists	50-Word Lists
3.3	100	98
0.0	100	98
1.7	100	96
3.3	96	96
5.0	96	96
6.7	96	94
8.3	96	94
10.0	96	92
11.7	92	92
13.3	92	90
15.0	92	90
16.7	88	88
18.3	88	86
20.0	88	86
21.7	84	84
23.3	84	82
25.0	80	80
26.7	80	78
28.3	76	76
30.0	76	74
31.7	72	72
33.3	72	70
35.0	68	68
36.7	68	66
38.3	64	64
40.0	64	62
41.7	60	60
43.3	56	58
45.0	56	56
46.7	52	52
48.3	52	50
50.0	48	48
51.7	48	46
53.3	44	44
55.0	44	42
56.7	40	40
58.3	40	38
60.0	36	38
61.7	36	36
63.3	32	34
65.0	32	32
66.7	32	30
68.3	28	30
70.0	28	28
71.7	24	26

From Dubno, Lee, Klein, Matthews, and Lam (1995), with permission.

speech recognition scores are low when the words are presented at very soft levels, and that the scores improve as the intensity increases. In this case, a maximum score of 100% is eventually achieved when the intensity reaches a level of 30 dB HL. The maximum score on the PI-PB function is traditionally called PB_{max}. Notice that the PI function flattens (or becomes asymptotic) as the intensity is raised above the level where PB_{max} is found. This plateau establishes the fact that PB_{max} has been reached, because it shows that the score does not improve any more when the intensity continues to be raised. (This is a moot point when 100% is reached, but it is a real issue when PB_{max} is lower than 100%.) This maximum score is used to express a patient's speech recognition performance. It is assumed that a patient's "speech recognition score" refers to PB_{max} unless otherwise indicated. Thus, we must be confident that PB_{max} has been obtained (or at least approximated).

Figure 8–6 shows some representative examples of PI functions. The normal PI-function from Figure 8–5 is shown as curve **a** for comparison with the others. Curve **b** shows what might happen if this normal patient were to develop a conductive hearing loss. Notice that this PI function is displaced to the right by 30 dB HL due to a conductive loss, but is otherwise the same as curve **a**. In other words, all the speech recognition scores would be the same as long as the intensity of the words is increased sufficiently to overcome the effects of the air-bone-gap. Performance-intensity function **c** is from a typical patient with a sensorineural hearing loss of cochlear origin. This patient's maximum speech recognition score is 30% and her PI function is essentially asymptotic above the level where PB_{max} is first obtained, as in curves **a** and **b**. Curve **d** is from another patient with a cochlear impairment, for whom PB_{max} is 76%. In this case raising the intensity above the level where PB_{max} was obtained results in speech recognition scores that fall somewhat below PB_{max}.

The PI function shown in curve **e** is from a patient with retrocochlear pathology. The maximum speech recognition score here is only 64%, which we will assume is atypically low for his audiogram. Atypically low speech recognition scores are considered a risk factor for retrocochlear pathology. In addition, notice that the speech recognition scores drop

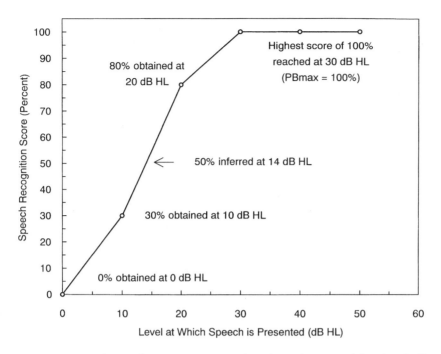

FIGURE 8–5   The performance-intensity function of a normal hearing individual whose maximum speech recognition score (PB$_{max}$) is 100%.

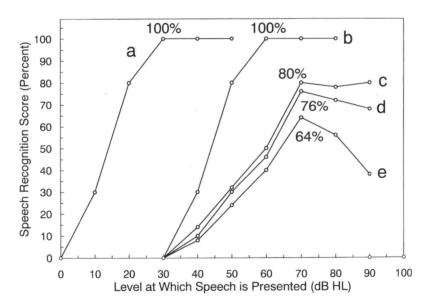

FIGURE 8–6   Several representative examples of various kinds of performance-intensity functions. (a) The same normal PI function from the prior figure. (b) The same normal PI function displaced rightward by 30 dB HL due to a conductive loss. (c) The PI function of a patient with sensorineural loss whose scores reach PB$_{max}$ of 30% at 70 dB HL and remain essentially the same at higher levels. (d) The PI function of a patient with sensorineural loss with PB$_{max}$ of 76% at 70 dB HL, which rolls over slightly at higher intensities. (e) A PI function with PB$_{max}$ of 64% and pathologic rollover in a patient with retrocochlear pathology.

substantially as the intensity is raised above the level where PB_{max} was obtained. This is an example of how the PI function provides diagnostic information in addition to the maximum speech recognition score, that is, by revealing the presence of abnormal PI rollover. **Rollover of the PI function** (or **PI rollover**) is defined as a reduction of speech recognition scores that occurs at intensities above the level where PB_{max} is obtained. Mild rollover as depicted in curve **d** is not considered abnormal; however, significant amounts of rollover as in curve **e** are pathologic and are associated with retrocochlear disorders (Jerger & Jerger, 1971; Dirks, Kamm, Bower, & Betsworth, 1977).

Curve **e** from Figure 8–6 is replotted in Figure 8–7 to show how to determine when rollover is clinically significant. In addition to PB_{max}, a second point is now highlighted on the PI function, labeled **PB_{min}**. This is the lowest speech recognition score obtained at intensity levels higher than where PB_{max} was obtained. These two scores are used to calcu-late a number called the **rollover index (RI)** (Jerger & Jerger, 1971), as follows:

$$RI = \frac{(PB_{max} - PB_{min})}{PB_{max}}.$$

Retrocochlear pathology is suggested when the rollover index is greater than 0.45 when using *PAL PB-50* materials (Jerger & Jerger, 1971; Dirks et al, 1977). When the *NU-6* test is used, the cutoff value has been reported to be from 0.25 (Bess, Josey, & Humes, 1979) to 0.35 (Meyer & Mishler, 1985). Abnormal rollover exists in this case because the rollover index is 0.41, which is significant for the NU-6 materials. Abnormal rollover also occurs in some elderly patients (Gang, 1976; Dirks et al, 1977; Shirinian & Arnst, 1980). These findings have been associated with neural presbycusis (Jerger & Jerger, 1976; Dirks et al, 1977; Shirinian & Arnst, 1980), and exemplify the concept that audiological tests reflect the site of the disorder (e.g., retrocochlear) rather than its etiology (e.g., acoustic tumor) (Jerger & Jerger, 1976).

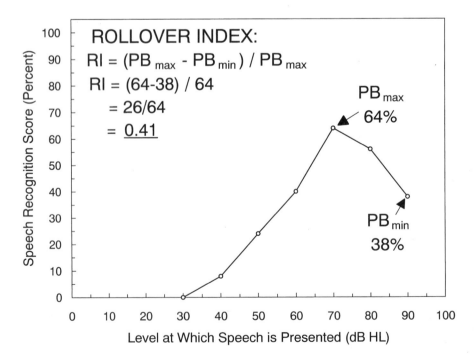

FIGURE 8–7 This is the same PI function with abnormal rollover from the prior figure, now indicating PB_{max}, PB_{min}, and how to calculate the rollover index.

Speech Recognition Testing Considerations

There are several considerations that must be addressed when choosing and administering speech recognition tests. Deciding which test to use for speech recognition assessment involves choosing the most efficient test for the purpose at hand. For most routine audiological evaluations this will be one of the widely accepted, open-set tests such as CID W-22 and NW-6. Other tests that might be used, as well as special purpose tests, are outlined later in this chapter and elsewhere in the text with respect to specific assessment issues. When and how to use masking is handled in Chapter 9. Here we will address several issues that pertain to the word recognition testing per se, such as lexical considerations, test forms and form equivalency, phonetic/phonemic balance, carrier phrases, choosing an initial testing level, whole-word versus phonemic scoring, foreign-language considerations, recorded versus monitored live-voice testing, and test size. The last two issues are controversial. About 82% of audiologists use **monitored live voice** instead of **recorded** speech recognition tests; and 56% use **shortened test lists** (typically 25-word "half-lists") instead of **full lists**, while 30% stop testing after 25 words unless the patient makes errors (Martin, Champlin, & Chambers, 1998).[2] These practices might maximize convenience and minimize testing time, but, as we shall see, the most cogent evidence supports the use of recorded materials and a larger test size. Wiley, Stoppenbach, Feldhake, Moss, and Thordardottir (1995) present an insightful discussion dealing with issues such as these that should be read by even the beginning audiology student.

LEXICAL CONSIDERATIONS

Speech recognition performance is affected by more than just how accurately the sounds of speech are heard. **Lexical considerations** come into play when the test materials are words, which is almost always the case in clinical speech recognition testing. **Word familiarity** has a substantial effect upon speech recognition performance (e.g., Owens, 1961b), and was addressed above in the discussion of how the traditional speech recognition tests were developed. Word familiarity must also be considered when deciding which test to use, especially when dealing with children.

Word familiarity is not the only lexical consideration involved in word recognition. There is a well-established effect of **word frequency**, with a significant bias favoring the recognition of words with a higher frequency of occurrence compared to lower frequency words (see, e.g., Luce & Pisoni, 1998). The ability to correctly repeat a test word is also affected by whether it has many or few similar sounding alternatives, that is, other possible words that could be confused with the test word if one of the phonemes is misheard. These similar sounding alternatives compose the **lexical neighborhood** of the test word. Test words with many similar sounding alternatives (*dense lexical neighborhoods*) are more difficult than words with a smaller number of similar sounding alternatives (*sparse lexical neighborhoods*). The manner in which these effects are involved in speech recognition is described by the **neighborhood activation model**[3] (Luce, 1990; Luce & Pisoni, 1998).

TEST FORMS AND EQUIVALENCY

The clinician must know about the alternative **test forms** that are available for each test she uses. More than one form of the same test

---

[2] Commenting that only 4% of audiologists attend to the relationship between sample size and measurement error, these surveyors implied that only 4% of clinicians use standard 50-word lists.

[3] The neighborhood activation model of spoken language recognition is outside the scope of this text. In oversimplified terms, the sound patterns of a stimulus word are compared to acoustic-phonetic representations in the listener's memory. On a probability basis, these representations are activated depending on how similar they are to the stimulus—the greater the similarity, the greater the degree of activation. This is followed by a lexical selection process among all words in memory that are potential matches to the stimulus, which is biased by word frequency. See Luce & Pisoni (1998) for a comprehensive discussion, and Kirk, Pisoni, and Osberger (1995) and Kirk, Eisenberg, Martinez, and Hay-McCutcheon (1999) for informative summaries.

is usually provided because more than one administration is almost always necessary. For example, we routinely test the speech recognition of each ear separately, and often have to do this at more than one hearing level. Different test forms are desirable for each of these administrations. The audiologist must also be aware of **test form equivalency**, which refers to how well various alternative forms of the same test agree with one another. The various forms of a given test tend to produce comparable results, but some forms are easier or harder than others for a given test, and the audiologist must be aware of these differences for the tests that she uses.

Not all speech recognition tests use a fixed set of alternative test forms. For example, the CASRA test (Gelfand, 1993, 1998), described below, produces one-time-use test forms that are balanced for difficulty by assigning equal numbers of high-, middle-, and low-difficulty words to each test list. These "difficulty ratings" are based on empirically obtained error rates, which in effect accounts for all factors affecting the recognition of the words in the pool. The unique test forms are used in the same order in which they were generated, so that any patient must hear all 450 words in the pool before any test word is repeated.

Phonetic/Phonemic Balance

The concept of **phonetic/phonemic balance** played a major role in the development of many speech recognition tests. However, phonetic/phonemic balance has been found to have little practical impact on the outcome of speech recognition tests, and its clinical relevance is at best questionable (Tobias, 1964; Carhart, 1970; Aspinall, 1973; Bess, 1983). In fact, attempts to achieve phonetic/phonemic balance have largely been abandoned over the course of time in the development of many speech recognition tests.

Carrier Phrases

Carrier phrase use also appears to be a minor issue during speech recognition testing. Some studies found statistically significant advantages for speech recognition scores obtained with a carrier phrase (Gladstone & Siegenthaler, 1971; Gelfand, 1975), but others found no significant differences (Martin, Hawkins, & Bailey, 1962; McLennan & Knox, 1975). Some patients are able to perform better with the carrier phrases, perhaps because they serve as alerting signals, whereas other patients are annoyed or even distracted by them. Thus, regardless of whether the audiologist uses carrier phrases as a matter of routine, she should be alert to the patient's responsiveness and be prepared to add, change, or omit carrier phrases as conditions warrant.

Initial Testing Level

Routine speech recognition testing is often done at one hearing level for each ear. Some audiologists add a second measurement at high levels to screen for the possibility of rollover, and the testing of speech recognition at more than one level is strongly encouraged. In any case, it is necessary to choose a level that will most likely result in the highest speech recognition score for the ear being tested. To accomplish this goal, routine speech recognition testing should be done at 30 to 40 dB SL (relative to the SRT) for those with essentially normal hearing, and at 40 dB SL for hearing impaired patients. Evidence for this recommendation is bountiful throughout the literature, but the findings of Maroonroge and Diefendorf (1984) are a nice example because they apply to three rather different speech recognition tests, as shown in Figure 8–8. Notice how the speech recognition scores in the figure flatten around 30 dB SL for the normal subjects, but continue to improve up to 40 dB SL for the hearing-impaired patients. Clearly, the hearing-impaired patients' scores would have been understated by a single test done below 40 dB SL. Even though many audiologists perform routine speech recognition testing at MCL, this is not desirable because the MCL is actually a range rather than a level, and the highest speech recognition score is often obtained at levels significantly above the MCL (Clemis & Carver, 1967; Ullrich & Grimm, 1976; Posner & Ventry, 1977; Dirks & Morgan 1983).

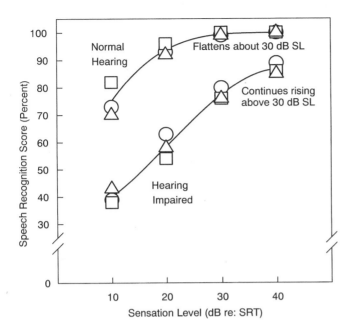

FIGURE 8–8 Speech recognition scores tend to improve up to about 30 dB SL for normals and 40 dB SL for patients with sensorineural losses. Data points are means for NU-6 (circles), Pascoe high frequency (triangles), and California Consonant Tests (squares) based on Maroonroge and Diefendorf (1984); best-fit curves are shown to highlight the general relationships.

WHOLE-WORD VERSUS PHONEMIC SCORING

Speech recognition tests that use words are usually scored on a whole-word basis. Whole-word scoring reflects the patient's correct reception of the intended word, but also misrepresents how well the patient is able to make use of the acoustical cues of speech. For example, a CNC word such as "cat" is correct only when the patient repeats "cat"; but whole-word scoring considers the response to be *equally* wrong regardless of whether the patient incorrectly repeats one, two, or all three of its phonemes (e.g., "pat," "pot," "pack," "tack," or "seed"), or cannot repeat any part of the word at all. An alternative approach is to score word recognition on a phoneme-by-phoneme basis, which has been done successfully for quite some time (Groen & Helleman, 1960; Boothroyd, 1968a,b, 1970, 1984; Markides, 1978; Duffy, 1983; Boothroyd & Nittrouer, 1988; Gelfand, 1993, 1998; Olsen, Van Tasell, & Speaks, 1997).

Compared to whole-word scoring, the use of phonemic scoring (1) provides a more precise and more valid measure of the correct reception of the acoustic cues of speech; (2) improves reliability by maximizing the num-

ber of scorable items; (3) makes it possible to obtain meaningful scores from patients whose whole word scores would have been zero; (4) gives a better idea of which speech sounds are misperceived; and (5) minimizes the effects of nonacoustic factors such as word familiarity, word-level predictability, context, and differences between word lists. Moreover, comparing word scores and phoneme scores makes it possible to estimate the benefit to speech recognition provided by taking advantage of lexical information (e.g., Boothroyd & Nittrouer, 1988; Nittrouer & Boothroyd, 1990; Olsen, Van Tasell, & Speaks, 1997).

The benefits of phonemic scoring are optimized by instructing the patient to repeat whatever he hears because partial credit is given for any part of a word or any individual sounds that are correct, even if the word itself is unintelligible (Markides, 1978). Also, the examiner should be able to see the patient's face and should ask for clarification of equivocal replies to minimize the chances of misperceiving the patient's intended response. Because of partial credit for any correct part of a "mix-heard" word, the phoneme score obtained on a test will be higher than the word score for the same test. (Exceptions occur when the score is 0% or 100%, and when all phonemes are wrong for every word that is wrong.) For this reason, one should state when phonemic scoring has been used.

Recorded versus Monitored Live-Voice Testing

The distinction between lists of test words and recorded tests is particularly relevant when testing speech recognition because the intelligibility of the same words is affected by speech differences among talkers, and even the same person does not produce a given word the same way each time it is spoken. In effect, one could propose that the same word list spoken by two different talkers constitutes two different tests (Kreul, Bell, & Nixon, 1969).[4] Significantly different speech recognition results are often obtained for the same test materials when they are administered by different talkers (Penrod, 1979; Gengel & Kupperman, 1980; Hood & Poole, 1980; Bess, 1983), and even when using different recordings made over time by the same speaker (Brandy, 1966). Clinicians also differ with regard to how they say test words, some using a conversational manner and others attempting to speak clearly. In fact, clinicians can inadvertently adjust their speech production depending on the nature of the patient's responses. This can be a significant factor because intelligibility is affected by the use of *conversational* versus *clear speech* (Picheny, Durlach, & Braida, 1985). These points provide a forceful argument for the use of recorded speech recognition materials whenever possible. Of course, monitored live-voice testing is often appropriate when the special needs of the patient call for a flexible approach and when a recorded version of the speech recognition test being used is not available.

Test Size

Even though most standard speech recognition tests include 50 monosyllabic words,

many attempts have been made to reduce the test size to 25 or even fewer words (for a review, see Bess, 1983). After determining the relative difficulty of the words on the W-22 lists, Runge and Hosford-Dunn (1985) suggested a speech recognition testing strategy that involves presenting the most difficult words first. They recommended presenting the 10 *most difficult words first*, and stopping if these are all correct. If any of the first 10 words are missed, then the next 15 words would be given, for a total of 25 words. Testing would then be terminated if there are no more than four errors based on the first 25 words. Otherwise, the entire 50-word list would be used. About 30% of audiologists stop testing after 25 words if the patient makes no errors (Martin, Champlin, & Chambers, 1998), suggesting that some aspects of this strategy have been adopted by many audiologists

The problem with reducing test size is that reliability depends on the size of the test. Shortening a test also makes it less reliable. Let us see why. The variability of speech recognition scores is largely defined by the binomial distribution (Boothroyd, 1968a; Hagerman, 1976; Thornton & Raffin, 1978; Raffin & Schafer, 1980; Raffin & Thornton, 1980; Gelfand, 1993, 1998). Specifically, the variability of a test score can be described in terms of its standard deviation, which depends on the percent correct *and* the number of scorable items in the test. For the math-minded, this relationship may be written as

$$SD = 100\sqrt{[(p)(1-p)/n]}$$

where SD is the standard deviation (in percent), p represents the test score (as a proportion from 0.0 to 1.0), and n is the number of scorable items.

This relationship is shown graphically in Figure 8–9. The y-axis shows the standard deviation of the test score in percent. A larger standard deviation means the score is more variable, or less reliable. The x-axis shows the test score in percent correct. The various curves show what happens when the test has

---

[4] In this context, one should also be aware that norms have been published for contemporary recordings of the various speech recognition tests (e.g., Heckendorf, Wiley, & Wilson, 1997; Wilson & Oyler, 1997; Stoppenbach, Craig, Wiley, & Wilson, 1999).

10 items, 25, 50, etc., up to 450 items. This figure depicts several principles: (1) Reliability improves as the number of test items increases and gets worse as the number of items gets smaller. Egan (1948) made this point in the original description of the PAL PB-50 test. (2) Speech recognition scores become more variable (less reliable) as they go from either extreme (100% or 0%) toward 50% correct. (3) The improvement in reliability that comes with adding more test items is greatest when the test has fewer items and gets progressively smaller as the test size increases, as shown by the convergence of the curves. The third curve from the top applies to the standard 50-item test list and the second curve from the top applies to a 25-word half-list. Notice how the test gets much more variable (less reliable) moving from the 50-word list to a 25-word half-list.

What does all this mean clinically? Consider the following. All tests have some degree of variability. Suppose we have two different tests for the same phenomenon. If the phenomenon is weight, the two different tests might be two different scales. The variability of scale A is ±2 pounds and the variability of scale B is ±4 pounds. Because scale A can vary by 2 pounds either way, a weight of 130 pounds really means 130 ± 2 pounds. On the other hand, 130 pounds on scale B really means 130 ± 4 pounds. If a dieter weighed 130 pounds two weeks ago, continued to follow the diet, and now weighs 127 pounds, can she really say that she lost weight? The answer is "yes" using scale A because the 3-pound change from 130 to 127 is larger than what could have been due to the variability of the scale (i.e., the test). However, the answer must be "no" (or, at

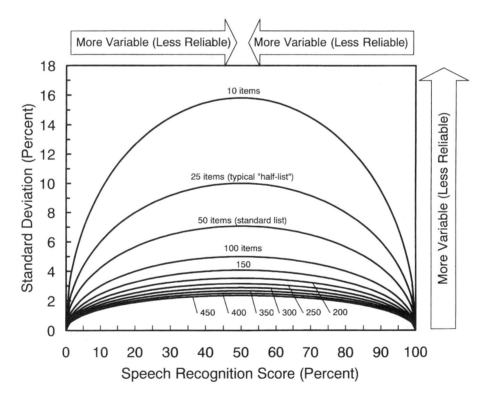

FIGURE 8–9 Test scores become more variable (less reliable) as (1) the number of tested items becomes smaller, and (2) when the percent correct approaches 50%. Notice how reducing the size of the test has a bigger effect when the test size is relatively small (e.g., going from 50 items to 25 or 10) compared to when it is relatively large (e.g., going from 450 items to 400 or 350). From Gelfand (1993), with permission.

least, "we can't confidently say yes") using the more variable scale B. The reason is that the 3-pound change could also have been due to the random fluctuations in the readings provided by the scale (i.e., the variability of the test).

Let us now extend this line of reasoning to speech recognition testing. The variability of a speech recognition test refers to the chance fluctuations of the scores obtained with that test. To be considered different, two scores must differ by an amount larger than what could have occurred by chance. Before we can confidently say that two speech recognition scores are different from each other, the difference must be wider than the size of the fluctuations associated with the test itself. In turn, the size of this variability depends on the size of the test: For any given score, variability is wider for a test with fewer items and narrower for tests with more items. Cutoff values that may be used to determine whether two word recognition scores are significantly different from one another take the form of **95% confidence limits** (Thornton & Raffin, 1978; Raffin & Schafer, 1980; Raffin & Thornton, 1980). These are shown in Table 8–2. To be considered a true difference the spread between two test scores must be *wider* than the applicable confidence limits shown in the table. If the difference between two test scores is *within* the applicable confidence limits, then it cannot be considered to reflect an actual performance difference because the same disparity could have occurred by chance (due just to the inherent variability of the test). For example, to be considered significantly different from a score of 80%, a second score must fall outside of the (1) 68 to 89% range on a 100-item test, (2) 64 to 92% range on a standard 50-word test, (3) 56 to 96% range on 25-word (half-list) test, and (4) 40 to 100% if only 10 words are used. Notice how a larger test size makes it possible to make finer distinctions between two test results.

FOREIGN LANGUAGE INFLUENCES AND IMPLICATIONS

It is often necessary to test a patient whose native language is not English or who may not speak English at all. This can be a problematic clinical issue because speech audiometry involves material that is inherently linguistic in nature, so the results may be influenced by such factors as differences in phonology and morphologic rules between languages, and are exacerbated by word familiarity effects. Hence, nonnative speakers of the language typically obtain lower scores on English speech recognition tests than do native speakers of the language (e.g., Gat & Keith, 1978), and speakers of Spanish score lower on a nonsense syllable test using English phonemes than do English or bilingual speakers (Danhauer, Crawford, & Edgerton, 1984). Audiologists everywhere face the same problem; only the local language changes.

Bilingual patients can usually be tested in English, but we must be mindful of linguistic influences when interpreting the results, especially if they are lower than expected. But what about the non–English-speaking patient? The perfect solution is for every patient to be tested in his native language by an audiologist who is also a native speaker or at least a fluent speaker of that language. This is often possible, but it is far from the norm. The opposite approach is simply to test foreign-language patients in English, which is the worst alternative because it confounds the results with the largest number of linguistic problems. A commonsense solution is for the English-speaking audiologist to use test materials in the patient's own language. In the United States this most often involves lists of Spanish bisyllabic words, which tend to yield results analogous to that found with English monosyllabic word lists (Weisleder & Hodgson, 1989). Several Spanish lists have been developed, some of which are listed in Appendix O. Recordings should be used so that the phonology of Spanish is actually embodied in the test words.

Linguistic limitations on the part of the clinician are a concern when English-speaking audiologists score verbal responses in a foreign language. However, Cokely and Yager (1993) found that English-speaking audiologists can competently score verbal responses in Spanish. It is hard to generalize their find-

TABLE 8–2 Lower and upper limits of the 95% critical differences for percentage scores; values within the range shown are not significantly different from the value shown in the percentage score columns (p>0.05)

% Score	n=50	n=25	n=10	% Score	n=100[a]
0	0–4	0–8	0–20	50	37–63
2	0–10			51	38–64
4	0–14	0–20		52	39–65
6	2–18			53	40–66
8	2–22	0–28		54	41–67
10	2–24		0–50	55	42–68
12	4–26	4–32		56	43–69
14	4–30			57	44–70
16	6–32	4–40		58	45–71
18	6–34			59	46–72
20	8–36	4–44	0–60	60	47–73
22	8–40			61	48–74
24	10–42	8–48		62	49–74
26	12–44			63	50–75
28	14–46	8–52		64	51–76
30	14–48		10–70	65	52–77
32	16–50	12–56		66	53–78
34	18–52			67	54–79
36	20–54	16–60		68	55–80
38	22–56			69	56–81
40	22–58	16–64	10–80	70	57–81
42	24–60			71	58–82
44	26–62	20–68		72	59–83
46	28–64			73	60–84
48	30–66	24–72		74	61–85
50	32–68		10–90	75	63–86
52	34–70	28–76		76	64–86
54	36–72			77	65–87
56	38–74	32–80		78	66–88
58	40–76			79	67–89
60	42–78	36–84	20–90	80	68–89
62	44–78			81	69–90
64	46–80	40–84		82	71–91
66	48–82			83	72–92
68	50–84	44–88		84	73–92
70	52–86		30–90	85	74–93
72	54–86	48–92		86	75–94
74	56–88			87	77–94
76	58–90	52–92		88	78–95
78	60–92			89	79–96
80	64–92	56–96	40–100	90	81–96
82	66–94			91	82–97
84	68–94	60–96		92	83–98
86	70–96			93	85–98
88	74–96	68–96		94	86–99
90	76–98		50–100	95	88–99
92	78–98	72–100		96	89–99
94	82–98			97	91–100
96	86–100	80–100		98	92–100
98	90–100			99	94–100
100	96–100	92–100	80–100	100	97–100

[a] If score is less than 50%, find % score = 100 − observed score and subtract each critical difference limit from 100.

From Thornton and Raffin (1978), with permission of American Speech–Language–Hearing Association.

ings to other languages. However, Cakiroglu and Danhauer (1992) found that different linguistic backgrounds do not seem to have a major impact on the results when English words are being used. They had talkers of Turkish, East Indian, and American origin record W-22 word lists, and then administered these tests to groups of listeners from each of these backgrounds. The only significant influence of talker background occurred for the Turkish subjects who heard the list recorded by the Indian talker. Overall, however, the linguistic backgrounds of the talkers and listeners did not pose a problem for clinical evaluation purposes.

The least biased approach to performing speech audiometry across languages is to use a closed-set test. In this way, recorded test items can be presented in the patient's language and her responses can be scored without being influenced by the perceptions of the clinician. Several tests have been developed in which the patient points to one of a choice of pictures corresponding to the test word, which was presented in a foreign language, such as Spanish or Russian. The pictures may be presented on paper (Spitzer, 1980; Comstock & Martin, 1984) or a computer screen (McCullough et al, 1994; Aleksandrovsky, McCullough, & Wilson, 1998).

Types of Speech Recognition Tests

The remainder of this chapter provides the student with a sample of the types of speech recognition tests that are available in addition to the traditional ones already described. Keep in mind that this is by no means an exhaustive listing—many fine tests and testing approaches are not included. Examples of tests intended principally for use with children are discussed in Chapter 12.

Many different kinds of speech recognition tests exist, which may be categorized in a variety of ways. Here we will distinguish between tests that use real words and those that use nonsense syllables, and between open- and closed-set formats.

Open-Set Tests

Open-set monosyllabic word tests are the most popular method for clinically assessing speech recognition, and the majority of practicing clinicians use the NU-6 and W-22 tests in day-to-day practice. Other tests involve different approaches to open-set word recognition testing, some of which are outlined in this section.

High-frequency word lists have been developed by Gardner (1971, 1987) and by Pascoe (1975) and are listed in Appendix N. These test lists concentrate on words that contain a preponderance of high-frequency consonants, which are frequently missed by patients with sensorineural hearing losses. They were originally designed to enhance the ability of speech recognition tests to distinguish performance differences between hearing aids, but can also be used for other clinical purposes. Pascoe's (1975) list includes 50 monosyllabic words, in which 63% of the consonants are voiceless. The two original 25-word Gardner (1971) lists included words composed of the consonants /p, t, k, s, f, θ, h/ with the vowel /I/. These were expanded to an alphabetical listing of 200 monosyllabic words using the same consonants with a variety of vowels (Gardner, 1987). An interesting variation of this approach are the **low-mid-high word lists** (Koike, Brown, Hobbs, & Asp, 1989; Koike, 1993). These 30-word lists have an equal number of words whose spectra emphasize the contribution of relatively low-frequency ("move"), midfrequency ("tag"), and high-frequency ("teeth") speech sounds.

The **AB isophonemic word lists** were developed by Boothroyd (1968a, 1984; Boothroyd & Nittrouer, 1988). The isophonemic word lists include CNC words drawn from a pool of 30 consonants. Each list includes 10 words that are presented in an open-set format and are scored phonemically, so that the resulting speech recognition score is based on 30 items. The original British English version of the test (Boothroyd, 1968a) included 15 lists, which were revised slightly for use in the United States at the Clark School for the Deaf (Boothroyd, 1984). This version of the isophonemic word lists is included in Appendix H. A subsequent revision includes 12 lists, and involves some modifications of the criteria used for word selection. (Boothroyd & Nittrouer, 1988). A computer program is available to facilitate the use of the isophonemic word lists (Boothroyd, 1999).

The **Computer-Assisted Speech Recognition Assessment (CASRA) test** (Gelfand, 1993, 1998) was developed (1) to minimize test variability by maximizing the number of scorable items, and (2) to enhance sensitivity for misperceived speech sounds by using phonemic scoring, while at the same time (3) retaining the major characteristics of a traditional word recognition test. These traditional test characteristics include the use of monosyllabic words, an open-set format, verbal responses, right/wrong scoring, and no more than 50 test presentations. A test size of 450 was chosen because the benefits of additional test items reach diminishing returns with about 450 scorable items, which is shown by the converging curves in Figure 8–9. This seemingly paradoxical combination of test characteristics is made possible by using an interactive computer program to administer 150 digitized CNC words in 50 three-word presentations, without a carrier phrase. The words are repeated by the patient and scored by the audiologist on a phoneme-by-phoneme basis, as illustrated in Figure 8–10. The outcome of this strategy is a test size of 450 scorable items (50 presentations × three words × three phonemes). The computer selects and presents the words, and is used to keep track of all the bookkeeping details. A test form generation program distributes a 450-word pool into three 150-word lists at a time, which are balanced for word difficulty. This program also minimizes semantic and syntactic cues within each three-word group. An added benefit of using digitized words and a computer in place of a tape recorder is that the intervals between word presentations automatically adjust to how long it takes the patient to respond.

The CASRA test optimizes reliability because the advantage of adding items becomes negligible by the time the test size reaches about 450. However, maximum reliability is not always needed clinically, providing the variability of the test is consistent with what the audiologist is trying to do with it. Thus, the size of the CASRA test can be reduced to what the clinician considers acceptable for the intended purpose, such as 25 (or even 10) presentations per test. Yet, using the CASRA test with 25 presentations still produces scores based on $25 \times 3 \times 3 = 225$ items, and even if it is administered with only 10 presentations, the scores are based on $10 \times 3 \times 3 = 90$ items. In either case, the CASRA test yields considerable improvements in reliability compared to the traditional approach with 50 items and dramatic improvements over 25-item testing.

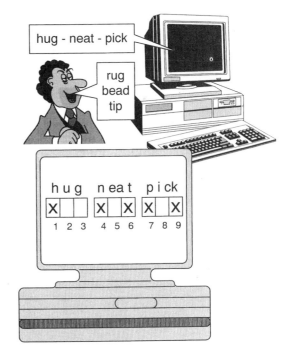

FIGURE 8–10 Example of a test item on the CASRA test. Three test words are presented to the patient (upper), who then repeats them as they were heard (middle). The errors are then scored phonemically, as shown on the computer screen (lower). From Gelfand (1993), with permission.

Closed-Set Tests

Closed-set speech recognition tests have several advantages over the open-set approach. Closed-set testing reduces (1) the effects of word frequency in the language, (2) the effects of a patient's familiarity with the test words and alternative choices, and (3) learning effects. An added advantage of closed-set tests is that they can focus on particular aspects of speech recognition by carefully arranging the choices for each stimulus, so the clinician can analyze the patient's errors and confusions in some detail.

Perhaps the most well-known closed-set word recognition tests are the Modified Rhyme Test and the California Consonant Test. There are certainly many other closed-set word tests, although the fundamental features are illustrated by these two. The **Modified Rhyme Test (MRT)** (House, Williams, Hecker, & Kryter, 1955; Kreul Nixon, Kryter, Bell, Lang, & Schubert, 1968) presents the patient with six alternatives for each stimulus word. Twenty-five of the 50 test words have choices that differ by their initial consonants, such as

bent went sent tent dent rent.

The other 25 test items involve final consonant distinctions, such as

mass mad mat map man math.

Several variations of the MRT are also available, such as the *Rhyming Minimal Contrasts Test* (Griffiths, 1967) and the *Distinctive Feature Discrimination Test* (McPherson & Pang-Ching, 1979). The **California Consonant Test (CCT)** (Owens & Schubert, 1977) has two 100-item test forms. Four closed-set choices are provided for each of the 36 initial consonant test items, such as

pin kin tin thin,

and for each of the 64 final consonant items, for example,

path patch pack pat.

The student should also be aware of the **University of Oklahoma Closed Response Speech Test (UOCRST)** (Pederson & Studebaker, 1972), which adds a medial vowel subtest to the initial and final consonant subtests, and also uses several replications of each test item. These two characteristics can be very useful, and are atypical of most other real-word tests.

The **Speech Pattern Contrast (SPAC) test** (Boothroyd, 1984, 1988) provides information about the patient's ability to perceive phonologically relevant distinctions, that is, those that affect the meaning of what is being said. This kind of information has many uses in aural rehabilitation, and when assessing needs and progress with various sensory aids (such as hearing aids, cochlear implants, and tactile devices). The SPAC test uses a closed-set format in which the patient is presented with a test word (or phrase), which must then be identified from choices that are written or that appear on a computer screen. The alternatives are contrasting in terms of particular characteristics of speech. Eight segmental contrasts and two suprasegmental contrasts are examined on the SPAC test: vowel height ("fall"–"fool"), vowel place ("feel"–"fool"), initial consonant voicing ("tip"–"dip"), initial consonant continuance ("tip"–"sip"), final consonant voicing ("do"–"too"), final consonant continuance ("fate"–"face"), initial consonant place ("big"–"dig"), final consonant place ("bid"–"big"), stress ("THESE new clocks"–"these NEW clocks"), and pitch rise/fall ("That's yours."–"That's yours?"). Separate subtests allow two segmental contrasts to be tested at a time by giving four alternatives for each item. For example, the four choices for "tip" are

zip sip dip tip.

If the response is "sip," then an error would be counted for *continuance* because /t/ and /s/ differ for this characteristic; however, *voicing* would be counted as correct because both /t/ and /s/ are unvoiced. The suprasegmental contrast subtests give two choices for each item. Two subtests that do not involve phonologically significant contrasts are also available. These assess the ability to distinguish between male and female voices (talker sex) and natural versus monotonous speech (pitch range).

Nonsense-Syllable Tests

Nonsense-syllable tests use meaningless syllables rather than real words to evaluate a patient's ability to accurately perceive speech sounds. They are probably the most sensitive approach for examining the details of a patient's speech recognition difficulties, but they are also the most abstract and are not as generally accepted as real-word tests in routine clinical practice. The **City University of New York Nonsense Syllable Test (CUNY-NST)** (Resnick, Dubno, Hoffnung, & Levitt, 1976; Levitt, & Resnick, 1978) and the **Nonsense Syllable Test (NST)** (Edgerton & Danhauer, 1979) are two carefully developed and widely known tests of this type. The CUNY-NST is a closed-set test made up of seven subtests that include between seven and nine consonant-vowel (CV) or vowel-consonant (VC) nonsense syllables, as shown in Table 8–3 (as well a some optional subtests). All of the syllables on a given subtest are offered as choices for each other. Each subtest of the CUNY-NST is composed of the consonants most likely to be confused by hearing impaired patients. A **Modified CUNY Nonsense Syllable Test (MNST)** (Gelfand, Schwander, Levitt, Weiss, & Silman, 1992) is also available for situations where it is necessary to test for all possible confusions among 16 CV syllables and 21 VC syllables. In contrast to the CUNY-NST, the Edgerton-Danhauer NST is an open-set test in which the patient must identify 25 nonsense bisyllables, that is, meaningless consonant-vowel-consonant-vowel (CVCV) items such as /ʃeθɑ/ or /sɛfɛ/.

Sentence Tests

Speech recognition testing can also be accomplished by presenting the test material in the form of sentences, which makes it possible to look at the patient's speech recognition ability in a variety of ways. The most straightforward approach is to determine the percentage of correctly recognized **key words** in a sentence. Key words are those that must be received to understand the full meaning of a sentence. The **CID Everyday Sentences** (Silverman & Hirsh, 1955; Davis & Silverman, 1978) include a total of 10 test lists, each of which is made up of 10 sentences that vary in length from 2 to 12 words. A total of 50 key words are contained in each of the lists, and the patient's speech recognition score is the percentage of key words that are correctly repeated. The CID sentences are rarely used in routine speech audiometry because they are too easy for most patients. However, they are often included in the assessment of patients with profound sensorineural hearing losses. A carefully constructed and standardized modern approach of this type is the **Connected Speech Test (CST)** (Cox, Alexander, & Gilmore, 1987; Cox, Alexander, Gilmore, & Pusakulich, 1988, 1989), which is available in both audio and audiovisual formats. The CST includes a total of 48 passages dealing with a variety of familiar topics. Each passage is composed of 10 test sentences which contain 25 scorable key words.

The test items are the last words of sentences in the **Speech Perception in Noise (SPIN) test** (Kalikow, Stevens, & Elliott, 1977; Bilger, 1984; Bilger, Nuetzel, Rabinowitz, &

TABLE 8–3   The CUNY Nonsense Syllable Test

Subtest	Stimuli and Response Alternatives								
1	ɑf	ɑʃ	ɑt	ɑk	ɑs	ɑp	ɑθ		
2	uθ	up	us	uk	ut	uf	uʃ		
3	iʃ	if	it	ik	is	iθ	ip		
4	ɑb	ɑð	ɑd	ɑm	ɑz	ɑg	ɑn	ɑŋ	ɑv
5	fɑ	tɑ	pɑ	hɑ	θɑ	tʃɑ	sɑ	ʃɑ	kɑ
6	lɑ	bɑ	dɑ	gɑ	rɑ	jɑ	dʒɑ	wɑ	
7	nɑ	vɑ	mɑ	zɑ	gɑ	bɑ	ðɑ	dɑ	

Modified from Levitt and Resnick (1978) with permission of *Scandinavian Audiology.*

Rzeczkowski, 1984). The SPIN test uses two kinds of sentences. The test word at the end of a **probability-high (PH-SPIN)** sentence is somewhat predictable from the information provided by the body of the sentence, such as

We shipped the furniture by TRUCK.

On the other hand, the test words at the end of a **probability-low (PL-SPIN)** sentence cannot be predicted from the sentence, as in

Mary could not discuss the TACK.

Comparing a patient's performance on the PI-SPIN and PH-SPIN allows us to assess the patient's ability to make use of contextual cues. The revised SPIN test (Bilger, 1984) includes eight lists of 50 sentences each. Each list contains 25 PL-SPIN sentences and 25 PH-SPIN sentences. As its name suggests, the SPIN can be presented in quiet or against a background noise (a 12-talker babble) which is provided on a second channel of the test. The **Synthetic Sentence Identification (SSI) test** (Speaks & Jerger, 1965; Jerger, Speaks, & Trammell, 1968) uses a different approach to speech recognition assessment with sentences, and has a wide range of clinical applications. The SSI uses sentences that are third-order approximations to English, which means they are composed of words selected at random except that every three-word sequence must be syntactically correct. This idea can be understood by analyzing each three-word sequence in a typical SSI test sentence *Women view men with green paper should*:

> Women view men
>   view men with
>   men with green
>   with green paper
>   green paper should.

Notice how the sentence is grammatically correct even though its meaning is irrational.

The SSI test is administered in a closed-set format. Before the test starts, the patient is provided with a written list of 10 numbered SSI sentences. After each sentence is presented, the patient responds by indicating its number on the list. The SSI recordings are provided with the test sentences on one channel of the recording and a story being read by the same talker on the other channel. The story is used as a competing message. In actual use, the SSI sentences are presented while the competing message is simultaneously being directed into the opposite ear (SSI with contralateral competing message, **SSI-CCM**) or into the same ear (SSI with ipsilateral competing message, **SSI-ICM**).

Speech Recognition Tests for Profound Hearing Impairments

The **Minimal Auditory Capabilities (MAC) Battery** (Owens, Kessler, Telleen, & Schubert, 1981; Owens, Kessler, Raggio, & Schubert, 1985) is a collection of tests used to assess profoundly hearing impaired patients who typically obtain scores around zero on standard speech recognition tests. It was originally designed for postlingually deafened adults, but parts of the MAC battery have been used with children as well. The MAC is one of several test batteries that are typically used to evaluate patients' candidacy for cochlear implants and/or tactile aids (Chapter 15), as well as to assess their progress. Other batteries are also available (e.g., Tyler, Preece, & Lowder, 1983; Osberger, Miyamoto, Zimmerman-Phillips, Kemink, Stroer, Firszt, & Novak, 1991; Beiter & Brimacombe, 1993), and it is common practice to pick and choose among these to formulate the optimum mix of tests for a particular clinical population.

To get a flavor for the range of tests that are used to assess profoundly impaired patients, we will go through the 13 auditory tests in the revised MAC battery in their relative order of difficulty (easiest to hardest) as reported by Owens et al (1985), followed by its visual enhancement test, which involves lipreading. Notice that several of its components have already been discussed in other contexts.

1. On the **spondee same/different test** the patient is presented with 20 pairs of spondee words and must indicate whether the two words in each pair are the same or different.
2. The patient must identify a spondaic test word from four multiple-choice alterna-

tives on the **four-choice spondee test**. It includes 20 items. Unlike the former discrimination task, this is a closed-set recognition test.

3. The **noise/voice test** includes 40 items made up of four noises with different spectra and temporal-intensity envelopes (i.e., how intensity varies over time) and five sentences spoken by different male and female talkers. The patient's task is to determine whether each item is a noise or the human voice.

4. The **final consonants test** is a 52-item closed-set word recognition test. Each item involves presenting the patient with a monosyllabic word that must be identified from four alternatives that have different final consonants (e.g., "rid / rip / rib / ridge").

5. The **accent test** deals with the perception of prosody. In each of its 20 items, a four-word phrase is presented in which one of the words is stressed or accented (e.g., "can you FIX it?"). The patient must select it from among four closed-set alternatives.

6. The **everyday sounds test** is an open-set task in which the patient must identify 15 familiar sounds (a doorbell, people talking, etc.).

7. The **initial consonants test** is a 52-item closed-set test similar to the final consonants test except that the four choices for each word have different initial consonants (e.g., "din/bin/fin/gin").

8. The **question/statement test** is a prosody perception task in which the patient must identify each of 20 phrases as a question (rising inflection) or a statement (falling inflection).

9. The **vowels test** is a 60-item closed-set test similar to the consonants tests except that the four choices for each word have different medial vowels or diphthongs (e.g., "fool/full/fall/foul").

10. The **CID Everyday Sentences test** involves presenting four CID sentences lists as a 40-sentence open-set test with 200 scorable key words.

11. The **spondee recognition test** is an open-set test in which the patient is asked to repeat each of 25 spondaic words. (Half credit is given when one of the two syllables are correct.)

12. The **words in context test** uses 50 PH-SPIN sentences. The results were originally scored in the standard way (i.e., based on the last word). However, the recommended scoring method was changed so that a sentence is considered correct when all of its key words are repeated correctly, and wrong if they are missed. (A key word is considered to be right as long as its root is correctly identified.) Key words considered essential for understanding the sentence were identified by Owens et al (1985) because they are not part of the standard SPIN test. Two examples are "Hold the baby on your lap" and "The cushion was filled with foam."

13. The **monosyllabic words test** is a standard monosyllabic word recognition task using the NU-6 materials.

The **visual enhancement test** is the lipreading component of the MAC battery. It includes 20 CID Everyday Sentences (100 key words) that are presented visually only (unaided lipreading) and 20 other sentences (100 key words) that are presented by lipreading plus amplified sound (aided lipreading). Both aided and unaided lipreading are tested to ascertain whether the patient's lipreading performance is enhanced by the auditory cues.

Information about the patient's ability to recognize differences in the temporal or rhythmic patterns of speech is provided by the **monosyllable-trochee-spondee (MTS) test** (Erber & Alencewicz, 1976), which is frequently used along with the MAC or as part of other speech perception batteries for those with profound hearing impairments. The MTS test involves three categories of words that are distinguishable on the basis of the number of syllables and the stress pattern: (1) **monosyllables** (e.g., "bed"); (2) **spondees**, which have two syllables with equal emphasis on both of them (e.g., "baseball"); and (3) **trochees**, which have two syllables with unequal emphasis on the first syllable (e.g., "button"). In this test, a test word is presented to the patient, who responds by making a selection from a choice of alternative words.

The **Lexical Neighborhood Test (LNT)** and the **Multisyllabic Lexical Neighborhood Test (MLNT)** were developed to facilitate the assessment of children with profound hearing losses with cochlear implants (Kirk, Pisoni & Osberger, 1995; Kirk, 1999; Kirk, et al, 1999). Because many of these children have limited vocabularies, the words on these tests were chosen from those known to be familiar to 3- to 5-year-olds based on Logan's (1992) analysis of the Child Language Data Exchange System (CHILDS) database (MacWinney & Snow, 1985). The LNT includes 25 lexically hard monosyllabic words and 25 lexically easy monosyllabic words. (Recall that words with a high frequency of occurrence and few similar sounding alternatives are lexically easy,

whereas low-frequency words with many alternatives are lexically hard.) Instead of using monosyllabic words, the MLNT involves presenting 24 two- and three-syllable words. As with the LNT, half of the words on the MLNT are lexically hard and half are lexically easy. The two LNT and MLNT lists are shown in Appendices I and J.

The stimuli and responses can be tallied on a matrix like the one in Figure 8–11. Examining the relationships between the stimulus words and responses reveals whether the patient can correctly identify words with different levels of difficulty, and also whether she is able to take advantage of temporal and/or stress patterns in speech. Let us consider several kinds of responses on the MTS test. We might find that a patient who cannot identify monosyllables (the conventional speech recognition stimuli) may still be able to correctly identify

STIMULUS

		monosyllables				trochees				spondees			
		bed	cat	duck	pig	button	chicken	doctor	turtle	baseball	birdhouse	popcorn	toothpaste
R E S P O N S E	bed					7							
	cat		1										
	duck	4											
	pig												
	button						5						
	chicken											8	
	doctor							2					
	turtle												
	baseball												
	birdhouse									6			
	popcorn							9					
	toothpaste												3

FIGURE 8–11 The MTS test allows us to analyze confusions among and between monosyllabic, trochaic, and spondaic words. Responses 1, 2, and 3 are correct word identifications; 4, 5, and 6 indicate incorrect word recognition but correct identification of the temporal patterns (i.e., monosyllable for monosyllable, trochee for trochee, spondee for spondee); 7, 8, and 9 are examples of word recognition errors that also involve temporal pattern errors: In 7, two syllables are identified as only one; in 8, equally stressed syllables are identified as unequal; and in 9, unequally stressed syllables are identified as having similar stress. Adapted from Erber and Alencewicz (1976), with permission of American Speech-Language-Hearing Association.

less difficult material such as two-syllable words. Errors like pointing to "popcorn" in response to "baseball" (both spondees) suggests that the patient correctly identified the stress pattern even though the word itself was not heard correctly. On the other hand, pointing to "duck" (a monosyllable) or "birdhouse" (a spondee) in response to "turtle" (a trochee) shows that the patient also has difficulty identifying temporal or stress patterns. The fundamental approach of the MTS test has been modified and expanded in various ways, such as increasing the number of words tested in each category (Geers & Moog, 1992), and the addition of three-syllable words (Erber, 1982).

REFERENCES

Aleksandrovsky IV, McCullough JA, Wilson RH. 1998. Development of suprathreshold word recognition test for Russian-speaking patients. *Am J Audiol 9*, 417–425.

American National Standards Institute (ANSI). 1996. *American National Standard Specifications for Audiometers*. ANSI S3.6-1996. New York: ANSI.

American Speech-Language-Hearing Association (ASHA). 1979. Guidelines for determining the threshold level for speech. *ASHA 20*, 297–301.

American Speech-Language-Hearing Association (ASHA). 1988. Guidelines for determining threshold level for speech. *ASHA 30*, 85–89.

Antablin McCullough J, Cunningham, LA, Wilson RH. 1992. Auditory-visual word identification test materials: Computer application with children. *J Am Acad Audiol 3*, 208–214.

Aspinall KB. 1973. The effect of phonetic balance on discrimination for speech in subjects with sensorineural hearing loss. Unpublished doctoral dissertation. Boulder, CO: University of Colorado.

Beattie RC, Edgerton BJ, Svihovec DV. 1975. An investigation of Auditec of St. Louis recordings of Central Institute for the Deaf spondees. *J Am Aud Soc 1*, 97–101.

Beattie, RC, Forrester PW, Ruby BK. 1976. Reliability of the Tillman-Olsen procedure for determination of spondee threshold using recorded and live voice presentations. *J Am Aud Soc 2*, 159–162.

Beattie, RC, Svihovec DV, Edgerton BJ. 1975. Relative intelligibility of the CID spondees as presented via monitored live voice. *J Speech Hear Dis 40*, 84–91.

Beiter AL, Brimacombe JA. 1993. Cochlear implants. In Alpiner JG, McCarthy PA (Eds.): *Rehabilitative Audiology in Children and Adults*, 2nd ed. Baltimore: Williams & Wilkins, 417–440.

Bess FH. 1983. Clinical assessment of speech recognition. In Konkle DF, Rintelmann WF (Eds.): *Principles of Speech Audiometry*. Baltimore: University Park Press, 127–201.

Bess FH, Josey AF, Humes LE. 1979. Performance intensity functions in cochlear and eighth nerve disorders. *Am J Otolaryngol 1*, 27–31.

Bilger RC. 1984. Speech recognition test development. In Elkins E. (Ed.): Speech Recognition by the Hearing Impaired. *ASHA Reports 14*, 2–15.

Bilger RC, Matthies ML, Meyer TA, Griffiths SK. 1998. Psychometric equivalence of recorded spondee words as test items. *J Speech Lang Hear Res 41*, 516–526.

Bilger RC, Nuetzel JM, Rabinowitz WM, Rzeczkowski C. 1984. Standardization of a test of speech perception in noise. *J Speech Hear Res 27*, 32–48.

Boothroyd A. 1968a. Developments in speech audiometry. *Sound 2*, 3–10.

Boothroyd A. 1968b. Statistical theory of the speech discrimination score. *J Acoust Soc Am 43*, 362–367.

Boothroyd A. 1970. Developmental factors in speech recognition. *Int Audiol 9*, 30–38.

Boothroyd A. 1984. Auditory perception of speech contrasts by subjects with sensorineural hearing loss. *J Speech Hear Res 27*, 134–144.

Boothroyd A. 1988. Perception of speech pattern contrasts from auditory presentation of voice fundamental frequency. *Ear Hear 9*, 313–321.

Boothroyd A. 1999. *Computer-Assisted Speech Perception Assessment (CASPA 2.2)*. San Diego: Arthur Boothroyd.

Boothroyd A, Nittrouer S. 1988. Mathematical treatment of context effects in phoneme and word recognition. *J Acoust Soc Am 84*, 101–114.

Brandy WT. 1966. Reliability of voice tests in speech discrimination. *J Speech Hear Res 9*, 461–465.

Cakiroglu S, Danhauer JL. 1992. Effects of listeners' and talkers' linguistic backgrounds on W-22 performance. *J Am Acad Audiol 3*, 186–192.

Cambron NK, Wilson RH, Shanks JE. 1991. Spondaic word detection and recognition functions for female and male speakers. *Ear Hear 12*, 64–70.

Carhart R. 1946a. Speech reception in relation to pattern of pure tone loss. *J Speech Hear Dis 11*, 97–108.

Carhart R. 1946b. Monitored live voice as a test of auditory acuity. *J Acoust Soc Am 17*, 339–349.

Carhart R. 1970. Discussion, questions, answers, comments. In Rojskjer C. (Ed.): *Speech Audiometry*. Denmark: Second Danavox Symposium, 229.

Carhart R. 1971. Observations on relations between thresholds for pure tones and for speech. *J Speech Hear Dis 36*, 476–483.

Carhart R, Porter LS. 1971. Audiometric configuration and prediction of threshold for spondees. *J Speech Hear Res 14*, 486–495.

Chaiklin JB. 1959. The relation among three selected auditory speech thresholds. *J Speech Hear Res 2*, 237–243.

Chaiklin JB, Font J, Dixon RF. 1967. Spondaic thresholds measured in ascending 5 dB steps. *J Speech Hear Res 10*, 141–145.

Chaiklin JB, Ventry IM. 1964. Spondee threshold measurement: A comparison of 2- and 5-dB steps. *J Speech Hear Dis 29*, 47–59.

Clemis J, Carver W. 1967. Discrimination scores for speech in Meniere's disease. *Arch Otolaryngol 86*, 614–618.

Cokely JA, Yager CR. 1993. Scoring Spanish word-recognition measures. *Ear Hear 14*, 395–400.

Comstock CL, Martin FN 1984. A children's Spanish word discrimination test for non-Spanish-speaking clinicians. *Ear Hear 5*, 166–170.

Conn M, Dancer J, Ventry IM. 1975. A spondee list for determining speech reception threshold without prior familiarization. *J Speech Hear Dis 40*, 388–396.

Cox RM, Alexander GC, Gilmore C. 1987. Development of the Connected Speech Test (CST). *Ear Hear 8* (suppl), 119S–126S.

Cox RM, Alexander GC, Gilmore C, Pusakulich KM. 1988. Use of the Connected Speech Test (CST) with hearing-impaired listeners. *Ear Hear* 9, 198–207.

Cox RM, Alexander GC, Gilmore C, Pusakulich KM. 1989. The Connected Speech Test version 3: Audiovisual administration. *Ear Hear* 10, 29–32.

Creston JE, Gillespie M, Krahn C. 1966. Speech Audiometry: Taped vs. live voice. *Arch Otolaryngol* 83, 14–17.

Danhauer JL, Crawford S, Edgerton BJ. 1984. English, Spanish and bilingual speakers' performance on a nonsense syllable test (NST) of speech sound discrimination. *J Speech Hear Dis* 49, 164–168.

Davis H, Silverman SR. 1978. *Hearing and Deafness*, 4th ed. New York: Holt, Rinehart & Winston.

Department of Veterans Affairs. 1998. *Speech Recognition and Identification Materials (disc 2.0)*. Mountain Home, TN: VA Medical Center.

Dewey, G. 1923. *Relative Frequency of English Speech Sounds*. Cambridge, MA: Harvard University Press.

Dirks DD, Kamm C, Bower D, Betsworth A. 1977. Use of performance-intensity functions for diagnosis. *J Speech Hear Dis* 42, 408–415.

Dirks DD, Morgan DE. 1983. Measures of discomfort and most comfortable loudness. In Konkle DF Rintelmann WF (Eds.): *Principles of Speech Audiometry*. Baltimore: University Park Press, 203–229.

Dubno JR, Lee F-S, Klein AJ, Matthews LJ, Lam CF. 1995. Confidence limits for maximum word-recognition scores. *J Speech Hear Res* 38, 490–502.

Duffy JK. 1983. The role of phoneme-recognition audiometry in aural rehabilitation. *Hear J* 37, 24–28.

Edgerton BJ, Danhauer JL. 1979. *Clinical Implications of Speech Discrimination Testing Using Nonsense Stimuli*. Baltimore: University Park Press.

Egan J. 1948. Articulation testing methods. *Laryngoscope* 58, 955–991.

Erber NP. 1982. *Auditory Training*. Washington, DC: AG Bell Association for the Deaf.

Erber NP, Alencewicz CM. 1976. Audiologic evaluation of deaf children. *J Speech Hear Dis* 41, 256–267.

Fletcher H. 1929. *Speech and Hearing in Communication*. Princeton: Van Nostrand Reinhold.

Fletcher H. 1950. A method for calculating hearing loss for speech from an audiogram. *J Acoust Soc Am* 22, 1–5.

Frank T. 1980. Clinical significance of the relative intelligibility of pictorally represented spondee words. *Ear Hear* 1, 46–49.

French NR, Carter CW Jr, Koenig W Jr. 1930. The words and sounds of telephone conversations. *Bell System Tech J* 9, 290–324.

Gang RP. 1976. The effects of age on the diagnostic utility of the rollover phenomenon. *J Speech Hear Dis* 41, 63–69.

Gardner HJ. 1971. Application of a high-frequency consonant discrimination word list in hearing-aid evaluation. *J Speech Hear Dis* 36, 354–355.

Gardner HJ. 1987. High frequency consonant word lists. *Hear Instr* 38, 28–29.

Gat IB, Keith RW. 1978. An effect of linguistic experience: Auditory discrimination by native and non-native speakers of English. *Audiology* 17, 339–345.

Gates GA, Cooper JC, Kannel WB, Miller NJ. 1990. Hearing in the elderly: The Framingham cohort, 1983–1985. Part I. Basic audiometric results. *Ear Hear* 15, 71–81.

Geers AE, Moog JS. 1992. Speech perception and production skills of students with impaired hearing from oral and total communication education settings. *J Speech Hear Res* 35, 1382–1393.

Gelfand SA. 1975. Use of the carrier phrase in live voice speech discrimination testing. *J Aud Res* 15, 107–110.

Gelfand SA. 1993. A clinical speech recognition method to optimize reliability and efficiency. Paper presented at Convention of American Academy of Audiology, Phoenix.

Gelfand SA. 1998. Optimizing the reliability of speech recognition scores. *J Speech Lang Hear Res* 41, 1088–1102.

Gelfand SA, Ross L, Miller S. 1988. Sentence reception in noise from one versus two sources: Effects of aging and hearing loss. *J Acoust Soc Am* 83, 248–256.

Gelfand SA, Schwander T, Levitt H, Weiss M, Silman S. 1992. Speech recognition performance on a modified nonsense syllable test. *J Rehabil Res Dev* 29, 53–60.

Gelfand SA, Silman S. 1985. Functional hearing loss and its relationship to resolved hearing levels. *Ear Hear* 6, 151–158.

Gelfand SA, Silman S. 1993. Relationship of exaggerated and resolved hearing levels in unilateral functional hearing loss. *Br J Audiol* 27, 29–34.

Gengel R, Kupperman GL. 1980. Word discrimination in noise: Effect of different speakers. *Ear Hear* 1, 156–160.

Gladstone VS, Siegenthaler BM. 1971. Carrier phrase and speech intelligibility score. *J Aud Res* 11, 101–103.

Griffiths JD. 1967. Rhyming minimal contrasts: A simplified diagnostic articulation test. *J Acoust Soc Am* 42, 236–241.

Groen JJ, Helleman AC. 1960. Binaural speech audiometry. *Acta Otolaryngol* 52, 397–314.

Hagerman B. 1976. Reliability in the determination of speech discrimination. *Scand Audiol* 5, 219–228.

Hagerman B. 1982. Sentences for testing speech intelligibility in noise. *Scand Audiol* 11, 79–87.

Heckendorf AL, Wiley TL, Wilson RH. 1997. Performance norms for the VA compact disc versions of CID W-22 (Hirsh) and PB-50 (Rush Hughes) word lists. *J Am Acad Audiol* 8, 163–172.

Hirsh IJ, Davis H, Silverman SR, Reynolds EG, Eldert E, Benson RW. 1952. Development of materials for speech audiometry. *J Speech Hear Dis* 17, 321–337.

Hood JD, Poole JP. 1980. Influence of the speaker and other factors affecting speech intelligibility. *Audiology* 19, 434–455.

House AS, Williams CE, Hecker MHL, Kryter KD. 1955. Articulation-testing methods: Consonantal differentiation with a closed-response set. *J Acoust Soc Am* 37, 158–166.

Hudgins CV, Hawkins JE Jr, Karlin JE, Stevens SS. 1947. The development of recorded auditory tests for measuring hearing loss for speech. *Laryngoscope* 57, 57–89.

Huff SJ, Nerbonne MA. 1982. Comparison of the American Speech-Language-Hearing Association and the revised Tillman-Olsen methods for speech threshold measurement. *Ear Hear* 3, 335–339.

Jahner JA, Schlauch RA, Doyle T. 1994. A comparison of American Speech-Language-Hearing Association guidelines for obtaining speech-recognition thresholds. *Ear Hear* 15, 324–329.

Jerger J, Jerger S. 1971. Diagnostic significance of PB word functions. *Arch Otolaryngol* 93, 573–580.

Jerger J, Jerger S. 1976. Comments on "The effects of age on the diagnostic utility of the rollover phenomenon." *J Speech Hear Dis* 41, 556–557.

Jerger J, Speaks C, Trammell J. 1968. A new approach to speech audiometry. *J Speech Hear Dis* 33, 318–328.

Johnson EW. 1977. Auditory test results in 500 cases of acoustic neuroma. *Arch Otolaryngol* 103, 152–158.

Kalikow DN, Stevens, KN, Elliott LL. 1977. Development of a test of speech intelligibility in noise using sentence materials with controlled word predictability. *J Acoust Soc Am* 61, 1337–1351.

Kirk KI. 1999. Assessing speech perception in listeners with cochlear implants: The development of the Lexical Neighborhood Test. *Volta Rev* 100, 63–85.

Kirk KI, Eisenberg LS, Martinez AS, Hay-McCutcheon. 1999. Lexical Neighborhood Test: Test-retest reliability and interlist equivalency. *J Am Acad Audiol* 10, 113–123.

Kirk KI, Pisoni DB, Osberger MJ. 1995. Lexical effects on spoken word recognition by pediatric cochlear implant users. *Ear Hear* 16, 470–481.

Koike KJM. 1993. Verifying speech amplification with low-mid-high frequency words. *Hear Instr* 44, 11–13.

Koike KJM, Brown B, Hobbs H, Asp C. 1989. New generation speech discrimination test: Tennessee Tonality Test. *Proc 6th Conf Rehab Eng* 11, 324–326.

Kreul EJ, Bell DW, Nixon JC. 1969. Factors affecting speech discrimination test difficulty. *J Speech Hear Res* 12, 281–287.

Kreul EJ, Nixon JC, Kryter KD, Bell DW, Lang JS, Schubert ED. 1968. A proposed clinical test of speech discrimination. *J Speech Hear Res* 11, 536–552.

Lehiste I, Peterson GE. 1959. Linguistic considerations in the study of speech intelligibility. *J Acoust Soc Am* 31, 280–286.

Levitt H, Resnick SB. 1978. Speech reception by the hearing impaired. *Scand Audiol* (suppl 6), 107–130.

Logan JS. 1992. *A Computational Analysis of Children's Lexicons*. (Research on Speech Perception Technical Report 8). Bloomington, IN: Indiana University.

Luce PA. 1990. *Neighborhoods of Words in the Mental Lexicon*. (Research on Speech Perception Technical Report 6). Bloomington, IN: Indiana University.

Luce PA, Pisoni DB. 1998. Recognizing spoken words: The neighborhood activation model. *Ear Hear* 19, 1–36.

MacWinney B, Snow C. 1985. The child language data exchange system. *J Child Lang* 12 271–296.

Markides A. 1978. Whole-word scoring versus phoneme scoring in speech audiometry. *Br J Audiol* 12, 40–46.

Maroonroge S, Diefendorf AO. 1984. Comparing normal hearing and hearing-impaired subjects' performance on the Northwestern Auditory Test Number 6, California Consonant Test, and Pascoe's High-Frequency Word Test. *Ear Hear* 5, 356–360.

Martin FN, Champlin, CA, Chambers JA. 1998. Seventh survey of audiological practices in the United States. *J Am Acad Audiol* 9, 95–104.

Martin FN, Hawkins RR, Bailey HA. 1962. The nonessentiality of the carrier phrase in phonetically balanced (PB) word testing. *J Aud Res* 2, 319–322

Martin FN, Stauffer ML. 1975. A modification of the Tillman-Olsen method for obtaining speech reception threshold. *J Speech Hear Dis* 40, 25–28.

McCullough JA, Wilson RH, Birck JD, Anderson LG. 1994. A multimedia approach for estimating speech recognition of multilingual clients. *Am J Audiol* 3, 19–22.

McLennan RO, Knox AW. 1975. Patient-controlled delivery of monosyllabic words in a test of auditory discrimination. *J Speech Hear Dis* 40, 538–543.

McPherson DF, Pang-Ching GK. 1979. Development of a distinctive feature discrimination test. *J Aud Res* 19, 235–246.

Meyer DH, Mishler ET. 1985. Rollover measurements with Auditec NU-6 word lists. *J Speech Hear Dis* 50, 356–360.

Meyer TA, Bilger RC. 1997. Effect of set size and method on speech reception thresholds in noise. *Ear Hear* 18, 202–209.

Nilsson M, Soli SD, Sullivan JA. 1994. Development of the Hearing In Noise Test for the measurement of speech reception thresholds in quiet and in noise. *J Acoust Soc Am* 95, 1085–1099.

Nittrouer S, Boothroyd A. 1990. Context effects in phoneme and word recognition of children and older adults. *J Acoust Soc Am* 87, 2705–2715.

Olsen WO, Matkin ND. 1991. Speech audiometry. In Rintelmann WF. (Ed.): *Hearing Assessment*, 2nd ed. Austin: Pro-Ed, 39–140.

Olsen WO, Noffsinger D, Kurdziel S. 1975. Speech discrimination in quiet and in white noise by patients with peripheral and central lesions. *Acta Otolaryngol* 80, 375–382.

Olsen WO, Van Tasell DJ, Speaks CE. 1997. Phoneme and word recognition for words in isolation and in sentences. *Ear Hear* 18, 175–188.

Osberger MJ, Miyamoto RT, Zimmerman-Phillips S, Kemink JL, Stroer BS, Firszt JB, Novak MA. 1991. Independent evaluation of the speech perception abilities of children with the Nucleus 22-channel cochlear implant system. *Ear Hear* 12, 66S–80S.

Owens E. 1961a. Development of the California Consonant Test. *J Speech Hear Res* 20, 463–474.

Owens E. 1961b. Intelligibility of words varying in familiarity. *J Speech Hear Res* 4, 113–129.

Owens E, Kessler DK, Raggio MW, Schubert ED. 1985. Intelligibility of words varying in familiarity. *Ear Hear* 4, 113–129.

Owens E, Kessler DK, Telleen CC, Schubert ED. 1981. The minimum auditory capabilities (MAC) battery. *Hear Aid J* 34, 9, 10, 32, 34.

Owens E, Schubert ED. 1977. Development of the California Consonant Test. *J Speech Hear Res* 20, 463–474.

Pascoe DR. 1975. Frequency responses of hearing aids and their effect on the speech perception of hearing impaired subjects. *Ann Otol Rhinol Laryngol* 23 (suppl), 1–40.

Pederson OT, Studebaker GA. 1972. A new minimal-contrasts closed-response-set speech test. *J Aud Res* 12, 187–195.

Penrod J. 1979. Talker effects on word discrimination scores of adults with sensorineural hearing impairment. *J Speech Hear Dis* 44, 340–349.

Peterson GE, Lehiste I. 1962. Revised CNC lists for auditory tests. *J Speech Hear Dis* 27, 62–70.

Picheny M, Durlach N, Braida L. 1985. Speaking clearly for the hard of hearing: I. Intelligibility differences between clear and conversational speech. *J Speech Hear Res* 28, 96–103.

Plomp R, Mimpin AM. 1979. Improving the reliability of testing the speech reception threshold for sentences. *Audiology* 18, 43–52.

Pollack I, Rubenstein H, Decker L. 1959. Intelligibility of known and unknown message sets. *J Acoust Soc Am* 31, 273–279.

Posner J, Ventry IJ. 1977. Relationships between comfortable loudness levels for speech and speech discrimination in sensorineural hearing loss. *J Speech Hear Dis* 42, 370–375.

Punch JL, Howard MT. 1985. Spondee recognition as a function of set size. *J Speech Hear Dis* 50, 120–125.

Raffin MJM, Schafer D. 1980. Application of a probability model based on the binomial distribution to speech discrimination scores. *J Speech Hear Res* 23, 570–575.

Raffin MJM, Thornton A. 1980. Confidence levels for differences between speech discrimination scores. *J Speech Hear Res* 23, 5–18.

Resnick SB, Dubno JR, Hoffnung S, Levitt H. 1976. Phoneme errors on a nonsense syllable test. *J Acoust Soc Am* 58 (suppl 1), 114.

Runge CA, Hosford-Dunn H. (1985). Word-recognition performance with modified CID W-22 word lists. *J Speech Hear Res* 28, 355–362.

Shirinian MJ, Arnst DJ. 1980. PI-PB rollover in a group of aged listeners. *Ear Hear* 1, 50–53.

Silman S, Silverman CA. 1991. *Auditory Diagnosis: Principles and Applications*. San Diego: Academic Press.

Silverman SR, Hirsh IJ. 1955. Problems related to the use of speech in clinical audiometry. *Ann Otol Rhinol Laryngol* 64, 1234–1244.

Smoorenburg GF. 1992. Speech reception in quiet and in noisy conditions by individuals with noise-induced hearing loss in relation to their tone audiogram. *J Acoust Soc Am* 91, 421–437.

Speaks C, Jerger J. 1965. Method for measurement of speech identification. *J Speech Hear Res* 8, 185–194.

Spearman C. 1908. The method of "right and wrong cases" ("constant stimuli") without Guass's formulae. *Br J Psych* 2, 227–242.

Spitzer JB. 1980. The development of a picture speech recognition threshold test in Spanish for use with urban U.S. residents of Hispanic background. *J Commun Dis* 13, 147–151.

Stoppenbach DT, Craig JM, Wiley TL, Wilson RH. 1999. Word recognition performance for Northwestern University Auditory Test No. 6 word lists in quiet and in competing message. *J Am Acad Audiol* 10, 429–435.

Thorndike DL. 1932. *A Teacher's Word Book of Twenty Thousand Words Found Most Frequently and Widely in General Reading for Children and Young People*. New York: Columbia University Press.

Thorndike DL, Lorge I. 1944. *The Teacher's Word Book of 30,000 Words*. New York: Columbia University Press.

Thornton A, Raffin MJM. 1978. Speech discrimination scores modeled as a binomial variable. *J Speech Hear Res* 21, 507–518.

Thurlow WR, Silverman SR, Davis H, Walsh TE. 1948. A statistical study of auditory tests in relation to the fenestration operation. *Laryngoscope* 58, 43–66.

Tillman TW, Carhart R. 1966. *An Expanded Test for Speech Discrimination Utilizing CNC Monosyllabic Words*. Northwestern University Auditory Test No. 6. Technical report SAM-TR-66-55. Brooks AFB, TX: USAF School of Aerospace Medicine.

Tillman TW, Carhart R, Wilber L. 1963. *A Test for Speech Discrimination Composed of CNC Monosyllabic Words*. Northwestern University Auditory Test No. 4. Technical Report SAM-TDR-62-135 Brooks AFB, TX: USAF School of Aerospace Medicine.

Tillman TW, Jerger JF. 1959. Some factors affecting the spondee threshold in normal-hearing subjects. *J Speech Hear Res* 2, 141–146.

Tillman TW, Olsen WO. 1973. Speech audiometry. In Jerger J. (Ed.): *Modern Developments in Audiology*, 2nd ed. New York: Academic Press, 37–74.

Tobias JV. 1964. On phonemic analysis of speech discrimination tests. *J Speech Hear Res* 7, 98–100.

Tyler RS, Preece JP, Lowder MW. 1983. The Iowa Cochlear-Implant Test Battery. Iowa City: Department of Otolaryngology–Head and Neck Surgery, University of Iowa.

Ullrich K, Grimm D. 1976. Most comfortable listening level presentation versus maximum discrimination for word discrimination material. *Audiology* 15, 338–347.

Versfeld NJ, Daalder L, Festen JM, Houtgast T. 2000. Method for the selection of sentence materials for efficient measurement of the speech reception threshold. *J Acoust Soc Am* 107, 1671–1684.

Wall LG, Davis LA, Myers DK. 1984. Four spondee threshold procedures: A comparison. *Ear Hear* 5, 171–174.

Weisleder P, Hodgson WR. 1989. Evaluation of four Spanish word-recognition-ability lists. *Ear Hear* 10, 387–392.

Wiley TL, Stoppenbach, DT, Feldhake LJ, Moss KA, Thordardottir ET. 1995. Audiologic practices: What is popular versus what is supported by evidence. *Am J Audiol* 4, 26–34.

Wilson RH, Antablin J. 1980. A picture identification task as an estimate of the word-recognition performance of non-verbal adults. *J Speech Hear Dis* 45, 223–237.

Wilson RH, Morgan DE, Dirks DD. 1973. A proposed SRT procedure and its statistical precedent. *J Speech Hear Dis* 38, 184–191.

Wilson RH, Oyler AL. 1997. Psychometric functions for the CID W-22 and NU Auditory Test No. 6 materials spoken by the same speaker. *Ear Hear* 18, 430–433.

Wilson RH, Strouse A. 1999. Psychometrically equivalent spondaic words spoken by a female speaker. *J Speech Lang Hear Res* 42, 1336–1346.

Yellin MW, Jerger J, Fifer RC. 1989. Norms for disproportionate loss in speech intelligibility. *Ear Hear* 10, 231–234.

Young LL, Dudley B, Gunter MB. 1982. Thresholds and psychometric functions of individual spondaic words. *J Speech Hear Res* 25, 586–593.

Clinical Masking

It seems reasonable to assume that sounds presented to the right ear are heard by the right ear, and that sounds presented to the left ear are heard by the left ear. However, this is not necessarily true. In fact, it is common to find that the sound being presented to one ear is actually being heard by the opposite ear. This phenomenon is called **cross-hearing** or **shadow hearing**. To avoid confusion it is customary to call the ear currently being tested the **test ear (TE)**, and to call the opposite ear, which is the one not being tested, the **nontest ear (NTE)**. Cross-hearing results in a false picture of the patient's hearing. Even the possibility that the sounds being presented to the TE are really being heard by the NTE causes the outcome of a test to be suspect, at best. This chapter explains why this situation occurs, how it is recognized, and the manner in which the NTE is removed from the test.

Cross-Hearing and Interaural Attenuation

Suppose we know for a fact that a patient's right ear is essentially normal and that his left ear is completely deaf. We would expect the audiogram to show air- and bone-conduction thresholds of perhaps 0 dB HL to 10 dB HL for the right ear and "no response" symbols for both air-conduction and bone-conduction at the maximum testable levels for the left ear, as in Figure 9–1a. However, this does not occur. Instead, the actual audiogram will be more like the one shown in Figure 9–1b. Here the thresholds for the right ear are just as expected. On the other hand, the left air-con-

duction thresholds are in the 55 to 60 dB HL range, and the left bone-conduction thresholds are the same as for the right ear. How can this be if the left ear is deaf?

Cross-Hearing for Air-Conduction

Let us first address this question for the air-conduction signals. Since the patient cannot hear anything in the left ear, the level of an air-conduction test tone presented to that ear will be raised higher and higher. Eventually, the tone presented to the deaf ear will be raised so high that it can actually be heard in the opposite ear, at which point the patient will finally respond. The patient's response to the signal directed to his deaf ear (the TE) is the result of hearing that signal in the other ear (the NTE). Thus, the left ear's threshold curve in Figure 9–1b is due to cross-hearing, and is often called a **shadow curve**.

For the tone to be heard in the NTE, it must be possible for a signal presented to one ear to be transmitted across the head to the other ear. This phenomenon is called **signal crossover**. The intensity of the sound reaching the NTE is less than what was originally presented to the TE because it takes a certain amount of energy to transmit the signal across the head. The number of dB that are "lost" in the process of signal crossover is called **interaural attenuation (IA)** (Chaiklin, 1967).

In Figure 9–1b, the patient's right air-conduction threshold at 1000 Hz is 10 dB HL. Even though his *left* ear is completely deaf, he also responded to a 1000 Hz tone presented from the *left* earphone at 60 dB HL. This means that the 60 dB HL tone presented

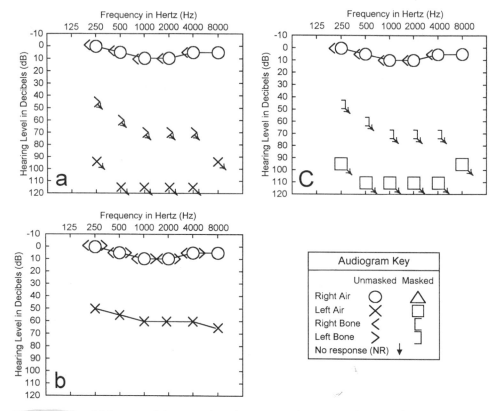

FIGURE 9–1   (a) Imagined (incorrect) audiogram without cross-hearing for a patient who is deaf in the left ear, showing "no response" for air-conduction or bone-conduction signals. (b) Actual audiogram for such a patient, reflecting the fact that the signals presented to the left side were heard in the right ear by cross-hearing. (c) Audiogram obtained when the left thresholds are retested with masking noise in the right ear.

to the left ear must have reached a level of 10 dB HL in the *right* ear. Consequently, IA at 1000 Hz in this case must be 50 dB (60 dB – 10 dB = 50 dB). Similarly, the amount of IA at 4000 Hz in this case is 55 dB (60 dB – 5 dB = 55 dB)

Crossover occurs when the signal is *physically present* in the opposite ear, whereas cross-hearing occurs only when it is *audible*. The distinction is clarified using the following example based on our hypothetical patient: The level of the 1000-Hz tone reaching this person's right (nontest) ear will always be 50 dB less than the amount presented from the left earphone due to IA. Consider three cases:

dB HL at Left Earphone	– IA	= dB HL Present at Right Cochlea
(a) 60 dB	– 50 dB	= 10 dB (at threshold)
(b) 80 dB	– 50 dB	= 30 dB (20 dB SL)
(c) 55 dB	– 50 dB	= 5 dB (5 dB below threshold)

These three examples are shown graphically in Figure 9–2. In (a) the tone reaches the right ear at 10 dB HL, and is heard because this is the right ear's threshold. In (b) the tone reaches the right ear at 30 dB HL and is heard because this level is 20 dB above the right ear's threshold (20 dB SL). In both of these cases signal crossover resulted in cross-

RIGHT EAR

LEFT EAR

(a)

50 dB
IA

60

10

Bone

Air

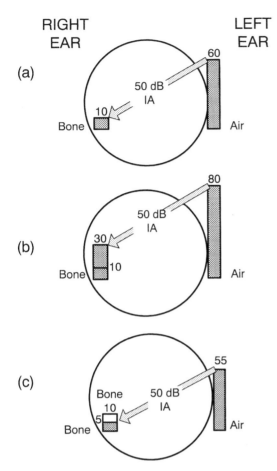

(b)

50 dB
IA

80

30

10

Bone

Air

(c)

Bone   50 dB
10   IA

55

5

Bone

Air

FIGURE 9–2 Three crossover conditions (see text).

hearing. However, the tone in (c) reaches the right ear at only 5 dB HL, which is 5 dB *below* threshold and is thus inaudible. Here, there is crossover because the signal is present in the NTE but there is no cross-hearing because it is below threshold.

Assuming the bone-conduction threshold remained at 10 dB HL, how would cross-hearing be affected if the IA was changed from 50 dB to another value, such as 40 dB or 60 dB? Some time with paper and pencil will reveal that the cross-hearing situation would change considerably.

Cross-Hearing for Bone-Conduction

The right and left bone-conduction thresholds are the same in Figure 9–1b even though

the right ear is normal and the left one is deaf. The implication is that the bone-conduction signal presented to the left side of the head is being received by the right ear. This should come as no surprise, since we found in Chapter 5 that a bone-conduction vibrator stimulates both cochleae about equally. From the cross-hearing standpoint, we may say that there is no interaural attenuation (IA = 0 dB) for bone-conduction. Thus, the right and left bone-conduction signals result in the same thresholds because they are both stimulating the same (right) ear.

Overcoming Cross-Hearing with Masking Noise

The above example demonstrates that there are times when the NTE is (or at least may be) responding to the signals intended for the TE. How can we stop the NTE from hearing the tones being presented to the TE? First, consider an analogy from vision testing. Looking at an eye chart with two eyes is akin to the cross-hearing issue. We all know from common experience that to test one eye at a time the optometrist simply blindfolds the nontest eye. In other words, one eye is tested while the other eye is **masked**. In effect, we do the same thing in audiology, except that the auditory "blindfold" is a noise that is directed into the NTE. The noise in the NTE stops it from hearing the sounds being presented to the TE. Just as the nontest eye is masked by the blindfold, so is the nontest ear masked by the noise.

Returning to our example, Figure 9–1c shows the results obtained when the air- and bone-conduction thresholds of the left (test) ear are retested with appropriate masking noise in the right (nontest) ear. The thresholds here are shown by different symbols than the ones in frames (a) and (b), to distinguish them as *masked* results. Because the left ear in this example is completely deaf, the masked thresholds have downward-pointing arrows indicating no response at the maximum limits of the audiometer. Notice that the **masked results** in frame (c) are at the same hearing levels as the ones in frame (a).

The important difference is that the **un-masked thresholds** in frame (a) could never have actually occurred because of cross-hearing. Note the dramatic difference between the unmasked results in frame (b) and the patient's real hearing status revealed by the masked thresholds in frame (c).

We see that when cross-hearing occurs it is necessary to retest the TE while directing a masking noise into the NTE. The purpose of the masking noise is to prevent the NTE from hearing the tone (or other signal) intended for the TE. Thus, the issue of whether cross-hearing might be occurring is tantamount to the question, Is masking (of the NTE) necessary?

Principal Mechanism of Crossover

Signal crossover (and therefore cross-hearing) for bone-conduction signals obviously occurs via a bone-conduction route, as depicted in Figure 9–3a. It occurs because a bone-conduction signal is transmitted to both cochleas.

Because crossover for air-conduction requires a reasonably substantial signal to be produced by the earphone (recall that interaural attenuation was about 50 dB in the prior example), common sense seems to suggest that air-conduction signals might reach the opposite ear by an air-conduction route. This might occur by sound escaping through the earphone cushion on the test side, traveling around the head, and then penetrating the earphone cushion on the nontest side. Alternatively, earphone vibration on the test side might be transmitted via the headset to the earphone on the nontest side. In either of these two scenarios, the signal from the test side would enter the ear canal of the NTE, that is, as an air-conduction signal. As compelling as these explanations may seem, they are not correct It has been shown repeatedly that the actual crossover route for air-conduction signals occurs principally by *bone-conduction* to the cochlea of the opposite ear (Sparrevohn, 1946; Zwislocki, 1953; Studebaker, 1962), as depicted in Figure 9–3b.

Interaural Attenuation for Air-Conduction

Cross-hearing of a test signal renders a test invalid. We must therefore identify cross-hearing whenever it occurs so that we can mask the NTE. The cost of failing to do so is so great that we want to employ masking every time that cross-hearing is even possible. Once we have obtained the unmasked audiogram, we are left with the following question: Is the air-conduction signal being

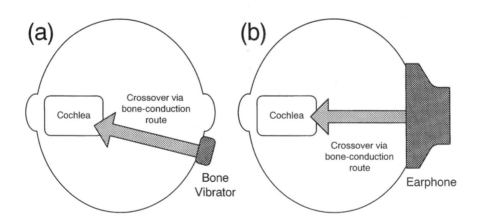

FIGURE 9–3 Signal crossover and cross-hearing occur via the bone-conduction route to the opposite cochlea, as indicated by the arrows for both (a) bone-conduction and (b) air-conduction.

presented to the TE great enough to cross the head and reach the bone-conduction threshold of the NTE? In other words, is this difference greater than the value of interaural attenuation? The corollary problem is to determine the IA value.

Interaural attenuation for air-conduction using supraaural earphones typical of the type used in audiological practice has been studied using a variety of approaches (Littler, Knight, & Strange, 1952; Zwislocki, 1953; Liden, 1954; Liden, Nilsson, & Anderson, 1959a; Chaiklin, 1967; Coles & Priede, 1970; Snyder, 1973; Smith & Markides, 1981; Sklare & Denenberg, 1987). Figure 9–4 shows the mean AI values found in four of these studies, as well as the maximum and minimum amounts of AI obtained across all four studies. Average IA values are about 50 to 65 dB, and there is a general tendency for IA to become larger with frequency. The range of IA values is very wide, and the means are much larger than the minimum IA values. Consequently, we cannot rely on average IA values as a red flag for cross-hearing in clinical practice because many cases of cross-hearing would be missed in many patients on the lower side of the IA range. For this reason it is common practice to use *minimum*

IA values to identify possible cross-hearing, that is, to decide when masking may be needed. As anticipated from the figure, the minimum IA value typically suggested to rule out crossover for clinical purposes is **40 dB** (Studebaker, 1967; Martin, 1974, 1980).

INTERAURAL ATTENUATION FOR INSERT EARPHONES

The IA values just described are obtained using typical supraaural audiometric earphones, such as Telephonics TDH-49 and related receivers. In contrast, insert earphones such as Etymotic ER-3A and EARtone 3A receivers provide much greater amounts of IA (Killion, Wilber, & Gudmundsen, 1985; Sklare & Denenberg, 1987). This occurs because the amount of IA is inversely related to the contact area between the earphone and the head (Zwislocki, 1953), and the contact area between the head and earphone is much less for insert receivers than it is for supraaural earphones. Figure 9–5 shows some of the results obtained by Sklare and Denenberg (1987), who compared the IA produced by TDH-49 (supraaural) and ER-3A (insert) earphones on the same subjects. They found that mean IA values were from 81 to 94+ dB

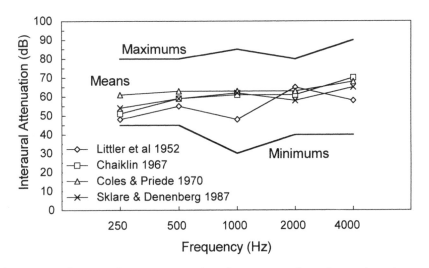

FIGURE 9–4 Interaural attenuation values for supraaural earphones from four representative studies. Lines with symbols are means for each study. The "minimum" and "maximum" lines show the smallest and largest IA values across all four studies.

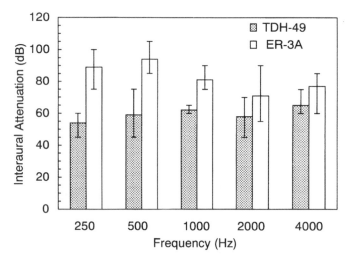

FIGURE 9–5   Interaural attenuation for TDH-49 (supraaural) versus ER-3A (insert) earphones. Bars show means and error lines show ranges. Some actual values were higher than shown. (This occurred because some individual IA values were higher than the limits of the equipment.) Based on the data of Sklare and Denenberg (1987).

up to 1000 Hz and 71 to 77 dB at higher frequencies, for insert receivers.

As already explained, we are most interested in the minimum IA values, which are shown by the bottoms of the error lines in the graph. Sklare and Denenberg found that insert receivers produced minimum IA values of 75 to 85 dB at frequencies up to 1000 Hz, and 50 to 65 dB above 1000 Hz. This is substantially greater than the minimum IA values found for the TDH-49 earphone, which ranged from 45 to 60 dB.

It should be noted that the IA values just described were obtained using insert receivers that were inserted to the proper depth into the ear canal. Insert receivers produce much less IA when their insertion into the ear canal is shallow compared to deep (Killion et al, 1985).

Interaural Attenuation for Bone-Conduction

It is commonly held that interaural attenuation is 0 dB for all bone-conduction signals, but this concept requires qualification. There is essentially no IA for bone-conduction signals presented by a bone-conduction vibrator using *frontal placement* (Studebaker, 1967). However, IA for the more commonly used

mastoid placement of the bone-conduction oscillator depends on the frequency being tested, and is also variable among patients (Studebaker, 1964, 1967). Interaural attenuation values for bone-conduction signals presented at the mastoid are about 0 dB at 250 Hz and rise to approximately 15 dB at 4000 Hz (Studebaker, 1967). The author's experience agrees with others' clinical observations that IA for bone-conduction varies among patients from roughly 0 to 15 dB at 2000 Hz and 4000 Hz (Silman & Silverman, 1991).

Clinical Masking

Recall that masking per se means to render a tone (or other signal) inaudible due to the presence of a noise in the same ear as the tone. Thus, masking the right ear means that a noise is put into the right ear, so that a tone cannot be heard in the right ear. *Clinical masking* is an application of the masking phenomenon used to alleviate cross-hearing. In clinical masking we put noise into the nontest ear because we want to assess the hearing of the test ear. In other words, the masking noise goes into the NTE, and the test signal goes into the TE. Also, the noise is delivered to the NTE by *air-conduction*, regardless of whether the TE is being tested by air- or bone-conduction. These rules apply in all but the most unusual circumstances. The kinds of masking noises used with various test signals are covered in a later section. In the meantime, it is assumed that the appropriate masking noise is always being used.

The meaning is clear when an audiologist says that she will "retest the left bone-conduction threshold with masking noise in the right ear." However, masking terminology is usually more telegraphic. As such, it suffers from ambiguity and can be confusing to the uninitiated. It is therefore worthwhile to familiarize oneself with typical masking phrases and what these really mean. *Unmasked air-conduction* (or just *unmasked air*) refers to an air-conduction threshold that was obtained without any masking noise. Similarly, *unmasked bone-conduction* (or *unmasked bone*) means a bone-conduction threshold obtained without any masking noise. For example, *unmasked right bone* means the bone-conduction threshold of the right ear that was obtained without any masking noise.

Masked air-conduction (or *masked air*) refers to an air-conduction threshold (in the TE) that was obtained with masking noise in the opposite ear. *Masked bone-conduction* (*masked bone*) denotes a bone-conduction threshold obtained with masking noise in the NTE. Thus, *masked right air* is referring to the air-conduction threshold of the right ear that was obtained while masking noise was being presented to the left (nontest) ear. By the same token, *masked left bone* means the bone-conduction threshold of the left ear that was obtained with masking noise in the right ear.

The process of *masking for air-conduction* (*masking for air*) means to put masking noise into the NTE while testing the TE by air-conduction. Likewise, the operation of *masking for bone-conduction* (*masking for bone*) means to put masking noise into the NTE while testing the TE by bone-conduction.

Instructions for Testing with Masking

The first step in clinical masking is to explain to the patient what is about to happen and what she is supposed to do. The very idea of being tested with "noise in your ears" can be confusing to some patients, especially when they are being evaluated for the first time. The author has found that most patients readily accept the situation when they are told that putting masking noise in the opposite ear is the same as an optometrist covering one eye while testing the other.

Noises Used for Clinical Masking

What kind of noise should be used to mask the nontest ear? The answer to this question depends on the signal being masked. If the signal being masked has a wide spectrum, such as speech or clicks, then the masker must also have a wide spectrum. (The student might wish to refer back to Chapter 1 to review the relevant physical concepts.) For example, masking for speech tests commonly uses white noise (actually broadband noise), pink noise, speech-shaped noise, or multitalker babble. Speech-shaped noise has a spectrum that approximates that of the long-term spectrum of speech. Multitalker babble is made by recording the voices of many people who are talking simultaneously, resulting in an unintelligible babble.

Complex noises (e.g., *sawtooth noise*), composed of a low fundamental frequency along with many harmonics, were also used in the past. These noises were poor and unreliable maskers, but one should be aware of them if only for historical perspective.

Pure tones can also be masked by wide-band noises, but this is not desirable. Recall from Chapter 3 that if we are trying to mask a given pure tone, only a rather limited band of frequencies in a wide-band noise actually contributes to masking that tone. This is the critical band (ratio). The parts of a wide-band noise that are higher and lower than the critical band do not help mask the tone, but they do make the noise sound louder. Thus, wide-band noise is a poor choice for masking pure tones because it is both inefficient and unnecessarily loud.

It would therefore seem that the optimal masking noises for pure tones would be critical bands. In practice, however, audiometers actually provide masking noise bandwidths that are wider than critical bands. This type of masking noise is called **narrow-band noise (NBN)**. Audiometric NBNs may approximate bandwidths that are one-third octaves, one-half octaves, or other widths, and also vary widely in how sharply intensity falls outside the pass band (i.e., the rejection rate or steepness of the filter skirts). If an NBN is centered around 1000 Hz, then we can call this a 1000-Hz NBN; if it is centered around 2000 Hz, then it is a 2000-Hz NBN, and so forth.

When to Mask for Bone-Conduction

It might seem odd to discuss the bone-conduction masking rule before the one for air-conduction (AC) because this is the reverse of the order used to obtain unmasked thresholds. However, masked thresholds are tested in the opposite order, bone-conduction (BC) before AC. This is done because the rule for determining when masking is needed for air-conduction depends upon knowing the true bone-conduction thresholds. This means that if masking is needed for BC, it must be done first.

Bone-conduction testing presents us with a peculiar dilemma if we take it for granted that we always need to know which ear is actually responding to a signal. This is so because there is little if any IA for BC, so we rarely know for sure which cochlea is actually responding to a signal, no matter where the vibrator is placed. (Although mastoid placement is assumed throughout this book unless specifically indicated, it should be noted that the bone oscillator and both earphones are usually in place from the outset when forehead placement is used.)

This situation might seem to imply that masking should always be used whenever bone-conduction is tested, but this is not encouraged. This approach has several serious problems in addition to being unnecessarily conservative at the cost of wasted effort (Studebaker, 1964, 1967). When bone-conduction thresholds are *always* tested with masking, the opposite ear would always be occluded with an earphone (both ears would probably be occluded with forehead place-

ment). Thus, one cannot know when or where an occlusion effect occurs, or how large it is. But you need to know the size of the occlusion effect in the first place to calculate how much noise is needed for bone-conduction masking. In addition, always having the headset in place denies the clinician the ability to cross-check for bone-conduction oscillator placement errors, which cause falsely elevated bone-conduction thresholds. Also, placement problems can be clouded by an occlusion effect and/or by unwittingly attributing a higher threshold to the masking. The headset itself only exacerbates vibrator placement problems.

Another questionable technique relies on the Weber test to determine which ear is hearing a bone-conduction signal. These results are not sufficiently accurate or reliable for this purpose. Even its proponents admit that it is best to disregard unlikely Weber results (Studebaker, 1967).

Because a given unmasked bone-conduction threshold could as likely be coming from either ear, a practical approach to deciding when to mask for bone-conduction is based on whether knowing which cochlea is actually responding affects how the audiogram is interpreted. In other words, when does it make a difference whether a given bone-conduction threshold is coming from one cochlea or the other?

A bone-conduction threshold should be retested with masking in the NTE whenever there is an air-bone-gap (ABG) within the test ear that is greater than 10 dB (i.e., ABG >10 dB). This principle is shown schematically in Figure 9–6a. The recommended rule is a slight modification of the one proposed by Studebaker (1964), who suggested masking whenever the ABG is ≥10 dB. The underlying concept is as follows: The variability of a clinical threshold is usually taken to be ±5 dB. Applying this principle to both the air- and bone-conduction thresholds for the same frequency allows them to be as much as 10 dB apart. Thus, for practical purposes an ABG ≤10 dB is too small to be clinically relevant.

With this in mind, consider the unmasked thresholds in the following example:

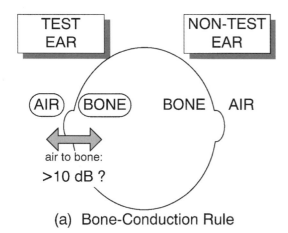

(a) Bone-Conduction Rule

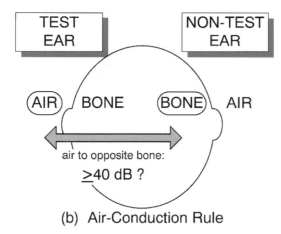

(b) Air-Conduction Rule

FIGURE 9–6 When to retest with masking for bone- and air-conduction. (a) The bone-conduction masking rule asks whether the air-bone-gap is >10 dB within the test ear. (b) The air-conduction masking rule asks whether there is a difference of ≥40 dB between the air-conduction threshold on the test side and the bone-conduction thresholds on the nontest side.

Right air-conduction	55 dB HL
Left air-conduction	70 dB HL
Bone-conduction	45 dB HL

We do not know which ear is really responsible for the bone-conduction threshold of 45 dB. First consider the situation from the standpoint of the *right* ear. If we assume that the unmasked bone-conduction threshold was heard in the right cochlea, then it would have a 10 dB ABG (55 − 45 = 10). It is therefore not necessary to retest the bone-conduction

of the right ear with masking noise in the left ear, because our rule says we should mask when the ABG is >10 dB. But one may say that we still do not know if the bone-conduction threshold is really from the right ear; how can this be acceptable? There are only two options:

1. If the tone was heard by the *right* cochlea, then the ABG is only 10 dB. This is too small to be clinically relevant and the 55 dB loss in the right ear would be interpreted as essentially sensorineural.
2. What if the bone-conduction threshold of 45 dB is really coming from the *left* ear? This option would mean the left cochlea must be more sensitive than the right one. This means the right ear's real bone-conduction threshold would be either 50 or 55 dB. If so, then the right ear is *still* sensorineural (because the air-conduction threshold is 55 dB HL). Thus, there is no reason to mask the opposite (left) ear in this case because the clinical outcome for the right ear is the same regardless of which cochlea really heard the tone.

The situation is different for the *left* ear, which has an air-conduction threshold of 70 dB. If we assume that the 45 dB bone-conduction threshold is from the *left* ear, then its ABG would be 70 − 45 = 25 dB. It would then be necessary to retest the left ear's bone-conduction threshold with masking in the opposite (right) because an ABG of 25 dB meets the ≥10-dB masking criterion. Consider some of the alternatives: Suppose we put the appropriate masking into the opposite (right) ear and find that the left ear's bone-conduction threshold really is 45 dB. This would mean that there really is a 25-dB ABG in the left ear, indicating the presence of a conductive component. In fact, with masking in the right ear, we might find that the real bone-conduction threshold of the left ear is anywhere between 45 and 70 dB. This would mean that the left ABG could be anywhere from 25 dB (a mixed loss) down to 0 dB (a sensorineural loss). Here, we *do* need to know which cochlea is really hearing the bone-conduction signal.

When to Mask for Air-Conduction

Recall that we must use masking whenever cross-hearing might occur. Cross-hearing for an air-conduction signal occurs via the bone-conduction route, and depends on three parameters: (1) the sound level in dB HL presented to the TE; (2) the amount of IA in dB, which determines how much of the signal crosses over; and (3) the *true bone-conduction threshold* in dB HL of the NTE, which determines whether this signal is audible in the NTE.

Consequently, one must mask for air-conduction whenever the sound (in dB HL) being presented to the TE is able to reach the bone-conduction threshold (in dB HL) of the NTE. Because we need to know the NTE's real bone-conduction thresholds, we must mask for bone-conduction before masking for air-conduction. This also means that the unmasked air- and bone-conduction thresholds should be obtained before any masking is accomplished.

The rule for when to mask for air-conduction is shown in Figure 9–6b, and may be stated in several ways. Using the minimum IA value of 40 dB as our criterion, masking is needed whenever the test ear's air-conduction threshold (AC_T) and the nontest ear's bone-conduction threshold (BC_N) differ by 40 dB or more. Some audiologists call the spread between AC_T and BC_N an **air-opposite-bone-gap (AOBG)** or an **air–contralateral-bone-gap (ACBG)**. Using this terminology, masking is necessary whenever the following relationship applies:

$$AOBG \geq 40 \text{ dB.}$$

For the mathematically minded it is necessary to retest an air-conduction threshold with masking whenever:

$$(AC_T - BC_N) \geq 40 \text{ dB.}$$

Of course, this comparison is done individually for each test frequency (usually between 250 and 4000 Hz), and one compares the two ears at the same frequency. [One should remember that the 40-dB figure being used here and elsewhere assumes that standard, supraaural audiometric earphones are being used. It should be replaced with the appropriate minimum IA value (Fig. 9–5) when testing with insert earphones.]

The rule just described is really simpler than it might seem. Suppose the *right air-conduction* threshold is 50 dB HL and the *left bone-conduction* threshold is 5 dB HL (at the same frequency, of course). Are they at least 40 dB apart? The answer is yes ($50 - 5 = 45$, and 45 dB is certainly ≥ 40 dB). Therefore, the right air-conduction threshold must be retested with masking noise in the left ear. In a second example, the *right air-conduction* threshold is 50 dB HL and the *left bone-conduction* threshold is 15 dB HL. Are they at least 40 dB apart? The answer is no ($50 - 15 = 35$, and 35 dB is less than the 40-dB criterion). Therefore, the right ear's air-conduction threshold does *not* need to be retested with masking noise in the left ear. In other words, the right ear's original air-conduction threshold of 50 dB HL is considered to be its true threshold. Consider one more example, in which the right ear's air-conduction threshold is 75 dB HL and the left ear's bone-conduction threshold is 35 dB HL. The right ear needs to be retested with masking because the AOBG is 40 dB, which meets the ≥ 40 dB criterion. It must be emphasized that the comparison made in the air-conduction masking decision is always between *air-conduction* on the *test* side and *bone-conduction* on the *nontest* side, because this is the crossover route. It cannot validly be based on a comparison between the air-conduction thresholds of the two ears. A logical exception occurs when air-conduction threshold of the NTE is better than its bone-conduction threshold at the same frequency; for example, when the air-conduction threshold is 10 dB HL and the bone-conduction threshold is 20 dB HL. Here, one uses the *better* air-conduction threshold (10 dB HL in this example).

Central Masking

As a scientific phenomenon, masking means a threshold shift for a signal that occurs when the noise and signal are presented to the *same* ear. Very technically, this is called "direct, ipsilateral masking," and it occurs because the noise and signal are present within the same cochlea. In *clinical* masking we are trying to cause direct, ipsilateral masking of the *non*test ear so that we can be sure that only the test ear is actually hearing the test signal.

Central masking can occur when the signal and noise are presented to different ears. Suppose that the right ear gets the tone and the left ear gets the noise. Let us also assume that we know for a fact that there is no crossover for either the signal or the noise. (We know this because both the tone and the noise levels being used are well below interaural attenuation.) Clearly, direct ipsilateral masking cannot occur because the signal is in one cochlea and the noise is in the other cochlea. We find that the right ear's threshold is consistently shifted (from, say, 5 dB HL to 10 dB HL) whenever there is noise in the left ear. The reason a noise in one ear can cause a threshold shift (masking) in the other ear is as follows. Even though the peripheral ears are physically separate, the neural signals that come from the two cochleae are combined in the central auditory nervous system (CANS). The noise in one ear can interfere with the ability to hear a tone in the other ear because they interact in the CANS.

Although central masking is a real phenomenon, it is not the effect of interest during clinical masking. In fact, central masking actually complicates matters in clinical masking. For this reason, the amount of central masking that occurs is of some importance when clinical masking is being done. Clinicians generally consider the central masking effect to be about 5 dB; however, threshold shifts as large as 15 dB have been reported (Liden, Nilsson, & Anderson, 1959b), and the effect increases with the magnitude of the masking noise (Studebaker, 1962; Dirks, 1964; Dirks & Malmquist, 1964). More information about the nature and parameters of central masking may be found in Gelfand (1998). We will follow the conservative practice of allowing for 5 dB of central masking during clinical masking procedures.

Effective Masking Calibration

If the audiometer is set up to produce a 1000-Hz pure tone, then an attenuator dial reading of 50 means that a 1000-Hz tone will be presented to the patient at 50 dB HL. If the patient can hear this, then we know her 1000-Hz tonal threshold is 50 dB HL or less. If we change the input selector from "tone" to "NBN," then most audiometers will produce a 1000-Hz NBN at 50 dB HL. This means a narrow band of noise is centered around 1000 Hz, which has an overall level equal to that of a 1000-Hz tone at 50 dB HL. If the patient can hear this, then we know her 1000-Hz NBN threshold is 50 dB HL or less.

However, suppose we want to mask a 50 dB HL 1000-Hz tone. It would seem that this could be done with a 50 dB HL 1000-Hz NBN, based on what we learned about the critical band for masking in Chapter 3, but the details of the narrow band noise spectrum coming from the audiometer rarely makes this work precisely.[1] Hence, if a noise has the same number of decibels as the tone, then it will be too weak to mask that tone. In other words, the level of an NBN noise needs to be increased in order to mask the tone. Audiometer standards (ANSI S3.6-1996 and ISO 389-4-1994) require these adjustments (shown in Table 9–1) to be built in to the audiometer's masking channel, so that the masking level dial is said to be calibrated in **decibels of effective masking (dB EM)**. However, it is up to the clinician to verify that these dial readings actually provide effective masking on her own equipment, and if necessary to determine the proper masking noise settings. Specifically, she must determine the difference in decibels between the level of a given tone and the level of the noise that just masks

---

[1] One reason why this may happen is that the pass band (i.e., the part of the band between the half power points, see Chapter 3) is usually wider than the critical band.

TABLE 9–1 Amounts in decibels (dB) to be added to the reference equivalent threshold sound pressure level (RETSPL) to achieve effective masking (dB EM) for one-third and one-half octave-band masking noises

Frequency (Hz)	125	250	500	750	1000	1500	2000	3000	4000	6000	8000
For one-third octave-band noise	4	4	4	5	6	6	6	6	5	5	5
For one-half octave-band noise	4	4	6	7	7	8	8	7	7	7	6

Based on ANSI S3.6-1996 and ISO 389-4-1994.

that tone. This difference is often called the **effective masking level (EML)**, but is more readily understood if it is called the **minimum effective masking correction (MEMC)** because it is the correction that must be added to the tone's level to arrive at a *minimum noise level* that will *effectively mask* that tone. For example, suppose it takes 55 dB HL of NBN to just mask a 50 dB HL tone. This means that to mask a tone, the noise has to be 5 dB higher than the tone, that is, the MEMC in this case is 55 dB − 50 dB = 5 dB.

The clinician arrives at a set of MEMCs for each audiometer by performing a simple biological (psychoacoustic) calibration study using normal-hearing subjects. There are various approaches to this approach, but the one about to be outlined is probably the simplest. The audiometer must have two channels. One channel will produce the tone, and the second channel will produce the masking noise. The output selector is set up so that both channels are directed into the same earphone, that is, both the tone and the noise are directed into the same ear because we want to find out how much noise is needed to mask the tone. Most audiometers automatically set the tone and the NBN to the same frequency. If the audiometer has separate frequency controls for the two channels, then they should both be set to the same frequency (we do not want to use a 4000-Hz NBN to mask a 1000-Hz tone).

We will go through the basic sequence at 1000 Hz. The noise attenuator is turned to a comfortable level, such as 40 dB HL, and the noise is set to the constantly on position. We now have a continuous 1000-Hz narrow

band noise at 40 dB HL. Next, we find the tone's threshold against the background of the continuously on noise. Many clinicians use a pulsing tone for this purpose because it makes the listening task somewhat easier. Having found the threshold for the tone (where it is *just audible* over the noise), the tone is then decreased in 5 dB steps until it is just *inaudible*. This is where the tone is *just masked* by the noise. Suppose we find that the tone's level is 35 dB HL at this point. We can now say that a 1000-Hz NBN at 40 dB will just mask a 35-dB 1000 Hz tone, or that a 35-dB tone is just masked by a 40-dB noise at 1000 Hz. Either way, the noise has to be 5 dB higher than the tone to just mask it in this example. This strategy is repeated several times to arrive at an average value, which represents that subject's MEMC at 1000 Hz. The procedure is then repeated at the remaining frequencies.

After testing at least 10 subjects, the clinician calculates a mean MEMC at each frequency. For example, the average correction at 500 Hz might be 8.5 dB, rounded to an MEMC of 10 dB; the mean at 1000-Hz MEMC might be 4.6 dB, rounded to 5 dB, etc. These MEMC values are then employed during clinical masking. For purposes of illustration, we will always assume that the MEMC is 5 dB.

This type of procedure can also be used to arrive at minimal effective masking levels on an individual patient basis (Veniar, 1965). Veniar's method involves presenting the tone at a constant level and increasing the noise (in the same earphone) until the patient no longer hears the tone. The student should also be aware that physical masking noise calibration methods based on electroacoustic measurements and/or calculations are also available (e.g., Sanders, 1972; Townsend & Schwartz, 1976), although most clinicians are probably best served by the psychoacoustic approach.

Some audiometers, such as portable instruments and those mainly intended for screening purposes, do not allow one to direct the tone and noise into the same channel. In this case, a simple mixing circuit must be built to properly combine the noise and tone into the same earphone (see Studebaker, 1967, p. 362). Fortunately, this is rarely necessary in modern practice.

The Initial Masking Level

Once we have decided to retest the TE with masking noise in the NTE, we must decide how much masking noise to use. The recommended approach is the initial masking level method described by Martin (1967, 1974, 1980). Other formulas have also been proposed (Liden, Nilsson, & Anderson, 1959b; Studebaker, 1964). However, they are more complex and have been shown to yield similar masking levels to the recommended approach (Martin, 1974). Obviously, we must start with enough noise to render the test tone inaudible in the NTE. It is important to remember at this juncture that we already have an unmasked threshold; we are just not sure about which ear is hearing it. If the threshold is really coming from the NTE, then we must start with enough noise to mask the NTE at threshold.

Initial Masking Level for Air-Conduction

We will assume that we have previously determined the average minimum effective masking correction for our audiometer to be 5 dB higher than the hearing level of the test tone at every frequency. In other words, the masking noise level must be 5 dB higher than the tone level. For example, the noise level would have to be set to 15 dB HL in order to mask a 10 dB HL tone, or 60 dB HL to mask a 55 dB HL tone. We must also add a 10-dB **safety factor** because the MEMC is an *average*. Adding a 10-dB safety factor means that

our starting masking level will have an attenuator (dB HL) dial reading that is 15 dB higher than the unmasked threshold in the NTE. For example, if the NTE's air-conduction threshold is 20 dB HL, then the initial masking level will be:

20 dB HL	(Air-conduction threshold of the tone we want to mask)
+ 5 dB	(MEM correction)
= 25 dB HL	(Average MEM level for a 20 dB HL tone)
+ 10 dB	(Safety factor)
= 35 dB HL	(Initial masking level)

In other words, if the air-conduction threshold of the NTE is 20 dB HL, we will use 35 dB HL of masking noise as the starting masking level. This value is the **initial masking level (IML)**. For the mathematically oriented, the initial masking level (in dB HL) directed into the NTE may be reduced to the formula

$$IML = HL_N + MEMC + SF \, ,$$

where HL_N is the air-conduction threshold hearing level of the NTE, MEMC is the minimum effective masking correction, and SF is the safety factor.

Initial Masking Level for Bone-Conduction and the Occlusion Effect

The IML for bone-conduction testing is similar to the one used for air-conduction with the important addition of a factor to account for the **occlusion effect (OE)**. This is done because the earphone covering the NTE can introduce an occlusion effect, which is an increase in the level of a bone-conduction signal due to occluding the ear canal.

A simple example will show how the OE affects a masked bone-conduction threshold. Suppose an unmasked bone-conduction threshold is 35 dB HL, and the test ear needs to be retested with masking. (To keep things simple, the NTE has a 35 dB HL sensorineural loss.) The 35 dB HL bone-conduction threshold was obtained without any earphones covering the ear canals, and is thus an *unoccluded* bone-conduction threshold. Here the NTE receives the tone at 35 dB HL (at the cochlea). When we retest this bone-conduction with masking, the NTE is covered with the earphone used to deliver the masking noise. In so doing, we change the bone-conduction test from *unoccluded* to *occluded*, which may cause an occlusion effect to occur. Let us assume that the OE is 15 dB. This means that a 35 dB HL bone-conduction signal from the audiometer will be boosted by 15 dB to 50 dB HL at the cochlea of the NTE. Consider what this means from the standpoint of the IML. If we use the above IML formula intended for air-conduction testing, we would be unsuccessfully trying to mask what is really a 50 dB HL signal with a noise that can only mask a tone as high as 35 dB HL. In other words, since occluding the NTE effectively boosted the tone level by 15 dB, we would also need to increase the amount of masking noise by 15 dB in order to account for the occlusion effect:

	35 dB HL	(AC threshold of the tone we want to mask)
+	5 dB	(MEM correction)
=	40 dB HL	(Average MEM level for a 35 dB HL tone)
+	10 dB	(Safety factor)
=	50 dB HL	(IML, unoccluded)
+	15 dB	(Correction for the OE)
=	65 dB HL	(Initial masking level accounting for the OE)

The initial masking level formula for bone-conduction testing accounts for the OE, and may be written as

$$IML = HL_N + MEMC + SF + OE \ .$$

DETERMINING THE OCCLUSION EFFECT

We need to know the size of the OE to determine the IML. Even though fixed OE values have been used to calculate masking levels (Studebaker, 1979; Goldstein & Newman, 1985), clinicians should determine the presence and magnitude of the OE on an individual patient basis. The reason is that we cannot assume any predetermined value because the occlusion effect (1) differs with frequency, (2)

is highly variable among people, and (3) is absent when there is a conductive pathology. Consequently, we must first perform an easy but important test to determine the presence and size of the OE before determining IMLs for BC.

The recommended procedure, sometimes called the **audiometric Bing test** (Martin, Butler, & Burns, 1974), is as follows: Having already obtained the unmasked bone-conduction thresholds, the audiologist places the earphone over the NTE and retests the bone-conduction *without any noise*. An OE is considered to be present if the occluded threshold is better (lower) than the unoccluded one; the size of the OE is simply the difference between them. In the case of the above example, the unoccluded bone-conduction threshold would be 35 dB and the occluded bone-conduction threshold would be 20 dB HL, revealing that the OE was 35 − 20 = 15 dB. The resulting OE value is then used in the calculation of the IML. The bone-conduction IML formula is the same as the air-conduction formula when the OE is zero. This is done for each frequency up to and including 1000 Hz, which is the region where OEs are expected to occur.

This procedure works because the OE increases the level of signal reaching the cochlea, so the dial reading of the threshold is lowered by the amount of the OE (which was 15 dB in our example).

There are at least two supplemental benefits of the audiometric Bing test. First, it provides supportive diagnostic information because the OE tends to be present in ears that are normal or have sensorineural impairments, and tends to be absent in ears with conductive or mixed losses. Second, the clinician can be alerted to the inadvertent displacement of the bone-conduction vibration by occluded thresholds which are poorer (higher) than the unoccluded thresholds.

Using the Initial Masking Level

Once we have determined that masking is necessary, the first step is to retest the threshold in question while masking noise is being presented to the NTE at the IML.

After instructing the patient and setting up the equipment for masked testing (see below), the masking noise is turned on. With the IML in the NTE, we now retest the threshold for the TE. As previously mentioned, we will allow for 5 dB of central masking during clinical masking procedures. If the patient responds within 5 dB of the same level obtained previously without masking, then we consider the original threshold to be confirmed as being derived from the test ear. This is so because the patient can still hear the tone even though the NTE is being masked; if the NTE is not hearing the tone, then it must have been heard in the TE. For example, suppose that the right ear's unmasked threshold was 40 dB HL. This threshold is considered to be true if it stays at 40 dB HL (or shifts only 5 dB to 45 dB HL) with the initial masking level in the left (nontest) ear. The 40 dB HL is now called a masked threshold, and the masking procedure is finished for this tone.

The alternative outcome is that the IML causes the threshold to shift by more than 5 dB from its original, unmasked value. For example, the right ear's unmasked threshold of 40 dB HL might shift to 50 dB HL with the IML in the left ear. In this case, even though the tone was directed into the right ear, the original (unmasked) threshold must have come from the left (nontest) ear. Why? Because if the tone was really heard in the right ear, then putting noise into the left would not have changed anything—it would still be heard in the right ear. If appropriate masking noise in the left ear stops the patient from hearing a tone from the right earphone, then the original threshold must have been originally picked up in the left ear via cross-hearing. Under these circumstances we must now move to the next phase of the masking procedure, which involves finding the actual threshold of the test ear using the **threshold shift or plateau method**.

We may summarize the use of the initial masking level as follows: (1) The original threshold is confirmed if it stays the same (within 5 dB) at the initial masking level. (2) An unmasked threshold was probably heard in the nontest ear if the initial masking level causes it to shift more than 5 dB.

The Plateau Method

The plateau method is a widely accepted strategy for finding the true masked threshold of the TE that was described by Hood (1960). Sometimes called the threshold shift method, the logic of the plateau strategy can be understood in terms of Figure 9–7, which shows the results of a hypothetical test. The abscissa shows the level of the masking noise being presented to the NTE, and the ordinate shows the threshold of the tone being presented to the test ear. Notice that the graph breaks down into three distinct ranges, labeled undermasking, plateau, and overmasking.

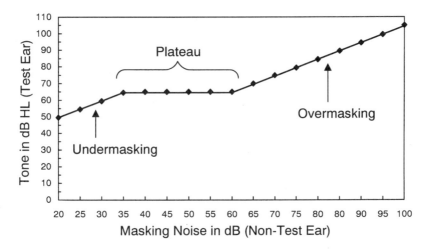

FIGURE 9–7   The masking plateau (see text).

Undermasking

When a tone is really being heard by the non-test ear via cross-hearing, then raising the level of the masking noise will cause the masked threshold to increase. This occurs because the noise and tone are both in the same (nontest) ear. For example, the left side of the graph in Figure 9–7 shows that raising the masking noise from 20 to 35 dB HL caused the apparent tonal threshold to rise from 50 to 65 dB HL. The one-for-one elevation occurs because masking increases linearly with masker level, as we learned in Chapter 3. This linear increase of apparent threshold with masking noise level indicates that the tone is still being picked up by the NTE. We call this **undermasking** because the amount of noise is not sufficient to exclude the NTE from the test. Thus, undermasking occurs when there is not enough masking noise, so that the tone is being heard by the nontest ear, as in Figure 9–8a.

The Plateau

The plateau occurs when the NTE is effectively masked by the noise so that the tone is heard by the test ear. Here the tone is picked up only by the test ear and the noise is picked up only by the nontest ear. When the tone is really being heard in the test ear, then raising the masking noise level will not cause the threshold to change. This is seen in the middle part of Figure 9–7 and conceptually in Figure 9–8b, where the threshold for the tone stays at 65 dB HL even though the masking noise is raised from 35 to 60 dB HL. The resulting plateau in the graph reveals the test ear's true masked threshold for the tone. The width of the plateau is the range of masking noise levels over which the threshold stays the same. In this example, the plateau is 65 dB HL, which is the test ear's threshold. The width of the plateau is from 35 to 60 dB HL of noise in the NTE, and is often called the range of **effective masking**.

The plateau occurs because the noise is effectively masking the nontest ear so that the test ear can hear the tone. Raising the noise in the NTE continues to keep it effectively

masked, thus the test ear remains free to respond to the tone at its own threshold. A visual analogy will make this clearer. Let us say that you can read the 20-20 vision line of an eye chart with both eyes. However, you can only read down to the 20-30 line if you cover (mask) your right eye with a small piece of paper. The left eye must have 20-30 vision because your right eye is covered. Now, what would happen if you were to cover the right eye with a larger piece of paper, then a bigger piece, and then an even larger one? You would find that the size of the paper would not make a difference as long as it covers just the right eye. The size of the paper used to mask the nontest eye is analogous to the level of the noise used to mask the nontest ear: Once the noise is effectively masking the nontest ear, you can add more noise without affecting the threshold because the amount of noise "covering" the NTE has nothing to do with the TE—at least within limits.

Overmasking

Overmasking occurs when so much noise is presented to the NTE that it crosses over and masks the test ear. Let us return to the vision example. If you keep increasing the size of the paper covering the right eye, it will eventually get big enough to cover the left eye as well, and this will have an obvious outcome. This is analogous to what would happen if we continue increasing the level of the masking noise. Eventually, the noise will become sufficiently intense to cross over to the test ear. Once this occurs, the threshold for the tone will start to rise again as the masking level is increased. This range on the plateau graph is aptly called **overmasking**, and is illustrated by the diagonal line on the right side of Figure 9–7 and also in Figure 9–8c. Overmasking will be covered further in a subsequent section.

Plateau Width

Masking plateaus become narrow when there is a conductive loss in the nontest (masked) ear: the wider the air-bone-gap, the smaller the plateau. The situation becomes

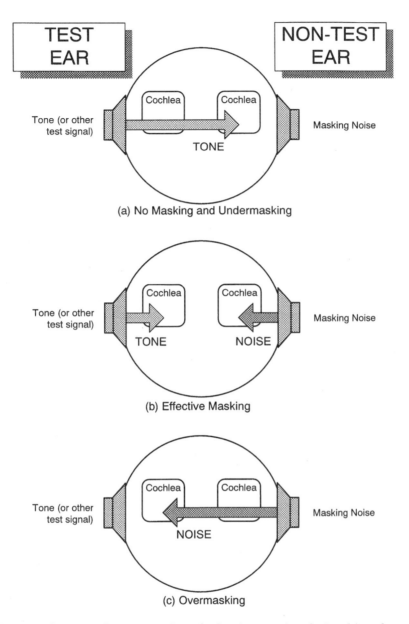

FIGURE 9–8 Conceptual representation of what is occurring during (a) undermasking, (b) effective masking along the plateau, and (c) overmasking. No arrow is shown for the noise in (a) because it is not preventing the NTE from hearing the tone (the same picture also describes cross-hearing without masking). No arrow is shown for the tone in (c) because the noise is preventing the TE from hearing it.

exacerbated when both ears have air-bone-gaps, as will be described below.

The width of the plateau is important for at least two reasons. First, the wider the plateau the more confidence you can have in the validity of the masked threshold. Audiol-ogists typically require a plateau to be at least 15 to 20 dB wide before accepting a masked threshold as valid. Second, a very nar-row plateau can be missed altogether during testing, in which case a masked threshold cannot be obtained. In fact, sometimes there is no plateau between the undermasking and overmasking ranges so that a usable masked threshold cannot be obtained. One must then indicate that obtaining a masked threshold was at least attempted, often with a phrase such as "no plateau" or "could not mask."

Factors that increase the likelihood of overmasking have the effect of making the masking plateau narrower. Everything else being equal, the plateau becomes smaller as (1) interaural attenuation values get smaller, (2) the test ear's bone-conduction threshold gets lower, (3) the masked ear's air-conduction threshold gets higher, and (4) the occlusion effect gets larger (when masking for bone-conduction). The first two factors increase the chances that a given amount of masking noise will reach and cause masking in the test ear's cochlea. The second pair makes it necessary for a higher masking noise level to be used.

Overmasking and the Maximum Masking Level[2]

Overmasking occurs when too much noise is presented to the NTE, so that the noise

---

[2] This section is rather advanced.

crosses the head and actually masks the tone in the TE. This is represented by the large arrow in Figure 9–9. In other words, the noise that was intended to prevent cross-hearing in the NTE is also stopping the test ear from hearing the signal. Since the patient can no longer hear the tone, the clinician will increase the tone level until the patient can hear it over the noise. The resulting threshold shift (represented by the small arrow in Fig. 9–9) is a false estimate of the threshold. Thus, a valid measurement cannot be obtained starting with the lowest noise level that causes overmasking, and for all higher noise levels. Clearly, the clinician must be constantly alert to the possibility of overmasking whenever masking is used.

Overmasking depends on the same cross-hearing effect that occurs when a tone is received by the NTE, except in the opposite direction. Because crossover occurs via the bone-conduction route, we must now think about how many decibels of the noise being delivered to the nontest ear reaches the cochlea of the test ear. This means that the noise level being presented to the NTE exceeds IA by an amount that reaches the bone-conduction threshold of the TE. For this reason it has been proposed (Martin, 1991)

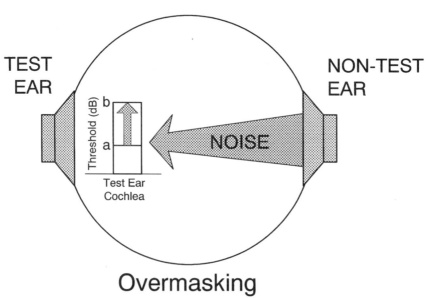

Overmasking

FIGURE 9–9 Overmasking occurs when the masking noise (large arrow) crosses to and masks the test ear. This causes a threshold shift in the test ear (small arrow), causing a false elevation of its threshold (from **a** to **b**).

that overmasking occurs when the level of the noise in the nontest ear (MN_N) is equal to or more than IA plus the bone-conduction threshold of the test ear (BC_T), or when

$$MN_N \geq (IA + BC_T).$$

For example, suppose that we present masking noise to the NTE of a patient whose TE has a bone-conduction threshold of 30 dB HL at 2000 Hz, and that her IA at this frequency is 50 dB. When will overmasking occur? To answer this important clinical question, we simply substitute these values into the formula:

$$MN_N \geq (IA + BC_T)$$

$$MN_N \geq (50 \text{ dB} + 30 \text{ dB HL})$$

$$MN_N \geq 80 \text{ dB HL}.$$

In other words, overmasking should occur in this case when the masking noise is 80 dB HL or more.

This commonly employed rule is actually too strict when the masking noise level just equals IA + BC_T. At this level what actually occurs is cross-hearing of the noise by the TE. The noise is at threshold (is just audible) in the TE, but this does not mean it can also cause masking in the TE. In terms of the example, the 80 dB HL noise presented to the NTE arrives at the TE's cochlea at 30 dB HL, which is the bone-conduction threshold. Hence, the noise is audible in the TE at 30 dB HL. However, it does not mean this 30-dB noise is capable of masking a 30-dB tone in that ear. This should not be surprising. Recall that we calibrated the MEML of our masking noise on a group of normal listeners, and found that the HL of a masking noise has to be an average of 5 dB higher than the HL of the tone it can mask (i.e., on average, it took 45 dB HL of noise to mask a 40 dB HL tone). For this reason, the 30 dB HL noise that reaches the test ear at threshold can be heard, but it will take an additional 5 dB (the minimum effective masking correction, MEMC) to actually mask the TE. For this reason, we can say that overmasking occurs when

$$MN_N \geq (IA + BC_T + MEMC).$$

Thus, overmasking in our example actually occurs when the noise presented to the NTE reaches 85 dB HL:

$$MN_N \geq (IA + BC_T + MEMC)$$

$$MN_N \geq (50 \text{ dB} + 30 \text{ dB HL} + 5 \text{ dB})$$

$$MN_N \geq 85 \text{ dB HL}.$$

Overmasking becomes problematic as early in the masking process as when one is deciding on the initial masking level. Once the IML is determined, the clinician must ask herself whether overmasking is already occurring at this starting level. This problem is particularly noticeable when the air-conduction threshold of the NTE is poorer than that of the TE. Consider the following example, where the thresholds (at some frequency) are:

Right AC:	50 dB HL (masked)
Right BC:	50 dB HL (masked)
Left AC:	25 dB HL (unmasked, masking not needed)
Left BC:	10 dB HL (*unmasked, masking needed*).

The right air- and bone-conduction thresholds have just been obtained with masking in the left ear.[3] The left bone conduction threshold still needs to be retested with masking. This involves putting the appropriate IML into the right ear, which is

	50 dB HL	(Threshold of the tone we want to mask)
+	5 dB	(Our MEM correction)
=	55 dB HL	(MEML for 50 dB HL)
+	10 dB	(Safety factor)
=	65 dB HL	(Initial masking level)

Assuming that IA = 40 dB, then the 65 dB starting noise level presented to the right ear will reach the left cochlea at 65 dB HL − 40 dB = 25 dB HL. Logically, overmasking occurs

---

[3] We are assuming that the right AC and BC are already established to simplify the illustration even though this implies a test order somewhat different from what was suggested earlier.

because 25 dB HL of noise in the left cochlea is more than sufficient to cause masking of its 10-dB bone-conduction threshold. This is confirmed with the overmasking formula, which shows that the 65 dB IML exceeds 55 dB, which is the level where overmasking begins in this case:

$$MN_N \geq (IA + BC_T + MEMC)$$

$$65\,dB \geq (40 + 10 + 5)$$

$$65\,dB \geq 55\,dB.$$

The chances of overmasking become even greater when bone-conduction is being tested with masking. This can occur because covering the NTE with the earphone can result in an occlusion effect, which would increase the level of the bone-conduction signal in the nontest ear. Suppose a 15-dB occlusion effect results when the right ear is covered with the earphone used to deliver the masking noise. If this occurs, then the IML must be increased to overcome the enhanced bone-conduction signal reaching the nontest cochlea at $65 + 15 = 80$ dB HL. Under these conditions, overmasking could occur even if IA was as high as 65 dB! This is so because $85\,dB \geq (65 + 10 + 5)$.

The maximum masking level (MML) is the highest masking noise level that can be used without causing overmasking to occur. Recall that the typical increment for an audiometric signal is 5 dB. It should thus make sense that the MML is simply 5 dB below the lowest noise level that causes overmasking. For example, if we determine that the lowest level for overmasking is 80 dB HL, then the MML is simple $80 - 5 = 75$ dB HL.

For the math-minded, overmasking occurs whenever

$$MN_N \geq (IA + BC_T + MEMC);$$

thus the lowest level at which overmasking occurs is

$$(IA + BC_T + MEMC).$$

Maximum masking occurs one attenuator step (5 dB) below this minimum overmasking value, or when

$$MN_N = (IA + BC_T + MEMC) - 5.$$

It is important to note that while one must always be on the alert for overmasking, one should not be too quick to write "could not mask," or "masking dilemma" on the audiogram without bothering to at least try to obtain a masked threshold. If the previously unmasked threshold is not shifted with the IML, then it has been confirmed as a masked threshold. If the unmasked threshold is shifted by the IML, then one should try to obtain a plateau beginning with lower masking levels. (This is actually what was called for in Hood's original description of the plateau.) At least sometimes an acceptable plateau (and therefore a masked threshold) is obtained. Of course, one's suspicions about overmasking will have been confirmed if no plateau is obtained. In that case, one can indicate "no plateau" on the audiogram, and know that this comment is *empirically* based.

The Masking Dilemma

A special case in which overmasking occurs at the initial masking level is aptly called the **masking dilemma** (Naunton, 1960). This problem occurs when the unmasked audiogram reveals large air-bone-gaps in both ears. Figure 9–10 shows a typical example of the masking dilemma in which the ABGs are approximately 55 dB wide. This situation is a dilemma because we must retest both ears with masking even though overmasking would occur at the initial masking levels. For example, the IML of a noise needed to mask the right ear at 1000 Hz would be $55 + 5 + 10 = 70$ dB HL, but the unmasked bone-conduction threshold is 0 dB HL. Overmasking occurs because presenting the IML to the right ear would cause masking at the left cochlea, which would shift the left ear's air- and bone-conduction thresholds. In such a case, we do not really know whether the left ear's threshold shifted because of (1) effective masking or (2) overmasking.

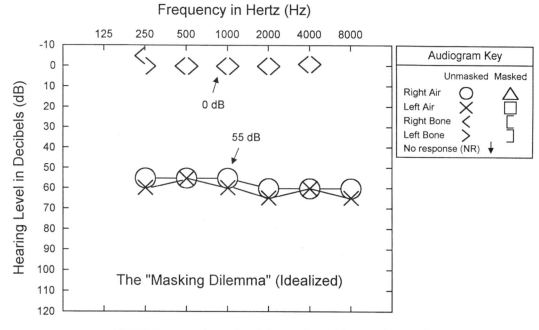

FIGURE 9–10 Example of the masking dilemma (see text).

Some Considerations for Bone-Conduction Masking

As already pointed out, masking is completed first for bone-conduction thresholds because these are needed to make air-conduction masking decisions. Unlike masking for AC, where the earphones are worn in the regular way, masking for bone-conduction involves a special arrangement of the bone vibrator and earphones. The transducer setup for masked bone-conduction testing is shown in Figure 9–11. The bone-conduction oscillator is placed on the test ear's mastoid process, and the nontest ear is covered with the earphone being used to deliver the masking noise. The test ear is left *uncovered*, and its earphone is placed on the side of the head between the test ear and eye as shown in the figure. It is very important to make sure that the bone vibrator and NTE earphone are properly placed. This is an important step because the earphone headset can easily interfere with the bone vibrator's headband. It is also important to tell the patient (1) that this peculiar arrangement is being done on

purpose; (2) to keep as still as comfortably possible to avoid jostling the equipment on her head; and (3) to let you know immediately if anything slips out of place. This setup is reversed when it is time to test for the other ear's masked bone-conduction thresholds.

The *unmasked* bone-conduction thresholds should be rechecked with the earphone headset in place before testing is done with masking noise. This is done for two purposes. One reason is to determine whether covering the NTE results in an occlusion effect, which constitutes administering the audiometric Bing test (Martin, Butler, & Burns, 1974). The size of the occlusion effect is noted for each frequency where it occurs (typically up to 1000 Hz) because this value must be added to the IML used for BC, as already described.

Another reason for rechecking the unmasked bone-conduction thresholds with the earphone in place is to assure that the bone-conduction vibrator placement has not been compromised by the addition of the headset. This is done by making sure that the bone-conduction thresholds with the earphone

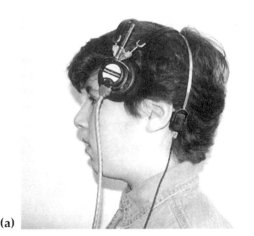

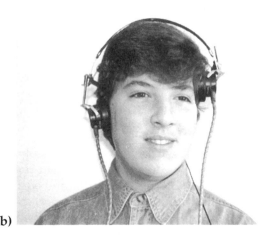

FIGURE 9–11 Typical arrangement of (a) the one vibrator and (b) earphones during masking for bone-conduction.

headset should be adjusted and rechecked if a placement problem is found.

Insert Earphones

Insert earphones such as EARtone 3A and ER-3A receivers are readily available for audiological use. Their use provides two significant advantages over standard supraaural audiometric earphones as far as masking is concerned. These advantages occur because properly used insert receivers (1) increase interaural attenuation (Zwislocki, 1953) and (2) alleviate the occlusion effect.

The interaural attenuation values provided by insert earphones were reported by Sklare and Denenberg (1987). These values were shown along with the values obtained with the more commonly used supraaural earphones in Figure 9–5. Recall that interaural attenuation is pivotal to the decision about when masking must be used. In fact, the rule to mask for air-conduction when the AOBG is ≥40 dB is based on the premise that IA is often as small as 40 dB. Using insert receivers makes the need for masking quite rare by increasing the amount of IA to the values shown in that figure, which are, on average, well over 70 dB (Killion, Wilber, & Gudmundsen, 1985). Moreover, using insert receivers to present the masking noise reduces the amount of noise reaching the test ear, thereby making overmasking less of a problem.

Masking for Suprathreshold Tonal Tests

The discussion of clinical masking so far has focused on pure-tone thresholds. Let us now address masking for tests that use pure tones presented at levels above threshold, for example, tone decay, SISI, etc. (see Chapter 10). It is readily apparent that if masking was required to obtain the threshold for a tone, then it will also be needed for tests performed above threshold. For example, suppose 35 dB of masking noise in the left ear was needed to obtain a 50 dB HL threshold in the right ear. We now want to assess the right ear with the Olsen-Noffsinger tone decay test (TDT), which begins at 20 dB SL (Chapter

headset in place are not worse than they were originally. Here one should use a frequency of at least 1000 Hz, preferably higher. The reason for using a higher frequency is that the occlusion effect can cloud the ability to detect a placement problem at frequencies up to about 1000 Hz. For example, suppose we retest at 500 Hz and find that the bone-conduction is unchanged by the addition of the headset. This could mean that the vibrator placement is fine and there is also no occlusion effect; but it can also mean that the bone-conduction threshold is 15 dB poorer because the vibrator moved, but that this was counteracted by a 15-dB occlusion effect. Needless to say, the vibrator and earphone

10). Clearly, if masking was needed to make sure that only the test ear was receiving a tone at 50 dB HL, then masking will also be needed if that same tone is presented at 70 dB HL. Moreover, the masking noise must be raised to account for the higher level of the tone now being presented to the test ear. In other words, even though the 35 dB HL noise (in the NTE) was fine when 50 dB HL was being presented to the test ear, it will not suffice when the test tone is raised to 70 dB HL. The noise needs to be 20 dB higher because the tone is now 20 dB higher.

Finally, since most special auditory tests are presented at *supra*threshold levels, they will often have to be administered with masking in the NTE even though masking was not needed when the threshold was obtained at the same frequency. This is so because cross-hearing will occur whenever the amount of the test signal that exceeds IA can reach the NTE's bone-conduction threshold. For example, suppose the air-conduction threshold of the right ear (TE) is 40 dB HL and the bone-conduction threshold of the left ear (NTE) is 10 dB HL. The right air-conduction threshold does not have to be retested with masking because the AOBG is 40 − 10 = 30 dB, which is less than the 40-dB AOBG criterion. Now consider what happens with a suprathreshold test such as the Olsen-Noffsinger TDT. This test begins at 20 dB above the 40 dB HL threshold, which means the test tone will be presented to the TE at 60 dB HL. If we properly extend the definition of the "A" ("air-") in AOBG to mean the *level at which the test tone is presented* to the TE (instead of just its threshold), then the AOBG in our example becomes 60 − 10 = 50 dB. The 50-dB AOBG exceeds the 40-dB AOBG criterion, indicating that cross-hearing is possible and therefore masking is indicated.

Thus, the rule for when masking is needed for any tonal suprathreshold test is simply a generalization of the already familiar concept, which is to mask whenever the AOBG is ≥40 dB *except* that "A" ("air-") now means the *presentation level* of the test tone (in dB HL). The 40-dB criterion can be replaced with the individual's actual IA value if it is known (see below). As before, this comparison is made separately at each test frequency where a suprathreshold tonal test is being considered.

Recall that the 40-dB criterion is used as a conservative rule of thumb because we usually do not know an individual's own IA for a given signal. In practice, we sometimes do know this value, especially after the threshold has been established. Here is how: Suppose a patient's thresholds at 1000 Hz are (1) 5 dB HL for both air- and bone-conduction in the right ear, and (2) 60 dB HL in the left ear. This patient's IA cannot be 40 dB because if it were, she would have responded at 45 dB HL in the left ear. Because she did not respond to the tone in the left ear until it reached 60 dB HL, then her actual minimum IA at this frequency must be 60 − 5 = 55 dB. In cases such as this we are able to replace the 40-dB value with the individually determined amount.

The amount of masking noise needed during suprathreshold tonal tests requires some calculations, which must account for several factors: (1) How much of the test signal reaches the nontest cochlea? This involves (a) the presentation level of the signal at the TE, (b) the bone-conduction threshold of the NTE, and (c) interaural attenuation. (2) How much of the masking noise presented to the NTE actually reaches its cochlea? This means that we must account for any air-bone-gap in the nontest ear. (3) Finally, we must remember to account for the effective masking ability of the noise, which involves the MEMC and safety factor. Thus, the amount of noise that must be presented to the NTE when masking for a suprathreshold tonal test is determined as follows:

$$
\begin{array}{ll}
& \text{Presentation level at the TE in dB HL} \\
& (P_T) \\
- & \text{Interaural attenuation (IA, 40 dB if unknown)} \\
\hline
= & \text{Level crossing over to NTE cochlea} \\
+ & \text{Air-bone-gap of the NTE (ABG}_N) \\
+ & \text{Minimum effective masking correction (MEMC)} \\
+ & \text{10-dB safety factor (SF)} \\
\hline
= & \text{Masking noise level in NTE in dB HL} \\
& (MN_N)
\end{array}
$$

This calculation can also be written as a formula:

$$MN_N = P_T - IA + ABG_N + MEMC + SF.$$

Just because one is able to calculate the correct masking level does not mean that it can be used blindly. One must first estimate whether overmasking is possible or likely, as described earlier. This is especially important when using masking with suprathreshold tests, which require the use of higher noise levels than those used for threshold measures.

A peculiar problem is encountered when masking is used during sweep-frequency Bekesy audiometry (see Chapter 10) because the frequency keeps changing over the course of the test instead of staying the same. For this reason, some audiometers which support Bekesy audiometry provide NBN maskers that change in frequency in synchrony with the changing test frequency, and some clinicians use broadband noise maskers. The problem does not stop here. Optimum masking noise levels (however one goes about determining what they should be) must also change "on the fly" as the test sweeps across the audiogram because the amount of hearing loss is rarely the same at every frequency. In fact, the author has never come across a truly adequate masking approach for sweep frequency Bekesy audiometry.

Effects of Masking on Test Results

The fact that central masking has already been considered highlights the fact that the noise in the NTE can have an impact on the test results. Even the beginning student should be aware of some of the effects that a contralateral masking noise can have on test outcomes, if only generally.

The presence of masking in the NTE can result in tone decay among subjects without threshold adaptation in the absence of the noise (Shimizu, 1969; Priede & Coles, 1975), and affects the results of the short increment sensitivity index (SISI) (Blegvad & Terkildsen, 1967; Blegvad, 1969; Shimizu, 1969; Swisher, Dudley, & Doehring, 1969). Even though effects vary widely among the subjects in these studies, SISI scores were typically higher with noise in the NTE compared to the scores obtained without masking. In fact, it was not uncommon for masking noise to cause SISI scores to change from one diagnostic category to another (e.g., a negative score might become questionable or positive).

A number of studies have also revealed that the outcome of Bekesy audiometry is affected by masking in the NTE (Dirks & Norris, 1966; Blegvad, 1967, 1968; Grimes & Feldman, 1969). Compared with unmasked results, the presence of masking noise in the NTE caused thresholds to become poorer (more so for continuous than pulsed tracings), narrowing of excursion widths, and widening of the separation between the pulsed and continuous tracings. In light of these specific effects, it is not surprising that masking caused the diagnostic classifications of Bekesy audiograms to change from Type I to Type II or IV, and from Type II to Type IV.

Masking for Speech Audiometry

The basic concepts already learned about masking for tonal tests can be applied to masking for speech audiometry (Chapter 8) with a few modifications.

Effective Masking Calibration for Speech

Minimum effective masking corrections can be determined for speech materials in a similar way to that described earlier for tones. Briefly, the masking noise and speech material are directed into the same earphone, with the noise turned on at a reasonably comfortable level (such as 40 dB HL or 50 dB HL) throughout the procedure. Beginning at a higher level than the noise, the subject is presented with a predetermined number of test words (e.g., six or eight), which are to be repeated. This procedure is continued in decreasing steps of 5 dB until a speech level is found where all of the words are missed by the listener. The difference between this speech level and that of the noise is the MEMC for that listener. The procedure is repeated using at least 10 normal hearing subjects, and the clinician then calculates an average. As we have already done for NBN masking, this average value is then used as the MEMC along with a safety factor for clinical masking.

The procedure just described actually applies to the kind of noise and speech materials used, for example speech noise and spondee words. Additional MEMC values can be arrived at in the same way for other materials and/or masking noises, for example, monosyllabic words, white noise, etc.

When to Mask During Speech Audiometry

We already know that the "when to mask" question involves three factors. The first factor is the level of the signal being presented to the TE. In speech audiometry this will typically be spondee words when obtaining the speech reception threshold (SRT) and monosyllabic words for speech recognition testing. Interaural attenuation is the second factor. Individual IA values for speech using standard audiometric earphones range from 48 to 68 dB across studies (Liden, 1954; Liden Nilsson, & Anderson, 1959a; Snyder, 1973; Smith & Markides, 1981; Sklare & Denenberg, 1987). The 48-dB minimum supports the use of 45 dB as the IA criterion for deciding when to mask for speech (assuming 5-dB test steps), as suggested by Konkle and Berry (1983) and Goldstein and Newman (1985). However, the author prefers using the more conservative value of 40 dB, at least under typical conditions. This concurs with others (e.g., Martin, 1991). Using insert receivers increases IA for speech up to the 68- to 84-dB range (Sklare & Denenberg, 1987).

The third factor to be considered is the bone-conduction threshold of the NTE. However, bone-conduction thresholds are rarely obtained for speech. It is therefore necessary to use one or more of the *pure-tone* bone-conduction thresholds of the NTE. ASHA (1988) guidelines suggest considering the frequencies between 500 and 4000 Hz with the most sensitive (lowest or best) bone-conduction threshold being used for this purpose. However, the author's experience

suggests that 250 Hz might also be considered, especially when thresholds are decidedly better at low frequencies compared with higher ones.

Thus, masking should be employed during speech audiometry when the speech level in the test ear (S_T) minus interaural attenuation equals or exceeds the "best" pure-tone bone-conduction threshold of the NTE (BC_N). For those who like formulas, masking for speech audiometry is indicated when

$$S_T - IA \geq BC_N .$$

Here, IA may be 40 or 45 dB, although 40 dB provides a more conservative margin of safety.

Masking for the Speech Reception Threshold

The masking procedure for SRT testing is analogous to the one used for pure-tone thresholds. To begin with, the initial masking level is equal to the SRT of the nontest ear plus the MEMC and a safety factor, or

$$IML_{SRT} = SRT_N + MEMC + SF.$$

The original SRT is considered to be confirmed if the SRT stays the same with the IML in the NTE, or if it shifts by only 5 dB, attributable to central masking (Martin, Bailey, & Pappas, 1965; Martin, 1966; Frank & Karlovich, 1975). If the IML causes the SRT to shift by ≥ 10 dB, then the SRT must be found using the plateau (threshold shift) method. The masking strategy is the same as that described for tonal testing, except one uses the test technique appropriate for obtaining an SRT rather than a pure-tone threshold (see Chapter 8).

Masking for Speech Recognition and Other Suprathreshold Speech Tests

A calculation is needed to determine the correct amount of masking noise to be used during speech recognition and other suprathreshold speech tests. This calculation is actually the same as the one described above for suprathreshold tonal tests, except the presentation level now refers to that of the speech material. By now the student already knows that one must be ever vigilant about the possibility of overmasking, especially when performing any suprathreshold test.

A nifty rule-of-thumb that often works to arrive at the needed amount of noise for masking during speech audiometry is to use a masking noise level (in the NTE) that is 20 dB less than the level of the speech material being presented to the test ear (Jerger & Jerger, 1971; Hannley, 1986; Yacullo, 1999). When properly used, this approach causes the masking noise in the NTE to be at least 20 dB greater than any speech signal that might cross over to it from the test ear. The author has found that this maneuver works especially well for symmetrical sensorineural hearing losses, and when masking the better ear while testing the poorer ear with asymmetrical sensorineural losses. However, after estimating how much masking noise to use with this technique, you *must* remember to consider whether either under- or overmasking might occur. Problems will arise if there is a conductive loss in the nontest ear.

Maximum Masking and Overmasking During Speech Audiometry

The maximum masking and overmasking rules for speech audiometry are similar to the ones already discussed, except that one attends to the *best* bone-conduction threshold of the test ear.

Masking for Speech Tests by Bone-Conduction

Speech testing by bone-conduction is relatively uncommon, but one must still be prepared to mask during these conditions should they arise. Here, the "when to mask" question follows the one used for tones, except that the comparison is made between the speech level and the best bone-conduction threshold. The issue of how much masking to use for bone-conduction speech stimuli must account for the occlusion effect. Even though the average occlusion effect for speech is approximately 6 dB

when the vibrator is at the mastoid (or 9 dB when stimulating from the forehead), individual values can be as large as 20 dB (Klodd & Edgerton, 1977). Because of this variability it is recommended that the size of the occlusion effect for speech be determined on an individual patient basis using the same approach already described for tonal signals.

REFERENCES

American National Standards Institute (ANSI). 1996. *American National Standard Specifications for Audiometers.* ANSI S3.6-1996. New York: ANSI.

American Speech-Language-Hearing Association (ASHA). 1988. Guidelines for determining threshold level for speech. *ASHA* 30, 85–89.

Blegvad B. 1967. Contralateral masking and Bekesy audiometry in normal listeners. *Acta Otolaryngol* 64, 157–165.

Blegvad B. 1968. Bekesy audiometry and clinical masking. *Acta Otolaryngol* 66, 229–240.

Blegvad B. 1969. Differential intensity sensitivity and clinical masking. *Acta Otolaryngol* 67, 428–434.

Blegvad B, Terkildsen K. 1967. Contralateral masking and the SISI-test in normal listeners. *Acta Otolaryngol* 63, 556–563.

Chaiklin JB. 1967. Interaural attenuation and cross-hearing in air-conduction audiometry. *J Aud Res* 7, 413–424.

Coles RRA, Priede VM. 1970. On the misdiagnoses resulting from incorrect use of masking. *J Laryngol Otol* 84, 41–63.

Dirks DD. 1964. Factors relating to bone-conduction reliability. *Arch Otolaryngol* 79, 551–558.

Dirks DD, Malmquist CW. 1964. Changes in bone-conduction thresholds produced by masking in the non-test ear. *J Speech Hear Res* 7, 271–278.

Dirks DD, Norris JD. 1966. Shifts in auditory thresholds produced by ipsilateral and contralateral maskers at low intensity levels. *J Acoust Soc Am* 40, 12–19.

Frank T, Karlovich RS. 1975. Effect of contralateral noise on speech detection and speech reception thresholds. *Audiology* 14, 34–43.

Gelfand SA. 1998. *Hearing: An Introduction to Psychological and Physiological Acoustics,* 3rd ed. New York: Marcel Dekker.

Goldstein BA., Newman CW. 1985. Clinical masking: A decision making process. In Katz J. (Ed.), *Handbook of Clinical Audiology,* 3rd ed. Baltimore: Williams & Wilkins, 170–201.

Grimes CT, Feldman AS. 1969. Comparative Bekesy typing with broad and modulated narrow-band noise. *J Speech Hear Res* 12, 840–846.

Hannley M. 1986. *Basic Principles of Auditory Assessment.* Boston: College-Hill.

Hood JD. 1960. The principles and practice of bone-conduction audiometry. *Laryngoscope,* 70, 1211–1228.

International Organization for Standardization (ISO). 1994. *Acoustics—Reference Zero for Calibration of Audiometric Equipment—Part 4: Reference Levels for Narrow-Band Masking Noise.* ISO 389–4. Geneva: ISO.

Jerger J, Jerger S. 1971. Diagnostic significance of PB word functions. *Arch Otolaryngol* 93, 573–580.

Killion MC, Wilber LA, Gudmundsen GI. 1985. Insert earphones for more interaural attenuation. *Hear Instr* 36, 34–36.

Klodd DA, Edgerton BJ. 1977. Occlusion effect: Bone conduction speech audiometry using forehead and mastoid placement. *Audiology* 16, 522–529.

Konkle DF, Berry GA. 1983. Masking in speech audiometry. In Konkle DF, Rintelmann WF (Eds.): *Principles of Speech Audiometry*. Baltimore: University Park Press, 285–319.

Liden G. 1954. Speech audiometry: An experimental study with Swedish language material. *Acta Otolaryngol Suppl* 114.

Liden G, Nilsson G, Anderson H. 1959a. Narrow-band masking with white noise. *Acta Otolaryngol* 50, 116–124.

Liden G, Nilsson G, Anderson H. 1959b. Masking in clinical audiometry. *Acta Otolaryngol* 50, 125–136.

Littler TS, Knight JJ, Strange PH. 1952. Hearing by bone conduction and the use of bone conduction hearing aids. *Proc R Soc Med* 45, 783–790.

Martin FN. 1966. Speech audiometry and clinical masking. *J Aud Res* 6, 199–203.

Martin FN. 1967. A simplified method for clinical masking. *J Aud Res* 7, 59–62.

Martin FN. 1974. Minimum effective masking levels in threshold audiometry. *J Speech Hear Dis* 39, 280–285.

Martin FN. 1980. The masking plateau revisited. *Ear Hear* 1, 112–116.

Martin FN. 1991. *Introduction to Audiology*, 4th Ed. Englewood Cliffs: Prentice-Hall.

Martin FN, Bailey H, & Pappas J. 1965. The effect of central masking on thresholds for speech. *J Aud Res* 5, 293–296.

Martin FN, Butler EC, Burns P. 1974. Audiometric Bing test for determination of minimum masking levels for bone-conduction tests. *J Speech Hear Dis* 39, 148–152.

Naunton RF. 1960. A masking dilemma in bilateral conductive deafness. *Arch Otolaryngol* 72, 753–757.

Priede VM, Coles RRA. 1975. Masking of the non-test ear in tone decay, Bekesy audiometry and SISI tests. *J Laryngol Otol* 89, 227–236

Sanders JW. 1972. Masking. In Katz J. (Ed.): *Handbook of Clinical Audiology*, 1st ed. Baltimore: Williams & Wilkins, 111–142.

Shimizu H. 1969. Influence of contralateral noise stimulation on tone decay and SISI tests. *Laryngoscope* 79, 2155–2164.

Silman S, Silverman CA. 1991. *Auditory Diagnosis: Principles and Applications*. San Diego: Academic Press.

Sklare DA, Denenberg LJ. 1987. Technical note: Interaural attenuation for Tubephone insert earphones. *Ear Hear* 8, 298–300.

Smith BL, Markides A. 1981. Interaural attenuation for pure tones and speech. *Brit J Audiol* 15, 49–54.

Snyder JM. 1973. Interaural attenuation characteristics in audiometry. *Laryngoscope* 83, 1847–1855.

Sparrevohn UR. 1946. Some audiometric investigations of monaurally deaf persons. *Acta Otolaryngol* 34, 1–10.

Studebaker GA. 1962. On masking in bone-conduction testing. *J Speech Hear Res* 5, 215–227.

Studebaker GA. 1964. Clinical masking of air- and bone-conducted stimuli. *J Speech Hear Dis* 29, 23–35.

Studebaker, GA. 1967. Clinical masking of the non-test ear. *J Speech Hear Dis* 32, 360–367.

Studebaker GA. 1979. Clinical masking. In Rintelmann WF (Ed.): *Hearing Assessment*. Baltimore: University Park Press, 51–100.

Swisher LP, Dudley JG, Doehring DG. 1969. Influence of contralateral noise on auditory intensity discrimination. *J Acoust Soc Am* 45, 1532–1536.

Townsend TH, Schwartz DM. 1976. Calculation of effective masking using one octave and one-third octave analysis. *Audiol Hear Ed* 2, 27–34.

Veniar FA. 1965. Individual masking levels in pure-tone audiometry. *Arch Otolaryngol* 82, 518–521.

Yacullo WS. 1999. Clinical masking in speech audiometry: A simplified approach. *Am J Audiol* 8, 106–116.

Zwislocki J. 1953. Acoustic attenuation between the ears. *J Acoust Soc Am* 25, 752–759.

Behavioral Tests for Diagnostic Assessment

This chapter deals for the most part with behavioral tests used for identifying the anatomical location ("site") of the abnormality ("lesion") causing the patient's problems—those traditionally referred to as site-of-lesion tests. **Site-of-lesion tests** have to do with *where* the abnormality probably resides. At this juncture it is wise to distinguish between medical and audiological diagnosis. Medical diagnosis involves determining the location of the abnormality and also its etiology, which involves the nature and cause of the pathology, and how it pertains to the patient's health. In this sense, audiological tests contribute to medical diagnosis in at least two ways, depending on who sees the patient first. When the patient sees the audiologist first, they can act as screening tests to identify the possibility of conditions that indicate the need for referral to a physician. If the patient has been referred to the audiologist by a physician, then these tests provide information that assist in arriving at a medical diagnosis. In contrast, audiological diagnosis deals with ascertaining the nature of the patient's auditory problems and their ramifications for dealing with the world of sound in general and communication in particular. Thus, there are areas of overlap and contrast between medical and audiological diagnosis, with each one contributing to the goals of the other.

Audiological site-of-lesion assessment was traditionally viewed in terms of certain special tests that are specifically intended for this purpose, and which were often administered during a follow-up visit called a "site-of-lesion evaluation." However, the student should know from the outset that solving the diagnostic puzzle really starts with the initial interview and case history. After all, this is when we begin to compare the patient's complaints and behaviors with the characteristics of the various clinical entities that might cause them. Moreover, *direct* site-of-lesion assessment is already under way with the pure-tone audiogram (Chapter 5) and routine speech audiometric tests (Chapter 8). To mention just the most overt example of why this is so, recall that we compare the pure-tone air- and bone-conduction thresholds to determine whether the hearing loss is conductive, sensorineural, or mixed. This is the same question as asking whether the problem is located in the conductive mechanism (the outer and/or middle ear), the sensorineural mechanism (the cochlea or eighth nerve), or a combination of the two. In addition, the acoustic immittance tests (Chapter 7) that are part of almost every routine evaluation constitute one of the most powerful audiological diagnostic batteries in and of themselves.

Most of this chapter addresses a class of traditional site-of-lesion tests that involve the patient's behavioral responses, mainly to tonal stimuli. A common thread among many of these tests is that they involve various aspects of the perception of intensity and how it is affected by pathology. They have been used in an attempt to help distinguish cases of sensorineural hearing loss into those where the site-of-lesion is in the cochlea (e.g., Meniere's disease) versus those where the lesion is retrocochlear (e.g., acoustic tumor). However, we shall see that the ability of these kinds of tests to confidently separate between cochlear and retrocochlear disorders is actually rather disappointing. It is therefore not surprising that only a small minority of audiologists routinely use many of these traditional site-of-lesion tests, and that their use has been steadily decreasing over the years (Martin, Champlin, & Chambers, 1998). Also covered in this chapter are behavioral audiological tests used in the assessment of central auditory processing disorders.

Threshold Tone Decay Tests

A continuous pure tone sounds less loud after it has been on for some time compared to when it was first turned on, or it may fade away altogether. The decrease in the tone's loudness over time is usually called **loudness adaptation**, and the situation in which it dies out completely is called **threshold adaptation** or **tone decay**. Adaptation is due to the reduction of the neural response to continuous stimulation over time, and is common to all sensory systems (Marks, 1974). Even though adaptation per se is a normal phenomenon, we shall see that excessive amounts of adaptation reflect the possibility of certain pathologies. It is for this reason that adaptation tests are often used as clinical site-of-lesion tests.

Clinical adaptation procedures are overwhelmingly **threshold tone decay tests**. In other words, they measure adaptation in terms of whether a continuous tone fades away completely within a certain amount of time, usually 60 seconds. The patient's task is easily understood in terms of these typical instructions: "You will hear a continuous tone for a period of time, which might be a few seconds or a few minutes. Raise your finger (or hand) as soon as the tone starts and keep it up as long as the tone is audible. Put your finger down whenever the tone fades away. Pick it up again if the tone comes back, and hold it up as long as you can still hear it. It is very important that you do not say anything or make any sounds during this test because that would interrupt the tone. Remember, don't make any sounds, keep

your finger raised whenever you hear the tone, and down whenever you don't hear it." Because the patient may be holding his hand or finger up for some time, it is a good idea to have him support his elbow on the arm of his chair. Many audiologists have the patient press and release a response signal button instead of holding up and lowering his finger or hand. The audiologist's task is then to present the tones according to the procedure involved in the specific test being done.

Even though Carhart (1957) suggested that tone decay tests (TDTs) be administered to each ear at 500, 1000, 2000, and 4000 Hz, the most common practice is for the audiologist to select the frequencies to be tested on a patient-by-patient basis. Whenever possible, it is desirable to test both ears at each frequency selected because this permits the clinician to compare the two ears as well as to determine whether abnormal tone decay is present bilaterally. Of course, each ear is tested separately.

Carhart Tone Decay Test

In the **Carhart threshold tone decay test** (1957), the continuous test tone is presented to the patient at threshold (0 dB SL) for 60 seconds. If the patient hears the tone for a full minute at the initial level, then the test is over. However, if the patient lowers his finger, indicating that the tone faded away before 60 seconds have passed, then the audiologist (1) increases the intensity by 5 dB without interrupting the tone, and (2) begins timing a new 60-second period as soon as the patient raises his hand. If the tone is heard for a full minute at 5 dB SL, then the test is over. However, if the tone fades away before 60 seconds are up, then the intensity is again raised 5 dB and a new minute is begun. This procedure continues until the patient is able to hear the tone for 60 seconds, or until the maximum limits of the audiometer are reached.

Tone decay test results are expressed as the *amount of tone decay*, which is simply the sensation level at which the tone was heard for 60 seconds. For example, if the tone was heard for one minute at threshold, then there would be 0 dB of tone decay; and if the tone was heard for 60 seconds at 5 dB SL, then there was 5 dB of tone decay. Similarly, if the tone could not be heard for a full minute until the level was raised to 45 dB SL, then there would be 45 dB of tone decay.

Normal individuals and those with conductive abnormalities are expected to have little or no threshold adaptation. Cochlear losses may come with varying degrees of tone decay, which may range up to perhaps 30 dB, but excessive tone decay of ≥35 dB is associated with retrocochlear pathologies (Carhart, 1957; Tillman, 1969; Morales-Garcia & Hood, 1972; Olsen & Noffsinger, 1974; Sanders, Josey, & Glasscock, 1974; Olsen & Kurdziel, 1976). Thus, if the TDT is viewed as a test for retrocochlear involvement, then ≤30 dB of tone decay is usually interpreted as "negative," and >30 dB of tone decay is "positive."

Tone decay test outcomes should be documented separately for each ear in terms of the number of decibels of tone decay at each frequency tested, to which one might add an interpretation (such as positive or negative). One should never record "positive" or "negative" without the actual results. You can always figure out whether a result was positive or negative from the amount of tone decay, but you could never go back and deduce the actual amount of tone decay from a record that says only "positive" or "negative." Moreover, not all clinicians agree on the cutoff point between positive and negative results. Once the actual results have been documented, the manner in which they are formally reported is another matter. Some audiologists report the actual data, others will give an interpretation, and others will give both. Even though these points are made in the context of the Carhart TDT, they apply to all diagnostic procedures.

Olsen-Noffsinger Tone Decay Test

The **Olsen-Noffsinger tone decay test** (1974) is identical to the Carhart TDT except that the test tone is initially presented at 20 dB SL instead of at threshold. Beginning at 20 dB SL is desirable for several reasons. It makes the

test simpler for the patient to take because a 20 dB SL test tone is much easier to detect than one given at threshold. It is also easier to distinguish it from any tinnitus that the patient may have. In addition, starting the test at 20 dB SL can shorten the test time by as much as 4 minutes for every frequency tested. Reducing the test time makes the experience less fatiguing for the patient, and saves clinician time, which is always at a premium. Of course, these benefits would be useless if diagnostic information would be lost. The Olsen-Noffsinger modification relies on the premise that amounts of tone decay up to 20 dB on the Carhart TDT are interpreted as being negative anyway. For this reason, omitting the test trials that would have been given at 0 to +15 dB SL should not change any diagnostic decisions. It has been found that the Carhart and Olsen-Noffsinger procedures yield similar results in terms of when the results are positive and negative (Olsen & Noffsinger, 1974; Olsen & Kurdziel, 1976).

The outcome of the Olsen-Noffsinger TDT is recorded as follows: If the patient hears the initial (20 dB SL) test tone for a full minute, then one records the results as "≤20 dB tone decay." Greater amounts of tone decay are recorded in the same way as for the Carhart TDT.

The Olsen-Noffsinger TDT is sometimes misconstrued as a tone decay "screening" test because most patients are able to hear the initial test tone for the full 60 seconds. It should be stressed that the reason why many patients do not have to be tested beyond the 20 dB SL starting level is simply that they do not have more than 20 dB of tone decay. One should remember that the Olsen-Noffsinger is a full-fledged TDT that yields the actual amount of significant tone decay >20 dB, just like the Carhart procedure.

Other Modifications
of the Carhart Tone Decay Test

There are several other modifications of the Carhart TDT of which the student should be aware. The **Yantis** (1959) **modification** differs from the original only in the sense that testing starts at 5 dB SL instead of at threshold. This modification is so commonly used that it is not distinguished from the Carhart by most clinicians. **Sorensen's (1960, 1962) modification** requires the patient to hear the test tone for 90 seconds instead of 60 seconds, and is only performed at 2000 Hz. This procedure is rarely used.

The **Rosenberg (1958, 1969) modified tone decay test** begins like the Carhart test but lasts only 60 seconds from start to finish. If the patient hears the tone for 60 seconds at threshold, then the test is over and there is 0 dB of tone decay. If the tone fades away before the end of one minute, then the clinician does the following: As with the Carhart TDT, she increases the intensity in 5-dB steps without interrupting the tone until the patient raises his hand. Every time the patient lowers his hand, the audiologist again raises the tone in 5 dB steps until the patient hears the tone again, and so on. However, unlike the Carhart TDT, she does *not* begin timing a new minute with every level increment. Instead, the clock keeps running until a total of 60 seconds has elapsed since the tone was originally turned on. The amount of tone decay is the sensation level reached at the end of 60 seconds. For example, if the threshold was 35 dB HL, the tone starts at this level and one begins timing for 60 seconds. If the attenuator has been raised by a total of 25 dB to 60 dB HL at the end of one minute, then there has been 25 dB of tone decay. Notice that the Rosenberg modification only considers the sensation level reached at the end of one minute, and ignores how long the tone was actually heard at any given level.

Green's (1963) modified tone decay test involves administering the Rosenberg one-minute test with a significant change in the instructions. The patient is told to lower his hand completely if the tone fades away and to lower his hand partially if the tone loses its tonal quality (even though it might still be audible). The modified instructions are based on the observation that some patients with retrocochlear pathologies hear a change

in the character of the tone in which it loses its tonal quality, becoming noise-like, before its audibility is completely lost (Pestalozza & Cioce, 1962; Sorensen, 1962; Green, 1963). This phenomenon of **atonality** is also called **tone perversion** (Parker & Dekker, 1971).

Owens Tone Decay Test

Owens (1964a) introduced a modification of a tone decay procedure originated by Hood (1955). Unlike the Carhart test and its modifications, which concentrate on the amount of adaptation, the **Owens tone decay test** focuses upon the *pattern* of tone decay. The test begins by presenting a continuous test tone at 5 dB SL. As with the Carhart TDT, the Owens test ends if the patient hears the tone for 60 seconds at this initial level. However, the Owens procedure differs from the Carhart TDT if the tone fades away before 60 seconds. When this happens, the tone is turned off for a 20-second rest (recovery) period. After the 20-second rest, the tone is reintroduced at 10 dB SL (i.e., 5 dB higher), and a new 60-second period is begun. If the tone is heard for a full minute at 10 dB SL, then the test is over. However, if the tone fades away before a full minute, then the tone is turned off for another 20-second rest period, after which it is given again at 15 dB SL. The same procedure is followed for the 15 dB SL tone. If necessary, the tone is presented for another one-minute period at 20 dB SL, but this is the last level tested regardless of whether the tone is heard for 60 seconds or less. The audiologist records the number of seconds that the tone was heard at each of the levels presented, and the test is interpreted in terms of the pattern of how many seconds the tone was heard at each of the four test levels.

Figure 10–1 shows the various patterns (types) of tone decay described by Owens (1964a). The type I pattern involves being able to hear the initial (5 dB SL) tone for a full minute, and is associated with normal ears and those with cochlear impairments.

There are five type II patterns, called II-A through II-E. As the lengths of the bars in the

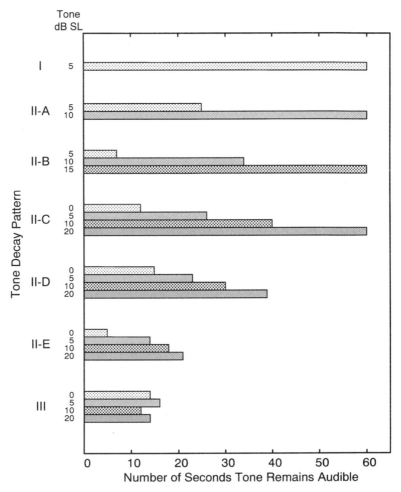

FIGURE 10–1 Tone decay patterns on the Owens tone decay test. Based on data by Owens (1964a).

figure show, the type II patterns share two characteristics: (1) the tone fades away before 60 seconds for at least the lowest sensation level, and (2) the tone is heard progressively longer at increasingly higher sensation levels. The tone is finally heard for a full minute at 10 dB SL in type II-A, at 15 dB in type II-B, and at 20 dB SL in type II-C. In the type II-D pattern, the patient is unable to hear the tone for a full minute at any of the four sensation levels tested, but it does remain audible for appreciably longer periods of time with each successively higher sensation level. Cochlear impairments are most commonly associated with types II-A through II-D.

In the type II-E pattern each 5-dB rise in sensation level produces only a small increase in how long the tone is heard (averaging 4 to 7 seconds per 5-dB level). This pattern is found in either cochlear or retrocochlear abnormalities.

The type III pattern is principally associated with retrocochlear disorders. Here, increasing the sensation level does not cause the tone to be heard for longer periods of time.

Rate of Tone Decay

Wiley and Lilly (1980) proposed a modification of the Owens TDT in which (1) the rest period between tones is reduced to 10 seconds, and (2) the test level continues to be raised until the tone remains audible for a full minute (or the audiometer's maximum level is reached). This modification allowed them to distinguish between the rates of tone decay in the two ears of a patient who had a cochlear disorder in one ear and an acoustic tumor in the other ear. The importance of looking at the rate of tone decay was also shown by Silman, Gelfand, Lutolf, and Chun (1981) in a patient whose hearing loss was so severe that the Owens TDT was the only usable tone decay method.

Overall Assessment of Threshold Tone Decay Tests

Tone decay appears to be the only classical site-of-lesion technique that is still routinely used by a majority of audiologists (Martin, Champlin, & Chambers, 1998). Several studies have compared the accuracy of threshold adaptation tests as indicators of retrocochlear pathology (e.g., Parker & Dekker, 1971; Olsen & Noffsinger, 1974; Sanders, Josey, & Glasscock, 1974). Overall, they have shown the Carhart TDT to be the most sensitive of these procedures. This appears to hold true whether the test is begun at threshold, or with the modifications that begin at 5 dB SL (Yantis, 1959) or 20 dB SL (Olsen & Noffsinger, 1974). This kind of tone decay test is thus the one of choice, with the Olsen-Noffsinger modification being the most efficient. The Owens TDT is particularly valuable when the severity of a hearing loss makes it impossible to determine the amount of tone decay using the Carhart or similar procedures (Silman, Gelfand, Lutolf, & Chun, 1981). In contrast, the Rosenberg one-minute TDT is not as effective in revealing the presence of retrocochlear lesions as the Carhart, Olsen-Noffsinger, or Owens procedures (Parker & Dekker, 1971; Olsen & Noffsinger, 1974), and is not recommended. Green's modification of the Rosenberg TDT has not been compared to other tests that do not use the atonality criterion, and we have just seen that the one-minute

approach itself is lacking in its ability to identify retrocochlear disorders compared to other tone decay tests. There is no clear answer to the question of whether atonality per se should be used as a criterion for tone decay testing in general because little if any research actually addresses this issue. It does appear that more tone decay can be obtained when the patient responds to either atonality or inaudibility compared to inaudibility alone, but this apparent advantage is not without cost. The experience of the author and his colleagues (see Silman & Silverman, 1991) has been that using the atonality criterion increases the number of false-positive TDT results, and this is especially problematic when testing elderly patients. Even though several earlier papers suggest accounting for the loss of tonal quality (e.g., Sorenson, 1962; Pestalozza & Cioce, 1962; Flottorp, 1963; Johnson, 1966; Sung, Goetzinger, & Knox, 1969; Olsen & Noffsinger, 1974), only about 10% of audiologists continue to use the atonality criterion (Martin, Woodrick Armstrong, & Champlin, 1994).

As a group, threshold TDTs have been reported to correctly indicate the presence of retrocochlear lesions among anywhere from 64 to 95% of the cases, and have correctly classified nonretrocochlear disorders about 77 to 96% of the time (Owens, 1964a; Gjaevenes & Sohoel, 1969; Tillman, 1969; Olsen & Noffsinger, 1974; Sanders, Josey, & Glasscock, 1974; Olsen & Kurdziel, 1976; Anatonelli, Bellotto, & Grandori, 1987; Josey, 1987). Part of the variability in these values comes from differences in which tone decay tests were used, how they were administered and interpreted, and also from differences in the patient populations. Turner, Shepard, and Frazer (1984) have shown that TDT results are correct in an average of 70% of retrocochlear cases and 87% for ears that do not have retrocochlear lesions, across studies.

Suprathreshold Adaptation Test

Jerger and Jerger (1975a) suggested a tone decay test performed at high levels instead of beginning at threshold, called the **supra-**

threshold adaptation test (STAT). The procedure of the STAT is remarkably simple. A continuous test tone lasting a total of 60 seconds is presented at 110 dB SPL. (This corresponds to about 105 dB HL when the test is done at 1000 Hz, and to 100 dB HL when testing at 500 Hz or 2000 Hz). As for threshold tone decay tests, the patient is told to keep her hand raised as long as she hears the tone, and to lower her hand if it fades away completely. If the high-intensity tone is heard for the full minute, then the test is over and the result is negative. The result is tentatively considered positive if the tone fades away before 60 seconds are up, in which case the patient is retested with a pulsing tone for confirmatory purposes. If the patient keeps her hand up for the full 60 seconds in response to the pulsing tone, then her failure to keep responding to the continuous tone is attributed to abnormal adaptation. The test is thus confirmed to be positive, and is considered to suggest a retrocochlear disorder. However, if she fails to respond to the pulsing tone for one minute, then the test result is not considered to be valid because tone decay should not occur with a pulsed tone. (Because of the high level used, the procedure also calls for presenting a 90 dB SPL broadband masking noise to the opposite ear.) The rates of correct identification for cochlear and retrocochlear cases, respectively, are 100% and 45% when the STAT is done at 500 and 1000 Hz, 95% and 54% at 500 to 2000 Hz, and 13% and 70% at 500 to 4000 Hz (Jerger & Jerger, 1975a; Turner, Shepard, & Frazer, 1984).

Loudness Recruitment and Loudness Balance Testing

Loudness Recruitment

We all have had the experience of being told to "speak up" by a hearing-impaired relative. Upon complying with this request, we are then told to "stop shouting." This common experience reveals an important facet of many cochlear impairments: Even though more intensity (i.e., a higher than normal

HL) is needed for a sound to be heard, once the sound is raised above this elevated threshold, the now higher-intensity sound is as loud to the patient as it would be to a normal-hearing person. Consider a normal person whose threshold for a tone is 0 dB HL and a patient whose threshold is 50 dB HL for the same tone. If the tone is raised to 80 dB HL, it will now be 80 dB above the normal person's threshold but only 30 dB above the patient's threshold. Yet, the tone will sound *as loud* to the patient (at 30 dB SL) as it does to the normal individual (at 80 dB SL). For this patient, the 30 dB level increase was perceived to have *increased in loudness* by an amount that took an 80 dB level increase for the normal person. In other words, the patient has experienced an abnormally rapid growth of loudness. This is called **loudness recruitment.**

When there is a sensorineural hearing loss, loudness recruitment is associated with a cochlear site-of-lesion, whereas the absence of loudness recruitment is associated with retrocochlear pathologies (Dix, Hallpike, & Hood, 1948; Hallpike & Hood, 1951, 1959; Jerger, 1961; Hallpike, 1965; Davis & Goodman, 1966; Hood, 1969; Priede & Coles, 1974; Coles & Priede, 1976).

Alternate Binaural Loudness Balance (ABLB) Test

The nature of the **Alternate Binaural Loudness Balance (ABLB) test** (Fowler, 1936) is described by its name. A tone is presented *alternately* between the two ears (*binaurally*). The level of the tone stays the same in one ear (the "fixed" ear), but is varied up and/or down in the other ear (the "variable" ear), as shown schematically in Figure 10–2. The patient is asked to report when the tone sounds louder in the right ear, when it is louder in the left ear, and when it sounds equally loud in both ears. We say that a loudness balance has been obtained when the patient indicates that the tones sound equally loud in both ears. The tester then records the two levels (in dB HL) where the loudness balance occurred.

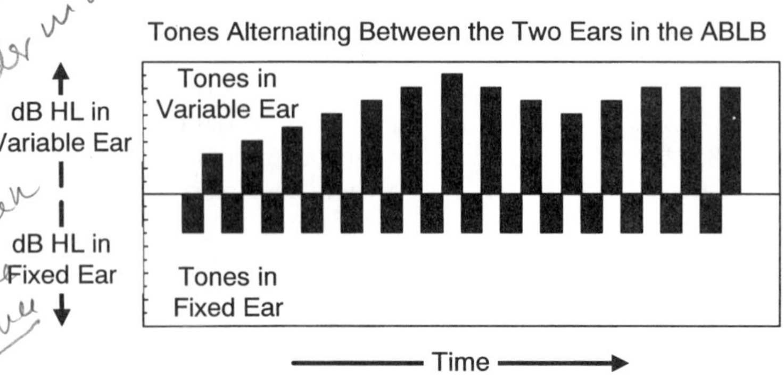

[handwritten margin notes: ABLB a tone to one ear when is louder in one ear. Till the person report equally balance then we obtain the balance ... louder]

Tones Alternating Between the Two Ears in the ABLB

FIGURE 10–2 Schematic representation of the Alternate Binaural Loudness Balance (ABLB) Test, showing a tone being presented alternately between the two ears. Its level is fixed in one ear and is variable in the other ear.

Because the ABLB compares one ear to the other, it is a good idea to see what happens in the situation where the two ears are exactly the same in a normal hearing person. Suppose we obtained a series of loudness balances at the same frequency in 20 dB intervals from a person with normal hearing. For purposes of discussion, the right ear was the fixed ear, and the left ear was the variable ear. The results might look something like this:

dB in Right	dB in Left	
0	0	(thresholds)
20	20	(loudness balance)
40	40	(loudness balance)
60	60	(loudness balance)
80	80	(loudness balance)
100	100	(loudness balance)

Notice that 20 dB HL in the right ear sounded as loud as 20 dB HL in the left ear, 40 dB HL in the right ear was just as loud as 40 dB HL in the left ear, etc. Also see that 0 dB HL in the right ear (its threshold) sounds as loud as 0 dB HL in the left ear (its threshold). We do not actually perform loudness balances at threshold. Instead, we simply assume that when the two ears are at threshold they must be equally loud.

Although ABLB results can be recorded numerically as just shown, it is more common to plot the results in one of the two ways shown in Figure 10–3. The diagram on the left side of the figure is called a **laddergram** for obvious reasons. Hearing level is shown

going down the y-axis just as on an audiogram. For each loudness balance, we draw a circle at the hearing level in the right ear and an X at the hearing level for the left ear, then join the two symbols with a line to show they are equally loud. Horizontal lines ("rungs") on the laddergram indicate equal loudness occurs at the same intensity for both ears. Another way to show the results is to plot them on an x-y graph such as the one shown on the right side of the figure. This is called a **Steinberg-Gardner plot**. Each point shows the coordinates of the levels in the two ears that sounded equally loud. In this case, all of the points fall along a diagonal line because there was a one-to-one relationship between the equally loud levels in the two ears. Whenever the points fall along this 45° line, it means that equal intensities sound equally loud.

CLINICAL USE OF THE ABLB

[handwritten note: use ABLB]

The ABLB is used clinically to determine whether loudness recruitment is present in the abnormal ear of a patient who has a unilateral hearing loss. Loudness balances are made between the patient's abnormal ear and his normal ear. Normal thresholds are needed in the better ear because the ABLB works by comparing loudnesses between the two ears. After all, if we are trying to find out whether loudness is growing at a faster than normal rate in the abnormal ear by comparing it to the other ear, then we must know

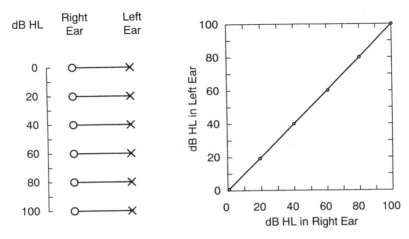

FIGURE 10–3   Loudness balance results for a normal hearing person shown on a ladder-gram (left) and on a Steinberg-Gardner plot (right). When equal intensities are equally loud, points are joined by a horizontal line on the laddergram and fall along the 45° line on the Steinberg-Gardner plot.

that loudness is growing at a normal rate in the other ear. The only way we can validly make this assumption is to require the threshold to be normal in the opposite ear at the frequencies being tested. Further, the threshold of the abnormal ear should be at least 35 dB HL at each frequency tested.

TYPES OF RECRUITMENT

Suppose a patient has a threshold of 0 dB HL in his normal right ear and 45 dB HL in his abnormal left ear at the frequency we are testing with the ABLB. Since we assume that loudnesses are equal at threshold, this means that 0 dB HL in the right ear sounds as loud as 45 dB HL in the left ear. For simplicity, this will be the starting point in all of our examples. The abnormal left ear will be used as the fixed ear and the normal right ear will be the variable ear, and we will do loudness balances in 20-dB increments. In other words, we will adjust the level of the tone in the right ear until it balances in loudness with a 65 dB HL tone in the left ear, after which we will repeat the procedure at 85 dB HL in the fixed ear, and finally at 105 dB in the fixed ear.

Complete Recruitment   Because the ABLB is principally a test for loudness recruitment, let us first see what the results are like when

recruitment is present. Complete recruitment occurs when the loudness balances at higher levels occur at the same intensities in both ears, that is, when equal intensities sound equally loud. This is what occurred in the earlier example, where the thresholds were 0 dB HL in the good ear and 50 dB HL in the bad ear, and yet 80 dB HL sounded equally loud in both ears.

Complete recruitment on the ABLB is shown in Figure 10–4a. Here, even though the thresholds are 0 dB HL and 45 dB HL, equal loudness is eventually obtained when both ears receive 105 dB HL. In practice, recruitment is generally considered complete if equal loudness occurs at equal hearing levels (dB HL) ±10 dB (Jerger, 1962). This is shown by the flattening of the rungs on the laddergram. In this example, a 60-dB rise (from 45 to 105 dB HL) in the abnormal ear sounds like a 105-dB rise (from 0 to 105 dB HL) in the normal ear. In terms of sensation level, 60 dB SL in the bad ear sounds as loud as 105 dB SL in the good ear (Fig. 10–5a).

Complete recruitment is easily seen on the Steinberg-Gardner plot (Fig. 10–4a), which plots the level in the abnormal ear on the x-axis and the equally loud level in the good ear on the y-axis. The normal one-to-one loudness-growth relationship is shown by a 45° line for comparison purposes. Any points

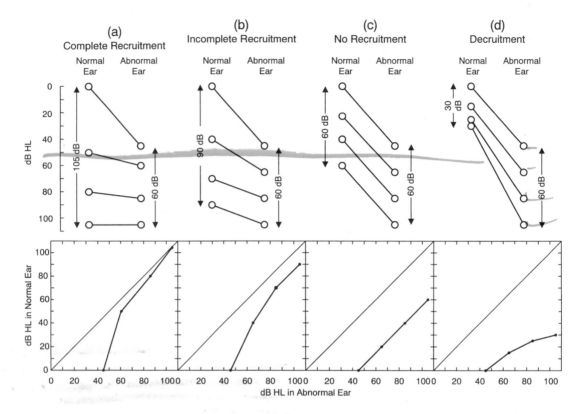

FIGURE 10–4 Laddergrams (above) and Steinberg-Gardner plots (below) for examples of (a) complete recruitment, (b) incomplete (partial) recruitment, (c) no recruitment, and (d) decruitment.

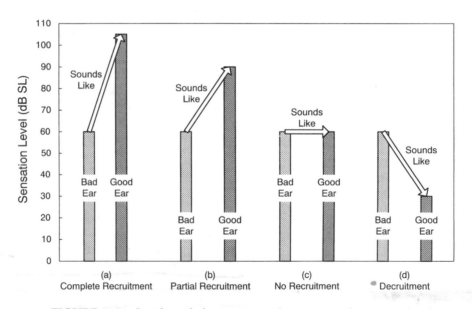

FIGURE 10–5 Loudness balance test results in terms of sensation levels.

that fall on this diagonal indicate that equal intensities sound equally loud. The plot of the test results begins 45 dB to the right (i.e., x = 45, y = 0) because the thresholds are 45 dB in the abnormal ear and 0 dB in the normal ear, but it rises at a sharp angle and eventually meets the 45° line at the point corresponding to 105 dB HL in both ears. The steeply rising line on the Steinberg-Gardner diagram gives a clear picture of what we mean when we say that recruitment is an abnormally rapid growth of loudness. As already pointed out, complete recruitment suggests a cochlear site-of-lesion.

Hyper-recruitment Some patients with Meniere's disease may exhibit a special case of recruitment in which the loudness in the abnormal ear not only catches up with the normal ear, but actually overtakes it (Dix, Hallpike, & Hood, 1948; Hallpike & Hood, 1959; Hood, 1977). This finding is called **hyper-recruitment (or over-recruitment)**, and is shown in Figure 10–6. Hyper-recruitment is revealed on the laddergram by rungs that first flatten and then reverse direction. In this example, 85 dB HL in the abnormal ear actually sounds as loud as 100 dB HL in the normal ear. The same effect is shown on the Steinberg-Gardner diagram when the line that shows the patient's equal loudness judgments crosses above the diagonal line. One

should note that hyper-recruitment is somewhat of a controversial issue, and the likelihood of finding it seems to be affected by how the ABLB test is carried out (Hood, 1969, 1977; Coles & Priede, 1976).

Incomplete Recruitment **Incomplete** (or **partial**) **recruitment** refers to results that fall between complete recruitment and no recruitment (discussed below). This is shown as a partial flattening of the laddergram or by a line that rises toward but does not quite reach the diagonal on the Steinberg-Gardner plot. An example is shown in Figures 10–4b and 10–5b. Audiologists are inconsistent about how they interpret incomplete recruitment, and it is not surprising that the diagnostic value of this result has been questioned (Priede & Coles, 1974).

No Recruitment **No recruitment** occurs when the relationship between the levels at the two ears is the same for the loudness balances as it is at threshold. An example is shown in Figures 10–4c and 10–5c. Here, same 45-dB spread that exists between the left and right thresholds is also found for each of the loudness balances. This is shown by the parallel lines on the laddergram. The situation is even clearer on the Steinberg-Gardner plot. In spite of the threshold differ-

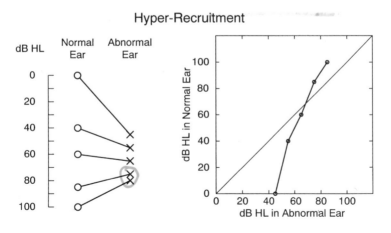

Hyper-Recruitment

FIGURE 10–6   An example of hyper-recruitment (over-recruitment).

ence between the ears, the line showing equally loud levels rises at a 45° angle just like the normal line. This shows that the spread between the two ears is maintained at high levels. It also means that a 20-dB-level increase in the abnormal ear sounds just as loud as a 20-dB-level increase in the normal ear, that is, loudness is growing at the same rate with intensity in both ears. Consequently, loudness must be growing at the normal rate in the abnormal ear. As a practical guideline, one might say that there is no recruitment if equal loudness occurs at equal sensation levels (dB SL) ± (10 dB (Jerger, 1962).

No recruitment is the expected result when the loss in the abnormal ear is conductive. In fact, Fowler (1936) originally conceived of the ABLB as a test to distinguish between otosclerosis (a conductive disorder) and sensorineural hearing losses. However, the ABLB is not used with conductive losses because its actual purpose is to help to distinguish between cochlear and retrocochlear disorders. Thus, finding no recruitment in a case of unilateral sensorineural loss is the same as failing to argue in favor of a cochlear disorder. By inference, this would lead us to suspect retrocochlear pathology.

Decruitment   In some cases, loudness grows at a slower than normal rate as intensity increases in the abnormal ear. This is called **decruitment** (Davis & Goodman, 1966) or **loudness reversal** (Priede & Coles, 1974), and is associated with retrocochlear pathology. In the example shown in Figure 10–4d, 105 dB HL in the bad ear sounds only as loud as 30 dB HL in the good ear. In other words, 60 dB SL in the abnormal ear sounds like only 30 dB SL in the normal ear (Fig. 10–5d). In effect, decruitment means that loudness is lost rather than gained as intensity is raised.

ABLB Testing Approaches

Different procedures have been suggested for administering the ABLB. Jerger's (1962) protocol has the following major components: The tone alternates between the ears automatically every 500 msec (as in Fig.

10–2), with the fixed level in the abnormal ear and the variable signal in the normal ear. The patient changes the intensity of the tone in the variable ear using the method of adjustment (see Chapter 3) until it sounds equal in loudness to the tone in the fixed ear. Loudness balances are made at 20-dB intervals above the bad ear's threshold, and are plotted on a laddergram.

One should note that because the tone alternates between the two ears every 500 msec, it will be off for 500 msec in each ear. This off-time ensures that the test tones will not be subject to adaptation. This requirement is met if the tone is off for at least a certain critical off-time, which is about 200 to 250 msec (Dallos & Tillman, 1966; Jerger & Jerger, 1966; Tillman, 1966).

In contrast to Jerger's approach, Hood (1969, 1977) suggested manual control over the presentation of the tones according to the method of limits (see Chapter 3), using the good ear as fixed-level ear, and plotting the results on a Steinberg-Gardner diagram. Others have suggested presenting the fixed level tone to the bad ear and testing according to Hood's method (Priede & Coles, 1974; Coles & Priede, 1976), or randomizing the use of the good and bad ears as the fixed-level ear under computer control (Fritze, 1978).

In the author's experience, ABLB techniques vary widely among audiologists, many of whom use one or more hybrid techniques. For example, one might use automatically alternating tones with the fixed level in the bad ear, a modified method of limits or bracketing, and have the patient respond with hand signals, or by saying "right," "left," or "equal."

An interesting ABLB modification was proposed by Miskolczy-Fodor (1964). In this approach, the level of the tone in the "fixed" ear increases over time, so that this ear may be considered a reference ear. The patient uses the Bekesy tracking method (see below) to keep the level in the variable ear equally loud as the one in the reference ear, and the results are automatically plotted on paper. Figure 10–7 shows an example. Carver (1970) and Gelfand (1976) found that accurate loudness

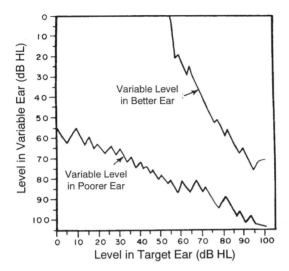

FIGURE 10–7 In Miskolczy-Fodor's modification of the ABLB, the level in the reference ("target") ear steadily rises instead of remaining fixed. The level in the variable ear is kept equally loud with the reference ear using a Bekesy tracking technique. Loudness balance tracings are shown here when the good ear is the reference, and when the poor ear is the reference. From Gelfand (1976), with permission.

balances with this method require combining two sets of results, one using the good ear as the reference and one using the bad ear. Otherwise, it over- or underestimates the loudness balance points that would be obtained using the fixed-level ABLB. Other variations have also been reported (Sung & Sung, 1976).

Simultaneous versus Alternate Loudness Balance The ABLB involves presenting the test tones alternately between the ears. This must be distinguished from presenting the tones to the two ears at the same time, which is called the **simultaneous binaural loudness balance test**. Jerger and Harford (1960) showed that the results of the alternate and simultaneous balance tests disagree in terms of which intensities are "equally loud" at the two ears. This happens because the two methods are testing two different things. The alternate balance yields the levels that sound equally loud at the two ears. In contrast, the

simultaneous test is really a lateralization task. In other words, presenting simultaneous tones to the two ears causes the patient to hear a single, fused image somewhere in the head between the left and right ears. Rather than showing the levels that cause the two sounds to be equally loud, the simultaneous test really shows the levels that cause the fused image to be lateralized in the middle of the head (a "median-plane localization"). Consequently, one should not use simultaneous balances to measure equal loudness between the ears.

Alternate Monaural Loudness Balance Test
The ABLB often cannot be done because (1) it requires a normal ear (or at least an ear with normal hearing at the frequency being tested), and (2) most people with sensorineural losses have bilateral impairments. This dilemma has been addressed with the **alternate monaural loudness balance (AMLB) test** (Reger, 1935). The AMLB is procedurally the same as the ABLB except that the loudness balance is done for *two different tones within the same ear*. Consider for example a patient with a bilateral loss that slopes sharply above 1000 Hz. The thresholds in one of her ears might be 0 dB HL at 500 Hz and 50 dB at 2000 Hz. In such a case, 500 Hz and 2000 Hz tones might be alternately presented to the same ear. The level would remain fixed at one frequency, and the level at the other frequency would be varied up and down until the two tones sound equally loud. Even though AMLB results are interpreted in the same general way as for the ABLB, a correction is needed to account for the loudness level differences (Chapter 3) that occur between frequencies (Denes & Naunton, 1950). Moreover, the interfrequency loudness balance task tends to be difficult for many patients. The AMLB is rarely used because of these problems.

DIAGNOSTIC ACCURACY OF THE ABLB

We can consider the ABLB from the standpoint of how well it distinguishes between cochlear disorders (where there should be recruitment) and retrocochlear pathologies (where there should be no recruitment or decruitment). The ABLB has been found to identify the correct site-of-lesion in about 90% for cochlear disorders and only about 59% for retrocochlear pathologies across studies (Turner, Shepard, & Frazer, 1984). These figures show that many acoustic tumor cases are misclassified as cochlear on the basis of having positive recruitment. It is possible that some retrocochlear cases might have recruitment or other characteristics of cochlear disorders (e.g., high SISI scores, see below) because of *secondary damage* to the cochlea (Dix & Hallpike, 1958; Benitez, Lopez-Rios, & Novon, 1967; Perez de Moura, 1967; Buus, Florentine, & Redden, 1982a). The basic concept involves these two steps: (1) the tumor damages the cochlea by putting pressure on its blood supply and/or adversely altering the chemistry of the cochlear fluids; and (2) the resulting cochlear disorder then produces positive recruitment. Also, there may well be a coexisting cochlear disorder having nothing to do with retrocochlear pathology. For example, a patient with an acoustic tumor may well have a noise-induced cochlear impairment. These points apply to the results of other site-of-lesion tests, as well.

Direct Loudness Scaling

The clinical use of direct scaling methods (see Chapter 3) such as magnitude estimation and magnitude production, as well as cross-modality matching, has been attempted by several researchers (Geller & Margolis, 1984; Knight & Margolis, 1984; Hellman & Meiselman, 1988, 1990). Even though these are advanced approaches that are not in general clinical use, the student should be aware of their existence because they appear to have promise as methods to assess loudness in patients with bilateral hearing losses.

Loudness Discomfort and Tolerance Tests

It has been known for a very long time that many patients with recruiting hearing losses complain that high-level sounds are uncomfortably loud. In the past, this relationship was sometimes assessed with a tuning fork test. After establishing the presence of a hearing loss, the clinician would strike the tuning fork very hard (so that it produced a high-intensity sound) and immediately place it near the impaired ear. If the patient perceived the sound to be extremely (uncomfortably) loud in spite of his hearing loss, then the test was considered to reflect "nerve deafness."

In the modern version of this approach, the clinician uses the patient's loudness discomfort level (LDL) to infer the presence of loudness recruitment. This can be done using tones, narrow-band noises, or speech. The audiologist obtains the patient's LDL and compares it to the normal range of LDLs, which is roughly 90 to 105 dB HL (Hood & Poole, 1966). Loudness recruitment is considered to be present if the LDL is obtained at these normal levels, in which case the result is considered to be consistent with a cochlear impairment. Obtaining the LDL at much higher levels is considered to indicate no recruitment, which would occur when the sensorineural loss is of retrocochlear origin. Another version of the test is to obtain the most comfortable listening level (MCL) as well as the LDL. In this case, recruitment is considered to be present when the LDL is close to the MCL.

Even though such tests of loudness tolerance do provide the audiologist with some insight into whether the patient has recruitment, they are gross assessments at best and are also subject to considerable amounts of variability. Perhaps more importantly, these tests rely on the faulty assumption that the LDL is not related to the amount of hearing loss. It has been shown that LDLs get higher as the amount of sensorineural hearing loss increases above approximately 50 dB HL (Kamm, Dirks, & Mickey, 1978). This means that the LDL is not an acceptable loudness recruitment test.

Intensity Difference Limen Tests

Recall from Chapter 3 that the smallest difference in intensity that can be perceived is called the **intensity difference limen (DLI)**. The DLI is smaller than normal in patients who also have loudness recruitment, and thus several DLI tests have found their way into and out of clinical use over the years. All of these tests assess one ear at a time, so they can be used with either bilateral or unilateral hearing losses.

The traditional DLI tests used one of two methods to test for the smallest perceptible intensity difference. In the **Lüscher-Zwislocki test** (1949) the patient heard an *amplitude modulated (AM) tone* at 40 dB SL. An AM tone is one that warbles or undulates in level at a regular rate such as twice per second, as represented in Figure 10–8a. The patient was asked to listen to this tone and to indicate whether it sounded continuous or if it seemed to undulate in level. This boils down to whether she can discern the intensity difference between the peaks and troughs of the undulating tone, which is called the amount of amplitude modulation. The smallest amount of AM that could be detected was thus the patient's difference limen for intensity. The DLIs were smaller for patients who had recruitment than for those without recruitment. This test was originally done at 40 dB SL, but modifications of the test have been done at ≤ 80 dB HL (Lüscher, 1951) and at 15 dB SL (Jerger, 1952).

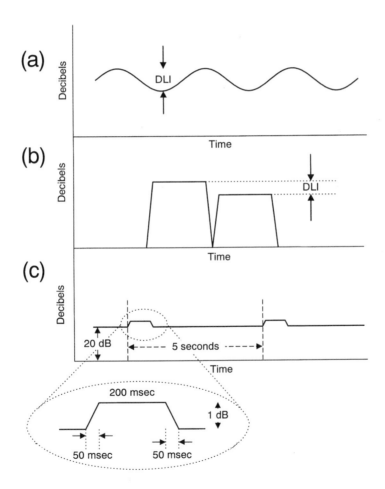

FIGURE 10–8 In the traditional difference limen tests, the intensity difference limen (DLI) was determined by finding the smallest perceptible difference between (a) the peaks and troughs of an amplitude modulated (AM) tone, or (b) the levels of two tones presented one after the other. (c) In the short increment sensitivity index (SISI) test, the patient has to detect 1-dB increments that are superimposed on a carrier tone.

The other approach to DLI testing was used in the **Denes-Naunton test** (1950). Here the patient was presented with a pair of tones, one after the other, and had to decide whether they were equal or if one was louder than the other (Fig. 10–8b). Many pairs of tones were presented to the patient. In order to find the DLI, the first tone was always kept at the same level, but the second tone would be changed in level (or vice versa). The procedure continued until the tester found the smallest level difference that the patient could detect. This was done for tone pairs presented at 4 dB SL and at 44 dB SL. Instead of concentrating on the absolute size of the DLI, the Denes-Naunton test was interpreted by comparing the relative sizes of the DLIs obtained at these two SLs. Intensity DLs were found to stay the same or get larger going from 4 dB SL to 44 dB SL in ears with recruitment. On the other hand, the DLIs were smaller at the higher SL in ears without recruitment. An interesting modification introduced by Jerger (1953) combined testing at two levels (10 and 40 dB SL) with the simpler-to-do AM procedure.

The use of these earlier DLI tests came to an almost abrupt halt after the appearance of a report by Hirsh, Palva, and Goodman (1954). They found similar DLIs among recruiting, nonrecruiting, and normal ears, and objected to the use of the DLI as a measure of recruitment on theoretical grounds. The discrepancies between their findings and those described above may partly be due to the fact that the different methods of measuring the DLI resulted in dissimilar results. [The interested student might see the discussions in Buus, Florentine, and Redden (1982a,b) or Gelfand (1998) in this regard.] There is also support for the distinction between the DLI and loudness recruitment (Lamore & Rodenburg, 1980). However, the DLI-recruitment controversy also diverted the focus of the diagnostic issue, which has more to do with distinguishing between cochlear and retrocochlear sites-of-lesion than with whether abnormally small DLIs are akin to loudness recruitment.

Short Increment Sensitivity Index

The DLI issue was refocused by Jerger, Shedd, and Harford (1959), who pointed out that the ability to detect small intensity differences is useful in the differential diagnosis among hearing disorders no matter what the DLI-recruitment relation may or may not be. They also substantially modified the nature of the intensity discrimination test, making the task easier for the patient to take, and easier for the clinician to administer and interpret. The result was a clinical test called the **short increment sensitivity index (SISI)**. Unlike the earlier tests, the SISI does not attempt to directly measure the size of the patient's DLI. Instead, it presents the patient with increments having a predetermined size of (usually) 1 dB, and simply asks the patient to indicate if she can hear them.

The basic structure of the SISI is depicted in Figure 10–8c, which shows that the stimulus in the SISI has two aspects. The first component is an ongoing tone that stays on for the entire duration of the test. This ongoing tone is called the carrier tone and is presented at 20 dB SL. The second element of the stimulus is a short-duration intensity increment of 1 dB that is superimposed on top of the carrier tone. Each 1-dB pulse is 200 msec long (between rise and fall times of 50 msec each). A total of 20 of these 1-dB pulses are superimposed on the carrier tone, spaced at 5-second intervals. The patient simply listens to the carrier tone and indicates whenever these brief pulses are heard. The patient responds with a hand signal or by pressing a button.

Several 5-dB pulses, which are easily detected by almost everybody, are also presented during the SISI test. They are used at the start of the test to demonstrate the stimulus and to ensure that the patient knows how to respond appropriately. It is sometimes helpful to use a familiarization/training strategy that begins with a 5-dB pulse, and then to reduce the sizes of the pips 1 dB at a time until reaching the 1-dB test increments (Harford, 1967). A few other 5-dB pulses are scattered among the 1-dB increments to make sure the patient continues to respond properly. This is especially important when a patient is missing many or all of the 1-dB increments. In addition, several "catch trials" are distributed among the 1-dB pips over the course of the test. A catch trial is the *absence* of a pulse that occurs at a 5-second interval where a 1-dB pulse would have been presented. This helps to ensure that the patient is responding to the increments and not to just the expectation of a pulse every 5 seconds. These "nonpulses" are especially important when the patient is responding to many or all of the 1-dB increments. The 5-dB and empty trials are important for the proper administration of the SISI test because they provide the clinician with guidance about the validity of the results, and often indicate when it is necessary to reinstruct the patient or to make some other change. However, it should be remembered that only the 20 one-dB pulses are used to score the test.

The SISI test is scored by simply counting how many of the 20 one-dB increments were heard, and expressing the result in percent. For example, a SISI score of 100% means that all 20 pulses were heard, and a score of 40% means that only 8 of them were detected. The percentage scoring system is straightforward and also recognizes that test outcomes usually fall along a continuum.

The fundamental principle of the SISI test is that a patient should be more or less likely to hear the 1-dB increments depending on the status of the ear being tested. Many of the pulses are expected to be heard if the ear being tested has a cochlear disorder. On the other hand, fewer of the increments should be detected if the test ear has a retrocochlear disorder, a conductive loss, or normal hearing. Presuming the test is done when there is a sensorineural hearing loss, this boils down to a distinction between cochlear and retrocochlear sites-of-lesion. Scores 70% on the SISI are usually considered "positive" or "high," and suggest a cochlear site-of-lesion. Scores that are ≤30% are called "negative" or "low," and suggest retrocochlear involvement if there is a sensorineural hearing loss. Results falling between these ranges are generally considered to be "questionable." How-

ever, the student should be aware that other cutoff values have been proposed over the years, none of which is universally accepted.

As expected, Jerger, Shedd, and Harford (1959) found that the SISI scores of eight patients with Meniere's disease were 70 to 100% at 1000 Hz and 95 to 100% at 4000 Hz, but were 0% at both frequencies for three retrocochlear cases. Also as expected, SISI scores were only 0% to 15% for conductive losses. A noteworthy configuration of SISI scores was found among patients who had high-frequency sensorineural losses due to noise exposure. They had low scores (0 to 40%) at 1000 Hz where their thresholds were normal, and high scores (95 to 100%) at 4000 Hz where their thresholds were elevated. In their case, the low scores at 1000 Hz were the correct outcomes associated with normal sensitivity and not a false indication of retrocochlear impairment. Presbycusic patients, whose thresholds ranged between 0 and 65 dB HL at 1000 Hz and 30 and 75 dB HL at 4000 Hz, had SISI scores anywhere from 0 to 100% at both frequencies. The wide range of scores for these patients with age-related hearing loss probably reflected the effects of both their widely disparate thresholds and also the variety of the underlying disturbances that can cause presbycusis.

The percentages of cochlear and retrocochlear disorders that are correctly identified by the SISI were calculated across studies by Buus, Florentine, and Redden (1982a) and by Turner, Shepard, and Frazer (1984). Their findings show that about 77 to 84% of cochlear impairments are correctly identified by high SISI scores, while 60 to 65% of retrocochlear disorders are correctly revealed by low SISI scores. Only about 5 to 10% of the ears with either site-of-lesion have SISI scores in the "questionable" range (Buus, Florentine, & Redden, 1982a).

High-Level SISI

Several reports have suggested that the SISI does a better job of revealing retrocochlear impairments when the test is given at higher intensity levels, typically at 75 to 90 dB HL

(Thompson, 1963; Harbert, Young, & Weiss, 1969; Sanders, Josey, & Glasscock, 1974; Cooper & Owen, 1976). When the test is administered at high-intensity levels, positive (high) SISI scores are expected in normal ears and those with cochlear disorders, and negative (low) scores are associated with retrocochlear pathology. In actuality, the high-level SISI correctly identifies an average of about 90% of cochlear disorders but only 69% of retrocochlear pathologies, across studies (Turner, Shepard, & Frazer, 1984). This is not much better than what we have just seen for the standard (20 dB SL) version of the test.

Bekesy Audiometry

Recall from Chapter 5 that Bekesy audiometry allows the patient to track his own threshold by pressing and releasing a button. The button controls a motor, which in turn controls the attenuator. The patient is told to hold the button down when he can hear the tone and to release it when he cannot hear the tone. Holding the button down causes the intensity to fall, and releasing the button causes the intensity to rise. The patient does not press the button whenever the tone is too soft to hear. In this case the motor causes the intensity to rise, so that the tone will eventually become audible. Upon hearing the tone, the patient presses (and holds down) the response button. This causes the motor to reverse so that the intensity decreases. The tone then becomes inaudible and the patient releases the button, which in turn causes the intensity to rise, and so on. This course of events will cause the level of the tone to rise and fall around the patient's threshold. At the same time, the motor also controls a pen that tracks the level of the tone on paper, resulting in a zigzag pattern around the patient's threshold, as shown in Figure 5–6 of Chapter 5. The width of the zigzags is often called the excursion width, and the patient's threshold is the midpoint of these excursions.

Conventional Bekesy Audiometry

Bekesy audiograms are obtained either one frequency at a time or while the test frequency slowly changes from low to high. During **sweep-frequency Bekesy audiometry** the patient tracks his threshold while the frequency of the test tone increases smoothly from 100 to 10,000 Hz at a rate of one octave/ second. During **fixed-frequency Bekesy audiometry**, the patient tracks his threshold at one frequency for a given period of time, such as 3 minutes. Intensity increases and decreases at a rate of 2.5 dB/second. Each Bekesy audiogram is tracked twice, once using a continuous tone and once using a tone that pulses on and off 2.5 times a second, and the results are interpreted by comparing the **continuous** and **pulsed** (or **interrupted**) **tracings**.

Jerger (1960a, 1962) classified Bekesy audiograms into four basic types. Several modifications of the original classification system have also been described (Owens, 1964b; Johnson & House, 1964; Hopkinson, 1966; Hughes, Winegar, & Crabtree, 1967; Erlich, 1971). The Bekesy types will be described principally in terms of the sweep-frequency patterns. These are shown in Figure 10–9. In the **type I** Bekesy audiogram the pulsed and continuous tone tracings are interwoven, following the pattern of the patient's audiogram. This type is associated with those who have normal hearing or conductive hearing losses.

Type II is associated with patients who have cochlear impairments. Here the pulsed and continuous tracings are interwoven for frequencies up to roughly 1000 Hz. Two things happened at higher frequencies. First, the continuous tracing falls below the pulsed tracing by an amount that is usually less than 20 dB, and then runs parallel to it. In addition, the excursions of the continuous tracing narrow considerably, becoming only about 3 to 5 dB wide.

The shifting of the continuous tracing in Bekesy audiograms is generally interpreted as revealing the effects of tone decay (e.g., Harbert & Young, 1964; Owens, 1965; Parker & Dekker, 1971; Silman et al, 1981), and we will see that larger shifts are seen in types III and IV. The narrowed excursion widths in the type II Bekesy audiogram reflect how intensity perception is affected by cochlear

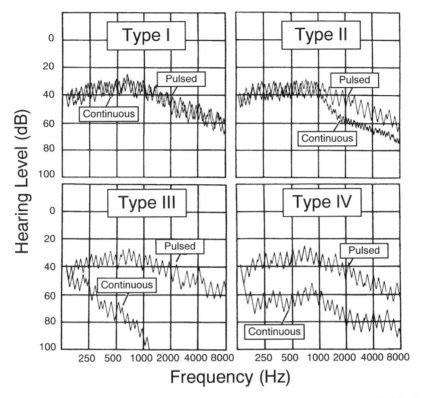

FIGURE 10–9   The classical Bekesy audiogram types (Jerger, 1960, 1962). Modified from Jerger (1962), with permission of American Speech-Language-Hearing Association.

impairments, but the mechanism is controversial (e.g., Bekesy, 1947; Denes & Naunton, 1950; Hirsh, Palva, & Goodman, 1954; Owens, 1965). It is probably related to the intensity DL around threshold, but it is not a test of loudness recruitment.

The **type III** Bekesy pattern is quite distinctive. Here, the continuous tracing diverts very quickly from the pulsed tracing, often shifting to the limits of the audiometer. Type III is associated with retrocochlear pathologies.

In **type IV** the continuous tracing quickly falls more than 20 dB below the pulsed audiogram, and then runs parallel to it. Even though type IV Bekesy audiograms may occur in patients with cochlear or retrocochlear disorders, they are often taken to suggest the possibility of the latter (e.g., Turner, Shepard, & Frazer, 1984).

A fifth Bekesy pattern, called **type V**, was described by Jerger and Herer (1961). It is distinctive because the pulsed tracing falls below the continuous one. The type V Bekesy

audiogram is associated with functional (or nonorganic) hearing loss and is described in greater detail in Chapter 14.

Forward-Backward Bekesy Audiometry

Rose (1962) reported that the difference between the continuous and pulsed tracings on sweep-frequency audiograms can be larger when the frequency sweep goes from high to low (backward) compared to the normal direction from low to high (forward). This difference is called the **forward-backward discrepancy**. Large forward-backward discrepancies are associated with retrocochlear pathologies (Karja & Palva, 1970; Palva, Karja, & Palva, 1970; Jerger, Jerger, & Mauldin, 1972; Jerger & Jerger, 1974a; Rose, Kurdziel, Olsen, & Noffsinger, 1975).

Figure 10–10 shows an example of the forward-backward discrepancy in a patient with an acoustic tumor. It was done using an approach like the one described by Jerger,

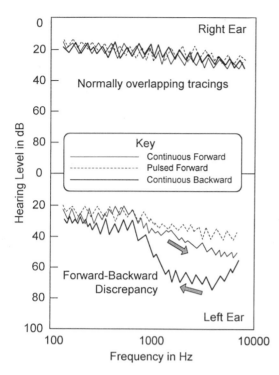

FIGURE 10–10 Forward-backward Bekesy audiograms in a patient with an acoustic tumor in the left ear. The upper frame shows *normal overlapping* of the three tracings in the unaffected right ear. The lower frame shows a *forward-backward discrepancy* in the pathological left.

Jerger, and Mauldin (1972). Notice that there are three Bekesy tracings in each frame, one pulsed and two continuous. The pulsed tracing goes in the forward direction (increasing in frequency from 200 to 8000 Hz). One of the continuous tracings goes in the forward direction (from 200 to 8000 Hz). However, the other continuous tracing goes in the backward direction (decreasing in frequency from 8000 to 200 Hz). This example demonstrates how the forward-backward discrepancy can reveal a retrocochlear site-of-lesion that would have been missed with standard sweep-frequency Bekesy audiometry. All three tracings are superimposed for the patient's normal right ear (upper panel). However, there is a forward-backward discrepancy for her left ear, which has an acoustic neuroma (lower panel). Notice that the backward continuous tracing falls far

below the pulsed tracing even though there is much less separation between the tracings for the pulsed tone and the forward continuous sweep (which would have been type II).

Bekesy Comfortable Loudness Testing

Bekesy Comfortable Loudness (BCL) testing was introduced by Jerger and Jerger (1974a). The BCL procedure is the same as for conventional sweep-frequency audiometry except the patient is instructed to press and release the Bekesy audiometer button to keep the tone "at a comfortable loudness level, neither too loud nor too soft" (p. 352).

Jerger and Jerger were able to identify six patterns of BCL results. Three BCL configurations were considered negative because they were associated with normal hearing and with conductive and cochlear impairments: The pulsed and continuous tracings were interwoven in type N1. The continuous tracing tracked above the pulsed in type N2 and below it in type N3. There were also three positive BCL patterns that were associated with retrocochlear disorders: The continuous tracings fell very far below the pulsed tracings at high frequencies in the type P1 pattern and at low and/or middle frequencies in type P2. The P3 pattern involved a forward-backward discrepancy for the BCL tracings. In other words, the BCL pattern was normal when the continuous tone was presented in the *forward* direction, but the *backward* continuous tracing descended well below the others. Not all ears could be classified as positive or negative. Nineteen percent of the retrocochlear cases and 8% of the other ears did not fit into the six categories.

Sensitivity and Specificity of Bekesy Audiometry

On average across studies, the correct identification rates for cochlear and retrocochlear disorders, respectively, are about 93% and 49% for conventional Bekesy audiometry, 95% and 71% for Forward-Backward Bekesy, and 92% and 85% for Bekesy Comfortable Loudness (Turner, Shepard, & Frazer, 1984).

Brief-Tone Audiometry

Brief-tone audiometry involves measuring the thresholds of tones having very short durations. It is the clinical application of **temporal summation (integration)**, which occurs when sounds are shorter than about one-third of a second. Recall from Chapter 3 that a normal hearing individual needs an intensity change of about 10 dB to compensate for the effect of a 10-times change in duration, as shown in Figure 10–11a. Clinical interest in brief-tone audiometry was based on the finding that patients with cochlear impairments typically need a smaller than normal intensity change to offset a 10-times change in duration (Sanders & Honig, 1967; Wright, 1968, 1978; Hattler & Northern 1970; Barry & Larson, 1974; Pedersen, 1976; Olsen, Rose, & Noffsinger, 1979; Chung & Smith, 1980). In other words, the intensity-duration relationship (called a temporal integration function) is typically shallower than normal when there is a cochlear impairment. This can be seen by comparing frames (a) and (b) in Figure 10–11.

The most common testing procedure in brief-tone audiometry involves Bekesy audiometry, which is why it is discussed at this point. However, other approaches have also been used. The basic testing method is quite simple. Bekesy audiograms are obtained using pulsing tones with various durations, and the resulting thresholds are compared to determine how much of a threshold change is needed to offset a duration difference. The clinician might test enough durations to plot a diagram such as those in the figure, or test at just two representative durations. Wright (1978) suggested that comparing the thresholds for tones having 20 and 500 msec durations is an efficient clinical approach.

Even though normal and cochlear-impaired ears are typically distinguished with brief-tone audiometry, the principal clinical question deals with the ability to differentiate between cochlear and retrocochlear disorders. In spite of optimistic early findings in this regard (Sanders, Josey, & Kemker, 1971), subsequent work showed that there is too much overlap between the results for cochlear and retrocochlear disorders for brief-tone audiometry to be a viable diagnostic test (Pedersen, 1976; Stephens, 1976; Olsen, Rose, & Noffsinger, 1979; Olsen, 1987).

Central Auditory Evaluation

Central auditory evaluation is used to assess abnormalities affecting the auditory nervous system and/or disorders of central auditory

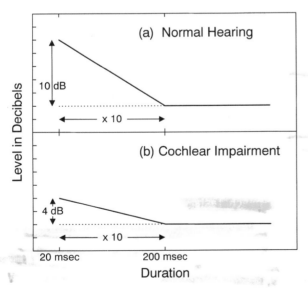

FIGURE 10–11 Idealized temporal integration functions showing the trade-off between intensity and duration needed to reach threshold for a tone when there is (a) normal hearing, and (b) cochlear impairment.

processes (see Chapter 6). Thus, central auditory disorders do not in and of themselves produce a hearing loss in the traditional sense of a threshold shift. This point is understandable when we consider the redundant "wiring diagram" of the central auditory nervous system described in Chapter 2. On the other hand, disorders of the auditory pathways will most certainly affect the processing of the auditory signals in myriad ways. As a result, central auditory tests use tasks that are sensitive to how sound perception is affected by abnormalities of the auditory nervous system, and are often quite subtle. As a result, it is not surprising that various kinds of behavioral measurements are used in central auditory assessment (ASHA, 1996), such as tests of perception of dichotic signals, temporal processes (discrimination, resolution, integration, and ordering), localization and lateralization, binaural interactions like masking level differences, and speech recognition using degraded (low-redundancy) materials. We will highlight some of the most commonly used approaches here. The interested student will find extensive coverages of the central auditory assessment in several advanced texts (e.g., Musiek & Rintelmann, 1999; Katz, 2000; Roeser, Valente, & Hosford-Dunn, 2000).

Tonal Tests

Most of the commonly used central auditory tests involve speech materials, although a number of tonal tests are also available. Two examples are the Pitch Pattern Sequence test and the masking level differences test. In the **Pitch Pattern Sequence Test** (Pinheiro, 1977; Pinheiro & Musiek, 1985), the patient is presented with "high" (1430 Hz) and "low" (880 Hz) brief tones at a readily audible level in groups of three. After hearing each sequence, the patient indicates the order of the tones (e.g., *high-low-low, high-low-high,* etc.) verbally or manually, and/or by humming the tonal sequence. It appears that patients with auditory cortex lesions on either side perform poorly for all response modes, while those with inter-hemispheric

lesions perform relatively better with the humming response. Musiek, Baran, and Pinheiro (1990) also described a test that uses sequences of longer (500 msec) and shorter (shorter) tone bursts instead of different pitches (e.g., *long-long-short, short-long-short*). They found that the duration patterns test is also sensitive to cerebral disorders, and that some patients with these disorders do poorly for duration patterns even if they have normal performance on the pitch patterns test.

Binaural **masking level differences (MLDs)** are useful clinically because they depend on the successful processing of binaural signals at the brainstem level. Recall from Chapter 3 that the MLD is obtained by comparing two measurements: One of them is the noise level needed to mask a signal when both the signal and the noise are in-phase at both ears, **SoNo**. The other value is the noise level needed to mask the signal when just the signal is out-of-phase at the two ears, but the noise is in-phase, $S_\pi N_o$ (or vice versa, $S_o N_\pi$). The MLD is equal to either $S_\pi N_o$ minus $S_o N_o$, or $S_o N_\pi$ minus $S_o N_o$. Clinical MLDs are usually done with a 500-Hz tone and/or with spondee words, and have been studied extensively (e.g., Noffsinger, Olsen, Carhart, Hart, & Sahgal, 1972; Olsen & Noffsinger, 1976, Olsen, Noffsinger, & Carhart, 1976; Lynn, Gilroy, Taylor, & Leiser, 1981; Hendler, Squires, & Emmerich, 1990). The essential findings are that MLDs are abnormally small or absent when there is multiple sclerosis or other disorders involving the brainstem, but tend to be unaffected by cortical lesions. However, one must be mindful that impaired MLDs are also caused by peripheral hearing losses. In fact, one must always consider the impact of a patient's hearing loss when interpreting central auditory tests because most of them are compromised by peripheral impairments to a greater or lesser extent.

Speech Tests

Monaural Tests   Monaural central auditory tests involve materials that are presented to just one ear. They are also known as **distorted, degraded,** or **low-redundancy speech** tests because the speech materials are degraded in some way to reduce the amount of information that can be derived from the signal (Bocca, 1958; Calearo & Lazzaroni, 1957; Jerger, 1960b; Bocca & Calearo, 1963). The speech materials are usually distorted by low-pass filtering, accelerating the speech rate (time compression), rapid interruptions, or by presenting the speech against a background of noise. An example of this approach is shown in the left panel of Figure 10–12, which illustrates the **low-passed filtered speech test**. Here, a filter is used to remove the higher frequencies, so the patient must rely on only the lower frequencies (usually below 500 or 750 Hz) to repeat the test words or sentences. Abnormally poor results in a given ear are typically associated with lesions of the auditory cortex on the *opposite side* of the brain, but can also be associated with brainstem disorders.

Why are degraded speech tests able to identify central auditory problems? Bocca and Calearo (1963) reasoned that successful speech recognition takes advantage of both the "intrinsic redundancy" that is built into the central auditory pathways and the "extrinsic redundancy" that is provided by the multiplicity of cues in the speech signal. Intrinsic redundancy is impaired by a central auditory lesion, and extrinsic redundancy is reduced by distorting the speech signal. Even though intrinsic redundancy is impaired in a patient who has a central lesion, he can often perform well with *un*distorted speech materials by relying on extrinsic redundancy. However, the patient's test performance breaks down when the extrinsic redundancy is also reduced, which is what happens when the speech is degraded. In contrast, the normal person can perform comparably well on distorted speech tests by relying on intrinsic redundancy, which is still intact.

Binaural Integration or Resynthesis Tests

Binaural integration tests involve presenting part of the speech signal to one ear and part of it to the other ear. Neither ear gets enough of the signal to allow adequate speech reception. As a result, the signals being presented to the two ears must be "put together"—"integrated" or "resynthesized"—by the central auditory nervous system. Several types of tests have been used. In the **Binaural Fusion Test** (Matzker, 1959; Ivey, 1969), filtering is used to produce a low-frequency band (e.g., 500 to 700 Hz) and a high-frequency band (e.g., 1900 to 2100 Hz) for each test word. The low-frequency band of a word goes to one ear and the high-frequency band of the same word simultaneously goes to the other ear, as represented in the middle panel

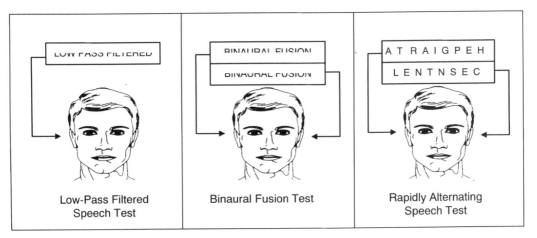

FIGURE 10–12 Illustrations of the Low-Pass Filtered Speech Test (left panel), Binaural Fusion Test (middle panel), and Rapidly Alternating Speech Test (right panel).

of Figure 10–12. The presentation of a low-pass filtered word to one ear and an unfiltered but very faint version of the same word to the other ear has also been used (e.g., Jerger, 1960b). Poor performance on the binaural fusion tests is generally associated with abnormalities affecting the brainstem.

In the **Rapidly Alternating Speech Perception Test** (Bocca & Calearo, 1963; Lynn & Gilroy, 1977) sentences are switched back and forth between the two ears at a quick rate, for example, every 300 msec, as illustrated in the right panel of Figure 10–12. At any given moment there is speech in one ear and silence in the other ear, but the whole message is present binaurally. The **Speech With Alternating Masking Index (SWAMI)** (Jerger, 1964) was a variation of this test in which a masking noise (instead of silence) was directed into the ear not receiving the speech at any given time. Difficulty on the rapidly alternating speech test is usually associated with brainstem abnormalities and also with diffuse cortical problems.

Dichotic Listening Tests In dichotic tests different speech signals are simultaneously presented to both ears, and the patient must repeat either one or both of them depending on which test is being used. The most common dichotic techniques include the Dichotic Digits test (Kimura, 1961; Musiek, 1983),

Dichotic Consonant-Vowel (CV) Syllables test (Berlin, Lowe-Bell, Jannetta, & Kline, 1972, Speaks, Gray, Miller, & Rubens, 1972; Berlin, Cullen, Hughes, Berlin, Lowe-Bell, & Thompson, 1975), Willeford's Competing Sentences test (Ivey, 1969), and the Staggered Spondaic Word test (Katz, 1962, 1968). Separate scores are obtained for each ear, and the principal clinical finding is that performance is lower in the ear opposite to a cortical lesion. This is consistent with the opposite ear effect already mentioned for the low-redundancy monaural tests. However, one must be careful about inferring the location of the disorder because dichotic test scores are also affected by brainstem disorders and by deep lesions of the higher pathways, in which the case opposite ear effect may not occur.

The test items on the **Dichotic Digits Test** are the numbers from "one" to "ten" (except "seven," which has two syllables). As represented in the left panel of Figure 10–13, each presentation includes one digit that goes to the right ear and a different digit that simultaneously goes to the left ear. The patient must repeat both digits, and receives a separate percent correct score for each ear. A similar approach is involved in the **Dichotic CV Test**, except that competing stimuli are CV monosyllables (usually /*pa, ta, ka, ba, da, ga*/), as shown in the right panel of Figure 10–13. The **Competing Sentences Test** simultane-

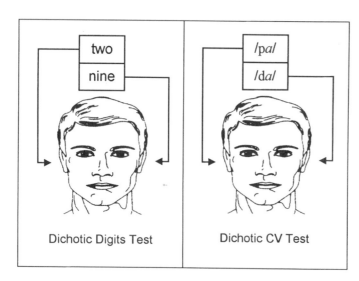

Dichotic Digits Test   Dichotic CV Test

FIGURE 10–13 Illustrations of the Dichotic Digits Test (left panel) and the Dichotic CV Test (right panel). In these tests, the patient is asked to repeat both stimuli.

ously presents different sentences to each ear, as illustrated in Figure 10–14. Separate scores are obtained for each, but two different scoring methods have been used. In one method, the patient is asked to repeat only the sentences presented to the right (or left) ear, while ignoring the sentence in the opposite ear. This is done twice, once for each ear. The alternate method involves having the patient repeat both of the sentences, which are scored separately for each ear.

The **Staggered Spondaic Word (SSW) Test** uses dichotically presented spondee words. However, the two words do not overlap completely in time. Instead, one of the spondees begins earlier than the other one so that (1) the second syllable of the spondee in one ear overlaps with the first syllable of the spondee in the other ear, but (2) the first syllable of one word and the second syllable of the other word are not overlapping. The right and left ears get an equal number of leading and trailing words. This paradigm sounds confusing but it is really quite simple, as shown in Figure 10–15. In effect, only the overlapping syllables ("light" and

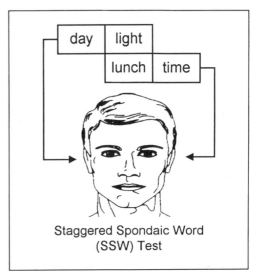

Staggered Spondaic Word
(SSW) Test

FIGURE 10–15 Illustration of Staggered Spondaic Word (SSW) Test. Notice how two of the syllables overlap in time ("light" and "lunch"), whereas the other two syllables do not overlap in time ("day" and "time").

"lunch" in the figure) are in dichotic competition, whereas the other two ("day" and "time") are noncompeting syllables. Even though we are addressing the SSW simply as a dichotic test in this introductory discussion, a complete interpretation actually considers several test findings, relationships, and nuances that appear to improve its ability to identify the location of a central disorder (see Katz & Ivey, 1994).

Synthetic Sentence Identification The **Synthetic Sentence Identification (SSI) Test** (Speaks & Jerger, 1965; Jerger, Speaks, & Trammell, 1968) involves identifying meaningless but syntactically correct sentences in the presence of a competing message (Chapter 8). The test is referred to as the SSI with an **ipsilateral competing message (SSI-ICM)** when the test sentences and competition (a continuous story) are in the same ear, and as the SSI with a **contralateral competing message (SSI-CCM)** when the message and competition are in opposite ears. These conditions are illustrated in Figure 10–16. The relative

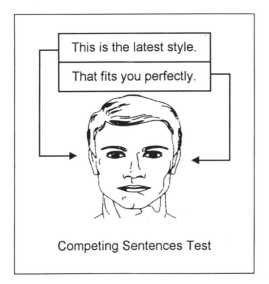

This is the latest style.

That fits you perfectly.

Competing Sentences Test

FIGURE 10–14 Illustration of the Competing Sentences Test. In this test, the patient may be asked to repeat both sentences, or to repeat one sentence while ignoring the other one.

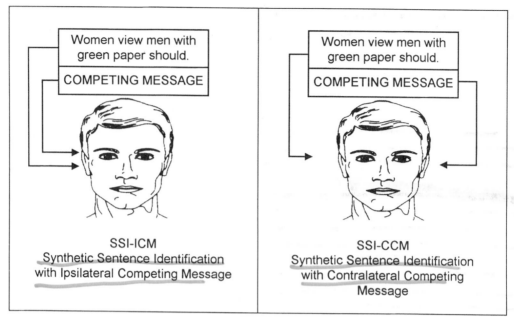

FIGURE 10–16 Illustration of Synthetic Sentence Identification Test with an ipsilateral competing message (SSI-ICM, left panel) and a contralateral competing message (SSI-CCM, right panel). Notice that the SSI-ICM is a monotic test, whereas the SSI-CCM involves a dichotic paradigm.

level between the SSI sentences and the competing message is called the **message to competition ratio (MCR),** which is analogous to signal-to-noise ratio. The SSI-ICM and SSI-CCM are done at various MCRs to obtain a performance-intensity function for the SSI (PI-SSI) for both conditions in each ear. The PI-SSI functions are compared with each other and also with the patient's PI-PB functions[1] (J. Jerger & S. Jerger, 1974a, 1975b; Jerger & Hayes, 1977; S. Jerger & J. Jerger, 1975, 1981). Brainstem disorders are associated with poorer SSI results when the competition is ipsilateral rather than when it is contralateral (SSI ICM is worse than SSI-CCM). In contrast, temporal lobe lesions are associated with poorer performance when the competing message is in the contralateral ear than when it is in the same ear (SSI-CCM is worse than SSI-ICM). As expected, the abnormally poor

results are usually found in the ear on the opposite side of the cortical disorder.

REFERENCES

American Speech-Language-Hearing Association Task Force on Central Auditory Processing Consensus Development (ASHA). 1996. Central auditory processing: Current status of research and implications for clinical practice. *Am J Audiol* 5, 41–54.

Anatonelli AR, Bellotto R, Grandori F. 1987. Audiologic diagnosis of central versus eighth nerve and cochlear hearing impairment. *Audiology* 26, 209–226.

Barry SJ, Larson VD. 1974. Brief-tone audiometry with normal and deaf school-age children. *J Speech Hear Dis* 39, 457–464.

Bekesy G. 1947. A new audiometer. *Arch Otolaryngol* 35, 411–422.

Benitez J, Lopez-Rios G, Novon V. 1967. Bilateral acoustic tumor: A human temporal bone study. *Arch Otolaryngol* 86, 51–57.

Berlin CI, Cullen JK, Hughes LF, Berlin JL, Lowe-Bell SS, Thompson CL. 1975. Dichotic processing of speech: Acoustic and phonetic variables. In Sullivan MD (Ed.): *Central Auditory Processing Disorders.* Omaha: University of Nebraska, 36–46.

Berlin CI, Lowe-Bell SS, Jannetta PJ, Kline DG. 1972. Central auditory deficits after temporal lobectomy. *Arch Otolaryngol* 96, 4–10.

---

[1] Review the section on PI-PB functions in Chapter 8 if these terms and concepts are not clear.

Bocca E. 1958. Clinical aspects of cortical deafness. *Laryngoscope* 68, 301–309.

Bocca E, Calearo C. 1963. Central hearing processes. In Jerger J. (Ed.), *Modern Developments in Audiology.* New York: Academic Press, 337–370.

Buus S, Florentine M, Redden RB. 1982a. The SISI test: A review. Part I. *Audiology* 21, 273–293.

Buus S, Florentine M, Redden RB. 1982b. The SISI test: A review. Part II. *Audiology* 21, 365–385.

Calearo C, Lazzaroni A. 1957. Speech intelligibility in relation to the speech of the message. *Laryngoscope,* 67, 410–419.

Carhart R. 1957. Clinical determination of abnormal auditory adaptation. *Arch Otolaryngol* 65, 32–40.

Carver WF. 1970. The reliability and precision of a modification of the ABLB test. *Ann Otol Rhinol Laryngol* 79, 398–412.

Chung DY, Smith F. 1980. Quiet and masked brief-tone audiometry in subjects with normal hearing and with noise-induced hearing loss. *Scand Audiol* 9, 43–47.

Coles RRA, Priede VM. 1976. Factors influencing the choice of fixed-level ear in the ABLB test. *Audiology* 15, 465–479.

Cooper JC Jr, Owen JH. 1976. In defense of SISIs. *Arch Otolaryngol* 102, 396–399.

Dallos PJ, Tillman TW. 1966. The effects of parameter variations in Bekesy audiometry in a patient with acoustic neuroma. *J Speech Hear Res* 9, 557–572.

Davis H, Goodman AC. 1966. Subtractive hearing loss, loudness recruitment, and decruitment. *Ann Otol Rhinol Laryngol* 75, 87–94.

Denes P, Naunton RF. 1950. The clinical detection of auditory recruitment. *J Laryngol Otol* 65, 375–398.

Dix MR, Hallpike CS. 1958. The otoneurological diagnosis of tumors of the VIII nerve. *Proc R Soc Med* 51, 689–897.

Dix MR, Hallpike CS, Hood JD. 1948. Observations upon the loudness recruitment phenomenon, with especial reference to the differential diagnosis of disorders of the internal ear and VIII nerve. *Proc R Soc Med* 41, 516–526.

Erlich CH. 1971. Analysis of selected fixed frequency Bekesy tracings. *Arch Otolaryngol* 93, 12–24.

Flottorp G. 1963. Pathological fatigue in part of the hearing nerve only. *Acta Otolaryngol Suppl* 188, 298–307.

Fowler EP. 1936. A method for the early detection of otosclerosis: A study of sounds well above threshold. *Arch Otolaryngol* 24, 731–741.

Fritze W. 1978. A computer-controlled binaural balance test. *Acta Otolaryngol* 86, 89–92.

Gelfand SA. 1976. The tracking ABLB in clinical recruitment testing. *J Aud Res* 16, 34–41.

Gelfand SA. 1998. *Hearing: An Introduction to Psychological and Physiological Acoustics,* 3rd ed. New York: Marcel Dekker.

Geller D, Margolis R. 1984. Magnitude estimation of loudness: I. Application to hearing aid selection. *J Speech Hear Res* 27, 20–27.

Gjaevenes K, Sohoel TH. 1969. The tone decay test. *Acta Otolaryngol* 68, 33–42.

Green DS. 1963. The modified tone decay test (MTDT) as a screening procedure for eighth nerve lesions. *J Speech Hear Dis* 28, 31–36.

Hallpike CS. 1965. Clinical otoneurology and its contributions to theory and practice. *Proc R Soc Med* 58, 185–196.

Hallpike CS, Hood JD. 1951. Some recent work on auditory adaptation and its relationship to the loudness recruitment phenomenon. *J Acoust Soc Am* 23, 270–274.

Hallpike CS, Hood JD. 1959. Observations on the neurological mechanism of loudness recruitment. *Acta Otolaryngol* 50, 472–486.

Harbert F, Young IM. 1964. Threshold auditory adaptation measured by tone decay test and Bekesy audiometry. *Ann Otol Rhinol Laryngol* 73, 48–60.

Harbert F, Young IM, Weiss B. 1969. Clinical application of intensity difference limen. *Acta Otolaryngol* 67, 435–443.

Harford ER. 1967. Clinical application and significance of the SISI test. In Graham AB (Ed.): *Sensorineural Hearing Processes and Disorders.* Boston: Little, Brown, 223–233.

Hattler K, Northern JL. 1970. Clinical application of temporal summation. *J Aud Res* 10, 72–78.

Hellman RP, Meiselman CH. 1988. Prediction of individual loudness exponents from cross-modality matching. *J Speech Hear Res* 31, 605–615.

Hellman RP, Meiselman CH. 1990. Loudness relations for individuals and groups in normal and impaired hearing. *J Acoust Soc Am* 88, 2596–2606.

Hendler T, Squires N, Emmerich D. 1990. Psychophysical measures of central auditory dysfunction in multiple sclerosis. *Ear Hear* 11, 403–416.

Hirsh IJ, Palva T, Goodman A. 1954. Difference limen and recruitment. *Arch Otolaryngol* 60, 525–540.

Hood JD. 1955. Auditory fatigue and adaptation in the differential diagnosis of end-organ disease. *Ann Otol Rhinol Laryngol* 64, 507–518.

Hood JD. 1969. Basic audiological requirements in neuro-otology. *J Laryngol Otol* 83, 695–711.

Hood JD. 1977. Loudness balance procedures for the measurement of recruitment. *Audiology* 16, 215–228.

Hood JD, Poole JP. 1966. Tolerance limits of loudness: Its clinical and physiological significance. *J Acoust Soc Am* 40, 47–53.

Hopkinson NT. 1966. Modifications of the four types of Bekesy audiograms. *J Speech Hear Dis* 31, 79–82.

Hughes RL, Winegar WJ, Crabtree JA. 1967. Bekesy audiometry: Type II versus Type IV patterns. *Arch Otolaryngol* 86, 424–430.

Ivey RG. 1969. Tests of CNS auditory function. Unpublished thesis, Colorado State University, Fort Collins, CO.

Jerger J. 1952. A difference limen test and its diagnostic significance. *Laryngoscope* 62, 1316–1332.

Jerger J. 1953. DL difference test. *Arch Otolaryngol* 57, 490–500.

Jerger J. 1960a. Bekesy audiometry in the analysis of auditory disorders. *J Speech Hear Res* 3, 275–287.

Jerger J. 1960b. Observations on auditory behavior in lesions of the central auditory pathways. *Arch Otolaryngol* 71, 797–806.

Jerger J. 1961. Recruitment and allied phenomena in differential diagnosis. *J Aud Res* 2, 145–151.

Jerger J. 1962. Hearing tests in otologic diagnosis. *ASHA* 4, 139–145.

Jerger J. 1964. Auditory tests for disorders of the central auditory mechanisms. In Fields WS, Alford BR (Eds.): *Neurological Aspects of Auditory and Vestibular Disorders.* Springfield, IL: CC Thomas, 77–93.

Jerger J, Harford ER. 1960. Alternate and simultaneous binaural balancing of tones. *J Speech Hear Res* 3, 15–30.

Jerger J, Hayes D. 1977. Diagnostic speech audiometry. *Arch Otolaryngol* 103, 216–222.

Jerger J, Herer G. 1961. Unexpected dividend in Bekesy audiometry. *J Speech Hear Dis* 26, 390–391.

Jerger J, Jerger S. 1966. Critical off-time in VIII nerve disorders. *J Speech Hear Res* 9, 573–583.

Jerger J, Jerger S. 1974a. Diagnostic value of Bekesy comfortable loudness tracings. *Arch Otolaryngol* 99, 351–360.

Jerger J, Jerger S. 1974b. Auditory findings in brainstem disorders. *Arch Otolaryngol* 99, 342–349.

Jerger J, Jerger S. 1975a. A simplified tone decay test. *Arch Otolaryngol* 101, 403–407.

Jerger J, Jerger S. 1975b. Clinical value of central auditory tests. *Scand Audiol* 4, 147–163.

Jerger J, Jerger S, Mauldin L. 1972. The forward-backward discrepancy in Bekesy audiometry. *Arch Otolaryngol* 96, 400–406.

Jerger J, Shedd J, Harford E. 1959. On the detection of extremely small changes in sound intensity. *Arch Otolaryngol* 69, 200–211.

Jerger J, Speaks C, Trammell J. 1968. A new approach to speech audiometry. *J Speech Hear Dis* 33, 318–328.

Jerger S, Jerger J. 1975. Extra- and intra-axial brain-stem disorders. *Audiology* 14, 93–117.

Jerger S, Jerger J. 1981. *Auditory Disorders*. Boston: Little, Brown.

Johnson EW. 1966. Confirmed retrocochlear lesions: Auditory test results in 163 patients. *Arch Otolaryngol* 84, 247–254.

Johnson EW, House WF. 1964. Auditory findings in 53 cases of acoustic neuromas. *Arch Otolaryngol* 80, 667–677.

Josey AF. 1987. Audiologic manifestations of tumors of the eighth nerve. *Ear Hear* 4 (suppl), 195–215.

Kamm C, Dirks DD, Mickey MR. 1978. Effect of sensorineural hearing loss on loudness discomfort level and most comfortable loudness judgments. *J Speech Hear Res* 21, 668–681.

Karja J, Palva T. 1970. Reverse frequency-sweep Bekesy audiometry. *Acta Otolaryngol Suppl* 263, 225–228.

Katz J. 1962. The use of staggered spondaic words for assessing the integrity of the central auditory nervous system. *J Aud Res* 2, 327–337.

Katz J. 1968. The SSW test: An interim report. *J Speech Hear Dis* 33, 132–146.

Katz J (Ed.). 2000. *Handbook of Clinical Audiology*, 5th ed. Baltimore: Lippincott Williams & Wilkins, in press.

Katz J, Ivey RG. 1994. Spondaic procedures in central testing. In Katz J (Ed.): *Handbook of Clinical Audiology*, 4th ed. Baltimore: Williams & Wilkins, 239–268.

Kimura D. 1961. Some effects of temporal lobe damage on auditory perception. *Can J Psychol* 15, 1157–1165.

Knight K, Margolis R. 1984. Magnitude estimation of loudness: II. Loudness perception in presbycusis listeners. *J Speech Hear Res* 27, 28–32.

Lamore PJJ, Rodenburg M. 1980. Significance of the SISI test and its relation to recruitment. *Audiology* 19, 75–85.

Lüscher E. 1951. The difference limen of intensity variations of pure tones and its diagnostic significance. *J Laryngol Otol* 65, 486–510.

Lüscher E, Zwislocki J. 1949. A simple method for indirect monaural determination of the recruitment phenomenon (difference limen in intensity in different types of deafness). *Acta Otolaryngol* 78, 156–168.

Lynn GE, Gilroy J. 1977. Evaluation of central auditory dysfunction in patients with neurological disorders. In Keith RW (Ed.): *Central Auditory Dysfunction*. New York: Grune & Stratton, 177–221.

Lynn GE, Gilroy J, Taylor PC, Leiser RP. 1981. Binaural masking-level differences in neurological disorders. *Arch Otolaryngol* 107, 357–362.

Marks LE. 1974. Sensory Processes. New York: Academic Press.

Martin FN, Champlin CA, Chambers JA. 1998. Seventh survey of audiological practices in the United States. *J Am Acad Audiol* 9, 95–104.

Martin FN, Woodrick Armstrong T, Champlin CA. 1994. A survey of audiological practices in the United States. *Am J Audiol* 3, 20–26.

Matzker J. 1959. Two new methods for the assessment of central auditory functions in cases of brain disease. *Ann Otol Rhinol Laryngol* 68, 1185–1197.

Miskolczy-Fodor F. 1964. Automatically recorded loudness balance testing: A new method. *Arch Otolaryngol* 79, 355–365.

Morales-Garcia C, Hood JD. 1972. Tone decay test in neuro-otologic diagnosis. *Arch Otolaryngol* 96, 231–247.

Musiek FE. 1983. Assessment of central auditory disfunction: The dichotic digit test revisited. *Ear Hear* 4, 79–83.

Musiek FE, Baran JA, Pinheiro ML. 1990. Duration pattern recognition in normal subjects and in patients with cerebral and cochlear lesions. *Audiology* 29, 304–313.

Musiek FE, Rintelmann WF (Eds.). 1999. *Contemporary Perspectives in Hearing Assessment*. Boston: Allyn & Bacon.

Noffsinger D, Olsen WO, Carhart R, Hart CW, Sahgal V. 1972. Auditory and vestibular aberrations in multiple sclerosis. *Acta Otolaryngol Suppl* 303, 1–63.

Olsen WO. 1987. Brief tone audiometry: A review. *Ear Hear* 8 (suppl), 13S–18S.

Olsen WO, Kurdziel SA. 1976. Extent and rate of tone decay for cochlear and for VIIIth nerve lesion patients. Paper presented at Convention of American Speech and Hearing Association, Houston.

Olsen WO, Noffsinger D. 1974. Comparison of one new and three old tests of auditory adaptation. *Arch Otolaryngol* 99, 94–99.

Olsen WO, Noffsinger D. 1976. Masking level differences for cochlear and brain stem lesions. *Ann Otol Rhinol Laryngol* 86, 820–825.

Olsen WO, Noffsinger D, Carhart R. 1976. Masking level differences encountered in clinical populations. *Audiology* 15, 287–301.

Olsen WO, Rose DE, Noffsinger D. 1979. Brief-tone audiometry with normal, cochlear, and eighth nerve tumor patients. *Arch Otolaryngol* 99, 185–189.

Owens E. 1964a. Tone decay in VIIIth nerve and cochlear lesions. *J Speech Hear Dis* 29, 14–22.

Owens E. 1964b. Bekesy tracings and site of lesion. *J Speech Hear Dis* 29, 456–468.

Owens E. 1965. Bekesy tracings, tone decay, and loudness recruitment. *J Speech Hear Dis* 30, 50–57.

Palva T, Karja J, Palva A. 1970. Forward vs reversed Bekesy tracings. *Arch Otolaryngol* 91, 449–452.

Parker WP, Dekker RL. 1971. Detection of abnormal auditory threshold adaptation. *Acta Otolaryngol* 94, 1–7.

Pedersen CB. 1976. Brief-tone audiometry. *Scand Audiol* 5, 27–33.

Perez de Moura L. 1967. Inner ear pathology in acoustic neurinomas. *J Speech Hear Dis* 32, 29–35.

Pestalozza G, Cioce C. 1962. Measuring auditory adaptation: The value of different clinical tests. *Laryngoscope* 72, 240–259.

Pinheiro ML. 1977. Auditory pattern reversal in auditory perception in patients with left and right hemisphere lesions. *Ohio J Speech Hear* 12, 9–20.

Pinheiro ML, Musiek FE. 1985. Sequencing and temporal ordering in the auditory system. In Pinheiro ML, Musiek FE (Eds.): *Assessment of Central Auditory Dysfunction*. Baltimore: Williams & Wilkins, 219–238.

Priede VM, Coles RRA. 1974. Interpretation of loudness recruitment tests. *J Laryngol Otol* 88, 641–662.

Reger S. 1935. Loudness level contours and intensity discrimination of ears with raised auditory threshold. *J Acoust Soc Am* 7, 73 (abstract).

Roeser, RJ, Valente M, Hosford-Dunn H. (Eds.). 2000. *Audiology: Diagnosis*. New York: Thieme.

Rose DE. 1962. Some effects and case histories of reversed frequency sweep in Bekesy audiometry. *J Aud Res* 2, 267–278.

Rose DE, Kurdziel S, Olsen WO, Noffsinger D. 1975. Bekesy test results in patients with eighth nerve lesions. *Arch Otolaryngol* 101, 573–575.

Rosenberg PE. 1958. Rapid clinical measurement of tone decay. Paper presented at Convention of American Speech and Hearing Association, New York.

Rosenberg PE. 1969. Tone decay. Maico Audiological Library Series, VII, report 6.

Sanders JW, Honig EA. 1967. Brief tone audiometry results in normal and impaired ears. *Arch Otolaryngol* 85, 640–647.

Sanders JW, Josey AF, Glasscock ME. 1974. Audiologic evaluation in cochlear and eighth nerve disorders. *Arch Otolaryngol* 100, 283–293.

Sanders JW, Josey AF, Kemker FJ. 1971. Brief-tone audiometry in patients with VIIIth nerve tumor. *J Speech Hear Res* 14, 172–178.

Silman S, Gelfand SA, Lutolf J, Chun TH. 1981. A response to Wiley and Lilly. *J Speech Hear Dis* 46, 217.

Silman S, Silverman CA. 1991. *Auditory Diagnosis: Principles and Applications*. San Diego: Academic Press.

Sorensen H. 1960. A threshold tone decay test. *Acta Otolaryngol* Suppl 158, 356–360.

Sorensen H. 1962. Clinical application of continuous threshold recordings. *Acta Otolaryngol* 54, 403–422.

Speaks C, Gray T, Miller J, Rubens A. 1972. Central auditory deficits and temporal lobe lesions. *J Speech Hear Dis* 40, 192–205.

Speaks C, Jerger J. 1965. Method for measurement of speech identification. *J Speech Hear Res* 8, 185–194.

Stephens SDG. 1976. Auditory temporal summation in patients with central nervous system lesions. In Stephens SDG (Ed.): *Disorders of Auditory Function, II*. London: Academic Press, 231–243.

Sung RJ, Sung GS. 1976. Study of the classical and modified alternate binaural loudness balance tests in normal and pathological ears. *J Am Audiol Soc* 2, 49–53.

Sung SS, Goetzinger CP, Knox AW. 1969. The sensitivity and reliability of three tone-decay tests. *J Aud Res* 9, 167–177.

Thompson G. 1963. A modified SISI technique for selected cases with suspected acoustic neurinoma. *J Speech Hear Dis* 28, 299–302.

Tillman TW. 1966. Audiologic diagnosis of acoustic tumors. *Arch Otolaryngol* 83, 574–581.

Tillman TW. 1969. Special hearing tests in otoneurologic diagnosis. *Arch Otolaryngol* 89, 51–56.

Turner RG, Shepard NT, Frazer GJ. 1984. Clinical performance of audiological and related diagnostic tests. *Ear Hear* 5, 187–194.

Wiley TL, Lilly DJ. 1980. Temporal characteristics of auditory adaptation: A case report. *J Speech Hear Dis* 45, 209–215.

Wright HN. 1968. Clinical measurement of temporal auditory summation. *J Speech Hear Res* 11, 109–227.

Wright HN. 1978. Brief tone audiometry. In Katz J (Ed.): *Handbook of Clinical Audiology*. Baltimore: Williams & Wilkins, 218–232.

Yantis PA. 1959. Clinical applications of the temporary threshold shift. *Arch Otolaryngol* 70, 779–787.

11

Physiological Methods in Audiology

An important aspect of audiology deals with the use of physiological tests in addition to the use of behavioral measurements. Physiological measurements provide powerful diagnostic tools that supplement the information obtained from the patient interview and behavioral tests, and make it possible to test patients who are too young or otherwise incapable of responding behaviorally. This chapter introduces the student to three types of physiological assessment approaches that are used in audiology: auditory evoked potentials, otoacoustic emissions, and vestibular assessment. Acoustic immittance methods are discussed in considerable detail in Chapter 7. Physiological techniques that are no longer used (such as psychogalvanic, respiration, and cardiac responses) are not covered; but the inquisitive reader may find discussions of these methods in Bradford (1975). In addition, the student should be aware that some audiologists perform physiological monitoring during surgical procedures (ASHA, 1992), and they may also use nonauditory physiological measurements such as facial nerve testing and the use of somatosensory evoked potentials. While intraoperative monitoring is not covered at the introductory level, several lucid discussions of the topic are readily available (Dennis, 1988; Hall, 1992; Beck, 1993; Musiek, Borenstein, Hall, & Schwaber, 1994; Jacobson, 1999; Møller, 2000).

Auditory Evoked Potentials

The activity of the nervous system produces electrical signals that can be picked up by electrodes placed on the head, and can then be displayed on the screen of a recording device and/or plotted on paper. A change in the activity of the nervous system occurs when it reacts to a stimulus (such as a sound). This change in neural activity also produces a change in the electrical signals picked up by the electrodes. As a result, the nervous system's reaction to a stimulus can be seen as a change in the electrical signals that are displayed on the recording device. These electrical responses of the nervous system that are elicited by a stimulus are called **evoked potentials**. When the stimulus is sound, they are called **auditory evoked potentials (AEPs)**. These auditory evoked potentials can be used to test the integrity of the auditory system and to make inferences about hearing. One of the great advantages of AEPs is that they are usually noninvasive, almost always being measured from outside the body with electrodes on the surface of the skin. The block diagram in Figure 11–1 illustrates a typical arrangement involved in recording AEPs from a patient. An example of an instrument used for evoked potentials testing is illustrated in Figure 11–2.

The nature and use of auditory evoked potentials have been described in considerable detail (e.g., Moore, 1983; Jacobson, 1985; Hall, 1992; Glattke, 1993; Kraus & McGee, 1994; Kraus, Kileny, & McGee, 1994; Chiappa, 1997). Figure 11–3 shows the three major AEPs in the form of a single composite picture. The time scale in the figure is labeled **latency**, which is simply the amount of time that has elapsed (or the delay) since the stimulus was presented. Each of the AEPs shown

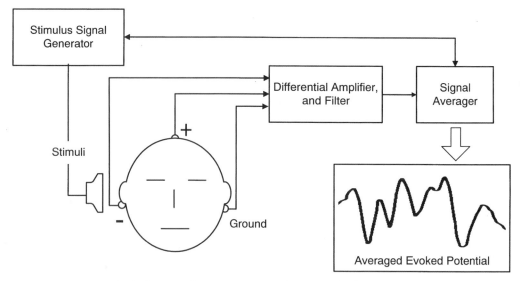

FIGURE 11–1   Block diagram for measuring auditory evoked potentials, using the auditory brainstem response as an example.

is made up of a characteristic grouping of peaks and troughs that occur within a certain range of latencies, and are for this reason identified as the short, middle, and long latency responses. Notice that a logarithmic time scale is used in this figure so that all three ranges of latencies can be shown. Each of these time frames is called a **time window** or **epoch**, and the ability to observe a given evoked potential is optimized by using the time window best suited for that response.

We will first briefly review some aspects of electrocochleography, and then concentrate on the auditory brainstem response (ABR), which is by far the most widely used of the various auditory evoked potentials. We will then go over some aspects of the later evoked potentials.

The electrodes are usually located at some distance from the structures that produce the signals. In addition, the electrodes will pick up all electrical signals that reach them,

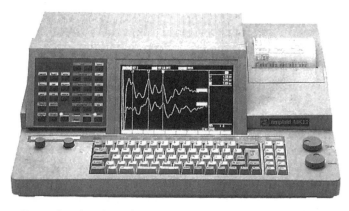

FIGURE 11–2   Example of a clinical instrument used for auditory brainstem responses and other evoked potentials tests. Picture courtesy of Amplifon div. Amplaid.

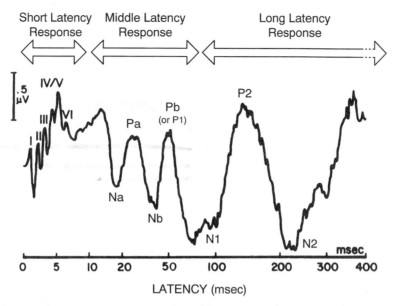

FIGURE 11–3 A composite representation of the major auditory evoked potentials. A logarithmic scale is used here so all of the different sets of waves can be shown on one graph. Modified from ASHA (1987), with permission of American Speech-Language-Hearing Association.

regardless of why they are there or where they are from. This means that the recording device receives all kinds of signals from the nervous system, muscles, and other physiological sources, as well as signals from electrical sources in the environment. All of these other signals are **noise**. As a result, we need to extract tiny evoked potential responses from an extraordinarily noisy background; for example, the ABR is *less than* 1 microvolt (μV) but the noise is often around 10 μV. This goal is accomplished with filtering, differential amplification, and averaging.

Filtering can be used to remove some low-frequency noises such as direct current (DC) signals from electronic equipment, 60-Hz hum from alternating current (AC) power sources, and background electroencephalographic (EEG) activity. **Differential amplification** is used to boost the level of the evoked potential response while at the same time removing noise. It involves using the signals picked up by two separate electrodes at different locations, such as the earlobe of the stimulated (ipsilateral) ear and the vertex of the skull. The differential amplifier then can-

cels ("rejects") noises that are similar ("in common") at the two electrodes. This process is called **common mode rejection** and is widely used in physiological measurements. A ground or common electrode is also necessary, and is usually located on the mastoid of the opposite ear or at midline on the lower forehead.

Recall that the responses we are looking for are tiny signals embedded in all kinds of noise. A great deal of noise still remains after filtering and differential amplification. **Averaging** is a technique that allows the responses (evoked potential) to be extracted from the noise, and is a central principle of many physiological methods. Averaging relies on a few fundamental notions. The first principle is that the evoked potential responses are *time-locked* to (or *synchronized* with) the stimulus. This means that the response will consistently appear in a certain way at the same latency, or point in time after the stimulus. On the other hand, noise is *random*. Suppose a certain evoked potential is positive in direction 3 msec after a click is presented to the ear, and is negative at a latency of 4 msec. In other words, the electrical response due to that click will be positive when measured 3 msec later and negative when measured 4 msec later. Now, suppose we present 1000 clicks, and measure the electrical signals picked up by the electrodes for a period lasting 10 msec following each one. A computer could be used to keep a "tally" of the electrical signals at 1-msec intervals after each click. More specifically, the computer will algebraically add the voltages in 1-msec intervals for all 1000 clicks. Thus, there would be an algebraic sum at latencies of 1 msec, 2 msec, 3 msec, 4 msec, etc. Even though any one of the responses might be very small, it will almost always be positive at a latency of 3 msec and negative at a latency of 4 msec. When these values are added algebraically (averaged) over a large number of trials (samples), then a relatively large *positive value will build up at 3 msec* and a relatively large *negative value will build up at 4 msec*, as illustrated in Figure 11–4. On the other hand, the electrical signals due to noise are random. Random events are as likely to be positive as negative, so that they will "average out" ("add up to zero" algebraically) over the long run, which is what happens when we add up a large number of samples. As a result of these principles, the averaging process causes the

real response to build up because it is consistent over time, and causes the noise to "cancel out" (actually add up to zero) because it is random over time.

Electrocochleography

Electrocochleography (ECochG) is the measurement of electrical potentials that are derived from the cochlear hair cells and the auditory nerve (ASHA, 1987; Ruth, Lambert, & Ferraro, 1988; Hall, 1992; Ferraro, 1992a,b, 1993a,b, 2000). The basic methodology of ECochG involves presenting clicks to the ear and monitoring the resulting electrical responses within a time frame of about 5 msec after each click. Averaging the responses to a large number of stimuli results in a waveform like the one illustrated in Figure 11–5, which will be described momentarily.

Electrocochleography typically uses click stimuli, although tone bursts are also used for various applications. The reason for using transient stimuli like clicks is that many neurons must be made to fire, or discharge, at essentially the same time (synchronously) in order to elicit a measurable action potential. This goal is accomplished by using stimuli that have abrupt onsets, very short

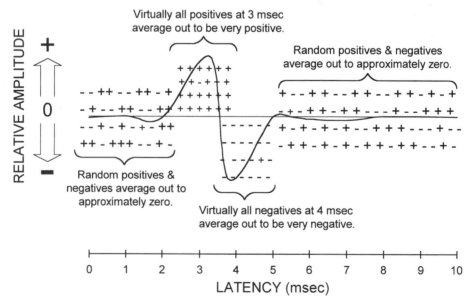

FIGURE 11–4   Illustration of the averaging concept (see text).

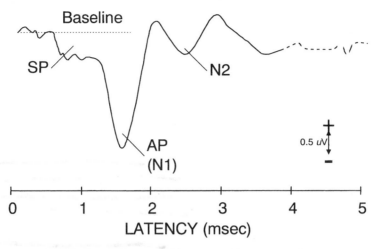

FIGURE 11–5 An idealized electrocochleogram. Negative voltage values are plotted downward. SP, summating potential; AP (N1), auditory nerve action potential; N2, second peak of auditory nerve action potential.

durations, and broad spectra, such as clicks. These characteristics enable clicks to almost simultaneously activate a large number of hair cells along the basal part of the cochlea, where the speed of the traveling wave is very fast. This, in turn, causes essentially simultaneous firing of the auditory nerve fibers associated with these basal turn hair cells.

Electrode location is a very important factor in ECochG because the magnitude and quality of the measured response deteriorates significantly with distance from the cochlea and auditory nerve. The highest quality clinical responses are obtained with an electrode on the cochlear promontory. This method is called the transtympanic approach because it involves using a needle electrode that must penetrate the tympanic membrane to get to the promontory, requiring medical participation. The **transtympanic approach** is thus an invasive procedure, which is its principal limitation. Less pristine but perfectly usable ECochG results are obtained with the alternative, *noninvasive* **extratympanic approach**. It uses various kinds of electrodes that are placed as close as possible to the tympanic membrane in the ear canal or on the eardrum itself. The extratympanic method avoids the limitations and potential complications of piercing the eardrum, and is the most com-

mon ECochG approach used in the United States.

The **electrocochleogram** (also abbreviated ECochG) is shown in Figure 11–5. It includes two major components, the **summating potential (SP)** derived from the cochlear hair cells, and the compound **action potential (AP)** of the auditory nerve. It is also possible to show a third component, the **cochlear microphonic**, which is an alternating current (AC) electrical response from the hair cells, although this is not always done clinically. The summating potential is a shift of the electrical baseline (a direct current, or DC, shift) that occurs when the hair cells are activated. This is followed by activation of auditory neurons, which produces the action potential. Figure 11–5 shows how these components are displayed on the electrocochleogram. Notice that the ongoing activity before the ECochG response is used as a *baseline*. The figure follows the convention of recording negative peaks downward, although some clinicians show negative values upward. The summating potential is usually seen as a displacement from the baseline just prior to the action potential, or as a hump on its leading edge, as shown in the figure. The AP is seen as a negative peak at a latency of roughly 1.5 msec after the click. It can include up to three peaks (**N1**, **N2**, and **N3**), but the AP refers to just the first peak (N1) for clinical purposes.

The ECochG response increases in amplitude (gets larger) and decreases in latency (occurs sooner) as the level of the stimulus is raised. In spite of this relationship, ECochG has not been found to be a reliable physiological method for estimating hearing thresholds, especially with extratympanic electrodes. On the other hand, ECochG has been shown to have at least three valuable clinical applications: (1) Electrocochleography is often used to help identify the first peak of the auditory brainstem response, which will be described in the next section. (2) It can also be used to monitor the status of the inner ear and auditory nerve during surgical procedures that place these structures at risk. Examples include acoustic tumor removal, and when endolymphatic sac surgery is used in an attempt to treat Meniere's disease (endolymphatic hydrops). (3) One of the most promising clinical uses of ECochG is in the diagnosis of Meniere's disease and for monitoring patients with this disorder (Ferraro & Krishnan, 1997; Ferraro & Tibbils, 1999). This application is possible because an abnormally large summating potential amplitude relative to the AP amplitude is a very good indicator of Meniere's disease. This finding is often described as an abnormally large **SP/AP amplitude ratio**. A potentially more sensitive measurement for detecting endolymphatic hydrops is the **SP/AP area ratio**, which compares the areas of the SP and the AP instead of their amplitudes.[1]

Auditory Brainstem Response

The group of waves identified as the "short latency response" in Figure 11–3 was originally described in detail by Jewett, Romano, and Williston (1970), as well as by Sohmer and Feinmesser (1967). They include up to seven peaks that normally occur within about 8 msec following the onset of a click stimulus. It is tempting to attribute these peaks to successive sites along the auditory pathway. However, it appears that the first two peaks are produced by the auditory nerve, whereas the subsequent peaks actually have multiple generators, meaning that they are due to the combined electrical activity of several nuclei in the auditory brainstem (Moller & Janetta, 1985; Scherg & vonCramon, 1985; Moore, 1987; Rudell, 1987). These short latency evoked potentials are generally known as the **auditory brainstem response (ABR)**, the **brainstem auditory evoked response (BSER or BAER),** or the **brainstem auditory evoked potential (BAEP).**

The auditory brainstem response is most commonly obtained using click stimuli for the same reason described above for electrocochleography. As a result, the ABR depends to a considerable extent on the status of the basal turn of the cochlea and principally involves the high frequencies. While their abruptness and broad spectra make clicks optimal stimuli for eliciting synchronous neural firings, these features also cause the ABR to be lacking in the ability to test on a frequency-by-frequency basis. The ability to distinguish among frequencies is often called **frequency specificity**. To improve the frequency specificity of the ABR, a number of compromise stimuli are available that involve switching a tone on and off very rapidly. These are described as tone bursts, tone pips, or logons, depending on their temporal details, although we will deal with them collectively. Stimuli of this type do not provide very much frequency specificity because they still contain broad spectra as a result of their rapid onsets and offsets. This lack of frequency specificity in ABR testing must always be kept in mind.

The frequency specificity problem may be partially addressed by using several advanced techniques, although they are not commonly employed in clinical practice. One class of approaches uses stimuli such as tone bursts in association with special masking techniques that prevent the cochlea from responding to the stimulus except within a certain frequency range. For example, a noise might be used to mask the high frequencies, so the response is more likely to come from lower frequencies

---

[1] The ECochGm shows amplitude (vertically) as a function of time (horizontally). The area of the SP is basically its amplitude (vertical size) times its duration (horizontal size), and the area of the AP is its amplitude times its duration.

(e.g., Kileny, 1981). Another masking method uses a noise that masks all frequencies except for those in a certain narrow frequency range where there is a "hole" or "notch" in the noise; thus, the ABR response is more likely to come only from the frequency range where the masking noise is missing (e.g., Stapells Picton, Durieux-Smith, Edwards, Morna, 1990; Stapells & Kurtzberg, 1991). The derived-response approach (e.g., Parker & Thornton, 1978; Don, Eggermont, & Brackmann, 1979) involves combining several ABRs that were obtained using various combinations of noises and signals. These various responses are, in effect, subtracted from one another to derive a frequency-specific response.

THE ABR WAVEFORM

An idealized ABR waveform is shown in Figure 11–6. This figure shows positive peaks that are recorded in the upward direction and numbered from I to VII, which is the most common convention in the United States.

However, other recording conventions also exist. As already mentioned, waves I and II are generated by the auditory nerve and correspond to the N1 (AP) and N2 peaks of the electrocochleogram. Even though these first two peaks were plotted downward in the ECochG, they are now flipped upward so they appear in the same direction as the rest of the ABR peaks. This inversion of waves I and II occurs during the process of differential amplification, and is very convenient because it causes all of the ABR peaks to be plotted in the same direction. Before proceeding, notice that only one curve is shown. In actual practice, two sets of tracings would be done because evoked potentials must be *replicated* to confirm that the results obtained are real.

Clinical ABR measurements are concerned with the first five peaks (I to V), and concentrate on peaks I, III, and V. The ABR waveform is usually described and interpreted in terms of the latencies and amplitudes of these peaks, as well as by its **morphology** or the overall configuration and appearance of the

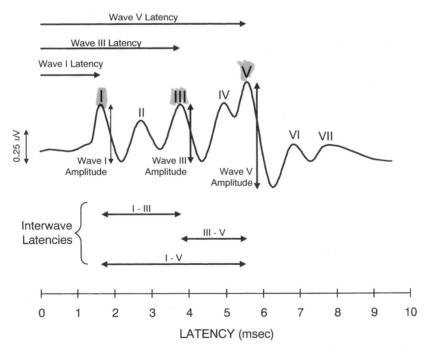

FIGURE 11–6 An idealized auditory brainstem response (ABR). Arrows indicate the wave I, II, and III absolute latencies and amplitudes, and the interwave latencies between waves I and V, I and III, and III and V.

waveform. A given wave's **absolute latency** is simply the time delay from 0 msec (where the click is presented) until its peak occurs.

Electrocochleography is sometimes used to locate wave I when it is not identifiable on the ABR. The time interval between two peaks is called an **interwave latency** or **relative latency**. Interwave latencies are usually measured between waves I and V, I and III, and III and V. These latency measurements are illustrated in the figure by the horizontal arrows. The vertical arrows show how to measure the **amplitudes** for waves I, II, and V. Wave V is the most prominent and robust of these peaks, and is so closely associated with wave IV that one must speak of a **IV/V complex**. There is, however, considerable variability in the morphology of normal ABR waveforms, particularly with respect to the configuration of the VI/V complex.

The ABR waveforms shown in the two previous figures were all obtained with clicks presented at fairly high intensity levels. They would have appeared differently if the clicks had been presented at progressively lower intensities, and would eventually disappear when the clicks were below threshold. In other words, the characteristics of the ABR depend on the level of the stimulus.

In the absence of a universally accepted standard, there has been a great deal of variability in the way that click levels have been described. The best way to specify the click level is in terms of its physical magnitude. Optimally, this involves measuring the click's **peak sound pressure level (peakSPL)**. This is done by directing the click from the earphone through the appropriate calibration coupler[2] into a precision sound level meter that is truly capable of measuring the peak level of a transient signal. Because sound level meters of this type are uncommon, an alternative approach is to describe the click's level in terms of the SPL of a pure-tone that has the same amplitude. This value is called the **peak-equivalent sound pressure level (peSPL)**. This method requires several steps: First, we direct

a click from the earphone into the appropriate calibration coupler and sound level meter and then to an oscilloscope. The click's peak amplitude is noted on the oscilloscope screen. The next step is to replace the click with a tone, and to adjust the level of the tone until its amplitude on the oscilloscope screen is the same as what we found for the click. We then read the tone's SPL on the sound level meter. The level of the tone that has the same amplitude on the screen as the peak amplitude of the click becomes the peSPL of the click. In other words, 40 dB peSPL means the peak level of the click has the same amplitude (on the oscilloscope screen) as that produced by a 40 dB SPL pure tone.

It is more common to find click intensities expressed in behavioral terms. This can be done on an individual patient basis by determining the patient's own behavioral threshold for clicks, and then to express the click intensity in **sensation level (dB SL)**. However, this approach is limited because it is difficult, at best, to assess hearing without knowing the physical level of the stimulus. Moreover, ABR testing is often done on patients who cannot be tested behaviorally, in which case the sensation level of the stimulus cannot be determined. The most widely used approach expresses click intensity in decibels of **normal Hearing Level (nHL)** based on a local norm corresponding to 0 dB HL for each ABR stimulus used (clicks, tone bursts, etc.). The procedure involves obtaining behavioral thresholds for a group of young, normal hearing individuals. Each person is tested to find the lowest intensity dial level on the ABR instrument where the clicks (or other stimulus) are just audible. This dial setting constitutes that person's click threshold, and the average for the group becomes 0 dB nHL. The mean physical level of 0 dB nHL for clicks appears to be between 36.4 and 40 dB peakSPL (Stapells, Picton, & Smith, 1982; Burkhard & Hecox, 1983).

Figure 11–7 shows a series of ABR results obtained from a normal individual with clicks presented at 80, 60, 40, and 20 dB nHL. Notice that the characteristics of the ABR waveform change considerably as the intensity of the clicks are decreased. Another series of ABR waveforms is shown across the upper part of

---

[2] A 6-cc coupler is used for standard audiometric earphones and a 2-cc coupler is used for insert earphones (see Chapter 4).

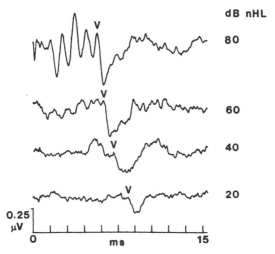

FIGURE 11–7 A series of click-evoked auditory brainstem responses from a normal adult obtained at various stimulus levels. Wave V indicated on each tracing. From Arnold (2000), with permission.

Figure 11–8, where intensity increases from left to right along the x-axis. *As the stimulus intensity gets lower, the peak latencies become longer and their amplitudes become smaller.* The latency shift is seen most vividly by the rightward shift of wave V as the intensity drops progressively from 80 dB nHL down to 20 dB nHL in Figure 11–7. Also, the earlier peaks become less distinctive and eventually disappear with progressively lower stimulus levels. Even though wave V becomes progressively smaller and later with decreasing intensity, it is generally still discernible at levels as low as the behavioral threshold for the click, which is typically down to 0 dB SL or 0 dB nHL, or roughly 35 dB peakSPL, for a normal person. The ABR is finally undetectable at levels below the behavioral threshold. Figure 11–8 also shows a graph that plots the latencies of waves I, III, and V as a function of stimulus (click) level. Such a graph is called a **latency-intensity function**, and it reveals the manner in which latency decreases as stimulus intensity increases.

CLINICAL USE OF THE AUDITORY BRAINSTEM RESPONSE

The ABR is a very valuable clinical tool for several reasons. (1) Auditory brainstem responses are measurable in everyone who is normal,

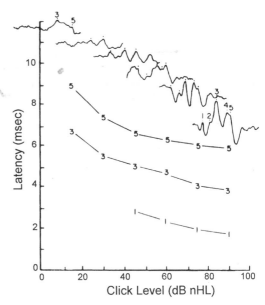

FIGURE 11–8 ABR waveforms obtained at increasing stimulus levels superimposed above the corresponding latency-intensity functions for waves I (1), III (3), and V (5). Adapted from ASHA (1987), with permission of American Speech-Language-Hearing Association.

including newborns. (2) The ABR is not affected by the patient's state of arousal, or by the use of sedation or anesthesia. As a result, ABR testing can be done with or without the cooperation of the patient, and even when the patient is unconscious or under general anesthesia. The ability to perform the ABR on a patient under sedation makes it possible to assess young and/or difficult-to-test children who could not otherwise be evaluated. It should be stressed, of course, that sedation is a medical responsibility. In addition, the ABR is also used in intraoperative monitoring during surgical procedures that jeopardize the eighth nerve, such as acoustic tumor removal. (3) The ABR can be used to assess hearing because it is affected by hearing loss. (4) Different abnormalities affect the ABR in different ways, so that it can be used for differential diagnosis.

Just because the ABR is ubiquitous does not mean that its characteristics are the same for everyone. On the contrary, maturation, gender, and aging need to be considered when developing norms and interpreting the results.

The ABR is present but not adult-like in newborns, and its character changes with the infant's maturation (Hecox & Galambos, 1974; Fria, 1980; Hall, 1992; Chiappa, 1997). For example, waves I, III, and V are observable in newborns, but the absolute latencies of waves III and V are prolonged relative to adult values, as are the interwave latencies. As the infant matures, the other peaks emerge, the latencies of the waves shorten, and their amplitudes change, eventually achieving adult characteristics by roughly 18 months of age.

Among adults, the ABR is affected by gender and aging (Stockard, Stockard, Westmoreland, & Corfits, 1979; Jerger & Hall, 1980; Jerger & Johnson, 1988). Compared to males, females tend to have shorter absolute latencies and larger amplitudes for waves III, IV, and V, as well as shorter interwave latencies. Also, it appears that the degree of cochlear impairment has a greater effect on wave V latencies for men than for women (Jerger & Johnson, 1988). The effect of aging is not as clear-cut, but its absolute latencies appear to become slightly longer with advancing age.

The earlier discussion about how the ABR is affected by stimulus intensity also reveals the procedure for estimating a patient's thresholds with the ABR. The basic procedure is to obtain a series of ABRs at progressively lower intensities until the level is reached where a replicable response is no longer discernible. This usually involves finding the lowest level where wave V can be identified. Normal hearing is implied when a response can be identified at stimulus levels as low as approximately 0 dB nHL. The word *implied* is used because physiological measures are not direct hearing tests in the sense that they do not reveal whether the patient is able to respond to sounds behaviorally. Rather, they are tests of the integrity of the structures and processes involved in hearing, and in the case of the ABR, these responses are coming from just the lower portions of the auditory pathways. In spite of these caveats, it is clear that ABR thresholds provide valuable information about the hearing of patients who cannot respond behaviorally, such as infants and the difficult-to-test. In fact, the ABR is widely used for infant screening purposes as well as

for the diagnostic assessment of this population (Chapters 12 and 13). In addition, even though ABR thresholds are obtained for clicks, they tend to be in good agreement with at least high-frequency behavioral thresholds.

An individual patient's latency-intensity functions are compared to normative values in order to make inferences about the nature and degree of her hearing loss. Several examples are shown in Figure 11–9. The normal range of wave V latencies is shown by a pair of curved lines in each panel. Each facility should develop a set of normal ranges that applies to its own equipment and procedures. The leftmost symbol of each individual latency-inten-

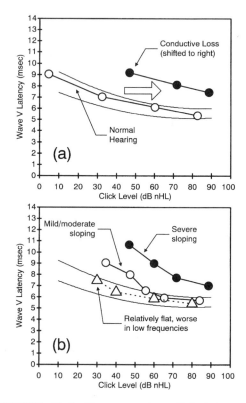

FIGURE 11–9 Representative clinical wave V latency-intensity functions. The paired curved lines in each panel are normal confidence limits. (a) Results for a normal ear and a case of conductive loss. Notice the conductive function is shifted to the right, represented by the arrow. (b) Functions for cochlear sensorineural loss generally converge toward the normal latency range as click intensity is raised, but this is affected by shape and degree of loss.

sity function is obtained from the lowest click level that produces a replicable ABR, and therefore also represents the threshold for clicks. These points occur at 5 dB nHL for the normal case and 45 dB nHL for conductive loss in the upper panel of the figure, and 30, 35, and 45 dB nHL for the examples of cochlear impairments in the lower panel.

The typical **wave V latency-intensity functions** associated with normal hearing, conductive losses, and sensorineural losses of cochlear origin are quite different. As we would expect, the *normal* latency-intensity function falls within the normal limit lines (open circles in Fig. 11–9a). *Conductive losses* reduce the amount of signal intensity reaching the cochlea. For this reason, they tend to have the latency-intensity functions that are essentially displaced horizontally to the right (higher click levels) by roughly the amount of the conductive loss (filled circles in Fig. 11–9a). On the other hand, *cochlear impairments* typically have wave V latencies that are elevated at and slightly above threshold, and then converge to the normal latency range as the click intensity is raised (circles in Fig. 11–9b). However, whether this pattern occurs depends on the configuration of the hearing loss because the ABR relies heavily on the basal (high-frequency) portion of the cochlea (Yamada, Kodera, & Yagi, 1979). Notice in Figure 11–9b that the wave V latency-intensity function is abnormal when the sensorineural hearing loss involves the high frequencies (circles), but can actually be within the normal range in cases of low frequency and relatively mild flat sensorineural loss, where the high frequencies are preserved (triangles). The different latency-intensity functions associated with conductive and cochlear impairments allow the ABR to help us discriminate between these two kinds of hearing losses. However, conductive losses may have to exceed 35 dB to be reliably distinguished from sensorineural impairments with the ABR (van der Drift, Brocaar, & van Zanten, 1988a,b).

Another way to use the ABR to identify the type of loss is to compare the results obtained when the clicks are presented by air-conduction versus bone-conduction. When bone-conduction ABRs are done, one must be mindful that (1) the highest usable click levels for bone-conduction ABR testing are limited to about 50 dB nHL, (2) bone-conduction wave V latencies are roughly 0.5 msec longer than they are by air-conduction, and (3) appropriate masking of the contralateral ear should be employed (Mauldin & Jerger, 1979; Weber, 1983; Schwartz, Larson, & DeChicchis, 1985; Gorga & Thornton, 1989).

Because the ABR reflects the activity of the auditory nerve and brainstem pathways, it is not surprising that it can be used to identify *retrocochlear pathologies* like acoustic tumors. The identification of retrocochlear disorders from the ABR involves interpreting peak measurements and waveform morphology, and has an overall sensitivity of about 95% (Turner, Shepard, & Frazer, 1984). The following ABR findings are associated with retrocochlear abnormalities, several of which may be found in Figure 11–10:

- *Prolonged latency* for wave V.
- *Prolonged interwave latency* for I to V (as well as for I to III and/or III to V).
- *Interaural latency differences.* Significant differences between the patient's two ears are considered for both the wave V latency and the interwave latencies.
- *Absence of the later waves.*
- *Absence of an ABR* even though hearing is normal or only mildly impaired.
- An ABR waveform that is *not replicable.*
- Abnormally low V:I amplitude ratio. The V:I amplitude ratio is simply the amplitude of wave V over the amplitude of wave I, and is expected to be ≥1.0 because wave V is normally larger. One becomes suspicious of a retrocochlear disorder when the V:I ratio is less than 1.0, but this criterion is not as sensitive as the latency measurements.
- Significant shifting of wave V latency when the clicks are presented at a faster rate, although the usefulness of this criterion is controversial.

An absent or grossly abnormal ABR with normal outer hair cell functioning demon-

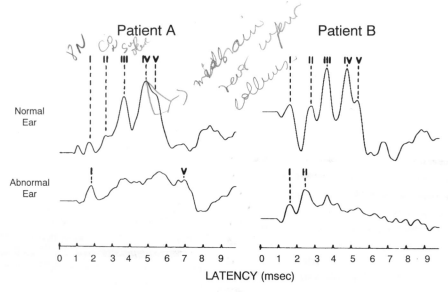

FIGURE 11–10 Two examples of abnormal ABR results in cases of retrocochlear pathology. Adapted from ASHA (1987), with permission of American Speech-Language-Hearing Association.

strated by otoacoustic emissions and/or cochlear microphonics (discussed elsewhere in this chapter) is also associated with *auditory neuropathy* (e.g., Starr, Picton, Sininger, Hood, & Berlin, 1996; see Chapter 6).

Later Auditory Evoked Potentials

The ABR is by far the class of auditory evoked potentials that is most widely used by audiologists, sometimes to the exclusion of all others. Yet, other kinds of AEPs are not only available but also provide information not obtainable with the ABR. Figure 11–3 identifies these as the **middle latency response (MLR)** and the **long latency response (LLR)** (Hall, 1992; Kraus, Kileny, & McGee 1994; Kraus & McGee, 1994; McPherson & Ballachanda, 2000). The major advantage of these responses is that they can provide frequency-specific information about hearing sensitivity. Their major disadvantage is that they are significantly affected by the state of the patient and are altered or obliterated by drugs (including sedatives and anesthetics), which curtails their usefulness with young children and other difficult-to-test patients.

The middle latency response is a series of negative (N) and positive (P) waves occur-

ring at latencies between 15 and 50 msec, identified as **Na, Pa, Nb,** and **Pb** (Fig. 11–3). It appears to reflect neural activity originating from several cortical and subcortical locations involving the midbrain, reticular formation, and the thalamocortical pathways. The principal clinical contribution of the MLR is that it can be elicited by relatively low-frequency tone bursts, such as 500 or 1000 Hz, which would not be successful stimuli with the ABR. As a result, the MLR can be used successfully to assess low-frequency hearing sensitivity. It is also useful in the diagnosis of central auditory nervous system abnormalities.

The long latency responses occur at latencies beyond approximately 75 msec, and have also been known as the **cortical evoked potentials**. The major LLR components are shown in Figure 11–3 as waves **N1, P2,** and **N2.** (Wave **P1** is generally considered to be the latest peak of the middle response, Pb.) It appears that the P2 and N2 components of the LLR are largely derived from activity from the auditory cortex, and that contributions are also made by the limbic system. Even though it is possible to obtain frequency-specific evoked response thresholds with the LLR, its susceptibility to the state of arousal and drugs means that its use is largely limited to awake and cooperative patients.

Event-Related Potentials Other kinds of late responses also occur that involve discriminations and various levels of processing for all kinds of signals from tones to speech. For example, **P3** (or **P300**) is a large positive wave that occurs at a latency of about 300 msec when the patient attends to and elicits a cognitive response to an atypical stimulus (e.g., Sutton, Barren, Zubin, & John, 1965; Kraus & McGee, 1994). Testing for the P3 wave involves an **odd-ball procedure** that uses two different signals, one that occurs frequently (the "frequent" signal) and another that occurs infrequently (the "rare" signal). The rare signal is also called an "odd-ball" because it differs from the frequent signal in some way, such as frequency. Different sets of evoked potentials are then obtained. "Frequent" test conditions have signals that are all the same. "Rare" test conditions include a relatively small percentage of odd-ball signals distributed randomly among the frequent signals. If the patient *ignores* the test stimuli, then the result will be a routine LLR regardless of whether the odd-ball was pres-

ent or absent (Fig. 11–11a,b). The situation is different if the patient *pays attention to the signals, listening particularly for the odd-balls.* Here the AEP is unchanged for the frequent-only signals (Fig. 11–11c); however, a clear P3 wave appears for the rarely included signals (Fig. 11–11d). In contrast, **mismatch negativity (MMN)** is a physiological measure of discrimination that occurs even *without attending* to the stimulus (Näätänen, 1995). It appears as a negative deflection that occurs at latencies between roughly 150 and 275 msec when the patient detects a signal that is different from those that came before it.

As one might expect, these and other event-related potentials are produced by neural activity extending well beyond just the auditory cortex, and provide us with physiological windows into the patient's ability to deal with almost every level of processing, from detecting and discriminating signals to processing them linguistically and cognitively.

Topographical Brain Mapping It is possible to record a particular potential, such as the P3 wave or a component of the MLR, simultaneously from many different locations on the

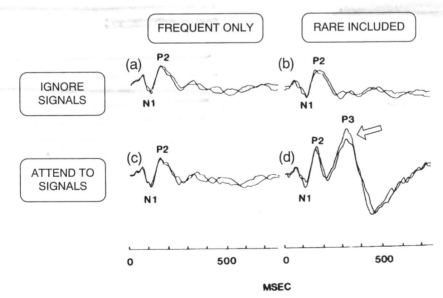

FIGURE 11–11 A P3 wave (arrow) is obtained when odd-ball signals are present and attended to by the patient. Modified from "Electrophysiological evaluation of higher level auditory processing" by Squires and Hecox (1983), with permission.

head. As one would expect, the amplitude of these responses will vary according to where they were picked up, being largest where the underlying neural activity is greatest and smallest at locations that are inactive. A computer program can then be used to "fill-in" the amplitudes that should occur between these sampled locations. The result can be drawn as contour lines or differently shaded areas depicting equally active locations on the scalp, just as geographical maps use contours to show equal land elevations. Other programs show equally active locations with different colors. We see the same kinds of pictures on television weather reports every day, representing regions of equal temperature or rain fall. Just as red means hot weather and other colors mean progressively less temperature, red areas on a topographical brain map are "hot" from the standpoint of neurologic brain activity and other colors represent progressively less active locations. Clinically, a patient's topographical brain map may be compared to normal patterns for such purposes as evaluating the physiological aspects of processing disorders and determining disordered anatomical sites.

Otoacoustic Emissions

One of the most fascinating characteristics of the cochlea is that it can produce sounds as well as receive them. These sounds that are elicited by the ear are called **otoacoustic emissions (OAEs)**, and can be measured with a sensitive microphone in the ear canal. Kemp (1978, 1979) demonstrated that OAEs are produced in response to signals presented to the ear, as well as spontaneously without any stimulation. The concept is best understood by imagining a simple experiment in which an OAE is produced as a result of presenting a click to the ear. We will need a probe assembly similar to the kind used for acoustic immittance testing (Chapter 7). For convenience, we will call this assembly the "probe tip." It contains a tiny loudspeaker ("receiver" or "earphone") to present the click stimulus, and a sensitive microphone to record the sounds in the ear canal, including the OAE.

The method involves measuring the sounds in the ear canal for a period of about 20 msec, beginning with the presentation of a click.

First, let us see what happens when the click is directed into an *inanimate cavity*. To do this, the probe tip is inserted into a Zwislocki coupler, which is a metal cavity that mimics the acoustics of the ear. The result is a damped oscillation lasting several milliseconds, as shown in the top frame of Figure 11–12. This damped oscillation is the acoustic waveform of the click itself. In contrast, presenting a click into a real ear results in the waveform shown in the middle frame of the figure. The most obvious aspects of this waveform are the same large, damped oscillations due to the click seen in the inert cavity. However, notice that this waveform, measured in a real ear canal, also contains a second group of tiny oscillations that begin several milliseconds later. These oscillations constitute the OAE or **cochlear echo (Kemp echo)** produced in the cochlea, transmitted back into the ear canal, and picked up by the probe tip microphone. The lower panel of the figure shows the OAE after it has been amplified, with the earlier click waveform removed. This kind of OAE is called a transient-evoked otoacoustic emission because it occurs in response to a click (transient) stimulus, and will be covered in greater detail below.

Otoacoustic emissions are the result of microscopic biomechanical activity (motility) associated with healthy outer hair cells. This activity produces a signal within the cochlea that is transmitted "backward" through the middle ear and into the ear canal, where it can be picked up by a microphone. The cochlear events that produce OAEs are said to be "preneural" because they occur before the signal is transmitted to the auditory nerve, and are related to the physiological processes underlying the sensitivity and the "fine tuning" of the normal cochlea (e.g., Kiang, Liberman, Sewell, & Guinan, 1986; Probst, Lonsbury-Martin, & Martin, 1991; Norton, 1992; Robinette, & Glattke, 1997; Gelfand, 1998). Our interest in OAEs is practical as well as theoretical because they are also useful clinical tools. Otoacoustic emissions are valuable clinically because they are

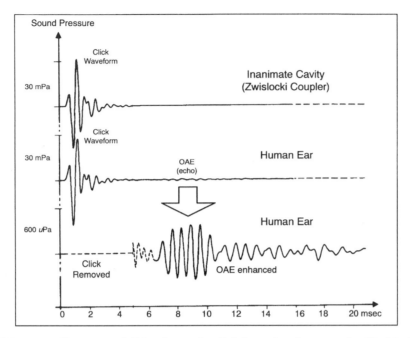

FIGURE 11–12 Upper panel: Waveform of a click in an inanimate cavity (Zwislocki coupler). Middle panel: Click waveform and resulting otoacoustic emission (OAE) or cochlear echo in a human ear canal. Lower panel: Same as middle panel, but with click waveform removed and otoacoustic emission enhanced. Adapted from Johnsen and Elberling (1982), with permission of *Scandinavian Audiology*.

(1) sensitive to the presence of hearing loss; (2) sensitive to problems affecting the integrity of the cochlea, particularly the outer hair cells; and (3) preneural in nature, which makes them different from measurements that involve neural activity, for example, the auditory brainstem response. In addition, OAEs are very practical because they are quick and easy to obtain without any invasive procedures. Otoacoustic emissions are the subject of extensive, ongoing research, and their clinical attributes and applications are provided in several extensive reviews (e.g., Probst, Lonsbury-Martin, & Martin, 1991; Lonsbury-Martin, Whitehead, & Martin, 1991; Dekker, 1992; Norton & Stover, 1994; Robinette & Glattke, 1997; Lonsbury-Martin, Martin, & Telischi, 1999; Glattke & Robinette, 2000).

As anticipated from the example just described, the equipment needed to measure OAEs includes a probe tip assembly that contains a microphone to measure sounds in the ear canal, as well as receivers to present various kinds of stimuli. The faint sounds picked up by the measurement microphone are amplified and filtered to minimize noises, and are then analyzed in one of several ways depending on what kind of OAE is being examined. The microphone is involved in all OAE measurements, regardless of whether the emissions are evoked by some kind of stimulus or occur spontaneously in the absence of stimulation. The receivers present the stimuli used to elicit the various kinds of evoked OAEs. Block diagrams describing the instrumentation involved in measuring various kinds of OAEs appear later in this chapter. An example of a clinical OAE instrument is shown in Figure 11–13.

Spontaneous Otoacoustic Emissions

Spontaneous otoacoustic emissions (SOAEs) are narrow band sounds emitted from the ear

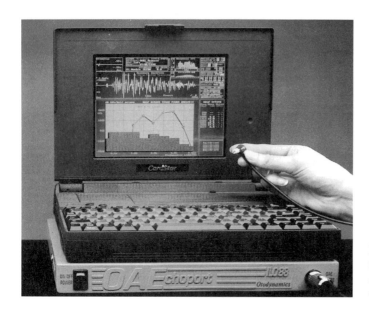

FIGURE 11–13 Example of an instrument used for otoacoustic emissions testing. Courtesy of Otodynamics, Ltd.

in the absence of stimulation. They are identified by examining the spectrum of the sound monitored by a probe microphone in the ear canal. The spectrum is the result of a spectral analysis performed by the OAE analysis system, as illustrated in the upper part of Figure 11–14. The lower part of the figure shows an example of the averaged spectrum from an ear with SOAEs at 1025, 1470, and 1895 Hz. The SOAEs are seen as narrow peaks extending above the background noise in the spectrum. They usually occur at one or several frequencies between 1000 and 3000 Hz, and occasionally as low as about 500 Hz. As indicated in the figure, SOAEs are very faint, typically ranging in size from roughly −10 to +20 dB SPL. For this reason, a number of spectra are averaged so that we are able to see the SOAEs above the background noise. This spectral averaging procedure is based on the same principles that were explained for auditory evoked potentials, except that averaging is done as a function of frequency instead of over time.

It was originally thought that SOAEs would be a useful clinical tool because they are relatively simple to measure, tend to occur at the same frequencies over time for a given ear, do not appear to be age related, and may be present at frequencies where

thresholds are in the normal range *but* are absent in frequency regions where the hearing loss exceeds 20 to 30 dB HL. However, the clinical usefulness of SOAEs is actually rather limited because of two different kinds of drawbacks. One set of restrictions involves the relatively low prevalence of SOAEs. Specifically, SOAEs occur in only about half of the normal-hearing population and are also less likely to occur in males than in females. The other clinical weaknesses of SOAEs pertain to the ears where they are found. These limitations are (1) just a few (or only one) SOAEs are found in an ear; (2) they occur at different frequencies in different ears; (3) SOAEs are found in a relatively restricted range of frequencies; and (4) their amplitudes can vary over time.

One cannot help but wonder whether SOAEs are the cause of tinnitus, or are at least a physiological manifestation of it. This is unlikely in most cases for a number of reasons. For example, tinnitus is more likely to be associated with hearing loss and/or disordered ears, whereas SOAEs are associated with normality. Most people who have SOAEs are not aware of them, and a rational association between tinnitus and SOAEs is found in no more than perhaps 9 to 12% of tinnitus

Spontaneous Otoacoustic Emissions (SOAE)

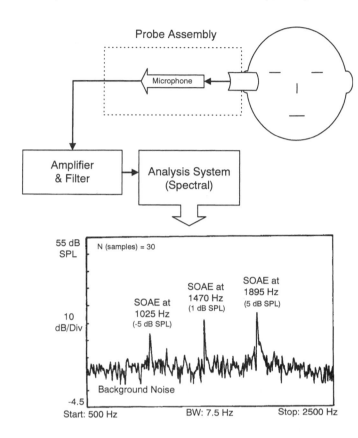

FIGURE 11–14 Instrumentation block diagram and an example of spontaneous otoacoustic emissions (SOAEs). These are seen as narrow peaks in the spectrum monitored in the ear canal. The ear in this example has SOAEs at 1025, 1470, and 1895 Hz. Adapted in part from Lonsbury-Martin, Whitehead, and Martin (1991), with permission of American Speech-Language-Hearing Association.

patients (Norton, Schmidt, & Stover, 1990; Penner, 1990).

Evoked Otoacoustic Emissions

Evoked otoacoustic emissions are sounds emitted from the ear as a result of stimulation. There are basically three different kinds of evoked otoacoustic emissions. **Stimulus-frequency otoacoustic emissions (SFOAEs)** are elicited by presenting a sweep-frequency tone to the ear. This class of OAEs may provide useful information, but complications in terms of technology and interpretation have prevented it from being a viable clinical tool at this point in time. We shall therefore concentrate on the two other types of evoked OAEs, which have considerable clinical utility and promise. These include transient evoked otoacoustic emissions and distortion product otoacoustic emissions.

TRANSIENT-EVOKED OTOACOUSTIC EMISSIONS

Transient-evoked otoacoustic emissions (TEOAEs) are produced in response to very brief stimuli, such as clicks. The TEOAE is also known as the **click-evoked otoacoustic emission, Kemp echo,** or **cochlear echo.** (Although not discussed here, more frequency-specific stimuli such as tone bursts can also be used.) Recall from the example used to introduce the concept of otoacoustic emissions earlier in this section that the TEOAE is seen as a waveform that is picked up in the ear canal several milliseconds after a click has been presented. The upper part of Figure 11–15 shows a block diagram of the equipment used to elicit and measure TEOAEs. The probe tip includes a loudspeaker to present the clicks and a microphone to monitor the sounds in the ear canal. The signals picked up by the microphone then

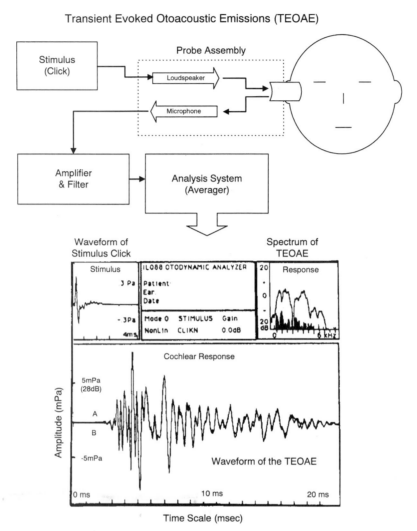

Transient Evoked Otoacoustic Emissions (TEOAE)

FIGURE 11–15 Instrumentation block diagram and an example of transient-evoked oto-acoustic emissions (TEOAEs). See text. Adapted in part from Lonsbury-Martin, Whitehead, and Martin (1991), with permission of American Speech-Language-Hearing Association.

go through an amplifier and filter to a signal analysis system. Because the OAEs have very small amplitudes that must be distinguished from background noise, a large number of clicks are presented in succession, and the sounds in the ear canal are monitored for a period of time (e.g., 20 msec) after each click. These responses are then averaged using the same basic approach described for auditory evoked potentials earlier in this chapter.

Clinical TEOAEs are usually elicited using clicks presented at about 82 to 83 dB peSPL.

An example of a normal TEOAE waveform is shown in the lower portion of Figure 11–15. The large frame shows the waveform of the TEOAE response. The time scale shows the latency of the response from when the click was presented. The first several milliseconds of the response appear flat so as to remove the waveform of the click stimulus, which is shown in a separate box (above left). Notice that two separate waveforms (A and B) were obtained and superimposed to establish the reliability of the results. The TEOAE waveform has latencies between about 5 and 20 msec. A given latency on this waveform reflects the "round trip" time it takes for the click to reach a particular location along the cochlear duct and for the returning TEOAE (cochlear echo) to be picked up by the probe microphone in the ear canal. This travel time is shortest for locations near the base of the cochlea and increases toward the apex. Hence, it appears that (1) the earlier parts of the TEOAE waveform (i.e., those at shorter latencies) are from locations toward the base of the cochlea, where higher frequencies are represented; and (2) the parts of the waveform at successively longer latencies are from locations successively closer to the apex, where lower frequencies are represented. The spectrum of this TEOAE is shown in the box above and to the right of the waveform. Normal TEOAEs are generally obtained at frequencies from about 400 to 500 Hz up to approximately 4500 Hz in adults and about 5000 to 6000 Hz in babies and young children. The decision about whether a TEOAE is present often depends on a visual assessment of the response along with certain objective criteria, such as the reproducibility of the waveform (in percent) and the signal-to-noise ratio (in decibels) of the response compared to the noise floor.

It is possible to point out several generalities about TEOAEs that have considerable clinical relevance. Transient-evoked OAEs can be obtained in almost all normal hearing individuals, including newborns. In fact, responses are larger in babies than they are in adults. Reduced or obliterated TEOAEs result from the same factors that are known to cause cochlear hearing losses, such as ototoxic agents, hypoxia, and noise exposure. Similarly, TEOAEs are absent in patients with cochlear sensorineural losses greater than about 30 to 50 dB HL, depending on the details of the test parameters. Conductive abnormalities can also interfere with the ability to obtain TEOAEs because they interfere with the ability of the OAE to be transmitted back to the probe microphone. These factors make TEOAEs very useful for detecting the presence of hearing loss, even in newborns. As a result, newborn hearing screening programs have been one of the most rapidly growing applications of TEOAEs, as discussed in Chapter 13. Because otoacoustic emissions are preneural events, it is not surprising that TEOAEs are usually not a particularly useful test for acoustic tumors per se (Bonfils & Uziel, 1988). However, they do contribute to differential diagnosis, improving the ability to distinguish cochlear and neural involvement, when used with tests that involve neural transmission, such as acoustic reflexes and the ABR (eg., Robinette, Bauch, Olsen, Hamer, & Beatty, 1992; Starr et al, 1996; Robinette & Glattke, 1997; Lonsbury-Martin, Martin, & Telischi, 1999).

DISTORTION PRODUCT OTOACOUSTIC EMISSIONS

Distortion product otoacoustic emissions (DPOAEs) are elicited by simultaneously presenting to the ear two stimulus tones with different frequencies, as shown in the block diagram at the top of Figure 11–16. The lower stimulus tone is called f_1 and the higher tone is called f_2. As a result of its normal nonlinear response to the two stimulus tones, the cochlea will generate another tone "of its own" at a different frequency, called a **distortion product**. The distortion product is then transmitted back to the ear canal as an otoacoustic emission. (This is why it is called a distortion product otoacoustic emission.) The probe microphone thus picks up three tones: the two original stimulus tones (often called primaries) plus the DPOAE that was produced in the cochlea. The OAE instrument then performs a spectral analysis similar to that described earlier for SOAEs, the result of which is exemplified in the lower part of Figure 11–16. Here we see the two original tones (f_1 and f_2) along with the much fainter DPOAE. The DPOAE is typically about 60 dB weaker than the primary tones (14 dB SPL for the DPOAE compared to 85 dB SPL for f_1 and f_2 in the figure). The frequency of the DPOAE will be equal to twice the frequency of the lower stimulus tone minus the frequency of the higher one, or $2f_1 - f_2$. The two stimulus tones shown in the figure are 3164 and 3828

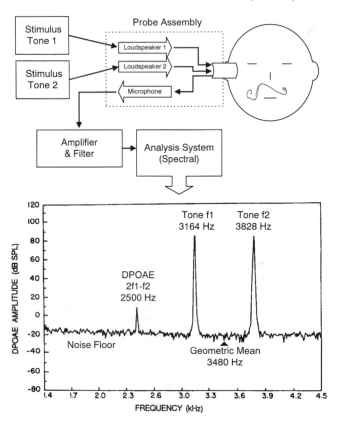

Distortion Product Otoacoustic Emissions (DPOAE)

FIGURE 11–16 Instrumentation block diagram and an example of distortion product emissions (DPOAEs). See text. Adapted in part from Lonsbury-Martin, Whitehead, and Martin (1991), with permission of American Speech Language-Hearing Association.

Hz; thus the DPOAE occurs at 2500 Hz. The arithmetic is as follows:

$$2f_1 - f_2 = (2 \times 3164) - 3828$$
$$= 6328 - 3828$$
$$= 2500 \text{ Hz}$$

As with other OAEs, DPOAEs are affected by various stimulus parameters. It appears that the strongest DPOAEs are obtained when f_1 and f_2 are between 1000 and 4000 Hz, and when the ratio of their frequencies (f_2/f_1) is about 1.2. In our example, this ratio is 3828/3164 = 1.21. Even though the DPOAE occurs at a frequency of $2f_1 - f_2$, the location in the cochlea and thus the frequency actually being tested is in the vicinity of the primary tones, and is usually taken to be the *geometric mean* of f_1 and f_2. The geometric mean is found by multiplying the two stimulus frequencies and then finding the square root of their product, or $\sqrt{(f_1 \times f_2)}$. In our example, this frequency is $\sqrt{(3164 \times 3828)} =$

$\sqrt{12,111,792)} = 3480$ Hz. The DPOAE is also affected by the levels of the two primary tones (L_1 and L_2), although the optimal relationship between them seems to depend on whether testing is done at overall higher versus lower stimulus levels. It seems best for levels of the two tones to be equal when using higher levels of stimulation (e.g., 75 dB SPL), but L_1 should be about 10 to 15 dB higher than L_2 for lower levels (e.g., $L_1 = 60$ dB SPL and $L_2 = 50$ dB SPL).

Distortion product OAEs are found in essentially all normal ears and are absent when there is a sensorineural loss of about 50 to 60 dB HL. The size of the DPOAE increases with the level of the primaries. In addition, DPOAEs can be obtained as a function of frequency. Two kinds of DPOAE measures based on these properties are the DP-gram[3]

---

[3] The DP-gram used to be called the DP audiogram or the DPOAE audiogram.

and the DPOAE input/output function. The **DP-gram** is obtained by presenting the stimulus tones at a fixed level (e.g., 65 SPL) across a range of (geometric mean) frequencies. In other words, it shows DPOAE amplitude as a function of frequency. The **DPOAE input/output function** is obtained by measuring DPOAE amplitude as a function of stimulus level at a given (geometric mean) frequency. Figure 11–17 shows normal results. The upper graph is a DP-gram obtained with 65 dB HL stimulus tones. Notice how the right and left ear data fall inside of the indicated "normal range." Results from an impaired ear would fall below this range at the frequencies where there is a hearing loss, as represented by the arrow labeled "hearing loss." The lower graph is a DPOAE input/output function, in which the test findings (labeled "DPE" for distortion product emissions) also fall within the "normal range." Abnormal results would be displaced rightward (represented by the arrow), indicating that more intensity is needed to obtain a DPOAE.

Vestibular Assessment

Audiologists are interested in the vestibular (balance) system because of its close association with the auditory system. The inner ear houses the sensory receptor organs for both hearing (the cochlea) and balance (the semicircular canals, utricle, and saccule). In addition, the auditory and vestibular systems both use the eighth nerve to send their signals to the central nervous system. It is therefore not surprising that at least some auditory problems are often accompanied by dizziness.

Vestibular disorders are associated with a kind of dizziness called **vertigo**, which is a sensation of rotation. The patient with vertigo

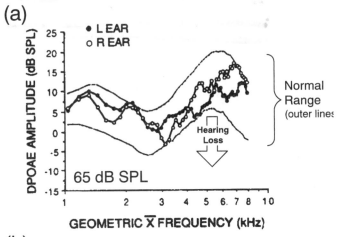

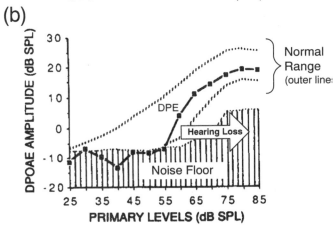

FIGURE 11–17 Examples of normal results on a DP-gram (above) and a DPOAE input/output function (below). See text. Adapted from Lonsbury-Martin, Whitehead, and Martin (1991), with permission of American Speech-Language-Hearing Association.

feels as though he is spinning or that the environment is spinning around him. Vertigo is accompanied by a kind of eye movement called **nystagmus**, in which the eyes move to one side and then bounce back to the center very rapidly. Nystagmus reflects what is going on in the vestibular system and is easily measured. Thus, vestibular evaluation involves measuring and interpreting the nystagmus.

The measurement of nystagmus is called **electronystagmography (ENG)**, which involves monitoring eye movements with electrodes placed around the eyes. The ENG electrodes pick up the **corneoretinal potential**, an electrical difference between the front and back of the eye. The front of the eye (cornea) has a positive electrical charge and the back of the eye (retina) has a negative charge. The orientation of the positive and negative "ends" changes according to which way the eyes are facing. For example, the more one gazes to the right the greater will be the electrical signal that is positive toward the right and negative toward the left. Alternatively, looking to the left makes the signal positive to the left and negative to the right. The resulting electrical signal can be picked up by electrodes at the outer edges of each eye. The electrodes transmit this information to the ENG recorder.

As shown in Figure 11–18, horizontal eye movements are measured by a pair of electrodes placed to the right of the right ear and to the left of the left eye. These electrodes are connected to one channel of an ENG recorder, which draws the right-left position of the eyes on a moving strip of graph paper. Specifically, the ENG recorder pen (actually a heat stylus) moves upward when the eyes move to the right and downward when the eyes move to the left, as shown in Figure 11–19. Vertical motion is picked up by a second pair of electrodes above and below one of the eyes, which leads to a second channel of the ENG recorder. On this channel upward eye movement is drawn upward on the recorder paper and downward eye motion is drawn downward. Finally, a ground electrode is placed in the middle of the forehead.

Nystagmus occurs in **beats**. The relatively slower motion is called the **slow phase**, and is due to the activity of the *vestibular system*. The very rapid movement back to the center is called the **fast phase** and is due to activity arising from within the *central nervous system*. Each complete set of eye movements to the side and back is a beat, and nystagmus is generally composed of a succession of beats one after the other. The direction of nystagmus is the direction of the fast phase. Its magnitude or strength is determined from the slow phase and is expressed in degrees of eye rotation per second. Figure 11–20 shows

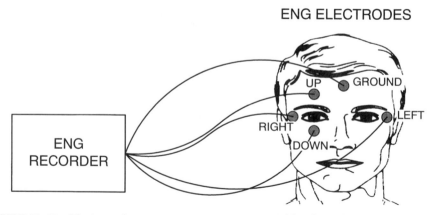

FIGURE 11–18 Horizontal eye movements are monitored by the right and left electrodes, and are depicted on one channel of the ENG recorder. Vertical eye movements are picked up by the electrodes above and below one eye, and are shown on the other channel of the recorder. The ground electrode is shown at the center of the forehead.

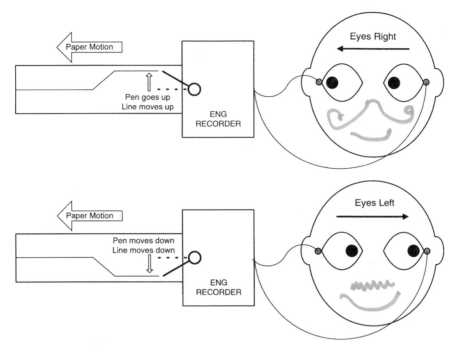

FIGURE 11–19 The pen (heat stylus) on the ENG recorder moves up on the recorder paper when the eyes move toward the right and down when the eyes move toward the left.

examples of right-beating and left-beating nystagmus.

The vestibular evaluation is unquestionably beyond the scope of a basic text, but it is worthwhile for even a beginning student to have a rudimentary idea of what the most commonly used ENG tests are and what the various outcomes imply. Many informative sources are available for students interested in more detailed coverages of this topic (e.g., Coats, 1975, 1986; Barber & Stockwell, 1980; Stockwell, 1983; Yellin, 2000).

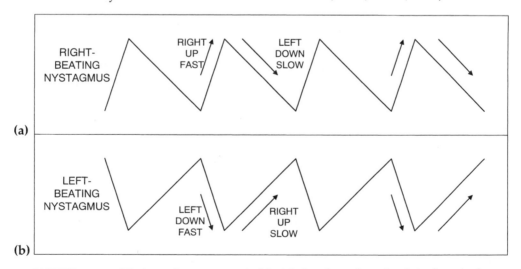

FIGURE 11–20 Horizontal nystagmus is (a) right-beating when the fast phase is drawn upward, and (b) left-beating when the fast phase is drawn downward. If these were vertical channel recordings, then (a) would be up-beating and (b) would be down-beating nystagmus.

The outcomes of vestibular tests are usually interpreted as normal or pathological. Pathological results are further delineated as (1) peripheral, (2) central, or (3) "nonlocalizing," that is, the abnormal result can be associated with either peripheral or central disorders.

The first procedure during an ENG evaluation is to calibrate the recorder to the patient's eye movements. The recorder paper is a strip of graph paper with 1-mm square boxes. The paper comes out of the recorder at 10 mm/sec, so that time is easily read horizontally. However, we want each millimeter vertically to represent 1° of eye rotation. This is easier than it sounds. The patient is asked to look back and forth between two points that are 10° to the right and left of center (a total of 20° of eye rotation). At the same time, the tester adjusts a control on the ENG recorder so that the pen moves up or down a total of 20 mm every time the eyes cover the 20° arc. The calibration procedure is also a clinical test. Normal people can do the task quite accurately. However, patients with pathologies of the cerebellum often overshoot the mark when trying to look back and forth between the two target points. Such a finding is called **calibration overshoot** or **ocular dysmetria**.

Gaze testing involves having the patient stare at a fixed point, and should not result in nystagmus. If it does, the result is called **gaze nystagmus**, which is associated with central involvement.

Two more tasks involve following a visual target and both of them are tests of central dysfunctions. One of these is a **smooth pursuit test**, in which the patient's eyes must follow a smoothly moving target, such as a pendulum. The motion of the target is sinusoidal, so that the normal eye motion should cause a smooth sine wave to be drawn on the ENG paper. The abnormal response, in which the sine-wave pattern is distorted and irregular, is called sinusoidal break-up or cogwheeling. The other procedure is called the **optokinetic nystagmus test**. The basic test involves having the patient follow a series of vertical bands moving from left to right, and then from right to left. The test mimics what happens when a passenger watches the rapid progression of telephone poles while looking out the window of a speeding train. This causes nystagmus in which the slow phase goes in the same direction as the moving bands. The normal result is for the nystagmus induced by the rightward bands to be a mirror image of the nystagmus induced by the leftward bands. The result is considered abnormal when the nystagmus is grossly asymmetric for the two different directions.

Nystagmus induced by being in a given position is called **positional nystagmus**. One test for this determines whether nystagmus is present on the ENG record while the patient is kept in each of several positions. The most typical positions tested are lying down supine, on the right and left sides, supine with the head hanging off the end of the table, and sitting erect. **Spontaneous nystagmus** is said to occur if nystagmus is present when the patient is in a "neutral" position, that is, sitting erect (Coats, 1975), or if the nystagmus has the same characteristics in several different positions (Barber & Stockwell, 1980). Both positional and spontaneous nystagmus are abnormal, but are most conservatively interpreted as nonlocalizing.

Many patients complain of vertigo associated with such quick movements as bending over, called paroxysmal vertigo. The clinical test for **paroxysmal vertigo** involves performing the **Dix-Hallpike maneuver**, which is basically as follows: The patient begins sitting erect. Under the control of the clinician, she is then rapidly moved down to a supine position with her head hanging off the end of the table and turned to one side or the other. One determines whether this manipulation results in nystagmus with particular characteristics. The maneuver may be repeated one or more times depending on whether the patient experiences vertigo and if there is nystagmus with a particular set of characteristics. The interpretation depends on the resulting constellation of findings.

The **bithermal** (two temperature) **caloric test** is used to stimulate the right and left semicircular canals separately, so that their responses can be compared. The patient lies supine with her head elevated 30°, which causes the horizontal semicircular canals to be in a vertical position. Then each ear canal is separately stimulated with cool water and then with warm water. Irrigating[4] with warm water heats the endolymph in that ear, causing it to flow upward and thus deflect the cupula. The result should be nystagmus that beats in the direction of the stimulated ear. Irrigating the ear with cool water will cool the endolymph, causing it to flow downward and thus deflect the cupula in the other direction, causing nystagmus that beats away from the stimulated ear.

The strength of the nystagmus caused by stimulating the right ear (right cool and right warm) is compared to the nystagmus due to stimulating the left ear (left cool and left warm). A difference of more than 20 to 25% between the ears is called a **unilateral weakness**, implying a peripheral disorder on the side with the smaller response. The strength of the bithermal caloric test is that we can recombine the nystagmus results into those that "beat toward the right" (right warm and left cool) and those that "beat toward the left ear" (left warm and right cool). We can thus distinguish between results due to a unilateral weakness and those due to a greater propensity for the eyes to beat in one direction relative to the other, called a **directional preponderance**.

A test for **fixation suppression** is performed during at least one of the caloric tests. Here we ask the patient to open her eyes and look at (fixate upon) a specified point. The normal response is a large reduction in the strength of the nystagmus. If the nystagmus does not get much weaker during fixation, the result is called **failure of fixation suppression** that suggests central pathology.

Other balance system tests may also be done, such as sinusoidal harmonic accelera-

tion and posturography. **Sinusoidal harmonic acceleration** (or **rotating chair**) testing involves a variety of nystagmus measurements on a patient who is rotated from side to side in a computer controlled chair. **Computerized dynamic posturography** involves assessing the patient's ability to maintain balance while standing. This is done by placing the patient on a platform in a booth, and measuring her responses while the platform is still or moves (which manipulates proprioceptive cues), and/or the surrounding booth stays still or moves (which manipulates visual cues).

REFERENCES

American Speech-Language-Hearing Association (ASHA). 1987. *The Short Latency Auditory Evoked Potentials.* Rockville Pike, MD: ASHA.

American Speech-Language-Hearing Association (ASHA). 1992. Neurophysiologic intraoperative monitoring. *ASHA* 34 (suppl 7), 34–36.

Arnold SA. 2000. The auditory brain stem response. In Roeser RJ, Valente M, Hosford-Dunn H (Eds.): *Audiology Diagnosis.* New York: Thieme, 451–470.

Barber HO, Stockwell CW. 1980. *Manual of Electronystagmograph,* 2nd ed. St. Louis, MO: Mosby.

Beck DL (Ed.). 1993. Audiology: Beyond the sound booth. *Semin Hear* 14, 1–214.

Bonfils P, Uziel A. 1988. Evoked otoacoustic emissions in patients with acoustic neuromas. *Am J Otol* 9, 412–417.

Bradford LJ. 1975. *Physiological Measures of the Audio-Vestibular System.* New York: Academic Press.

Burkhard R, Hecox K. 1983. The effect of broadband noise on the human brainstem auditory evoked response: I. Rate and intensity effects. *J Acoust Soc Am* 74, 1204–1213.

Chiappa KH (Ed.). 1997. *Evoked Potentials in Clinical Medicine,* 3rd Ed. New York: Lippincott-Raven.

Coats AC. 1975. Electronystagmography. In Bradford IJ (Ed.): *Physiological Measures of the Audio-Vestibular System.* New York: Academic Press, 37–85.

Coats AC. 1986. ENG examination technique. *Ear Hear* 7, 143–150.

Dekker TN (Ed.): 1992. Otoacoustic emissions. *Semin Hear* 13, 1–104.

Dennis JM. (Ed.). 1988. Intraoperative monitoring with evoked potentials. *Semin Hear* 9, 1–164.

Don M, Eggermont JJ, Brackmann DE. 1979. Reconstruction of the audiogram using brain stem responses and high-pass noise masking. *Ann Otol Rhinol Laryngol Suppl* 57, 1–20.

Ferraro JA. 1992a. Electrocochleography: What and why. *Audiol Today* 4, 25–26.

Ferraro JA. 1992b. Electrocochleography: How—part I. *Audiol Today* 4, 26–28.

Ferraro JA. 1993a. Electrocochleography: How—part II. *Audiol Today* 5, 31–33.

Ferraro JA. 1993b. Electrocochleography: Techniques. *Audiol Today,* 5, 36–38.

---

[4] Instead of having water flow into the canal, other systems use a "closed loop" system in which the water heats (or cools) a plastic balloon in the ear canal. Other systems use air instead of water.

Ferraro JA. 2000. Electrocochleography. In Roeser RJ, Valente M, Hosford-Dunn H (Eds.): *Audiology Diagnosis*. New York: Thieme, 425–450.

Ferraro JA, Krishnan G. 1997. Cochlear potentials in clinical audiology. *Audiol Neur-Otol* 2, 241–256.

Ferraro JA, Tibbils RP. 1999. SP/AP area ratio in the diagnosis of Meniere's disease. *Am J Audiol* 8, 21–28.

Fria TJ. 1980. The auditory brainstem response: Background and clinical applications. *Monogr Contemp Audiol* 2, 1–44.

Gelfand SA. 1998. *Hearing: An Introduction to Psychological and Physiological Acoustics*, 3rd ed. New York: Marcel Dekker.

Glattke TJ. 1993. *Short-Latency Auditory Evoked Potentials*. Austin: Pro-Ed.

Glattke TJ, Robinette MS. 2000. Otoacoustic emissions. In Roeser RJ, Valente M, Hosford-Dunn H (Eds.): *Audiology Diagnosis*. New York: Thieme, 503–526.

Gorga MP, Thornton AR. 1989. The choice of stimuli for ABR measurements. *Ear Hear* 10, 217–230.

Hall JW. 1992. *Handbook of Auditory Evoked Potentials*. Boston: Allyn & Bacon.

Hecox K, Galambos R. 1974. Brain stem auditory evoked responses in human infants and adults. *Arch Otolaryngol* 99, 30–33.

Jacobson GP. 1999. Otoacoustic emissions in clinical practice. In Musiek FE, Rintelmann WF (Eds.): *Contemporary Perspectives in Hearing Assessment*. Needham Heights, MA: Allyn & Bacon, 273–303.

Jacobson JT. 1985. *The Auditory Brainstem Response*. San Diego: College-Hill.

Jerger J, Hall J. 1980. Effects of age and sex on the auditory brainstem response. *Arch Otolaryngol* 106, 387–391.

Jerger J, Johnson K. 1988. Interactions of age, gender, and sensorineural hearing loss on ABR latency. *Ear Hear* 9, 168–176.

Jewett DL, Romano MN, Williston JS. 1970. Human auditory evoked potentials: Possible brainstem components detected on the scalp. *Science* 167, 1517–1518.

Johnsen NJ, Elberling C. 1982. Evoked acoustic emissions from the human ear. *Scand Audiol* 11, 3–12.

Kemp DT. 1978. Stimulated acoustic emissions from within the human auditory system. *J Acoust Soc Am* 64, 1386–1391.

Kemp DT. 1979. Evidence of mechanical nonlinearity and frequency selective wave amplification in the cochlea. *Ann Otol Rhinol Laryngol* 224, 37–45.

Kiang NYS, Liberman MC, Sewell WF, Guinan JJ. 1986. Single unit clues to cochlear mechanisms. *Hear Res* 22, 171–182.

Kileny P. 1981. The frequency specificity of tone-pip evoked auditory brain stem responses. *Ear Hear* 2, 270–275.

Kraus N, Kileny P, McGee T. 1994. Middle latency auditory evoked potentials. In Katz J (Ed.): *Handbook of Clinical Audiology*, 4th ed. Baltimore: Williams & Wilkins, 387–405.

Kraus N, McGee T. 1994. Auditory event-related potentials. In Katz J (Ed.): *Handbook of Clinical Audiology*, 4th ed. Baltimore: Williams & Wilkins, 406–423.

Lonsbury-Martin BL, Martin GK, Telischi FF. 1999. Otoacoustic emissions in clinical practice. In Musiek FE, Rintelmann WF (Eds.): *Contemporary Perspectives in Hearing Assessment*. Needham Heights, MA: Allyn & Bacon, 167–196.

Lonsbury-Martin BL, Whitehead ML, Martin GK. 1991. Clinical applications of otoacoustic emissions. *J Speech Hear Res* 34, 964–981.

Mauldin L, Jerger J. 1979. Auditory brainstem evoked responses to bone-conduction signals. *Arch Otolaryngol* 105, 656–661.

McPherson DL, Ballachandra B. 2000. Middle and long latency auditory evoked potentials. In Roeser RJ, Valente M, Hosford-Dunn H (Eds.): *Audiology Diagnosis*. New York: Thieme, 471–502.

Møller AR. 2000. Intraoperative neurophysiological monitoring. In Roeser RJ, Valente M, Hosford-Dunn H (Eds.): *Audiology Diagnosis*. New York: Thieme, 545–570.

Møller AR, Janetta PJ. 1985. Neural generators of the auditory brainstem response. In Jacobson JT (Ed.): *The Auditory Brainstem Response*. San Diego: College Hill, 13–31.

Moore EJ. 1983. *Bases of Auditory Brain-Stem Evoked Responses*. New York: Grune & Stratton.

Moore JK. 1987. The human auditory brainstem as a generator of auditory evoked potentials. *Hear Res* 29, 33–43.

Musiek FE, Borenstein SP, Hall JW, Schwaber MK. 1994. Auditory brainstem response: Neurodiagnostic and intraoperative applications. In Katz J (Ed.): *Handbook of Clinical Audiology*, 4th ed. Baltimore: Williams & Wilkins, 351–374.

Näätänen R (Ed.). 1995. Special issue: Mismatch negativity as an index of central auditory function. *Ear Hear* 16, 1–146.

Norton SJ. 1992. Cochlear function and otoacoustic emissions. *Semin Hear* 13, 1–14.

Norton SJ, Schmidt AR, Stover LJ. 1990. Tinnitus and otoacoustic emissions: Is there a link? *Ear Hear* 11, 159–166.

Norton SJ, Stover LJ. 1994. Otoacoustic emissions: An emerging clinical tool. In Katz J (Ed.). *Handbook of Clinical Audiology*, 4th ed. Baltimore: Williams & Wilkins, 448–462.

Parker DJ, Thornton ARD. 1978. Derived cochlear nerve and brainstem evoked responses of the human auditory system. *Scand Audiol* 7, 73–80.

Penner MJ. 1990. An estimate of the prevalence of tinnitus caused by spontaneous otoacoustic emissions. *Arch Otolaryngol* 116, 418–423.

Probst R, Lonsbury-Martin BL, Martin GK. 1991. A review of otoacoustic emissions. *J Acoust Soc Am* 89, 2027–2067.

Robinette MS, Bauch CD, Olsen WO, Hamer SG, Beatty CW. 1992. Use of TEOAE, ABR and acoustic reflex measures to assess auditory function in patients with acoustic neuroma. *Am J Audiol* 1, 66–72.

Robinette MS, Glattke TJ (Eds.). 1997. *Otoacoustic Emissions: Clinical Applications*. New York: Thieme.

Rudell AP. 1987. A fiber tract model of auditory brainstem responses. *EEG Clin Neurophysiol* 62, 53–62.

Ruth RA, Lambert P, Ferraro JA. 1988. Electrocochleography: Methods and clinical applications. *Am J Otol* 9, 1–11.

Scherg M, vonCramon D. 1985. A new interpretation of the generators of BAEP waves I–V: Results of a spatio-temporal dipole model. *EEG Clin Neurophysiol* 62, 290–299.

Schwartz DM, Larson VD, DeChicchis AR. 1985. Spectral characteristics of air and bone conduction transducers used to record the auditory brainstem response. *Ear Hear* 6, 274–277.

Sohmer H, Feinmesser M. 1967. Cochlear action potentials recorded from the external ear in man. *Ann Otol Rhinol Laryngol* 76, 427–435.

Squires KC, Hecox KE. 1983. Electrophysiological evaluation of higher level auditory processing. *Semin Hear* 4, 415–433.

Stapells DR, Kurtzberg D. 1991. Evoked potential assessment of auditory integrity in infants. *Clin Perinatol* 18, 497–518.

Stapells DR, Picton TW, Durieux-Smith A, Edwards CG, Morna LM. 1990. Thresholds for short-latency auditory-evoked potentials to tones in notched noise in normal-hearing and hearing-impaired subjects. *Audiology* 29, 262–274.

Stapells DR, Picton TW, Smith AD. 1982. Normal hearing thresholds for clicks. *J Acoust Soc Am* 72, 74–79.

Starr A, Picton TW, Sininger YS, Hood LJ, Berlin CI. 1996. Auditory neuropathy. *Brain* 119, 741–753.

Stockard JE, Stockard JJ, Westmoreland BF, Corfits JL. 1979. Brainstem auditory-evoked response: Normal variation as a function of stimulus and subject characteristics. *Arch Neurol* 36, 823–831.

Stockwell CW. 1983. *ENG Workbook*. Austin: Pro-Ed.

Sutton S, Barren M, Zubin J, John JE. 1965. Evoked-potential correlates of stimulus uncertainty. *Science* 150, 1187–1188.

Turner RG, Shepard NT, Frazer GJ. 1984. Clinical performance of audiological and related diagnostic tests. *Ear Hear* 5, 187–194.

van der Drift JFC, Brocaar, MP, van Zanten GA. 1988a. Brainstem response audiometry: I. Its use in distinguishing between conductive and cochlear hearing loss. *Audiology* 27, 260–270.

van der Drift JFC, Brocaar, MP, van Zanten GA. 1988b. Brainstem response audiometry: II. Classification of hearing loss by discriminant analysis. *Audiology* 27, 271–278.

Weber BA. 1983. Pitfalls in auditory brain stem response audiometry. *Ear Hear* 4, 179-184.

Yamada O, Kodera K, Yagi T. 1979. Cochlear processes affecting wave V latency of the auditory evoked brainstem response: A study of patients with sensory hearing loss. *Scand Audiol* 8, 67–70.

Yellin MW. 2000. Assessment of vestibular function. In Roeser RJ, Valente M, Hosford-Dunn H (Eds.): *Audiology Diagnosis*. New York: Thieme, 571–592.

12

Assessment of Infants and Children

This chapter is concerned with the audiologic evaluation of children. Here, we are concerned with audiological procedures that have been modified or specially developed for use with infants and children at various levels of development, and with the clinical considerations that pertain to this population. The student should notice more than a few similarities between what is discussed here and what is covered in the context of audiologic screening for children in Chapter 13. This is not surprising because screening tests are usually simplified and/or abbreviated clinical procedures. In fact, some procedures used for screening purposes are equally useful clinically. For example, the acoustic immittance methods used to screen for the presence of middle ear fluid are also used as part of the clinical immittance assessment and are often used to monitor a patient's middle ear status over time. However, the greater depth and scope involved in clinical assessment and the knowledge and expertise demanded of those who accomplish it should be readily apparent, as well. For example, the auditory brainstem response is used on a "pass/fail" basis for screening purposes, but its clinical use involves extensive and sophisticated testing procedures. Similarly, the screening use of the hearing loss risk factors enumerated in Chapter 13 is to indicate the need for a referral, but they are also used clinically as part of the case history that contributes to the diagnostic assessment of the child.

By convention, children are considered infants from birth to three years old, of which the first 28 days of life is the neonatal period. They are preschoolers from ages three to five, and school-aged from then through high school. We will use these terms loosely because phrases like "two-week-old infant" and "14-month-old child" are self-explanatory. However, we must be aware of certain *kinds* of ages that have specific meanings and that are pertinent when dealing with children. For example, we are all aware that **chronological age** means age since birth, and that **mental age** expresses an individual's cognitive ability (usually as measured on an intelligence test) in terms of the age when an average normal person achieves the same level of performance. **Gestational age** is the time period between conception and birth, and is conventionally measured from the time of the last menstruation until the time when the baby is born. **Conceptional age** is the child's age measured from the date of conception; in other words, it includes the gestational age plus the time since the baby was born. Consider two babies born on the same day, one following a full-term pregnancy, and the other who was born one month early. Even though their chronological ages will be the same on the day when they eat their first birthday cakes, they will be one month apart in conceptional age (21 and 20 months). This difference brings us to the notion of **developmental age**, which is the individual's age in terms of his level of maturation; for example, if a 12-month-old (chronologically) functions in a manner that is typical of the average normal eight-month-old, then his developmental age would be eight months. For audiological purposes, it is often helpful to consider an infant's **prematurity-adjusted** or **corrected age**, which is determined by subtracting the number of weeks of prematurity from his chronological age (e.g., Moore, Wilson, & Thompson, 1977; ASHA, 1991; Moore, Thompson, & Folsom, 1992).

The initial aspects of the audiological evaluation of a child involve obtaining a case history, a physical inspection of the ears and related structures, and taking the time to observe and informally interact with the child to develop a clinical impression of her developmental level and communicative abilities. The physical inspection of the ears and related structures is necessary to identify anomalies that affect audiological procedures, suggest the possibility of hearing-related abnormalities, and/or indicate the need for medical referral. The child's case history is generally obtained from the parents or other caregivers, and should address the child's medical history, physical and neuromotor development, and her communicative behavior and development. As pointed out in Chapter 6, the specific material to be covered in the case history should come from a knowledge and understanding of auditory and related disorders (Chapter 6), risk factors (Chapter 13, Tables 13–1 to 13–3), and a firm background in child development in general and speech-language in particular (e.g., Linder, 1990; Nelson, 1993). In addition to providing diagnostic insight, the history is used in combination with an informal observation of and interaction with the child to help determine what kinds of audiological testing methods might be most appropriate to use with her.

Behavioral Assessment

It is so obvious that nobody expects an infant to raise her hand every time she hears a tone, that it seems ridiculous to say so. Yet, what makes such a statement preposterous or humorous is a common albeit general understanding that there is a developmental sequence for *what* sounds babies will respond to and *how* they will go about responding. The details of this developmental sequence form the foundation for the audiological evaluation of infants and young children.

Table 12–1 is an **Auditory Behavior Index** (Northern & Downs, 1991) that summarizes many of the responses to sound expected from infants during the first two years of life, along with the levels of various kinds of sounds expected to elicit these responses. Before proceeding to the details, it is a good idea to peruse this chart for several important general principles. First, notice that the earliest responses are gross, reflexive behaviors and that they become finer and more specific with the infant's development. The behavioral assessment of hearing depends on knowing which responses to look for at which age range in the child's development. In addition, the audiologist must also be alert for responses that are characteristic of children who are appreciably younger than the one being tested, indicating the possibility of mental retardation or other developmental disorders and the need for an appropriate referral. An example of such a developmentally delayed response would be an 18-month-old who can localize sounds to one side or the other, but not above or below eye level.

Second, comparing the stimulus intensities needed for a normal infant to respond to warble tones versus speech or noisemakers reveals that infants are not equally responsive to all kinds of sounds. Third, looking down any of the three representative stimulus columns shows that normal infants elicit developmentally appropriate responses to sounds at progressively lower intensity levels with increasing age. This does *not* mean that the normal infant's hearing sensitivity improves with age. Rather, it highlights the fact that we are often looking at the infant's responsiveness to the *presence* of a sound, which must be distinguished from the *threshold* of hearing for that sound. Similarly, the lowest levels at which infants respond also tend to improve with increasing age, as shown in Figure 12–1. In recognition of these points, the lowest level at which an infant produces a behavioral response at a given time is often called the **minimum response level (MRL)** rather than the threshold (Matkin, 1977).

TABLE 12–1 Responses to sounds from developmentally normal infants at various ages, and typical stimulus levels expected to elicit these responses in behavioral observation audiometry

Age Range	Types of Behavioral Responses	Warble Tones (db HL)	Speech[a] (db HL)	Noisemakers (dB SPL, approximate)
0 to 6 weeks	Eye-blink Eye-widening Startle Arousal/stirring from sleep	78	40–60	50–70
6 weeks to 4 months	Eye-blink Eye-widening Eye shift Quieting Rudimentary head turn starts by 4 months	70	47	50–60
4 to 7 months	Head turn laterally toward sound Listening attitude	51	21	40–50
7 to 9 months	Directly localizes to side Indirectly localizes below ear level	45	15	30–40
9 to 13 months	Directly localizes to side and below ear level Indirectly localizes above ear level	38	8	25–35
13 to 16 months	Directly localizes to side/below/ above ear level	32	5	25–30
16 to 21 months	Directly localizes to side/below/ above ear level	25	5	25
21 to 24 months	Directly localizes to side/below/ above ear level	26	3	25

[a]A startle response to speech is typically expected at 65 dB HL for all of the age groups shown.

Adapted from J.L. Northern and M.P. Downs. 1991. Hearing in Children, 4th Edition. Baltimore, MD: Williams and Wilkins, with permission.

Behavioral Observation Audiometry

Behavioral observation audiometry (BOA) involves watching the baby's responses to relatively sudden and intense stimulus sounds presented in the soundfield, such as a speech signal (e.g., "bah-bah-bah"), warble tones, narrow band noises, and various hand-held noise makers. Remember that soundfield testing means that we do not know whether a response resulted from hearing in both ears or just one of them. The stimulus levels expected to elicit responses from normal infants at various ages are shown in Table 12–1. Because wide band stimuli are being used, any information we might get about hearing in different frequency regions is limited at best. In addition, we must keep in mind that many of the toys used as noisemakers for BOA are unstandardized sound sources, the characteristics of which are unknown to us unless we actually measure their spectra (which is done with embarrassing rarity). This is not a minor point because, for example, an apparently "high-frequency" toy may have a very complex spectrum including considerable energy at much lower frequencies than we might think.

Behavioral observation audiometry should involve two examiners, typically one with the infant and the other in the control room with the audiometer, who observes the patient through the control room window. It is preferable for both examiners to be audiologists,

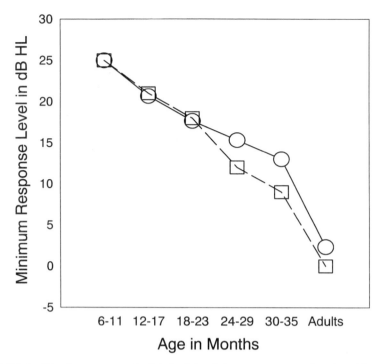

FIGURE 12–1 The improvement of infants' minimum response levels with maturation from 6 to 35 months of age using visual reinforcement audiometry and adult thresholds for comparison. Based on data by Matkin (1977).

but one audiologist and a knowledgeable and experienced assistant is a commonly used alternative. The infant should be placed on an examining table so that his whole body is clearly seen by both examiners. Depending on the infant's age and state, it may be necessary for him to be held by a parent or an assistant, but it is essential for the person holding the child to not respond during testing.

During the first four months of life the infant's response may be any of several reflexes or a change in its state, either alone or in combination. **Startle reflexes** are often seen as a body shudder and/or considerable gross movements of the arms, legs, and/or the body. The startle response is often called the **Moro reflex** when the body is thrown into a hugging or embracing posture. Eye-related reflexes are often seen as well, and include eye blinks, opening, or widening of the eyes. The reflexive contraction of the muscles around the eyes, producing a blink, is known as the **auropalpebral reflex (APR)**. The startle and APR reflexes habituate rather quickly with

repeated presentations of the stimulus sounds. **Habituation** means that the child stops responding after a number of stimulus presentations. The most typical changes in state that we watch for are arousal from sleep or stirring in response to the stimulus sound. Later during this period (between roughly 6 weeks and 4 months), we can observe quieting in response to the stimulus, eye shifts toward the sound source (the **cochleo-oculogyric** or **auro-oculogyric reflex**), and some rudimentary head turning toward the sound source.

Several sources of variability and subjectivity in behavioral observation audiometry have been outlined by Widen (1993). First, examiner judgments are subject to bias because the nature of the response itself can be elusive in the sense that it varies depending on such factors as the infant's state and age, and with the nature of the stimulus. For example, decisions about the infant's responses are biased by whether the examiner knows when the stimulus was presented (Ling, Ling, & Doehring, 1970; Gans & Flexer, 1982).

Second, it is the infant's responsiveness to the presence of sound rather than his threshold that is being measured, and this responsiveness differs for different kinds of sounds. Third, the intensity levels at which responses occur and the nature of those responses vary with the age of the infant. The fourth issue is that habituation leads to variability in the responses obtained from the same child. The fifth source of variability is that normal infants respond over such a wide range of levels that the examiner can be hard pressed to tell when a given child's responses are within or beyond the normal range.

Visual Reinforcement Audiometry

During the four- to seven-month period, the infant becomes more interested in softer sounds, an active listening attitude becomes apparent, and her neuromotor control matures to the extent that she begins to develop a localization response that involves turning her head toward the sound source. As shown in Table 12–1, these responses begin as horizontal localizations at ear level, and then mature to include localizations below (at about 9 to 13 months) and finally above ear level around 13 to 16 months. Testing approaches that make use of these localization responses are sometimes referred to as "localization audiometry." When the infant reaches about five to six months of age, the localization responses are robust enough for us to move from BOA, which involves the observation of *unconditioned* behaviors, to the use of *conditioned* responses.

Hearing measurement using a conditioned localization response and a visual reinforcer is generally known as **visual reinforcement audiometry (VRA)** (Liden & Kankkunen, 1969). The basic approach was described by Suzuki and Obiga (1961), who called it the **conditioned orientation reflex (COR)**. In their method, the child is placed in the test room with loudspeakers off to each side, as in Figure 12–2. Presenting a sound from one of the loudspeakers elicits an orientation or localization response from the child, which involves looking toward the stimulus speaker.

This response is followed by the illumination of a visually appealing object that is associated with that loudspeaker, serving as a reward or **reinforcer**. This visual reinforcer is shown on top of each speaker in the figure; it is often placed next to it. This process constitutes **conditioning** because the visual reinforcer increases the chances that the child will continue responding to subsequent stimulus presentations.

Various visual reinforcement audiometry approaches and testing protocols are available (e.g., Haug, Baccaro, & Guilford, 1967; Liden & Kankkunen, 1969; Moore, Thompson, & Thompson, 1975; Matkin, 1977; Diefendorf & Gravel, 1996; Gravel & Hood, 1999), of which the one developed by Moore, Thompson, and Thompson (1975) is the most extensively documented and studied. The major characteristics of this VRA method are as follows:

1. A single loudspeaker and associated visual reinforcer are used.
2. The reinforcement device is a toy that is illuminated *and* moves in place. Typical examples include mechanical stuffed animals or a clown that plays the drums or cymbals (silently) when activated. The same switch activates the mechanical toy and the light. The toy is mounted inside a dark Plexiglas box so that it is not visible until it is lit up for reinforcement purposes. A selection of several different animated toy reinforcers may be used instead of just one (e.g., Merer & Gravel, 1997).
3. To be acceptable, the infant's response must be a clear head turn toward the loudspeaker/reinforcer.
4. Responses are judged by two examiners.
5. There are clearly defined criteria for when the patient is considered to be conditioned (e.g., three correct responses in a row) and habituated (e.g., four no responses out of five consecutive trials).

Depending on the infant's age, neuromotor status, and state, she is seated on a chair (or on a parent's lap), held, or placed on an examining table. The examiner with the infant usually manipulates quiet toys or pictures on

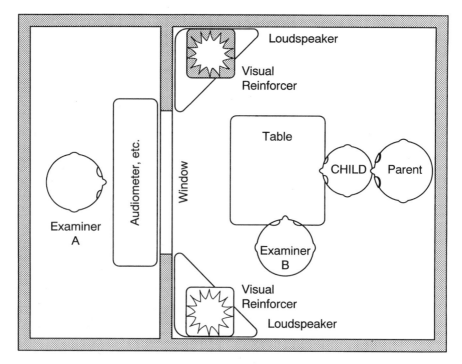

FIGURE 12–2 Typical testing arrangement for visual reinforcement audiometry, with the child sitting on its parent's lap at a table. The reinforcer devices in this diagram are on top of the two corner loudspeakers. Some approaches like COR use two loudspeakers and reinforcers, but many modern VRA methods use only one, which is represented by the filled (upper) box.

a table in front of the child to keep her passively attendant and facing forward. The person holding the child should not respond during testing, and parents in particular must be instructed not to participate in the testing process.

Thresholds may be obtained using modifications of conventional threshold search approaches, or with sophisticated programmed approaches (e.g., Bernstein & Gravel, 1990). Unlike the usual "up 5-dB/down 10-dB" threshold method used in routine pure-tone audiometry, visual reinforcement audiometry often involves an "up 10-dB/down 10-dB" or an "up 10-dB/down 20-dB" technique (Gravel, 1989; Gravel & Hood, 1999; Tharpe & Ashmead, 1993). On the basis of findings obtained using computer simulations, Tharpe and Ashmead (1993) suggested that a very efficient threshold testing strategy for visual reinforcement audiometry involves the following characteristics: (1) beginning the test

without conditioning (i.e., training) trials in which the test tone and reinforcer are paired, (2) an initial test level of 30 dB HL (which is raised in 20-dB steps if there is no response at 30 dB HL), and (3) the use of an "up 10-dB/ down 20-dB" technique.

The characteristics of effective reinforcers were investigated by Moore, Wilson, and Thompson (1977). They found that the highest rate of responses among 12- to 18-month old infants occurs when using complex visual reinforcers such as toys that were lit up and moved in place. Progressively lower response rates are obtained with a simple visual reinforcer such as a flashing light; social reinforcers such as verbal praise, a pat on the shoulder, and/or smiling; and without any reinforcement at all.

Visual reinforcement audiometry can be effective with full-term infants who are at least five to six months old (Moore, Wilson, & Thompson, 1977). Babies who were born prematurely can be expected to respond effectively to VRA at a corrected age of eight months (Moore, Thompson, & Folsom, 1992). Recall that the corrected age is the child's chronological age minus the estimated number of weeks of prematurity. One- and two-year-olds tend to be conditioned for visual reinforcement audiometry quickly and easily, and are similar in terms of the rate of conditioning (how quickly they learn to perform the task) and the consistency of their responses (Primus & Thompson, 1985). Unfortunately, however, infants do not continue responding to the stimulus forever. Instead, their responses habituate, or die out, as the stimulus trials are repeated over the course of the testing session. Habituation occurs more quickly for two-year-olds than for one-year-olds (Primus & Thompson, 1985; Thompson, Thompson, & McCall, 1992).

Habituation is a major consideration with young children because the amount of information we can get about the child's hearing depends on how many times he will respond. The number of responses obtained before habituation occurs can be increased by using different animated reinforcers instead of using just one (Primus & Thompson, 1985; Thompson, Thompson, & McCall, 1992). Giving the child a 10-minute break after habituation has occurred and then beginning a second test session significantly increases the total number of responses obtained from one-year-olds, but not from two-year-olds (Thompson, Thompson, & McCall, 1992). Culpepper and Thompson (1994) showed the number of responses from two-year-olds before habituation increased as the duration of the reinforcer was reduced from four seconds to a half-second.

Tangible and Visual Reinforcement Operant Conditioning Audiometry

Tangible reinforcement operant conditioning audiometry (TROCA) (Lloyd, Spradlin, & Reid, 1968) is a highly structured testing approach originally described for use with **difficult-to-test** patients, such as the mentally retarded. *Difficult-to-test* is a general term

used to mean those who cannot be readily assessed with conventional behavioral tests, so that special methods are needed. Patients may be difficult-to-test due to physical, developmental, perceptual, cognitive, emotional, or other problems, or to any combination of these factors. Approaches like TROCA, which were developed for the difficult-to-test, are also effective with normal, young children. Upon hearing a tone (or other test signal), the child is required to push a response button or to make another simple but specific motor response within his range of neuromotor capabilities. Correct responses are reinforced by the delivery of a tangible reward, which might be cereal, candy, tokens, and other small trinkets. False-positive responses are discouraged because they are followed by time-out periods. The entire procedure is accomplished with instrumentation programmed to present the stimuli, monitor the responses, and deliver the reinforcers according to a predefined operant conditioning schedule.

In **visual reinforcement operant conditioning audiometry (VROCA)** (Wilson & Thompson, 1984; Thompson, Thompson, & Vethivelu, 1989) the child is required to press a response button (which is a large, bright box) instead of turning toward the loudspeaker, after which a visual reinforcer is presented. The visual reinforcer itself is the same kind used in visual reinforcement audiometry. When VROCA is employed with soundfield testing, the loudspeaker is kept in front of the child so he is not distracted from the response box, as opposed to being placed off to one side as is done for a head turning response.

Play Audiometry

Play audiometry, or **conditioned play audiometry**, involves training the child to listen for stimuli and then make a specific motor response within the framework of a game, usually in combination with social reinforcement such as smiles, praise, etc. For example, the child might be trained to place a peg into a pegboard after each test sound. Other commonly used games include stacking blocks or cups, placing small items into a container (or taking them out), or just about any other simple activity that can be repeated over and over gain. Play audiometry is often appropriate for children between about two to five years of age (Northern & Downs, 1991). However, one should keep in mind that this is a wide age range as far as child development is concerned, and it is not surprising to find that the successful use of conditioned play audiometry improves with age, especially beyond the second year (e.g., Nielsen & Olsen, 1997). Hence, we should not expect that all youngsters will be ready to be conditioned for play audiometry at age two (Thompson, Thompson, & Vethivelu, 1989).

If at all possible, the mother and father should not be in the room during play audiometry. Parents in the control room are also undesirable, especially if the child can see them through the observation window. A parent who simply must be in the room should be seated quietly out of the child's direct line of sight, and instructed not to interact with the child or participate in the testing process in any way.

Play audiometry employs two clinicians who communicate by intercom and visually through the window between the control and test rooms. One of them operates the audiometer and the other stays with the child. The child is generally seated at a small table, which is the play surface, either next to or opposite one of the examiners. A collection of games should be kept on hand so when the child gets bored with one activity you can quickly and smoothly replace it with another. Keep the backup games out of sight so they do not distract the child from the task at hand. If accepted by the child, earphone testing may be attempted from the start, or at least as soon as possible. Some children accept earphones immediately. In other cases, getting the child to accept earphones is a challenge in which the audiologist's personal "way with kids" comes to the fore. A knowledge of the most current children's cartoon series and action toy fads is a valuable asset in this context. Earphone acceptance is sometimes facilitated if the clinician first puts on

her own headset (which houses the intercom and permits her to monitor the test signals). A reasonable amount of good-natured firmness and confident tenacity often works, but keep in mind that "winning" means getting the child to cooperate sufficiently so that valid and reliable audiological information can be obtained, which will not happen if he is crying hysterically. If earphones are simply out of the question, then in the most matter-of-fact manner try the bone-conduction vibrator or insert earphones. If all reasonable attempts fail, simply place the headset on the table where the child can see them, and start the test in soundfield.

The goal is to condition the child to perform a specific, observable action every time he hears a tone, and then to manipulate the level of the tone to find the child's threshold. The basic game used in conditioned play audiometry involves having the child hold a peg up to his ear while listening for a tone, and then placing it into a hole in the pegboard when a tone is heard (or to add it to a pile, etc.). *Tell and demonstrate* what to do. Then tell the child it is now his turn. It is often necessary to take the child's hand and *lead him through* the task physically at first while verbalizing what he is doing. Then let him try. *Praise* the child for doing the task correctly. Reinstruct the child if necessary (this usually involves reminding him to wait for the tone before responding), but keep the emphasis on reinforcing the desired behavior.

Once the child has learned the task, we need to obtain thresholds efficiently before habituation occurs. Northern and Downs (1991) recommend starting in the 40-dB HL to 50-dB HL range and descending in 10- or 15-dB steps, and then to use ascending presentations to find the threshold, using two responses as the criterion; or one may use the threshold-search methods described earlier in the section on visual reinforcement audiometry. Habituation will most likely limit the number of thresholds that can be obtained in any one session, which means we must begin testing at the frequencies that will provide the most information about the child's audiogram as quickly as possible. For this reason it is usually desirable to obtain thresholds at 500 and 2000 Hz for both ears first. The other frequencies can then be filled in as long as the child remains "on task." Northern and Downs recommended that these frequencies should generally be added in the following order: 1000 Hz, 250 Hz, and 4000 Hz.

Physiological Measures

Physiological methods are playing an increasing role in the audiological evaluation of infants and young children. These allow us to assess neonates and younger infants in ways that cannot be done by behavioral observation audiometry because they (1) do not require the child's cooperation, (2) allow us to test each ear individually, or (3) directly assess the physiological integrity of at least the lower portions of the auditory system. On the other hand, we must keep in mind that physiological measurements give us a limited perspective of the infant's world of sound because they do not involve a behavioral response. As previously indicated, physiological tests are often useful even with children who can be tested with behavioral methods, because they provide us with valuable cross-checks on the behavioral results (Jerger & Hayes, 1976; ASHA, 1991), and also provide additional differential diagnostic information.

The physiological tests regularly used in pediatric audiology include the auditory brainstem response (ABR), otoacoustic emissions (OAEs), and acoustic immittance tests. For example, Figure 12–3 shows an infant whose hearing is being evaluated with the auditory brainstem response. The later evoked potentials (see Chapter 11) are not routinely used with infants and younger children because they are affected by sleep and sedation. This is a significant factor because it is often necessary for young children and difficult-to-test patients to be asleep or sedated for results to be obtained. (This involves the participation of a physician because sedation and other forms of anesthesia are medical activities.) However, the later evoked responses cannot be totally discarded for use with young children. For example, Shimizu (1992)

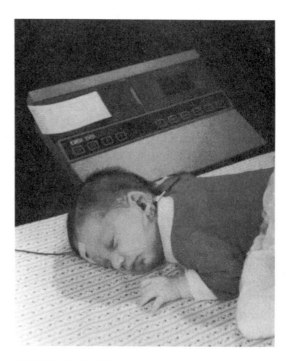

FIGURE 12–3 Physiological testing methods are well established in pediatric audiology. In the example shown here, the auditory brainstem responses are obtained from an infant. Notice the electrodes on the child's earlobe and forehead, as well as the insert receiver in his ear. Photograph courtesy of Grason-Stadler, Inc.

pointed out that it is possible to obtain cortical evoked potentials from young children during certain sleep stages, and that this can provide important information particularly in children with absent ABRs. Other physiological approaches have also been used in the past. Examples include the monitoring of respiratory and/or cardiac responses to sound (Bradford, 1975; Eisenberg, 1975) and the psychogalvanic skin response (PGSR) (Ventry, 1975). These methods were more cumbersome and less practical than modern approaches, in addition to which the PGSR was unnecessarily traumatic for the child.

Auditory Brainstem Response

Although there are maturational effects that must be considered, the auditory brainstem response has numerous characteristics that make it well suited for use in pediatric audiology (Jacobson, 1985; ASHA, 1991; Hall, 1992): Very young as well as seriously disabled children can be tested by ABR because it does not involve a behavioral response and it is reasonably unaffected by sleep and sedation. Separate results can be obtained from each ear. Although the ABR certainly does not produce an audiogram, we can get some idea of the degree and general configuration of a hearing loss by using clicks to estimate sensitivity in the higher frequencies and tone-pips to estimate lower-frequency sensitivity. An ABR obtained with bone-conduction stimuli gives us some insight about the type of hearing loss. In addition, ABR results also provide information about the child's neurologic integrity at the brainstem level.

Otoacoustic Emissions

Otoacoustic emissions, described in Chapter 11, have considerable value in pediatric audiological assessment. In contrast to the ABR, acoustic reflexes, and other tests that rely on both sensory and neural activity, otoacoustic emissions are "preneural," depending on the integrity of the cochlea before the auditory nervous system gets involved in the processing of a signal; hence, they can be measured even when there are neurological deficits that affect other measures. Otoacoustic emissions do not require a behavioral response, are reliably obtained in normal infants and young children, are very sensitive to hearing loss, are obtained separately for each ear, and can provide information at different frequencies.

Acoustic Immittance

Tympanometry and acoustic reflex tests are a central part of the evaluation of infants and young children. The use of acoustic immittance tests with infants and children is covered in Chapter 7. Acoustic immittance measurements allow us to monitor middle ear conditions over time, and also can provide us with information about the status of the middle ear when reliable masked thresholds cannot be obtained, as is often the case with very young children. Acoustic reflex measurements provide information about the integrity of

several aspects of the peripheral ears and lower parts of the auditory pathway, and also help us distinguish between the presence and absence of significant amounts of hearing loss.

Speech Audiometry

Threshold for Speech

Speech signals are used in the behavioral testing of infants and children from birth onward. The initial use of speech may be to elicit a startle response from a neonate; months later, speech signals may be used to elicit localizing behavior.

Olsen and Matkin (1991) have suggested some guidelines for determining the threshold for speech depending on the child's overall level of functioning, which is effectively her developmental age. As with other aspects of assessment in pediatric audiology, there is no clear line of demarcation between the times when one type of method or the other should be used, which is implied by Olsen and Matkin's subtle use of overlapping age ranges. They recommended that a **speech detection threshold (SDT)** using a repetitive speech utterance should be obtained from children who are functioning below the three-year level. The speech detection threshold is obtained using the same kinds of techniques described earlier in this chapter. Unconditioned responses are used for those functioning at the lowest developmental levels, whereas conditioned responses can be obtained from children who can be tested by VRA, play audiometry, TROCA, or VROCA.

A modified **speech recognition (reception) threshold (SRT)** can be obtained from many children from about 30 months to roughly 6 years old. This can be accomplished by, for example, presenting a group of easily recognizable objects or pictures that depict words selected to be within the child's receptive vocabulary (e.g., a toy airplane, baseball, cowboy, toothbrush, etc.), and having her identify them as they are named by the examiner. It is also possible to have a child respond by pointing with an eye gaze in the direction of a selected picture (Byers & Bristow, 1990). This kind of technique can be used for testing either speech thresholds or word recognition performance, and is useful with some children regardless of age (and adults, for that matter) who have cerebral palsy or other disorders that prevent them from pointing manually. Older children within this range are often able to give a verbal response to selected spondee words.

A conventional SRT can often be obtained from children who function in the five- to ten-year range, although a children's spondee list is recommended for them. A list of spondee words considered to be within the receptive vocabularies of most children (ASHA, 1988) is included in Appendix E. A conventional SRT based on standard spondee word lists is expected from children functioning at the level of 10 years and above.

Testing the speech recognition threshold by bone-conduction and comparing it to the air-conduction SRT can provide insights about the type of hearing loss, which can be quite valuable if reliable tonal results have yet to be obtained (Olsen & Matkin, 1991; Northern & Downs, 1991). However, calibration values for speech presented via the bone-conduction vibrator must be determined empirically before this procedure is used.

Speech Recognition

In general, speech recognition tests (Chapter 8) are used to reveal the accuracy of the patient's auditory reception and processing of speech material, usually in terms of a percent correct score for monosyllabic words. This can be problematic when testing children because their speech recognition scores are affected by their level of language development as well as by their auditory capabilities. As a result, normal children's speech recognition scores on many tests increase as they get older, eventually becoming comparable to adult scores at roughly 10 to 12 years of age, when they are familiar with most if not all of the test words. The situation is exacerbated in patients who have speech-language disorders, or other problems that impair either the level of linguistic functioning or the ability to respond during the test. In addition, we must remember that speech-language disorders are common among children with significant amounts of hearing impairment. Consequently, we should try to use speech recognition tests that include words within the child's receptive vocabulary and employ responses that she is capable of making, at least to the extent that this is possible. Moreover, in light of the fact that practical tests often cannot realize these lofty goals, we must consider the individual child's receptive vocabulary and response limitations when interpreting and reporting speech recognition test results.

OPEN-SET TESTS

A number of open-set tests are available for children who are not ready for adult speech recognition measures. Recall from Chapter 8 that the open-set format is essentially the same as a fill-in test. The speech recognition ability of children who are about 6 to 9 years old can often be tested with the **Phonetically-Balanced Kindergarten** or **PBK-50 lists** (Haskins, 1949). The PBK-50 test is made up of 50-word lists based on a kindergarten-level vocabulary, and the word recognition score is simply the percent of the words that were repeated correctly. The four PBK-50 lists are included in Appendix K. Although PBK-50 lists 1, 3, and 4 are usually considered to be equivalent, list 2 is rarely used clinically because Haskins found it to be easier than the other three. Meyer and Pisoni (1999) demonstrated that compared to the words in the other three "equivalent" lists, the words in the easier list 2 have a higher frequency of occurrence and are less likely to be confused with other words. Recall from Chapter 8 in this context that the **Lexical Neighborhood Test (LNT)** may be used to obtain word recognition scores for lexically easy and lexically hard words (Kirk, Pisoni, & Osberger, 1995; Kirk, 1999: Kirk, Eisenberg, Martinez, & Hay-McCutcheon, 1999).

Boothroyd's **isophonemic word lists** (Boothroyd, 1968, 1970, 1984; Boothroyd &

Nittrouer, 1988) can also be used with children in this age range. The isophonemic words test was discussed in Chapter 8, and may also be found in Appendix H. Each isophonemic word test list includes 10 consonant-vowel-consonant (CVC) words that are scored on a phoneme-by-phoneme basis. In other words, scores on the isophonemic word test are based on 30 phonemes.

CLOSED-SET TESTS

Several closed-set or multiple-choice format monosyllabic word recognition tests are available for children who are at least about three years of age. The most widely used tests of this type are the **Word Intelligibility by Picture Identification (WIPI) Test** (Ross & Lerman, 1970, 1971), the **Northwestern University Children's Perception of Speech (NU-CHIPS) Test** (Kalikow, Stevens, & Elliot, 1977; Elliot & Katz, 1980), and the **Pediatric Speech Intelligibility (PSI) Test** (Jerger, Lewis, Hawkins, & Jerger, 1980; Jerger, Jerger, & Lewis, 1981; Jerger & Jerger, 1984), although others are also available. In the WIPI test, the child points to a picture that corresponds to the stimulus word from a choice of six color pictures. Each set of six pictures is arranged on the same page of a test book. An administration of the WIPI includes 25 items, and there are four test lists. Figure 12–4 shows an example of a response plate from the WIPI test, and the test words are listed in Appendix L.

The NU-CHIPS test is made up of 50 words that are within the receptive vocabularies of inner city three-year-olds, which are listed in Appendix M, including four recorded randomizations of these words. The child is pre-

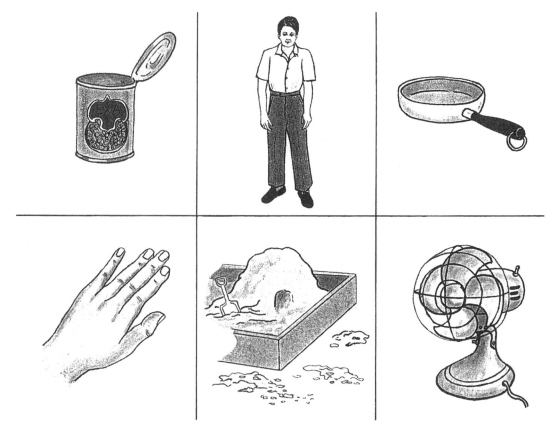

FIGURE 12–4   An example of a WIPI test response plate. From Ross and Lerman (1971), with permission.

sented with a page showing four picture choices for each test word, as in Figure 12–5, and responds by pointing to the picture that corresponds to the test word.

The material in the PSI test was derived from the vocabularies and sentence structures used by normal three-to-six year-old children. The test words are 20 monosyllabic nouns. The child responds by pointing at the picture corresponding to the test word or sentence. Two sentence formats may be used on the PSI test, depending on the child's language level, which are referred to as Format I (e.g., "Show me a bear combing his hair") and Format II (e.g., "A bear is combing his hair").

Other speech recognition tests have also been developed for use with children. For example, the **Auditory Perception of Alphabet Letters (APAL) Test** can be used for younger children who are familiar with the alphabet even though their vocabularies are inadequate for word recognition testing (Ross & Randolf, 1988). Robbins and Kirk (1996) described a technique for assessing speech recognition in preschoolers with limited vocabularies by having them follow verbal directions to assemble the familiar Mr. Potato Head toy. Weber and Redell (1976) devised a modification of the WIPI test in which the test items are presented in a sentence format. Another children's sentence test was developed by Bench, Koval, and Bamford (1979) called the **BKB Sentences Test**. One version of the BKB test is composed of 16 sentences that are presented to older children in an open-set format, and the test is graded on the basis of how many key words are repeated correctly. The other version is intended for use with younger children and involves a picture pointing response. The **Hearing in Noise Test for Children (HINT-C)** (Nilsson, Soli, & Gelnett, 1996) is a pediatric version of the Hearing in Noise Test (HINT) (described in Chapter 8), and is used to measure the SRT for sentences.

INNOVATIVE TESTS AND TECHNIQUES

Other speech recognition testing approaches for children are also available that are different from those already described. Several tests involve the **change/no change** or **go/no go task**, in which the child is trained to respond to a *change* in the stimulus. The **Visual Reinforcement Infant Speech Discrimination (VRISD) Test** uses *visual reinforcement audiometry* with the change/no change task

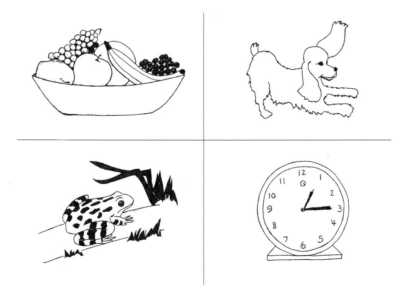

FIGURE 12–5 An example of a NU-CHIPS test response plate. From Elliot and Katz (1980), with permission.

to test an infant's ability to discriminate between pairs of syllables (Eilers, Wilson, & Moore, 1977). Instead of being conditioned to respond to the presence of a stimulus sound, the infant is trained to respond when a train of syllables that are all the same (e.g., /va va va . . . va/) *changes* to another, contrasting syllable (e.g., (/sa sa . . ./). A modification of the VRISD method, using real words instead of syllables and pointing instead of head turning, has been used to test speech discrimination in four-year-olds (Menary, Trehub, & McNutt, 1982). The **Speech Feature Test (SFT)** uses *conditioned play audiometry* with the change/no change task to test discrimination between pairs of syllables, and can be employed successfully with many three- and four-year-olds, as well as some two-year-olds (Dawson, Nott, Clark, & Cowan, 1998)

Recall from Chapter 8 that the **Speech Pattern Contrast (SPAC) Test** provides information about the patient's ability to correctly perceive the acoustic information needed to make phonologically relevant distinctions (Boothroyd, 1984, 1988). Similar information is often needed for young children who do not have the vocabulary or reading ability required for the SPAC test, and may be obtained with the **Three-Interval Forced-Choice Test of Speech Pattern Contrast Perception (THRIFT)** (Boothroyd, Springer, Smith, & Schulman, 1988). On the THRIFT the child must simply identify the location of the **"odd-ball"** in a sequence like "pea–*bee*–pea" or "*sue*–zoo–zoo." The odd-ball is distinguished from the other two stimuli based on the same kinds of contrasts used in the SPAC test. The THRIFT can be used with prelingually deaf children because it does not require the child to have any preexisting phonological knowledge, vocabulary, or reading skills, but the motivational demands of the test limit its use to children who are at least seven years old (Boothroyd, 1991). The imitative version of the SPAC test **(IMSPAC)** makes it possible to test children too young for the THRIFT (perhaps as young as two to three years of age) because the response mode involves imitating the stimuli, although performance does improve with increasing age (Boothroyd, 1991;

Boothroyd, Hanin, Yeung, & Eran, 1996). A video-game variation of the speech contrasts test **(VIDSPAC)** appears to be useful with children as young as three years of age (Boothroyd, 1991; Boothroyd, Hanin, Yeung, & Chen, 1992). On this test an animated character says a stimulus sound and then hides. The following scene shows two hiding places. Two sounds are produced in sequence, one of them matches the sound produced by the animated character and the other is a contrasting sound. One of these sounds is represented as coming from a hideout on the left side of a computer screen and the other coming from a hideout on the right. The child then points to where the character is hiding. A tangible reinforcer is provided after a certain number of correct responses.

The **Five and Six Sounds Tests** (Ling, 1976, 1989; Ling & Ling, 1978) employ an informal approach to obtain information about the child's ability to make use of spectral cues in speech reception. In the **Five Sounds Test**, the child is asked to detect the five sounds, /a, u, i, s, ʃ/, which are presented separately by the examiner. Hearing the vowels implies that the child has usable residual hearing up to roughly 1000 Hz and that she can also hear the suprasegmental features of speech. If /ʃ/ is also audible, it is inferred that the child's usable residual hearing extends up to about 2000 Hz and at least several vowel discriminations are possible. The ability to hear /s/ implies usable residual hearing as high as about 4000 Hz. The /m/ sound may be added to assess residual hearing for the lower frequencies, constituting the **Six Sounds Test**.

Other types of tests are also needed under certain circumstances. Consider, for example, the case of a child with a severe-to-profound hearing loss whose conventional speech recognition score is very low or even zero, or "chance" on a closed-set test. Chance performance means that the score could have occurred from random guessing. For example, guessing would yield the "right" answer one-fifth of the time on a closed-set test with five alternatives per item, so that chance performance in this case would be 20%. In these cases, useful information might be obtained by determining how well the child is able to recognize words containing more than one syllable, which is done with tests such as the **Multisyllabic Lexical Neighborhood Test (MLNT)** (Kirk, Pisoni, & Osberger, 1995; Kirk, 1999; Kirk et al, 1999), described in Chapter 8.

When dealing with very limited speech recognition ability, it often becomes important to know whether the child can at least recognize differences in the temporal or rhythmic patterns of speech. This type of information is provided by the **monosyllable-trochee-spondee (MTS) test**, which was originally described as the **Children's Auditory Test (CAT)** (Erber & Alencewicz, 1976). Recall from Chapter 8 that the MTS test uses three kinds of stimulus words that differ with respect to the number of syllables and the stress pattern, including (1) monosyllabic words; (2) spondaic words, which have two equally stressed syllables (e.g., "baseball"); and (3) trochaic words, which have two unequally stressed syllables (e.g., "button"). The test words are presented to the child, who responds by pointing to corresponding pictures. Examining the relationships between the stimulus words and responses reveals whether the child can correctly identify words with different levels of difficulty, and also whether she is able to take advantage of temporal and/or stress patterns in speech.

Similar information may be obtained with the **Early Speech-Perception (ESP) Test** (Geers & Moog, 1989; Moog & Geers, 1990), which employs pointing responses to pictures and toys with children as young as three years of age. The **Auditory Numbers Test (ANT)** is a simplified approach designed to obtain information about the ability to use the spectral versus temporal patterns of speech in young children whose vocabularies are too limited for the MTS test; it can be used with three-year-olds who can count from one to five (Erber, 1980). Here the examiner says a number and the child points to the corresponding one of five cards that illustrates the number in the form of numerals and pictures of groups of ants. Analyzing the nature of errors provides insight about whether the child can make use of spectral cues and temporal patterns.

Tests such as the **Sound Effects Recognition Test (SERT)** (Finitzo-Hieber, Matkin, Cherow-Skalka, & Rice, 1975; Finitzo-Hieber, Matkin, Cherow-Skalka, & Gerling, 1977) can often be used with children who cannot respond adequately to verbal stimuli. On the SERT, the child listens to a familiar environmental sound and then points to the corresponding picture from a choice of four alternatives. Some examples of the test stimuli used included a dog barking, splashing water, a father's voice, and a doorbell. This kind of information reveals how well a child can make use of spectral and temporal information to identify complex stimuli.

The tests outlined in this section are by no means the only ones available to assess the speech reception abilities of children, neither do they represent the only approaches that can be used. They do, however, reveal the diversity of approaches available to us as we try to construct a picture of the child's auditory ability.

Because of the differences among the test instruments, the meaning of a given speech recognition score is unclear unless the clinician also specifies which test instrument was used and the conditions of testing. These differences are quite substantial even for "conventional" tests such as the PBK-50, WIPI, and NU-CHIPS. This notion is illustrated in Figure 12–6, which shows the average speech recognition scores of normal children who took these three tests under the same conditions. It is clear that the three tests yield three different speech recognition scores. In addition, closed-set tests like the WIPI and NU-CHIPS result in considerably higher scores than the PBK-50, which is an open-set test. Also notice that the ten-year-olds have higher scores than the five-year-olds, which highlights the importance of considering the effects of language development when interpreting children's speech recognition scores. Differences among the test instruments are complicated when the clinician must modify the "standard" procedures in order to test a particular child.

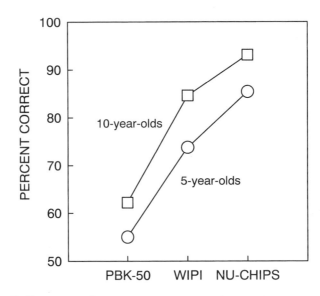

FIGURE 12–6 Different speech recognition tests result in different speech recognition scores. The graph compares the mean speech recognition scores obtained by normal 5- and 10-year-old children on three different tests (PBK-50, WIPI, and NU-CHIPS) presented at 12 dB sensation level. Based on data reported by Elliot and Katz (1980).

Testing Approaches at Various Ages

In this section we will review the kinds of testing procedures that are typically appropriate at different stages of the child's development. The first three age ranges described here (birth to four months, four to 24 months, and 25 to 36 months) are used to be consistent with guidelines suggested by the ASHA Committee on Infant Hearing (1991), although other age breakdowns would also be appropriate. The 1991 ASHA guidelines recommended that assessment protocols for young children should strive to achieve the following goals:

1. The audiological assessment should be individualized and carried out in a timely manner.
2. The assessment should be ear specific, so that we know the status of each ear.
3. The test stimuli should be frequency specific, so hearing sensitivity is estimated on a frequency-by-frequency basis, that is, to approximate the audiometric configuration as closely as possible.

4. Bone-conduction thresholds and acoustic immittance measurements should be used so that the status of the middle ear can be assessed.

In addition, the student should be aware that a central principle in pediatric audiology is that no single test should be used to define a child's auditory status (Jerger & Hayes, 1976; Gravel, Kurtzberg, Stapells, Vaughan, & Wallace, 1989; ASHA, 1991; Hall, 1992; Stach, Wolf, & Bland, 1993). Instead, modern approaches involve the judicious use of both behavioral and physiological testing methods to complement and supplement one another. The use of one type of measure to corroborate the results of another is often called the **cross-check principle** (Jerger & Hayes, 1976).

Birth to Four Months

The assessment of infants' hearing during the first four months of life (adjusted for prematurity) is principally based on physiological tests. The main assessment tool at this time is the auditory brainstem response (ABR), and involves obtaining latency-intensity functions and ABR thresholds (Chapter 11) separately for each ear. Air-conduction clicks are used to estimate high-frequency sensitivity and tone-pips are used to estimate lower frequency hearing to get an idea of the infant's general audiometric configuration. If the air-conduction ABR thresholds are elevated (worse than normal), then the ABR is repeated with bone-conduction signals as well. Comparing the air-conduction and bone-conduction ABR thresholds permits us to determine whether there is an air-bone-gap, and hence the type of hearing loss. Published in 1991, the ASHA guidelines focused on the ABR and could only intimate that otoacoustic emissions would probably play a significant role in the future. It is now clear that OAEs are highly sensitive to hearing loss and provide complementary information because they reflect preneural cochlear integrity. In addition, results can be obtained as a function of frequency.

Behavioral assessment for infants in the birth to four-month age range is not used for the purpose of estimating the infant's hearing sensitivity, but rather is used to assess the qualitative aspects of the infant's auditory behavior, and to corroborate what has been reported by the parents or caregiver.

The acoustic immittance assessment recommended by ASHA (1991) includes tympanograms and acoustic reflex thresholds for both ears, and the use of probe-tone frequencies above 226 Hz (or 220 Hz) should be considered. Broadband noise acoustic reflex measures that can be used for hearing loss identification/prediction purposes may also be useful during the early months, although the ASHA (1991) guidelines do not actually recommend this until the 5- to 24-month period. Acoustic immittance measures are explained in Chapter 7.

Five to Twenty-Four Months

The audiological evaluation approach changes from physiological testing to a behavioral focus when the child is approximately five or six months old. At this stage, the infant's neuromotor development has matured to the extent that visual reinforcement audiometry is feasible. Hence, audiological evaluations for infants in the 5- to 24-month corrected-age range concentrate on behavioral methods combined with acoustic immittance tests. From now on the ABR is reserved for cases in which the behavioral results are questionable or inadequate, or when there are reasons to question the integrity of the lower auditory pathways. It is too soon to tell whether the same can be said for otoacoustic emissions. At least some OAK tests may become part of the routine protocol for all young children as an efficient cross-check of the behavioral results.

The behavioral testing battery recommended by ASHA (1991) involves visual reinforcement audiometry to estimate the infant's sensitivity in the 500- to 4000-Hz range and for speech signals. Once the infant is responding appropriately in soundfield, it is desirable to obtain results for both ears using appropriate earphones. An attempt should be made to obtain bone-conduction thresholds if the air-conduction thresholds are elevated, but the limitations of unmasked bone-conduction thresholds should be kept in mind. An estimate of speech recognition ability should be made as early as possible, albeit informally, within the constraints imposed by the infant's language abilities.

Along with tympanometry and conventional acoustic reflex testing, ASHA (1991) also suggests that broadband noise reflex testing may be beneficial in this age range. When used, the ABR protocol is the same as the one described for younger infants.

Twenty-Five to Thrity-Six Months

The audiological evaluation of children in the 25- to 36-month age range is principally composed of behavioral methods combined with acoustic immittance tests. The indications and testing protocols for physiological measures are the same as they were for 5- to

24-month-olds. The type of behavioral testing used during this period depends on the individual characteristics of the child, and may involve play audiometry, VRA, TROCA, VROCA, or a hybrid technique. Thus, the audiologist must take the time to interact with the child, not only to establish a sense of rapport but also to estimate the child's developmental level and ability to perform the tasks involved with each of the behavioral approaches being considered.

The findings of Thompson, Thompson, and Vethivelu (1989) are very instructive in this context. They compared the performance of two-year-olds using visual reinforcement audiometry, VROCA, and play audiometry. All of the children could be conditioned to respond for VRA, compared to 83% for VROCA and only 68% for play audiometry. However, among the two-year-olds who could be conditioned, the average number of responses given before habituation was highest (28.3) for play audiometry and smallest (11.4) for VRA, with VROCA occupying a position between them.

Regardless of the methodology used, or whether the testing can be completed within a single session or must be spread over several visits, the goal is to obtain an audiological picture of the child that is as complete as possible. As before, we hope to obtain air-conduction thresholds for each ear between at least 500 and 4000 Hz, bone-conduction thresholds where the air-conduction thresholds are elevated, and acoustic immittance measurements.

Speech audiometry for children in this age range should include a measure of the threshold for speech, usually with a closed-set approach such as pointing to the named picture or object, or by repeating the words. Whenever possible, speech recognition scores should be obtained using an age-appropriate standardized test, such as the WIPI (Ross & Lerman, 1971), NU-CHIPS (Elliot & Katz, 1980), and the PSI (Jerger & Jerger, 1984). If standardized tests are not appropriate for a child, then her speech recognition ability should be assessed informally, as described earlier. However, the results of informal testing should be expressed in the form of a descriptive statement about the child's speech recognition performance instead of using a percentage score.

Four to Five Years

Developmentally normal children in the four- and five-year-old range can usually be tested with play audiometry and standardized children's speech recognition tests like WIPI, NU-CHIPS, and the PSI.

Six Years and Beyond

Children become candidates for more standard audiometric testing procedures (Chapter 5) somewhere in the vicinity of five or six years old. However, just because a child can perform the task does not mean she will be a self-motivated responder. If anything, this is a period when the audiologist must provide the child with encouragement, direction, and praise to keep the child "on task." Open-set speech recognition testing using a vocabulary within the child's range, such as the PBK-50 (Haskins, 1949), can also be used around this time. Otherwise normal children are responding in an almost adult-like manner by roughly 10 to 12 years old, and standard speech recognition tests (Chapter 8) can be used providing the material is within the child's receptive vocabulary.

REFERENCES

American Speech-Language-Hearing Association (ASHA). 1988. Guidelines for determining threshold level for speech. *ASHA* 30, 85–89.

American Speech-Language-Hearing Association (ASHA). 1991. Guidelines for the audiologic assessment of children from birth through 36 months of age. *ASHA* 33 (suppl 5), 37–43.

Bench J, Koval A, & Bamford J. 1979. The BKB (Bamford-Koval-Bench) sentence lists for partially-hearing children. *Br J Audiol*, 13, 108–112.

Bernstein R, Gravel JS. 1990. A method for determining hearing sensitivity in infants: The interweaving staircase procedure (ISP). *J Am Acad Audiol* 1, 138–145.

Boothroyd A. 1968. Developments in speech audiometry. *Sound* 2, 3–10.

Boothroyd A. 1970. Developmental factors in speech recognition. *Int Audiol* 9, 30–38.

Boothroyd A. 1984. Auditory perception of speech contrasts by subjects with sensorineural hearing loss. *J Speech Hear Res* 27, 134–144.

Boothroyd A. 1988. Perception of speech pattern contrasts from auditory presentation of voice fundamental frequency. *Ear Hear* 9, 313–321.

Boothroyd A. 1991. Speech perception measures and their role in the evaluation of hearing aid performance in a pediatric population. In Feigin J, Stelmachowicz P (Eds.): *Pediatric Amplification*. Omaha: Boys Town National Research Hospital, 78–91.

Boothroyd A, Hanin L, Yeung E, Chen Q. 1992. Videogame for speech perception testing and training of young hearing-impaired children. Proceedings of the Johns Hopkins National Search for Computing Applications to Assist Persons with Disabilities, Laurel, MD, 25–28.

Boothroyd A, Hanin L, Yeung E, Eran O. 1996. Speech perception and production in hearing-impaired children. In Bess FH, Gravel JS, Tharpe AM (Eds.): *Amplification for Children with Auditory Deficits*. Nashville: Billy Wilkerson Center Press, 55–74.

Boothroyd A, Nittrouer S. 1988. Mathematical treatment of context effects in phoneme and word recognition. *J Acoust Soc Am* 84, 101–114.

Boothroyd A, Springer N, Smith L, Schulman J. 1988. Amplitude compression and profound hearing loss. *J Speech Hear Res* 31, 362–376.

Bradford LJ. 1975. Respiration audiometry. In Bradford LJ (Ed.): *Physiological Measures of the Audio-Vestibular System*. New York: Academic Press, 249–317.

Byers VW, Bristow DC. 1990. Audiological evaluation of nonspeaking, physically challenged populations. *Ear Hear* 11, 382–386.

Culpepper B, Thompson G. 1994. Effects of reinforcer duration on the response behavior of preterm 2-year-olds in visual reinforcement audiometry. *Ear Hear* 15, 161–167.

Dawson PW, Nott PE, Clark GM, Cowan RSC. 1998. A modification of play audiometry to assess speech discrimination ability in severe-profound deaf 2- to 4-year old children. *Ear Hear* 19, 371–384.

Diefendorf AO, Gravel JS. 1996. Behavioral observation and visual reinforcement audiometry. In Gerber S (Ed.): *Handbook of Pediatric Audiology*. Washington, DC: Gallaudet University Press, 55–83.

Eilers RE, Wilson WR, Moore JM. 1977. Developmental changes in speech discrimination in infants. *J Speech Hear Res* 20, 766–780.

Eisenberg RB. 1975. Cardiotachometry. In Bradford LJ (Ed.): *Physiological Measures of the Audio-Vestibular System*. New York Academic Press, 319–347.

Elliot L, Katz D. 1980. *Northwestern University Children's Perception Speech (NU-CHIPS)*. St. Louis: Auditec.

Erber NP, 1980. Use of the Auditory Numbers Test to evaluate speech perception abilities of hearing-impaired children. *J Speech Hear Dis* 45, 527–532.

Erber NP, Alencewicz CM. 1976. Audiologic evaluation of deaf children. *J Speech Hear Dis* 41, 256–267.

Finitzo-Hieber T, Matkin ND, Cherow-Skalka E, Gerling IJ. 1977. *Sound Effects Recognition Test*. St. Louis: Auditec.

Finitzo-Hieber T, Matkin ND, Cherow-Skalka E, Rice C. 1975. A preliminary investigation of a sound effects recognition test. Paper presented at American Speech and Hearing Association Convention, Washington, DC.

Gans DP, Flexer C. 1982. Observer bias in the hearing testing of profoundly involved multiply handicapped children. *Ear Hear* 3, 309–313.

Geers AE, Moog JS. 1989. Evaluating speech perception skills: Tools for measuring benefits of cochlear implants, tactile aids and hearing aids. In Ownes E, Kessler D (Eds.): *Cochlear Implants in Children*. Boston: College-Hill.

Gravel JS. 1989. Behavioral assessment of auditory function. *Semin Hear* 10, 216–228.

Gravel JS, Hood LJ. 1999. Pediatric audiologic assessment. In Musiek FE, Rintelmann WF (Eds.): *Contemporary Perspectives in Hearing Assessment*. Needham Heights, MA: Allyn & Bacon, 305–326.

Gravel JS, Kurtzberg D, Stapells D, Vaughan H, Wallace IF. 1989. Case studies. *Semin Hear* 10, 272–286.

Hall JW. 1992. *Handbook of Auditory Evoked Responses*. Boston: Allyn & Bacon.

Haskins HA. 1949. A phonetically balanced test of speech discrimination for children. Masters thesis, Northwestern University, Evanston, IL.

Haug O, Baccaro P, Guilford F. 1967. A pure-tone audiogram on the infant: The PIWI technique. *Arch Otolaryngol* 86, 435–440.

Jacobson, JT. (Ed.). 1985. *The Auditory Brainstem Response*. San Diego: College-Hill.

Jerger J, Hayes D. 1976. The cross-check principle in pediatric audiology. *Arch Otolaryngol* 102, 614–620.

Jerger S, Jerger J. 1984. *Pediatric Speech Intelligibility Test—PSI*. St. Louis: Auditec.

Jerger S, Jerger J, Lewis S. 1981. Pediatric speech intelligibility test: II. Effect of receptive language and chronological age. *Int J Pediatr Otolaryngol* 3, 101–118.

Jerger S, Lewis S, Hawkins J, Jerger J. 1980. Pediatric speech intelligibility test: I. Generation of test materials. *Int J Pediatr Otolaryngol* 2, 217–230.

Kalikow DN, Stevens DN, Elliot LL. 1977. Development of a test of speech intelligibility in noise using sentence materials with controlled word predictability. *J Acoust Soc Am* 61, 1337–1351.

Kirk KI. 1999. Assessing speech perception in listeners with cochlear implants: The development of the Lexical Neighborhood Test. *Volta Rev* 100, 63–85.

Kirk KI, Eisenberg LS, Martinez AS, Hay-McCutcheon. 1999. Lexical Neighborhood Test: Test-retest reliability and interlist equivalency. *J Am Acad Audiol* 10, 113–123.

Kirk KI, Pisoni DB, Osberger MJ. 1995. Lexical effects on spoken word recognition by pediatric cochlear implant users. *Ear Hear* 16, 470–481.

Liden G, Kankkunen A. 1969. Visual reinforcement audiometry. *Arch Otolaryngol* 89, 865–872.

Linder TW. 1990. *Transdisciplinary Play-Based Assessment: A Functional Approach to Working with Young Children*. Baltimore: Brooks.

Ling D. 1976. *Speech for the Deaf Child*. Washington, DC: AG Bell Association for the Deaf.

Ling D. 1989. *Foundations of Spoken Language for Hearing-Impaired Children*. Washington, DC: AG Bell Association for the Deaf.

Ling D, Ling AH. 1978. *Aural Habilitation*. Washington, DC: AG Bell Association for the Deaf.

Ling D, Ling AH, Doehring DG. 1970. Stimulus response and observer variables in the auditory screening of newborn infants. *J Speech Hear Res* 13, 9–18.

Lloyd LL, Spradlin JE, Reid MJ. 1968. An operant audiometric procedure for difficult-to-test patients. *J Speech Hear Dis* 33, 236–245.

Matkin N. 1977. Assessment of hearing sensitivity during the preschool years. In Bess F (Ed.): *Childhood Deafness*. New York: Grune & Stratton, 127–134.

Menary S, Trehub SE, McNutt J. 1982. Speech discrimination in preschool children: A comparison of two tasks. *J Speech Hear Res* 25, 202–207.

Merer DM, Gravel JA. 1997. Screening infants and young children for hearing loss: Examination of the CAST Procedure. *J Am Acad Audiol* 8, 233–242.

Meyer TA, Pisoni DB. 1999. Some computational analyses of the PBK test: Effects of frequency and lexical density on spoken word recognition. *Ear Hear* 20, 363–371.

Moog JS, Geers AE. 1990. *Early Speech Perception Test*. St. Louis: Central Institute for the Deaf Publications.

Moore JM, Thompson G, Folsom RC. 1992. Auditory responsiveness of premature infants using visual reinforcement audiometry. *Ear Hear* 13, 187–194.

Moore JM, Thompson G, Thompson M. 1975. Auditory localization of infants as a function of reinforcement conditions. *J Speech Hear Dis* 40, 29–34.

Moore JM, Wilson WR, Thompson M. 1977. Visual reinforcement of head-turn responses in infants under 12 months of age. *J Speech Hear Dis* 42, 328–334.

Nelson NW. 1993. *Childhood Language Disorders in Context: Infancy Through Adolescence*. New York Merrill.

Nielsen SE, Olsen SØ. 1997. Validation of play-conditioned audiometry in a clinical setting. *Scand Audiol* 26, 187–191.

Nilsson MJ, Soli SD, Gelnett D. 1996. *Development of the Hearing in Noise Test for Children*. Los Angeles: House Ear Institute.

Northern JL, Downs MP. 1991. *Hearing in Children*, 4th ed. Baltimore: Williams & Wilkins.

Olsen WO, Matkin ND. 1991. Speech audiometry. In Rintelmann WF (Ed.): *Hearing Assessment*, 2nd ed. Austin, TX: Pro-Ed, 39–140.

Primus M, Thompson G. 1985. Response strength of young children in operant audiometry. *J Speech Hear Res* 28, 539–547.

Robbins AM, Kirk KI. 1966. Speech perception assessment performance in pediatric cochlear implant users. *Semin Hear* 17, 353–369.

Ross M, Lerman J. 1970. A picture identification test for hearing-impaired children. *J Speech Hear Res* 13, 44–53.

Ross M, Lerman, J. 1971. *Word Intelligibility by Picture Identification WIPI*. Pittsburgh: Stanwix House.

Ross M, Lerman J. 1988. *Auditory Perception of Alphabet Letters (APAL) Test*. St. Louis: Auditec.

Ross M, Randolf K. 1988. *Auditory Perception of Alphabet Letters Test (APAL)*. St. Louis: Auditec.

Shimizu H. 1992. Childhood hearing impairment: Issues and thoughts on diagnostic approaches. *AAS Bull* 17, 15–37.

Stach BA, Wolf SJ, Bland L. 1993. Otoacoustic emissions as a cross-check in pediatric hearing assessment. *J Am Acad Audiol* 4, 392–398.

Suzuki T, Obiga Y. 1961. Conditioned orientation audiometry. *Arch Otolaryngol* 74, 192–198.

Tharpe AM, Ashmead DH. 1993. Computer simulation technique for assessing pediatric auditory test protocols. *J Am Acad Audiol* 4, 80–90.

Thompson G, Thompson M, McCall A. 1992. Strategies for increasing response behavior of 1- and 2-year-old children during visual reinforcement audiometry (VRA). *Ear Hear* 13, 236–240.

Thompson M, Thompson G, Vethivelu S. 1989. A comparison of audiometric test methods for 2-year-old children. *J Speech Hear Dis* 54, 174–179.

Ventry IM. 1975. Conditioned galvanic skin response audiometry. In Bradford LJ (Ed.): *Physiological Measures of the Audio-Vestibular System*. New York: Academic Press, 215–247.

Weber S, Redell RC. 1976. A sentence test for measuring speech discrimination in children. *Audiol Hear Educ* 2, 25–30, 40.

Widen JE. 1993. Adding objectivity to infant behavioral audiometry. *Ear Hear* 14, 49–57.

Wilson WR, Thompson G. 1984. Behavioral audiometry. In Jerger J (Ed.): *Pediatric Audiology*. San Diego: College-Hill, 1–44.

13

Audiological Screening

Screening Principles

Screening programs are used to identify those individuals who have a particular disorder or group of disorders. Screening is warranted when a disorder has appreciable adverse effects on those who have it, and if it can be treated once it has been identified. In addition, the problem should be reasonably widespread in its occurrence, and there must be a test for it that is quick, reliable, and acceptable to those who receive it. These criteria are undeniably met by hearing impairments, disorders, and disabilities, which may be defined as follows (ASHA, 1997).[1] A **disorder** is an anatomical *abnormality* (e.g., an ear deformity) or a *pathology* (e.g., a middle ear infection). An **impairment** means that physiological and/or psychological *functioning* is lost or abnormal (e.g., a hearing loss). A **disability** occurs when a person's *ability to perform* is adversely affected (e.g., when a hearing loss impedes academic performance or social interactions). These areas are addressed by **audiological screening** (AAA, 1997a,b; ASHA, 1997; NIH, 1993; Mauk & Behrens, 1993; JCIH, 2000). The term **identification audiometry** is sometimes used to refer to screening for hearing impairment, and is often encountered in the older literature.

Hearing screening programs should be supervised by a qualified audiologist, but it is generally agreed that cost-effective mass screening programs entail testing procedures that do not require an audiologist's expertise (NIH, 1993; AAA, 1997a,b; ASHA, 1997; JCIH, 2000). Thus, the goal is for the day-to-day screening activities to be carried out by support personnel hired for this purpose, or by nonaudiologist professionals who are in the right place at the right time to perform the tests. Although we will not directly address financial factors in detail here, one must also be aware that the costs of personnel, instrumentation, space, etc., cannot be overlooked, and often play a central role in real-world decisions about screening programs. For these reasons, the clinician may be asked to provide such information as the cost of a screening program on a per child basis. A formula that can be used for this purpose (Cooper, Gates, Owen, & Dickson, 1975) is provided here so that it can be readily available:

$$\text{Cost per child} = \frac{S}{R} + \frac{C + (M \times L)}{(N \times L)}$$

Here, S is the hourly salary of the screening personnel, R is the rate of screening (children tested per hour), C is the cost of the equipment, M is the annual equipment maintenance cost, N is the number of children screened in a year, and L is the lifetime (in years) of the equipment.

The fundamental goal of a screening test is to identify the individuals in a population who have a specified disorder or group of disorders. People who actually have the targeted disorder are said to be "abnormal" and those who really do not have that disorder are "normal." It is important to remember that normality or abnormality here pertains

---

[1] For consistency, these terms as defined in the ASHA (1997) guidelines will be employed throughout this chapter.

only to the particular disorder(s) being screened. In a perfect screening test every abnormal person would fail and every normal case would pass. In spite of our best intentions, no screening test (or any test for that matter) can separate all normal and abnormal individuals with complete accuracy. For this reason we must consider the screening process in terms of the percentages of correct and incorrect results. Complicating matters is the issue of what constitutes the **"gold standard"** used to determine the patient's "real status." This is often established by another test, which itself may not be perfect.

To understand the principles involved in assessing a screening test, let us make up a population to be screened for a particular disorder. It is represented by the upper box of Figure 13–1, and includes nine individuals who really have the disorder (filled squares) who are intermingled among 31 people who are actually normal (open squares). This disorder has a **prevalence** of 22.5% because it occurs in nine out of 40 people ($9/40 = 0.225$).

A person who *passes* a screening test is considered to be free of the problem, whereas one who *fails* is thought to have the problem. For example, a hearing screening test might involve listening for a tone. People who *can hear* the tone will *pass* the screening test, but those who *cannot hear* the tone will *fail*. Hence, on a perfect screening test, everyone who is really normal would pass and everyone who is really abnormal would fail. The results of our hypothetical screening test are represented by the two lower boxes in the figure, labeled "pass" and "fail." Notice that the screening test outcome is not perfect: 27 of the 31 normal people passed the screening, but four of them failed; and seven of the nine abnormal individuals failed, but two of them passed. Hence, even though screening tests seem to have two results (pass and fail), there are really four possible outcomes from the standpoint of whether the pass and fail results are right or wrong.

The four possible outcomes of a screening test are often shown in the form of a matrix such as the one shown in Figure 13–2. The two correct outcomes are called sensitivity

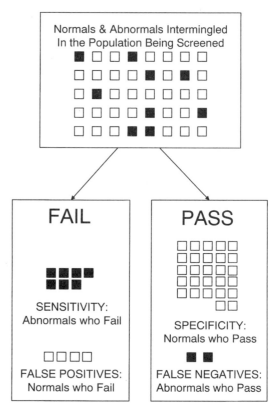

FIGURE 13–1 The upper box represents a hypothetical population being screened for some disorder, and the two lower boxes represent those who pass and fail the screening test. Open squares represent people who are actually normal; filled squares are those who really have the disorder (see text).

and specificity. **Sensitivity** is the proportion of *abnormal* people who *fail* the screening test, and is also known as the **hit rate**. It is obtained by dividing the number of abnormals who fail by the total number of abnormals. The sensitivity of our hypothetical screening test is $7/9 = 0.78$, or 78%. Figure 13–3 shows the sensitivity and other values obtained in our hypothetical example. **Specificity** is the proportion of *normal* individuals who *pass* the screening test. It is calculated by dividing the number of normals who pass by the total number of normal cases, which is $27/31 = 0.87$, or 87%, in our example.

The two incorrect screening outcomes are false-negatives and false-positives. A **false-negative** result, or a **miss**, occurs when an

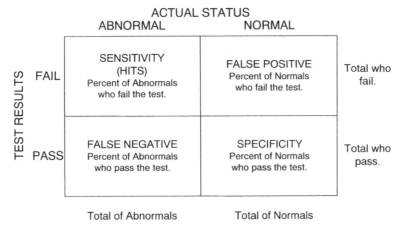

FIGURE 13–2 The outcomes of screening tests are shown as a matrix that plots the test results (passes or failures) against the true condition of the patient (normal or abnormal).

abnormal person *passes* the screening test. In contrast, a **false-positive** result occurs when a *normal* person *fails*. Passing the screening test is a "negative" result because it implies the person does *not* have the problem, and failing the screening test is a "positive" result because it suggests the person *does* have the problem. The false-negative rate is the proportion of abnormal cases who pass the test, that is, the number of misses divided by the total number of abnormals. For our hypo-

thetical data the false-negative rate is 2/9 = 0.22, or 22%. The false-positive rate is the proportion of normals who fail the screening test. It is obtained by dividing the number of false-positives by the total number of normals, which is 4/31 = 0.13, or 13%.

In summary, sensitivity (or the hit rate) tells us how well the screening test correctly identifies people who have the problem, and specificity shows how well the test correctly identifies those who are normal. The false-

a

| | ACTUAL STATUS | |
	ABNORMAL	NORMAL
FAIL	7	4
PASS	2	27
	9	31

TEST RESULTS

b

| | ACTUAL STATUS | |
	ABNORMAL	NORMAL
FAIL	78% Sensitivity	13% False Positive
PASS	22% False Negative	87% Specificity
	100%	100%

TEST RESULTS

FIGURE 13–3 (a) Number of patients in each category from the screening test example in Figure 13-1. (b) Sensitivity, specificity, false-positive, and false-negative rates for this example.

negative (miss) and false-positive rates are the errors associated with sensitivity and specificity, respectively. The goal is to have a screening test with both good sensitivity and good specificity. Even a very sensitive screening test would be useless if it is also failed by too many people who are normal, and a test with great specificity would be useless if it is also passed by too many people who are abnormal.

Audiological Screening in Infants and Children

Prevalence of Hearing Impairment. The need for hearing screening in infants and children becomes clear when we consider, the high prevalence of hearing loss, the impact of hearing impairment, and the importance of early intervention. An analysis of 10 large-sample studies by Mauk and Behrens (1993) revealed the prevalence of hearing losses ≥50 dB hearing level (HL) is about 1 per 1000 live births, and roughly 2.5 per 1000 for hearing losses of at least 20 dB HL, which is commonly accepted as the nominal level where

communication becomes adversely affected. Based on empirical data emanating from large-scale newborn screening programs, Stein (1999) estimated the prevalence of hearing loss to be about 1 per 1000 births for bilateral losses, rising to about 5 to 6 per 1000 if moderate losses and unilateral losses are included, and reaching a rate of about 2 to 4% for at-risk babies such as those in neonatal intensive care units.

Estimates of the prevalence of hearing loss among school children vary widely among studies between roughly 3 and 33%, depending on how "hearing loss" is defined and a host of methodological and sampling differences (e.g., Sarff, 1981; Axelsson, Aniansson, & Costa, 1987; Lundeen, 1991; Montgomery & Fujikawa, 1992; Bess, Dodd-Murphy, & Parker, 1998; Niskar, Kieszak, Holmes, Esteban, Rubin, & Brody, 1998). However, the comprehensive, large-sample studies by Bess et al (1998) and Niskar et al (1998) suggest the overall prevalence among American school children is approximately 11 to 15%. Some details of their prevalence findings are summarized in Figures 13–4 and 13–5. Niskar et

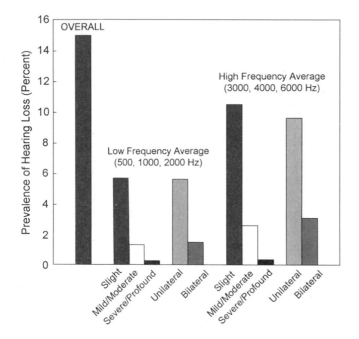

FIGURE 13–4 Prevalence of average hearing losses of ≥16 dB HL for low frequencies (500, 1000, and 2000 Hz) and high frequencies (3000, 4000, and 6000 Hz) among 6166 children between 6 and 19 years old. Based on Niskar, Kieszak, Holmes, Esteban, Rubin, and Brody (1998).

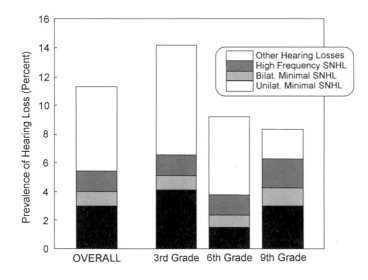

FIGURE 13–5 Prevalence of hearing losses among 1218 children in the 3rd, 6th, and 9th grades according to the categories defined in Table 13–1. SNHL, sensorinerual hearing loss. Based on Bess, Dodd-Murphy, and Parker (1998).

al (1998) categorized losses as slight, mild/moderate, and severe/profound based on a low-frequency average (500, 1000, 2000 Hz) and a high-frequency average (3000, 4000, 6000 Hz). Bess et al (1998) distinguished between *minimal sensorineural hearing losses* and other types and degrees of hearing loss (see Table 13–1). Niskar et al (1998) found that *slight losses* (16 to 25 dB HL) are more prevalent than greater degrees of hearing loss (Fig. 13–4); and Bess et al (1998) found a prevalence of 5.4% for various types of *minimal sensorineural hearing loss* and 5.9% for other categories of hearing loss (Fig. 13–5). Both studies found that unilateral hearing losses are more prevalent than bilateral losses among school age children. High-frequency hearing loss is clearly found among school age children but its prevalence is hard to establish, with 3% reported by Bess et al

TABLE 13–1 Characteristics of minimal and other hearing loss categories used in Figure 13–5[a]

Minimal Sensorineural Hearing Loss (SNHL) Categories[b]	
Bilateral minimal SNHL	500–2000 Hz PTA 20–40 dB HL in both ears
Unilateral minimal SNHL	500–2000 Hz PTA ≥20–40 dB HL in poorer ear 500–2000 Hz PTA ≤15 dB HL in better ear
High-frequency SNHL	≥2 thresholds ≥25 dB HL among 3000, 4000, 6000, and 8000 Hz One or both ears
Other Hearing Loss Categories[c]	
Conductive hearing loss	Average air-conduction thresholds ≥25 Hz Average air-bone-gap ≥10 dB HL Type B tympanogram One or both ears
Other hearing loss	Hearing losses not falling into the other groups (e.g., greater than minimal sensorineural losses, mixed losses)

[a]As defined by Bess, Dodd-Murphy, and Parker (1998).

[b]Normal hearing defined as average thresholds ≤15 dB HL in both ears and no more than one threshold >25 dB HL in either ear.

[c]Combined in Figure 13–5.

PTA, pure-tone average.

(1998) compared to 12.7% by Niskar et al. (1998).[2] Prevalence rates like those just described make it clear that we need a strategy to identify hearing impaired infants as early as possible and to continue screening efforts in children through the school years.

The adverse impact of hearing impairment on speech and language, literacy and academic performance, and psychosocial factors is substantial and well-established (see, e.g., Schow & Nerbonne, 1996; Alpiner & McCarthy, 2000). Even children with minimal sensorineural hearing loss and unilateral hearing loss experience educational and psychosocial difficulties (Bess et al, 1998). The key to mitigating these effects lies in early identification leading to early intervention. Particularly impressive is the finding of significantly better language skills among hearing-impaired children who were identified by the time they were 6 months old compared to those who were identified later than this (Yoshinaga-Itano, Sedey, Coulter, & Mehl, 1998).

Infant Hearing Screening

Universal newborn hearing screening refers to the systematic screening for hearing loss of as close as possible to all babies before leaving the hospital, along with follow-up measures that will be described below. It has

been endorsed by major professional organizations, state and federal legislation, and international groups, and is the subject of extensive clinical and research efforts.[3]

A variety of techniques are available for identifying hearing loss in infants. In the broadest terms, these include the use of public awareness campaigns, risk indicators, behavioral tests, and physiological tests. The public awareness approach uses such methods as mass media campaigns, brochures, and checklists to educate the public about the danger signs of hearing loss in children. The idea is to make parents and other caregivers aware of the problem and able to identify it so they can refer the child for diagnosis and treatment. There is no question that public awareness campaigns are a valuable adjunct to hearing loss identification in general, but they are not effective by themselves because there is great uncertainty about who actually receives and responds to these efforts, and because many primary care health providers often discount parental suspicions (Elssmann, Matkin, & Sabo, 1987; Mauk, White, Mortensen, & Behrens, 1991).

Risk Indicators for Hearing Impairment

One approach to the early identification of hearing-impaired babies involves determining whether the child meets any of several criteria associated with hearing loss. Infants identified by this **high-risk** register are then referred for evaluation and their cases are followed over time. The list of **risk factors** or **indicators** for hearing loss in neonates has evolved over the years. Tables 13–2 through 13–4 summarize the risk factors identified by

---

[2] Let's use this difference as an opportunity to illustrate why it is important to pay attention to how terms are defined and how subjects are placed into groups. Niskar et al's (1998) prevalence figures for high-frequency losses are close to those for older children and teenagers by Axelsson, Aniansson, and Costa (1987) and Montgomery and Fujikawa (1992). However, those studies found prevalence rates of about 6% for 7 year olds and second graders, whereas Niskar et al (1998) found similar percentages for 6 to 11 year olds (12.2%) and 12 to 19 year olds (13%). Niskar et al's (1998) 6 to 11 year old age range included 7 year olds (who had a lower prevalence in the earlier studies) and 10 year olds (who had a high prevalence rate). Also, Bess et al (1998) commented that their prevalence rates were similar to or higher than the ones by Axelsson et al (1987) and Montgomery and Fujikawa (1992) when they recalculated their data using the definitions of high-frequency loss from those studies. Thus, some of the prevalence discrepancies may be due to differences in how high-frequency hearing losses are defined, and possibly to how children are grouped according to age.

---

[3] Developments in universal newborn hearing screening are occurring at an extraordinary pace. The interested student should consult Internet sites such as those maintained by the Center for Disease Control and Prevention (www.cdc.gov/nceh/programs/CDDH/ehdi.htm), Marion Downs National Center for Infant Hearing (www.colorado.edu/slhs/mdnc/), American Academy of Audiology (www.audiolog.org), and the American Speech-Language-Hearing Association (www.asha.org). Here will be found up-to-date information and Internet links pertaining to all aspects of newborn screening, details about particular screening programs, state and federal legislation, instrumentation, etc.

TABLE 13–2 Hearing loss risk indicators for neonates from birth to 28 days of age

(a) Risk Indicators based on the JCIH (2000) Position Statement

- Neonatal condition requiring care in the neonatal intensive care unit for ≥48 hours
- Familial history of permanent sensorineural hearing loss in childhood
- Infections during pregnancy (e.g., rubella, cytomegalovirus, herpes, toxoplasmosis)
- Craniofacial anomalies, including pinna and ear canal abnormalities
- Stigmata (or other findings) associated with syndromes involving sensorineural and/or conductive hearing impairments

(b) Risk Indicators included in JCIH (1994) but omitted from JCIH (2000)

- Low birth weight (<1500 grams or <3.3 pounds)
- Hyperbilirubinemia requiring transfusion
- Ototoxic medications (aminoglycoside antibiotics or others) in multiple courses or combined with loop diuretics
- Bacterial meningitis
- Low Apgar scores[a] (0–4 at 1 minute, or 0–6 at 5 minutes)
- Mechanical ventilation for ≥5 days

[a]Many earlier listings referred to asphyxia and/or anoxia.

TABLE 13–3 Hearing loss risk indicators for rescreening infants from 29 days to two years old

(a) Risk Indicators based on the JCIH (2000) Position Statement

- Concern about hearing, speech, language, and/or developmental delay by parent and/or caregiver
- Infections during pregnancy (e.g., syphilis, toxoplasmosis, rubella, cytomegalovirus, herpes)
- Postnatal infections (including bacterial meningitis) associated with sensorineural hearing loss
- Neonatal conditions such as hyperbilirubinemia requiring transfusion, persistent pulmonary hypertension of the newborn with mechanical ventilation, and those requiring extracorporeal membrane oxygenation
- Familial history of permanent sensorineural hearing loss in childhood
- Syndromes associated with progressive hearing loss (e.g., neurofibromatosis, Usher's syndrome, osteopetrosis)
- Neurodegenerative disorders (e.g., Hunter syndrome) or sensory motor neuropathies (e.g., Charcot-Marie-Tooth syndrome, Friedreichs's ataxia)
- Stigmata (or other findings) associated with syndromes that involve sensorineural or conductive hearing impairments, or Eustachian tube dysfunction
- Head trauma
- Persistent or recurrent otitis media with effusion lasting ≥3 months

(b) Risk Indicators included in JCIH (1994) but omitted from JCIH (2000)

- Ototoxic medications (aminoglycoside antibiotics or others) in multiple courses or combined with loop diuretics

TABLE 13–4 Risk indicators for auditory neuropathy based on the Joint Committee on Infant Hearing Position Statement (JCIH, 2000)

- Compromise during the neonatal period with care in the neonatal intensive care unit
- Familial history of hearing loss in childhood
- Hyperbilirubinemia

the Joint Committee on Infant Hearing (JCIH, 1994, 2000). Differences between the risk factors recommended by the JCIH in 1994 and in 2000 reflect accumulating epidemiological evidence, and are identified in these figures. Notice that risk factors such as a family history of hearing loss and, to some extent, infections during pregnancy are based on historical information as opposed to being observable entities at the time of birth or while the baby is still in the newborn nursery. Other indicators are based on factors observable during or soon after birth, such as low birth weight, low Apgar scores, and certain structural anomalies. Some risk indicators are based on phenomena that may occur over the course of the postnatal hospital stay, such as hyperbilirubinemia, ototoxic agents, and mechanical ventilation. The characteristics of syndromes related to hearing losses might be noticed soon after delivery or may not become apparent for quite some time, perhaps years later.

High-risk registers are a relatively inexpensive approach to hearing loss identification, but they are subject to difficulties involved in gathering the needed information, and many children are lost to follow-up. For example, the information used to decide whether a baby should be placed on the high-risk register is usually based on birth certificate information or maternal questionnaires. However, the major weakness involved in relying on high-risk registers is that about half of all hearing-impaired newborns are missed by the risk indicators (Pappas, 1983; Elssman, Matkin & Sabo, 1987; Mauk et al, 1991; NIH, 1993).

Behavioral Observation

Behavioral methods have been used for infant hearing screening for quite some time (Wedenberg, 1956; Downs & Sterritt, 1967). These screening procedures may use **behavior observational audiometry (BOA)**, including automated methods such as the Crib-O-Gram. Recall from Chapter 12 that BOA involves presenting a stimulus to the child and watching for responses, which are

changes in behavior appropriate for her stage of development. In the case of newborns, behavioral observation screening techniques involve determining whether rather intense stimuli (typically 60 dB SPL or more) delivered from a handheld instrument are able to evoke gross responses such as a startle reflex, auropalpebral reflex, or arousal from sleep. Determining whether an infant responded to the presented signal involves subjective judgments about subtle behaviors. For this reason, the personnel who perform behavioral observation audiometry screenings require a fair amount of training, and two observers are preferred over a single tester.

Screening with the **Crib-O-Gram** (Simmons & Russ, 1974) involves the use of a crib fitted with motion detectors that monitor the infant's movements in response to a 3000-Hz stimulus at 90 dB SPL. Similarly, the **neonatal auditory response cradle** (Bennett, 1975; Shepard, 1983) monitors respiratory changes as well as body movements in response to a 2600- to 4300-Hz noise band at 85 dB SPL. The techniques are more objective than manual BOA screening because they are automated, and the relationship of the stimuli and responses are recorded and judged according to explicit criteria. In addition, the personnel requirements are less demanding and do not interfere as much with the routine of the newborn nursery. However, behavioral observation approaches have important limitations (Northern & Gerkin, 1989; Durieux-Smith & Jacobson, 1985; Durieux-Smith, Picton, Edwards, Goodman, & MacMurray, 1985; Shimizu, Walters, Proctor, Kennedy, Allen, & Markowitz, 1990; Hall, 1992; Mauk & Behrens, 1993). For example, they use high-level stimuli so that mild and moderate losses cannot be confidently identified; it is impossible to tell whether a response was due to hearing the sound in one or both ears because the signals are presented from a loudspeaker, and the results have reliability problems as well as many false-positive and false-negative results. Hence, it is not surprising that behavioral methods are now considered inappropriate for newborn screening purposes (ASHA, 1997). Behavioral screening in older infants and toddlers may employ visual reinforcement audiometry and conditioned play audiometry (see Chapter 12), as described below.

Physiological Screening

Physiological measures are becoming the standard means of testing in neonatal hearing screening programs. The principal techniques are the auditory brainstem response and evoked otoacoustic emissions (NIH, 1993; ASHA, 1997; JCIH, 2000), which are explained in Chapter 11. In addition to greater sensitivity and objectivity, the physiological methods can be used when the infant is sleeping, and permit us to screen each ear separately. These methods require more costly instrumentation than behavioral approaches, tend to be limited in their ability to detect low-frequency hearing losses, and reflect the integrity of the peripheral and lower auditory system rather than the notion of "hearing" that is inferred from a behavioral response.

The **auditory brainstem response (ABR)** is well established as a neonatal hearing screening test, and has impressive rates of sensitivity, specificity, and reliability (Hall, 1992; Mauk & Behrens, 1993; NIH, 1993; ASHA, 1997; Finitzo, Albright, & O'Neil, 1998; Vohr, Carty, Moore, et al, 1998). **Evoked otoacoustic emissions (EOAEs)** have been used for newborn hearing screening since the late 1980s. Most of this work to date has involved **transient-evoked otoacoustic emissions (TEOAEs)**, which have been used with great success and for which an extensive body of empirical information has been compiled (Bonfils, Uziel, & Pujol, 1988; Uziel & Piron, 1991; Maxon, White, Behrens, & Vohr 1995; Prieve, 1997; Thompson, 1997; Finitzo, Albright & O'Neill, 1998; Vohr et al, 1998; Gravel et al, 2000; Dalzell et al, 2000; Prieve et al, 2000; Prieve & Stevens, 2000; Spivak et al, 2000). Successful screening experience with **distortion product otoacoustic emissions (DPOAEs)** is also steadily accumulating (Bonfils, Avan, Martine, Trotoux, & Narcy, 1992; Lafreniere, Smurzynski, Jung,

Leonard, & Kim, 1994; Brown, Sheppard, & Russell, 1994; Bergman, Gorga, Neely, Kaminski, Beauchaine, & Peters, 1995). The EOAE shares excellent sensitivity with the ABR for detecting hearing loss in infants, although its specificity may not be quite as high as that obtained with the auditory brainstem response.

Universal newborn hearing screening becomes simpler, quicker, and more cost efficient when **automated auditory brainstem response (AABR)** and **automated otoacoustic emissions (AOAE)** screening devices are used in place of clinical ABR and OAE instrumentation. These instruments employ statistical criteria to determine if an acceptable response is present, leading to a "pass" versus "refer" recommendation instead of an ABR or OAE record that must be professionally interpreted. As a result, the routine aspects of carrying out the screening program do not require highly trained professionals to perform the tests. Considerable experience has accumulated with the use AABR instruments, such as the Natus ALGO-1 and ALGO-2 newborn hearing screeners. The AABR produces outcomes that are in good agreement with conventional ABR results and has been used successfully in large-scale newborn screening programs (Jacobson, Jacobson & Spahr, 1990; Herrmann, Thornton, & Joseph, 1995; Prieve, 1997; Thompson, 1997; Mason & Herrmann, 1998; Mason, Davis, Wood, & Farnsworth, 1998). Several automated OAE screeners are available and hold promise for successful use, although large-scale screening outcomes based on their use are not yet available.

Numerous proposed guidelines and position statements have been published over the years in an evolutionary attempt to arrive at the optimal strategy for identifying hearing-impaired infants. Let us briefly outline some of the more current approaches to the issue, being mindful that (1) we are dealing with an evolutionary process in the development of strategies for the early identification of hearing impairment, and (2) no single protocol can be expected to be the best one for every screening program and setting. These caveats are not limited to hearing screening in babies; they also apply to screening approaches used for children and adults, discussed later in this chapter.

NIH Consensus Statement (1993)

A consensus statement on the early identification of hearing impairment was prepared by a multidisciplinary panel convened by the National Institutes of Health (NIH, 1993). It calls for the universal screening for hearing impairment of all neonates regardless of whether they are at high-risk or low-risk for hearing impairment. This screening should occur within 3 months of the infants' birth, and preferably before they have been discharged from the hospital because accessibility is greatest while babies are in the newborn nursery. Recognizing that many hearing losses develop or worsen after the neonatal period, the NIH panel also recommended that surveillance for hearing impairment should continue through early childhood. They also pointed out that another opportunity for universal screening presents itself when children enter school.

The newborn screening approach suggested by the NIH panel involves (TEOAE) and ABR testing according to the following protocol:

1. First, TEOAE screening for all babies.
2. Then, ABR screening for babies who fail the TEOAE screen.

The TEOAE screening is done first because it is very sensitive to the presence of hearing loss, it is fast, and it does not require the use of electrodes. Neonates who pass the TEOAE screen are considered normal. Those who fail the TEOAE screen proceed to the next step to minimize the number of false-positive results. Babies who fail the ABR screen are referred for diagnostic evaluations. Those who pass the ABR screen are discharged, but they should be rescreened in 3 to 6 months. Although the NIH panel estimated that the two-tier TEOAE/ABR protocol is more cost-effective, it encouraged institutions that have been successfully using the ABR alone for universal newborn screening to continuing doing so.

An important suggestion made by the NIH panel is that primary caregivers and health care providers need to be educated about hearing loss and its identification in young children. These educational efforts should highlight (1) neonatal risk factors, (2) acquired hearing impairment risk factors, (3) the early behavioral signs of hearing loss, and (4) the fact that crude "measures" of hearing ability (e.g., hand clapping) do not work and are misleading.

Joint Committee on Infant Hearing Position Statement (2000)

The Joint Committee on Infant Hearing (JCIH)[4] developed position statements on the identification of hearing loss in infants in 1982, 1990, 1994, and 2000. The current JCIH (2000) position statement calls for (1) universal newborn hearing screening using physiological measures (otoacoustic emissions and/or auditory brainstem responses), (2) confirmation of the hearing loss by 3 months of age, and (3) commencement of an interdisciplinary intervention program by the time the infant is six months old.

The JCIH (2000) position statement also involves a significant role for the use of high-risk indicators. Table 13–2 shows the indicators recommended for neonates from birth to 28 days old, and was suggested for use when a universal screening program is not available. It is quite possible for hearing losses to develop or become progressively worse *after* the neonatal period, so an infant who correctly passed the neonatal screening may become significantly hearing impaired at a later point in time. For this reason, the JCIH (2000) suggested the risk indicators listed in Table 13–3 for use with infants and toddlers from 29 days to two years old even if they had passed the newborn screening test. It

---

[4] The JCIH includes the American Academy of Audiology; the American Academy of Otolaryngology-Head and Neck Surgery; the American Academy of Pediatrics; the American Speech-Language-Hearing Association; the Council on Education of the Deaf; and the Directors of Speech and Hearing Programs in State Health and Welfare Agencies.

was recommended that children with any of these risk indicators should undergo audiological monitoring every 6 months through three years of age. Tables 13–2 and 13–3 also show several indicators that were included in the previous JCIH (1994) position statement, but were omitted from the current one on the basis of accumulating epidemiological findings. The JCIH also recommended monitoring of children who have risk indicators for *auditory neuropathy* (see Chapter 6), which are enumerated in Table 13–4.

ASHA (1997) Infant Screening Guidelines

Newborn to Six Months The American Speech-Language-Hearing Association (ASHA, 1997) infant screening guidelines cite the JCIH (1994) goal of hearing impairment detection by 3 months old and intervention under way by 6 months of age. The ASHA guidelines call for newborns and younger infants up to 6 months of age be screened for hearing impairment using either ABR *and/or* otoacoustic emissions testing. The OAE test may use either transient-evoked or distortion-product otoacoustic emissions. Passing the ABR test requires a response at 35 dB nHL in both ears; and passing the OAE test requires an acceptable TEOAE or DPOAE in both ears. In addition to these screening tests, the ASHA guidelines also call for surveillance

based on the kinds of indicators listed in Tables 13–2 through 13–4, which continue to be considered as the child gets older.

Seven Months to Two Years There are many reasons to screen babies after the sixth month. Regardless of our goals and efforts to effect universal screening within the newborn period, there will always be at least some infants who have not been screened by the time they reach 6 months old. Other babies will require rescreening based on risk indicators (often at regular intervals), suspicions that develop over time, and various screening mandates that might apply. In fact, phrases like "as needed, requested, or mandated" appear as screening indicators throughout the guideline.

In the 7 months to 2 years range, *pure-tone screening* should be done at *1000, 2000,* and *4000 Hz* using *conditioned response methods*. Each ear should be tested separately using earphones. Stimuli lacking in frequency specificity such as noisemakers, music, speech, and other broad-band signals, are considered inappropriate at every age (except, of course, for ABR and TEOAE). The test tones should be presented at a screening level of *30 dB HL* using *visual reinforcement audiometry (VRA)* or at *20 dB HL* using *conditioned play audiometry* (Table 13–5). These

TABLE 13–5 Summary of the major components of hearing impairment screening protocols throughout the age range recommended by ASHA (1997) guidelines

Population (Testing Method)	Frequencies Tested (Hz)	Screening Level (dB HL)	Pass Criteria
Newborn–6 months			ABR at ≤35 dB nHL, or TEOAE or DPOAE, in both ears
7 months–2 years (visual reinforcement audiometry)	1000,	30	Respond at all frequencies in both ears
7 months–2 years (conditioned play audiometry)	2000,	20	
3–5 years (conditioned play audiometry	and 4000	20	Respond to at least two of three presentations at all frequencies in both ears
5–18 years		20	Respond at all frequencies in both ears
Adults		25	

methods require the screening to be done by audiologists rather than by support personnel. The inability to hear any tone in either ear constitutes a failure, leading to rescreening or an audiological evaluation. Soundfield testing is an acceptable modification for children who refuse earphones, keeping in mind that we do not know which ear(s) are responsible for a response to a soundfield stimulus. However, unconditioned methods like BOA are not considered acceptable. Of course, there will be children in this age range who cannot be reliably tested with conditioned audiometric techniques, in which case ABR and OAE should be used.

Screening for Hearing Impairment in Preschool and School Children

The screening approach for preschool children (3- to 5-year-olds) recommended by ASHA (1997) involves testing under earphones at *1000, 2000,* and *4000 Hz* at *20 dB HL* using *conditioned play audiometry.* To pass the screening, the child must respond to at least two out of three tone presentations at all frequencies in both ears (Table 13–5). Visual reinforcement audiometry can be used if conditioned play audiometry is unsuccessful. Soundfield testing is acceptable for children who refuse earphones, being mindful of the limitations already mentioned. A preschooler who fails the screening should be referred for an audiological evaluation, although she may be rescreened using procedures for younger children if the failure is attributed to an inability to condition the child.

The ASHA (1997) hearing impairment screening guidelines for school children (5- to 18-year-olds) are intended to identify hearing impairments that could negatively affect the child's communication, development, education, or health—generally accepted as thresholds poorer than 20 dB HL. The ASHA guidelines call for hearing screenings to be administered

- when the child enters school;
- annually in kindergarten through the third grade; and
- in grades 7 and 11.

In addition to these "regularly scheduled" times, screening is also indicated when risk factors are present or when special circumstances exist. Risk factors for hearing impairment indicating the need for screening during other school years include

- concern about the child's hearing, speech, language, or learning;
- history of delayed and/or late-onset hearing loss in the family;
- signs of syndromes that include hearing loss;
- craniofacial and/or ear anomalies;
- persistent or recurrent otitis media with effusion for more than 3 months;
- head trauma with unconsciousness;
- exposure to ototoxic drugs; and
- exposure to potentially harmful noise levels.

Other circumstances under which hearing screenings should take place are when a child

- initiates special education;
- repeats a grade;
- was absent for the last "regularly scheduled" screening; or
- enters a new school system without evidence of having passed the previous scheduled hearing screening.

The ASHA screening protocol involves determining whether the child can hear pure tones of *1000, 2000,* and *4000 Hz* presented by air-conduction at a screening level of *20 dB HL* in each ear. Each child is tested individually using conventional pure-tone audiometry or conditioned play audiometry. Group testing and nonstandard instruments (e.g., hand-held devices) are not appropriate. To pass, the child must respond to all of the tones presented to both ears (Table 13–5). Missing one or more of the tones in either ear constitutes a failure. Those failing the screening test should be *rescreened* during the same session. Children who fail the rescreening (or could not be conditioned for the screening test) should be referred for audiological evaluations, to be followed by the appropriate kind of management.

In 1997, the American Academy of Audiology issued a report and position statement recommending issues to be considered when designing and implementing screening programs for preschool and school age children (AAA, 1997a,b). The AAA (1997b) position statement recommends pure-tone screening for all children at least once during the preschool period, and when a child is being considered for special education, or if a parent or caregiver suspects a hearing loss. Similar to ASHA (1997), the AAA recommends determining whether the child can respond to *1000-, 2000- and 4000-Hz* pure tones presented at *20 dB HL* in each ear. Each child should be screened individually using a manual method, although a specific technique (e.g., visual reinforcement, conditioned play, or conventional audiometry) is not specified. Missing any tone in either ear constitutes a failure, in which case the child should be referred for an audiological evaluation.

Survey data by Penn (1999) revealed that 44 states and the District of Columbia have hearing screening programs that are legally mandated or have some type of statewide coordination. State recommended hearing screening is commonplace in the elementary school grades, and decreases in the middle and high school years. Of the 40 states with written screening guidelines, 23 screen at 1000 to 4000 Hz (as recommended by ASHA and AAA), 12 use 500 to 4000 Hz, and five use other frequency combinations. All but two of the state guidelines recommend a 20 or 25 dB HL screening level, but at least some of the survey respondents mentioned that levels are raised to as high as 35 dB HL to deal with ambient noise in screening rooms. The implications of room noise and the practice of raising screening levels to overcome it are discussed later in the chapter.

Screening for Outer and Middle Ear Disorders in Children

The ASHA screening guidelines include the following procedures to screen for outer and middle ear disorders in children: (1) *case history* obtained from the child's parent or guardian; (2) *otoscopic inspection* for obvious

structural anomalies and obstructions of the ear canal and tympanic membrane; and (2) low frequency (220 or 226 Hz) *tympanometry*. (See Chapter 7 for a discussion of tympanometry and other aspects of acoustic immittance assessment.) Pure-tone screening is not employed by contemporary protocols for identifying outer and middle ear disorders (ASHA, 1997; AAA, 1997a,b).[5]

The child should be referred directly for a medical examination if any of the following conditions are identified for either ear:

- drainage from the ear (otorrhea);
- ear pain (otalgia);
- structural anomalies of the ear that were not previously identified;
- ear canal abnormalities (e.g., impacted cerumen, foreign body, blood or other secretion, atresia, stenosis, otitis external); or
- eardrum abnormalities or perforations.

A medical referral is also indicated if there is a flat tympanogram with ear volume exceeding 1.0 cm^3 (suggesting perforation of the tympanic membrane) *unless* the excessive normal volume is explained by the presence of a tympanostomy tube and/or the child has a perforation that is under medical care.

The tympanograms are also evaluated in terms of *static acoustic admittance* (Y^{TM} in mmhos), and *tympanometric width* (TW, which is the pressure interval, or how wide the tympanogram is in daPa, when measured halfway down from its peak). The criteria for failure are (1) static acoustic admittance that is too low; and/or (2) tympanometric width that is too wide, using the criteria shown in Table 13–6. A screening failure on this basis should result in referral for a rescreening, and failure

---

[5] Pure-tone screening at 20 dB HL may identify middle ear effusions with a sensitivity of 85% if the frequency range is extended to 500 to 4000 Hz, compared to only 54% for 1000 to 4000 Hz (Silman, Silverman, & Arick, 1994). The implication is that a 20 dB pure-tone screening at 500 to 4000 Hz might be used when immittance testing is not possible. A major problem is that room noise usually precludes testing at 500 Hz under typical screening conditions.

TABLE 13–6   ASHA (1997) tympanometry screening failure criteria based on static middle ear admittance (Y_{TM}) and tympanometric width (TW)

Age Group	Tympanometric Failure Criteria
Infants[a]	$Y_{TM} < 0.2$ mmho *or* TW > 235 daPa
One year through school age[b]	$Y_{TM} < 0.3^c$ mmho *or* TW > 200 daPa

[a] Based on Roush, Bryant, Mundy, Zeisel, and Roberts (1995).

[b] Based on Nozza, Bluestone, Kardatzke, and Bachman (1992, 1994).

[c] $Y_{TM} < 0.4$ mmho if ear canal compensation is based on ±400 daPa for children older than 6 years of age.

of the tympanometric rescreening should result in a referral for a medical examination.

The AAA (1997b) position statement recommends screening for middle ear disorders in association with pure-tone screening, and emphasizes the importance of screening for middle ear disorders for children at increased risk for the effects of otitis media with effusion. Those at-risk groups are children with (1) preexisting sensorineural hearing losses, (2) developmental disabilities, (3) developmental delays in speech and language, (4) learning disabilities, (5) craniofacial syndromes, (6) cleft palate and/or lip, (7) Down syndrome, (8) histories of recurrent or chronic otitis media with effusion, (9) native American background; as well as (10) children who attend group day care centers and (11) those who have failed pure-tone screenings. The screening techniques recommended by the AAA include *otoscopic inspection* to identify obvious indications of outer and middle ear disease, obstructions of the ear canal, and the presence of tympanostomy tubes; and low frequency (220 or 226 Hz) *tympanometry,* interpreted in terms of total ear volume, Y_{TM}, and TW.

Similar to the ASHA (1997) guidelines, the AAA recommends immediate medical referrals if any of the follow conditions are identified: (1) otalgia, (2) otorrhea, (3) external ear disease, and (4) flat tympanogram with ear volume >1.0 cm^3 (suggesting eardrum perforation) *unless* there is a tympanostomy tube.

The AAA position statement recommends that each screening program should arrive at specific pass/fail criteria based on norms that are most appropriate for its own population. The ASHA (1997) guidelines also point out that different screening guidelines may sometimes be appropriate depending on the nature of the population being screened (ASHA, 1997). For example, Nozza, Bluestone, Kardatzke, and Bachman (1992, 1994) found different 5 to 95% normal ranges for the general population of children and those from a subpopulation who were at risk for middle ear effusion. Several examples of these differences are shown in Table 13–7. Thus, different pass-fail criteria my be appropriate depending on whether the children

TABLE 13–7   Ranges (5–95%) for several tympanometric measures from an unselected group of children with normal otoscopy versus a group of at-risk children found to have no middle ear effusion during surgery

	Static Admittance (mmhos)	Tympanometric Width (daPa)	Tympanometric Peak Pressure (daPa)
Unselected children/ no effusion by otoscopy	0.4 to 1.4	60 to 168	−207 to +15
At-risk children/ no effusion at surgery	0.2 to 1.2	84 to 394	−325 to +30

Based on Nozza, Bluestone, Kardatzke, and Bachman (1992, 1994).

being screened are from the general ("unse-lected") population or from a subgrouping known ("selected") to have a higher than average risk for middle ear effusion.

With these points in mind, the AAA (1997b) suggests that typical criteria for a screening failure for middle ear dysfunction in children would be (1) Y_{TM} <0.2 mmho, and/or (2) TW >250 daPa. Screening failures based on these criteria should lead to a *rescreen* after an inter-val (typically about 4 to 6 weeks) to distin-guish between persistent cases and those that are self-limiting or transitory. Failure of the rescreening indicates a persistent prob-lem, and results in a medical referral. Chil-dren who pass the rescreen should be considered "at risk" for middle ear effusion, and should be seen again after an appropri-ate interval. Failure of the second rescreening should also lead to a medical referral. Audio-logical evaluations or rescreening should be done after medical intervention has been com-pleted to ascertain whether the previously identified middle ear dysfunction and/or hearing loss has been resolved.

Tympanometric Peak Pressure and Acoustic Reflex in Screening for Middle Ear Effusion. The ASHA and AAA screening guidelines do not include the use of tympanometric peak pressure (TPP) because it was judged to have little value in the identification of middle ear effusion (e.g., Nozza, et al, 1992; ASHA, 1997; AAA, 1997a,b). They also omit ipsilateral acoustic reflex testing[6] because it is associ-ated with unacceptably high false-positive rates, that is, over-referrals due to absent reflexes in normal ears (e.g., Lucker, 1980; Lous, 1983; Roush & Tait, 1985; ASHA, 1997; AAA, 1997a,b). In contrast, Silman, Silver-man, and Arick (1992) reported very high

sensitivity (90%) and specificity (92.5%) for a middle ear effusion immittance screening protocol[7] that includes ipsilateral acoustic reflex testing. They recommend the follow-ing referral criteria:

1. *Either*
   a. TW >180 daPa and/or Y_{TM} <0.35 mmhos *plus*
   b. absent 1000-Hz ipsilateral acoustic reflex at 110 dB HL;
2. *Or*
   a. TPP ≤100 daPa *plus*
   b. absent 1000-Hz ipsilateral acoustic reflex at 110 dB HL.

The underlying reason for the inconsis-tencies about the usefulness of ipsilateral acoustic reflexes in screening for middle ear effusion appear to have been identified by Sells, Hurley, Morehouse, & Douglas (1997). Using the same subjects, they found a 31% false-positive rate for ipsilateral acoustic reflexes when the immittance device was set to its "screening mode" compared to its "diagnostic mode." The high false-positive rate for ipsilateral reflex screening has to do with how the screening mode differs from the diagnostic mode. In the diagnostic mode (1) the probe and stimulus tones are rapidly alternated so they are less likely to interact and produce artifacts, and (2) the clinician can use small immittance changes to deter-mine whether a reflex has occurred. In the screening mode, however, (1) the probe and stimulus tones can interact and produce arti-facts because they are on at the same time, and (2) the criterion for a reflex response is a relatively large preset immittance change. The implication of these findings is that screening protocols might include ipsilateral reflex testing using the appropriate instru-mentation and measurement parameters.

[6] The AAA (1997b) position paper does not completely exclude acoustic reflexes. It states that their use "in a first-tier screening protocol using currently available instrumentation for screening should be undertaken cautiously." (p. 21). This point will make sense when considered in light of the findings by Sells, Hurley, Morehouse, and Douglas (1997), discussed below.

[7] This protocol assumes the use of an immittance device with a multiplexing circuit that alternates the probe tone and stimulus tone to minimize artifact responses during ipsilateral acoustic reflex testing, as well as a pump speed of 50 daPa/sec during tympanometry.

Effect of the Gold Standard   Before proceeding with the next topic, it is important to emphasize that the success of a screening protocol for middle ear effusion is affected by the validity of the eventual diagnosis. A conclusive diagnosis of middle ear effusion depends on whether fluid is actually found surgically (by myringotomy)—a true gold standard for effusion (Stool et al, 1994). However, real-world screening outcomes are usually judged by whether they are validated by otoscopic examinations—an assumed gold standard. The problem is that middle ear effusion is not reliably diagnosed by regular otoscopy (e.g., Roeser, Soh, Dunckel, & Adams, 1978; Stool, 1984; Nozza et al, 1994; Stool et al, 1994), and that otoscopic errors will affect both the apparent sensitivity and false-positive rates of the screening program. Otoscopic errors may be minimized with pneumatic and/or microscopic otoscopy. The Agency for Health Care Policy and Research *Clinical Practice Guideline* specifies the use of pneumatic otoscopy in the diagnosis of otitis media with effusion in young children (Stool et al, 1994) although it too is far from infallible (e.g., Toner & Mains, 1990; Kaleida & Stool, 1992).

Screening for Hearing Disability in Children

A distinction is drawn between hearing disorders and impairments on the one hand and hearing disability on the other. As a result, current philosophy also encourages screening for audiologically relevant disabilities, such as problems in speech and language development, academic progress, and behavior and adjustment. The ASHA (1997) audiological screening guidelines recommend disability screening as part of all pediatric well-care visits and audiological evaluations for children up to 5 years of age[8], as well as for children with hearing impairments and

those with risk factors, and when concerns arise. The AAA (1997b) position statement on audiological screening encourages audiologists to refer a child to a speech-language pathologist if delays in speech/language development are suggested by the case history, results on developmental screening instruments, or direct observation.

Disability screening may employ any of a wide variety of age-appropriate measures having published data about their validity, reliability, and pass/fail criteria. Several examples of tests that might be used for this purpose are listed in Table 13–8. Obviously, the criteria for what constitutes a "pass" or "refer" decision depend on the specific instrument used, and the nature of the problem will determine the kind of professional to whom the referral should be made.

Follow-Up Diagnosis and Intervention

Few things are more disturbing than to find that a hearing-impaired infant or child has been "lost to follow-up." It is universally accepted that infants and children who are identified by a hearing screening program should be referred for diagnostic evaluation and a comprehensive program of early intervention (e.g., NIH, 1993; ASHA, 1997; JCIH, 2000). The assessment and management program for the hearing-impaired infant or child should be multidisciplinary, and the child's parents or other caregivers should be integrated into the process from the start. The professionals involved in the diagnostic and management team will depend on many individual aspects, but will always involve the audiologist and physician, and often the speech-language pathologist, special and/or deaf educators, genetic counselor, and family support counselors. These details of diagnosis and intervention are discussed elsewhere throughout the text.

Audiological Screening in Adults

Except for occasional community health fairs and similar events, there has long been a lack

---

[8] More specifically, during the regular well-care visits at 1, 2, 4, 6, 9, 12, 15, 18, 24, 36, 48, and 60 months recommended by the American Academy of Pediatrics (AAP, 1995).

TABLE 13–8   Examples of instruments that may be used for disability screening for different age groups

Infants and toddlers	
Physician's Developmental Quick Screen for Speech Disorders	Kulig and Bakler (1973)
Fluharty Preschool Speech and Language Screening Test	Fluharty (1974)
Communication Screen	Striffler and Willis (1981)
Early Language Mildstone (ELM) Scale	Coplan (1983)

Preschool children	
Physician's Developmental Quick Screen for Speech Disorders	Kulig and Bakler (1973)
Compton Speech and Language Screening Evaluation	Compton (1978)
Fluharty Preschool Speech and Language Screening Test	Fluharty (1974)
Communication Screen	Striffler and Willis (1981)
Texas Preschool Screening Inventory	Haber and Norris (1983)
Preschool SIFTER	Anderson and Matkin (1996)

School-Age children	
Revised Behavior Problem Checklist (RBPC)	Quay (1983)
Screening Instrument for Targeting Educational Risk (SIFTER)	Anderson (1989)
Dartmouth COOP Functional Health Assessment Charts	Nelson, Wasson, Johnson, and Hays (1996)

Adults	
Self-Assessment for Communication (SAC)	Schow and Nerbonne (1982)
Hearing Handicap Inventory for the Elderly/Screening Version (HHIE-S)	Ventry and Weinstein (1983)

Based in part on ASHA (1997).

of ongoing, formal hearing screening programs for adults in the general public, and the common omission of hearing from routine medical examinations is a disturbing reality. This has been so in spite of the fact that the prevalence of hearing impairments rises through adulthood, as shown in Figure 13–6, from roughly 5% among young adults to over 40% for those 75 years of age and older. Happily, attention to the issue of hearing screening for the adults is growing, at least within the audiological community, and particularly with respect to the elderly.

The ASHA (1997) guidelines call for screening adults for hearing disorders using case history information and visual inspec-

tion, pure-tone screening for hearing impairment, and the use of hearing disability measures (typically self-assessment instruments) to screen for hearing disability.

Hearing Disorders Screening in Adults

The case history portion of the ASHA (1997) hearing disorders screening protocol for adults involves asking whether the individual has any of the following problems, and whether they have received medical attention:

• hearing loss;
• unilateral hearing loss;

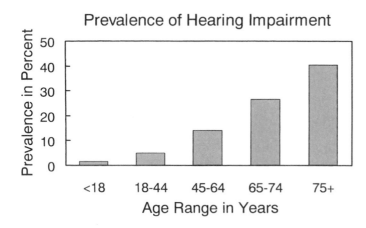

FIGURE 13–6 Estimated prevalence of hearing impairments through the adult years. Based on National Health Interview Survey data by Adams and Benson (1991).

- sudden-onset or rapidly progressing hearing loss;
- dizziness;
- unilateral tinnitus;
- recent ear pain or discomfort;
- recent ear drainage.

In addition to case history information, hearing disorders screening in adults also includes identifying outer ear and ear canal abnormalities, and impacted cerumen, by visual inspection and otoscopy. The screening is passed if no problems are identified by the case history and physical inspection. An immediate medical examination or cerumen management should be recommended if any problems are detected.[9]

Hearing Impairment Screening in Adults

Screening for hearing impairments in the adult population is not a straightforward problem and involves controversial practical and theoretical considerations. Much of the difficulty is related to the fact that the prevalence and degree of hearing loss increases with increasing age. The problem might be stated this way: A 20 or 25 dB HL screening criterion is needed to identify hearing losses that adversely affect communication. Yet so many older adults will fail at these levels that

the very use of a screening test to identify those who are hearing impaired could become a superfluous exercise. However, just because hearing problems are common among the elderly does not mean they are any less impairing (Gelfand & Silman, 1985). Happily, the current ASHA (1997) screening guidelines for adults indicate that a 25 dB is appropriate for adults because hearing losses greater than this level "can affect communication regardless of age" (p. 51).

The ASHA (1997) guidelines recommend pure-tone screening for hearing impairment and for hearing disability (see below) in adults at least every 10 years up to age 50 and every 3 years thereafter. Pure-tone screening for adults is done at *25 dB HL at 1000, 2000, and 4000 Hz for both ears.* The inability to hear any tone in either ear constitutes a failure, and leads to a referral in the form of a brief counseling session about hearing impairment. Recommendations for further testing are considered in the context of the hearing disability screening, discussed below.

Hearing Disability Screening in Adults

The ASHA (1997) screening proposal for hearing disability involves the administration of disability measures (or self-assessment scales, see Chapter 15) with known validity, reliability, and pass/fail criteria, such as the **Self-Assessment for Communication (SAC)** (Schow & Nerbonne, 1982) or the **Hearing Handicap Inventory for the Elderly/Screening Version (HHIE-S)** (Ventry

---

[9] The ASHA (1997) guidelines exclude immittance screening for adults, citing a low incidence of middle ear disorders and a negligible diagnostic yield.

& Weinstein, 1983). These self-assessment scales are included in the screening guidelines and are shown in Tables 13–9 and 13–10. Scores based on the patient's responses are associated with various degrees of handicap[10] or disability, as shown in Table 13–11. Higher scores indicate greater degrees of self-assessed disability, and scores outside the normal range (≥19 on the SAC or ≥10 on

the HHIE-S) are considered screening failures. Those who fail the disability screening are counseled so that they understand that their responses fall outside of the norms that are established for the screening scale.

The outcomes of the hearing impairment and the hearing disability screenings are considered together for the purpose of making follow-up recommendations. Audiological evaluations are recommended for those who fail both the impairment and disability screenings. Discharge may be recommended if the individual fails the impairment screening and passes the disability screening (or vice versa) *and* declines an audiological evaluation.

---

[10]As in the ASHA (1997) guidelines, the term *handicap* is employed here to be consistent with the terminology used in the research references.

TABLE 13–9   Self-Assessment of Communication (SAC) (Schow & Nerbonne, 1982)[a]

Please respond by circling the appropriate number ranging from 1 to 5, to the following questions:
   (1) almost never (or never)
   (2) occasionally (about 1/4 of the time)
   (3) about half of the time
   (4) frequently (about 3/4 of the time)
   (5) practically always (or always).

If you have a hearing aid, please fill out the form according to how you communicate when the hearing aid *is not* in use.

Various Communication Situations
   1. Do you experience communication difficulties in situations when speaking with one other person? (For example: at home, at work, in a social situation, with a waitress, a store clerk, a spouse, a boss, etc.)
   1   2   3   4   5
   2. Do you experience communication difficulties in situations when conversing with a small group of several persons? (For example: with friends or family, co-workers, in meetings or casual conversations, over dinner or while playing cards, etc.)
   1   2   3   4   5
   3. Do you experience communication difficulties while listening to someone speak to a large group? (For example, at church or in a civic meeting, in a fraternal or women's club, at an educational lecture, etc.)
   1   2   3   4   5
   4. Do you experience communication difficulties while participating in various types of entertainment? (For example: TV, radio, plays, night clubs, musical entertainment, etc.)
   1   2   3   4   5
   5. Do you experience communication difficulties when you are in an unfavorable listening environment? (For example: at a noisy party, where there is background music, when riding in an auto or a bus, when someone whispers or talks from across the room, etc.)
   1   2   3   4   5
   6. Do you experience communication difficulties when using or listening to various communication devices? (For example: telephone, telephone ring, doorbell, public address system, warning signals, alarms, etc.)
   1   2   3   4   5

continued

TABLE 13–9   Self-Assessment of Communication (SAC) (Schow & Nerbonne, 1982) *(continued)*

Feelings About Communication

7. Do you feel that any difficulty with your hearing limits or hampers your personal or social life?

1 2 3 4 5

8. Does any problem or difficulty with your hearing upset you?

1 2 3 4 5

Other People

9. Do others suggest that you have a hearing problem?

1 2 3 4 5

10. Do others leave you out of conversations or become annoyed because of your hearing?

1 2 3 4 5

Raw score (total of circled numbers): _____ (Normal range: 10–18)

[a]Adapted from Considerations in screening adults/older persons for handicapping hearing impairments. *ASHA* 34, 81–87 (1992), with permission.

TABLE 13–10   Hearing Handicap Inventory for the Elderly/Screening Version (HHIE-S) (Ventry & Weinstein, 1983)[a]

Please check "yes," "no," or "sometimes" in response to each of the following items. Do not skip a question if you avoid a situation because of a hearing problem. If you use a hearing aid, please answer the way you hear without the aid.

		Yes	No	Sometimes
E	1. Does hearing problem cause you to feel embarrassed when you meet new people?			
E	2. Does a hearing problem cause you to feel frustrated when talking to members of your family?			
S	3. Do you have difficulty hearing when someone speaks in a whisper?			
E	4. Do you feel handicapped by a hearing problem?			
S	5. Does a hearing problem cause you difficulty when visiting friends, relatives, or neighbors?			
S	6. Does a hearing problem cause you to attend religious services less often than you would like?			
E	7. Does a hearing problem cause you to have arguments with family members?			
S	8. Does a hearing problem cause you difficulty when listening to TV or radio?			
E	9. Do you feel that any difficulty with your hearing limits or hampers your personal or social life?			
S	10. Does a hearing problem cause you difficulty when in a restaurant with relatives or friends?			

S, social-situational; E, emotional.

"No" = 0, "sometimes" = 2, "yes" = 4. To score, count the number of "yes" responses and multiply by 4; count the number of "sometimes" responses and multiply by 2; then add the two products:

"Yes" responses   _____ × 4 = _____ (a)

"Sometimes" responses   _____ × 2 = _____ (b)

Score equals sum of (a) + (b): _____ (normal range 0–8)

[a]Adapted from Ventry, I., & Weinstein, B. 1983. Identification of elderly people with hearing problems. *Asha* 25, 37–47, with permission.

TABLE 13–11 Handicap interpretations for raw scores on the SAC and the HHIE-S

	SAC Raw Score	*HHIE-S Raw Score*
Normal / no handicap / no referral	10–18	0–8
Disability Screening Referral Criterion (ASHA, 1997)	≥19	≥10
Slight handicap	19–26	
Mild-to-moderate handicap	27–38	10–24
Severe handicap	39–50	26–40

Based on Schow, Smedley, and Longhurst (1990) and Lichtenstein, Bess, and Logan (1988).

Ambient Noise Levels in the Screening Environment

Recall from Chapter 4 that the lowest stimulus levels that can be used in a hearing test depend on the ambient noise levels in the testing environment. This is so because ambient noise can prevent the test signals from being heard due to **masking** (Chapter 3). Hearing screening tests are usually done in rooms or offices that were not designed for hearing testing. Even though the quietest available room should be used, it is not realistic to expect the sound isolation provided by an audiometric chamber. As a result, ambient noise is always a major consideration in hearing screening programs. Clearly, we cannot legitimately test hearing in a room unless its noise levels are known.

We have seen that the ASHA (1997) screening guidelines involve screening with 1000-to 4000-Hz pure tones presented at 20, 25, or 30 dB HL, depending on the individual's age and the testing method used. The maximum allowable ambient noise octave-band levels appropriate for these screening levels are shown in the upper part of Table 13–12. Maximum allowable noise levels at 250 and 500 Hz are also shown because of upward spread of masking, which effectively means that lower-frequency noises in the room can potentially mask higher frequency test tones (Chapter 3). The lower part of the table shows how these maximum allowable levels are calculated, using a 20-dB HL screening level as an example.

The ambient noise issue has several practical considerations that interact with the intended goals of a screening program. Once we decide on the test level that accomplishes the intended goals of our screening program, then we must find a room in which the noise

TABLE 13–12 Maximum permissible ambient noise levels in the testing room when performing air-conduction screening tests with earphones at 20, 25, and 30-db HL for the frequencies 500 to 4000 Hz or 1000 to 4000 Hz; also shown are examples of how maximal allowable room noise levels are calculated assuming a 20-db HL screening level; values are in dB octave band level

Octave Band Center Frequency (Hz)	*250*	*500*	*1000*	*2000*	*4000*
a. Maximum allowable noise level to screen at					
20 dB HL	53.5	39.5	46.5	48.0	54.5
25 dB HL	58.5	44.5	51.5	53.0	59.5
30 dB HL	63.5	49.5	56.5	58.0	64.5
b. Examples of how maximum noise levels are calculated (using a 20 dB HL screening level)					
ANSI (1991) value for 0 dB HL	33.5	19.5	26.5	28.0	34.5
+20 dB screening level	20	20	20	20	20
= Maximum allowable noise level	53.5	39.5	46.5	48.0	54.5

Based on ANSI (1991).

levels are low enough to permit testing at that level. What if the quietest available room has noise levels too high to permit screening at the level appropriate for our purposes? Then we must (1) consider changing the screening levels and/or frequencies so they are testable in that room; and (2) grapple with the question of whether these practical, compromised screening criteria are justifiable within the goals of our screening program.

REFERENCES

Adams PF, Benson V. 1991. Current estimates from the National Health Interview Survey. National Center for Health Statistics, Vital Health Statistics, series 10(184).

Alpiner JG, McCarthy PA (Eds.). 2000. *Rehabilitative Audiology: Children and Adults*, 3rd ed. Philadelphia: Lippincott Williams & Wilkins.

American Academy of Audiology Task Force on Audiologic Screening (AAA). 1997a. Identification of hearing loss and middle-ear dysfunction in children. *Audiol Today* 9, 18–20.

American Academy of Audiology Position Statement (AAA). 1997b. Identification of hearing loss and middle-ear dysfunction in preschool and school-age children. *Audiol Today* 9, 21–23.

American Academy of Pediatrics Committee on Practice and Ambulatory Medicine (AAP). 1995. Recommendations for preventive pediatric health care. *Pediatrics* 96.

American National Standards Institute (ANSI). 1991. *Maximum Permissible Ambient Noise Levels for Audiometric Test Rooms.* ANSI S3.1-1991. New York: ANSI.

American Speech-Language-Hearing Association (ASHA). 1991. Guidelines for the audiologic assessment of children from birth through 36 months of age. *ASHA* 32 (suppl 5), 37–43.

American Speech-Language-Hearing Association (ASHA). 1992. Considerations in screening adults/older persons for handicapping hearing impairments. *ASHA* 34, 81–87.

American Speech-Language-Hearing Association (ASHA). 1997. *Guidelines for Audiologic Screening.* Rockville Pike, MD: ASHA.

Anderson KL. 1989. *Screening Instrument for Targeting Educational Risk (SIFTER).* Austin: Pro-Ed.

Anderson KL, Matkin ND. 1996. *Preschool SIFTER: Screening Instrument for Targeting Educational Risk in Pre-school Children (Age 3–Kindergarten).* Tampa: Ed. Audiol. Assn.

Axelsson A, Aniansson G, Costa O. 1987. Hearing loss in school children. *Scand Audiol* 16, 137–143.

Bennett MJ. 1975. The auditory response cradle: A device for the objective assessment of auditory state in the neonate. *Symp Zool Soc Lond* 37, 291–305.

Bergman BM, Gorga MP, Neely ST, Kaminski JK, Beauchaine KL, Peters J. 1995. Preliminary descriptions of transient-evoked and distortion-product otoacoustic emissions from graduates of an intensive care nursery. *J Am Acad Audiol* 6, 150–162.

Bess FH, Dodd-Murphy J, Parker RA. 1998. Children with minimal sensorineural hearing loss: Prevalence, educational performance, and functional status. *Ear Hear* 19, 339–354.

Bonfils P, Avan P, Martine M, Trotoux J, Narcy P. 1992. Distortion-product oto-acoustic emissions in neonate: Normative data. *Acta Otolaryngol* 112, 739–744.

Bonfils P, Uziel A, Pujol R. 1988. Screening for auditory dysfunction in infants by evoked oto-acoustic emissions. *Arch Otolaryngol* 114, 887–890.

Brown AM, Sheppard SL, Russell PT. 1994. Acoustic distortion products (ADP) from the ears of term infants and young adults using low stimulus levels. *Br J Audiol* 28, 273–280.

Compton A. 1978. *Compton Speech and Language Screening Evaluation.* San Francisco: Carousel House.

Cooper JC, Gates GA, Owen JH, Dickson HD. 1975. An abbreviated impedance bridge technique for school screening. *J Speech Hear Dis* 40, 260–269.

Coplan J. 1983. *EML Scale: The Early Language Mildstone Scale.* Tulsa: Modern Education Corp.

Dalzell L, Orlando M, MacDonald M, et al. 2000. The New York State newborn hearing screening demonstration project: Ages of hearing loss identification, hearing aid fitting, and enrollment in early intervention. *Ear Hear* 21, 118–130.

Downs M, Sterritt G. 1967. A guide to newborn and infant hearing screening programs. *Arch Otolaryngol* 85, 15–22.

Durieux-Smith A, Jacobson JT. 1985. Comparison of auditory brainstem response and behavioral screening in neonates. *J Otolaryngol* 14, 47–52.

Durieux-Smith A, Picton T, Edwards C, Goodman JT, MacMurray B. 1985. The Crib-O-Gram in the NICU: An evaluation based on brain stem electric response audiometry. *Ear Hear* 6, 20–24.

Elssman S, Matkin, N, Sabo M. 1987. Early identification of congenital hearing loss. *Hear J* 40, 13–17.

Finitzo T, Albright K, O'Neil J. 1998. The newborn with hearing loss: Detection in the nursery. *Pediatrics* 102, 1452–1460.

Fluharty NB. 1974. *Fluharty Preschool Speech and Language Screening Test.* Boston: Teaching Resources.

Gelfand SA, Silman S. 1985. Future perspectives in hearing and aging: Clinical and research needs. *Semin Hear* 6, 207–219.

Gravel J, Berg A, Bradley M, et al. 2000. The New York State newborn hearing screening demonstration project: Effects of screening protocol on inpatient outcome measures. *Ear Hear* 21, 131–140.

Haber JS, Norris ML. 1983. The Texas preschool screening inventory: A simple screening device for language and learning disorders. *Children's Health Care* 12, 11–18.

Hall JW. 1992. *Handbook of Auditory Evoked Responses.* Boston: Allyn & Bacon.

Herrmann BS, Thornton AR, Joseph JM. 1995. Automated infant hearing screening using the ABR: Development and validation. *Am J Audiol* 4, 6–14.

Jacobson JT, Jacobson CA, Spahr RC. 1990. Automated and conventional ABR screening techniques in high-risk infants. *J Am Acad Audiol* 1, 187–195.

Joint Committee on Infant Hearing (JCIH). 1994. Position statement. *Audiol Today* 6, 6–9.

Joint Committee on Infant Hearing (JCIH). 2000. Year 2000 position statement: Principles and guidelines for early hearing detection and intervention programs. *Am J Audiol* 9, 9–29.

Kaleida PH, Stool SE. 1992. Assessment of otoscopists' accuracy regarding middle-ear effusion. *Am J Dis Child* 146, 433–435.

Kulig SG, Bakler K. 1973. *Physician's Developmental Quick Screen for Speech Disorders.* Galveston: University of Texas Medical Branch.

Lafreniere D, Smurzynski J, Jung M, Leonard F, Kim, DO. 1994. Otoacoustic emissions in full-term neonates at risk for hearing loss. *Laryngoscope* 103, 1334–1341.

Lichtenstein MJ, Bess FH, Logan SA. 1988. Diagnostic performance of the Hearing Handicap Inventory for Elderly (Screening Version) against different definitions of hearing loss. *Ear Hear* 10, 250–253

Lous J. 1983. Three impedance screening programs on a cohort of seven-year-old children. *Scand Audiol* Suppl 17, 60–64.

Lucker JR. 1980. Application of pass fail criteria to middle-ear screening results. *ASHA* 22, 839–840.

Lundeen C. 1991. Prevalence of hearing impairment among school children. *Lang Speech Hear Services in Schools* 22, 269–271.

Mason JA, Herrmann KR. 1998. Universal infant hearing screening by automated auditory brainstem response measurement. *Pediatrics* 101, 221–228.

Mason S, Davis A, Wood S, Farnsworth A. 1998. Field sensitivity of targeted neonatal hearing screening using the Nottingham ABR Screener. *Ear Hear* 19, 91–102.

Mauk GW, Behrens TR. 1993. Historical, political and technological context associated with early identification of hearing loss. *Semin Hear* 14, 1–17.

Mauk GW, White KR, Mortensen LB, Behrens TR. 1991. The effectiveness of screening programs based on high-risk characteristics in early identification of hearing impairments. *Ear Hear* 12, 312–319.

Maxon AB, White KR, Behrens TR, Vohr BR. 1995. Referral rates and cost efficiency in a universal newborn hearing screening program using transient evoked otoacoustic emissions. *J Am Acad Audiol* 6, 271–277.

Montgomery J, Fujikawa S. 1992. Hearing thresholds of students in the second, eighth, and twelfth grades. *Lang Speech Hear Services in Schools* 23, 61–63.

National Institute on Deafness and Other Communicative Disorders (NIDOCD). 1989. *A Report of the Task Force on the National Strategic Research Plan.* Bethesda: National Institutes of Health.

National Institutes of Health (NIH). 1993. Early identification of hearing impairment. *NIH Consens Statement* 11, 1–24.

Nelson EC, Wasson JH, Johnson D, Hays R. 1996. Dartmouth COOP functional health assessment charts: Brief measures for clinical practice. In Spilker B (Ed.): *Quality of Life and Pharmacoeconomics in Clinical Trials*, 2nd ed. Philadelphia: Lippincott-Raven, 161–168.

Niskar AS, Kieszak SM, Holmes A, Esteban E, Rubin C, Brody DJ. 1998. Prevalence of hearing loss among children 6 to 19 years of age: The third national health and nutrition examination survey. *JAMA* 279, 1071–1075.

Northern JL, Gerkin KP. 1989. New technology in infant hearing screening. *Otolaryngol Clin North Am* 22, 75–87.

Nozza RJ, Bluestone CD, Kardatzke D, Bachman R. 1992. Towards the validation of aural acoustic immit-

tance measures for diagnosis of middle ear effusion in children. *Ear Hear* 13, 442–453.

Nozza RJ, Bluestone CD, Kardatzke D, Bachman R. 1994. Identification of middle ear effusion by aural acoustic admittance and otoscopy. *Ear Hear* 15, 310–323.

Pappas DG. 1983. A study of the high-risk registry for sensorineural hearing impairment. *Arch Otolaryngol* 91, 41–44.

Parving A. 1993. Congenital hearing disability: Epidemiology and identification: A comparison of two health authority districts. *Int J Pediatr Otolaryngol* 27, 29–46.

Penn TO. 1999. School-based hearing screening in the United States. *Audiol Today* 11, 20–21.

Prieve BA. 1997. Establishing infant hearing programs in hospitals. *Am J Audiol* 6 (suppl), 84–87.

Prieve B, Dalzell L, Berg A, et al. 2000. The New York State newborn hearing screening demonstration project: Outpatient outcome measures. *Ear Hear* 21, 104–117.

Prieve B, Stevens F. 2000. The New York State newborn hearing screening demonstration project: Introduction and overview. *Ear Hear* 21, 85–91.

Quay HC. 1983. A dimensional approach to children's behavioral disorder: The revised behavior problem checklist. *School Psych Rev* 12, 244–249.

Roeser RJ, Soh J, Dunckel DC, Adams RM. 1978. Comparison of tympanometry and otoscopy in establishing pass/fail referral criteria. In Harford ER, Bess FH, Bluestone CD, Klein JO (Eds.): *Impedance Screening for Middle Ear Disease in Children.* New York: Grune & Stratton, 135–144.

Roush J, Bryant K, Mundy M, Zeisel S, Roberts J. 1995. Developmental changes in static admittance and tympanometric width in infants and toddlers. *J Am Acad Audiol* 6, 334–338.

Roush J, Tait C. 1985. Pure-tone and acoustic immittance screening of preschool aged children: An examination of referral criteria. *Ear Hear* 6, 245–249.

Sarff CS. 1981. An innovative use of free-field amplification in regular classrooms. In Roeser RJ, Downs MP (Eds.): *Auditory Disorders in School Children.* New York: Thieme, 263–272.

Schow RL. 1991. Considerations in selecting and validating an adult/elderly hearing screening protocol. *Ear Hear* 12, 337–348.

Schow RL, Nerbonne MA. 1982. Communication screening profile: Use with elderly clients. *Ear Hear* 3, 135–147.

Schow RL, Nerbonne MA (Eds.). 1996. *Introduction to Audiologic Rehabilitation*, 3rd ed. Boston: Allyn & Bacon.

Schow RL, Smedley TC, Longhurst TM. 1990. Self-assessment and impairment in adult/elderly hearing screening: Recent data and new perspectives. *Ear Hear* 11, 17S–27S.

Sells JP, Hurley RM, Morehouse CR, Douglas JE. 1997. Validity of the ipsilateral acoustic reflex as a screening parameter. *J Am Acad Audiol* 8, 132–136.

Shepard NT. 1983. Newborn hearing screening using the Linco-Bennett Auditory Response Cradle: A pilot study. *Ear Hear* 4, 5–10.

Shimizu H, Walters RJ, Proctor LR, Kennedy DW, Allen MC, Markowitz RK. 1990. Identification of hearing impairment in the neonatal intensive care unit population: Outcome of a five-year project at the Johns Hopkins Hospital. *Semin Hear* 11, 150–160.

Silman S, Silverman CA, Arick DS. 1992. Acoustic-immittance screening for detection of middle-ear effusion. *J Am Acad Audiol* 3, 262–268.

Silman S, Silverman CA, Arick DS. 1994. Pure-tone assessment and screening of children with middle-ear effusion. *J Am Acad Audiol* 5, 173–182.

Simmons FB, Russ FN. 1974. Automated newborn hearing screening, the Crib-O-Gram. *Arch Otolaryngol* 100, 1–7.

Spivak L, Dalzell L, Berg A, et al. 2000. The New York State newborn hearing screening demonstration project: Inpatient outcome measures. *Ear Hear* 21, 92–103.

Stein L. 1999. Factors influencing the efficacy of universal newborn hearing screening. In Roizen NJ, Diefendorf AO (Eds.): *Hearing Loss in Children. Pediat Clin North Am* 46, 95–105.

Stool SE. 1984. Medical relevancy of immittance measurements. *Ear Hear* 4, 309–313.

Stool SE, Berg AO, Berman S, et al. 1994. *Otitis Media with Effusion in Young Children: Clinical Practice Guideline.* AHCPR publ. no. 94–0622. Rockville, MD: Agency for Health Care Policy & Research, Public Health Service, US Department of Health & Human Services.

Striffler N, Willis S. 1981. *Communication Screen.* Tucson: Communication Skills Builders.

Thompson V. 1997. The Colorado newborn hearing screening project. *Am J Audiol* 6 (suppl), 74–77.

Toner JG, Mains B. 1990. Pneumatic otoscopy and tympanometry in the detection of middle ear effusion. *Clin Otolaryngol* 15, 121–123.

Uziel A, Piron JP. 1991. Evoked otoacoustic emissions from normal newborns and babies admitted to an intensive care baby unit. *Acta Otolaryngol* Suppl 482, 85–91.

Ventry I, Weinstein B. 1983. Identification of elderly people with hearing problems. *ASHA* 25, 37–47.

Vohr BR, Carty LM , Moore PE, et al. 1998. The Rhode Island hearing assessment program: Experience with statewide hearing screening (1993–1996). *J Pediatr* 133, 353–357.

Wedenberg 1956. Auditory test in newborn infants. *Arch Otolaryngol* 46, 446–461.

Yoshinaga-Itano C, Sedey AL, Coulter DK, Mehl AL. 1998. Language of early- and later-identified children with hearing loss. *Pediatrics* 102, 1161–1171.

14

Nonorganic Hearing Loss

Routine audiological tests rely on the patient's behavioral responses to the stimuli presented to her. If she can hear a tone as soft as 0 dB HL, then she will respond to tones down to 0 dB HL, and if the softest tone she can hear is 50 dB HL, then she will respond to all tones down to 50 dB HL. Her thresholds represent her actual hearing sensitivity, and any hearing loss revealed by these thresholds will be due to some kind of real, physical disorder, or anomaly. Here we may say that the hearing loss is of *organic origin* because it is the result of anatomical and/or physiological abnormalities. In contrast, another patient might not respond as directed. Instead of responding to the softest sound she can hear, she might wait until the sounds are well above her actual threshold before she is willing to volunteer a response. For example, she might hold off on responding until a tone reaches 55 dB HL even though she could really hear it as low as 0 dB HL. In this case, her 55 dB HL threshold gives the false impression that she has a hearing loss even though she is actually normal. This exaggerated loss is not due to an organic cause, and may therefore be called a **nonorganic hearing loss**. Nonorganic hearing losses are also known as **functional** or **exaggerated hearing losses**, or **pseudohypacusis**, and these terms will be used interchangeably here.

A functional loss involves *questionable test results*. In operational terms, a nonorganic hearing loss is identified on the basis of observable discrepancies in the audiological tests and/or between the patient's behavior and the test results, which are not accounted for by an organic disorder (Ventry & Chaiklin,

1965). On the other hand, a functional loss is not indicated by test results that are better than expected from the patient's complaints, or when subjective problems cannot be verified by routine audiological tests. In fact, subjective complaints that are not accounted for by the audiogram may suggest the possibility of abnormalities requiring more advanced diagnostic efforts (e.g., Saunders & Haggard, 1989; Baran & Musiek, 1994).

Not all patients with exaggerated hearing losses actually have normal hearing. In fact, most adults with functional impairments have at least some degree of underlying organic hearing loss (Chaiklin & Ventry, 1963; Coles & Priede, 1971; Coles & Mason, 1984; Gelfand & Silman, 1985, 1993; Gelfand, 1994). For example, a functional patient whose real threshold is 35 dB HL might not respond until 65 dB HL. In this case, 35 dB of the loss is organic (real) and the remaining 30 dB is nonorganic. Hence, we often distinguish between (1) the overall nonorganic loss, which is represented by the patient's voluntary thresholds, and (2) the **functional component** or **overlay**, which is the *nonorganic part* of the loss. The nonorganic component is simply the difference between the exaggerated thresholds volunteered by the patient and the underlying organic loss.

The literature is unclear about the relative incidences of bilateral and unilateral nonorganic hearing loss, but clinical experience suggests that it is more common bilaterally. For example, among 88 patients whose nonorganic losses were eventually resolved, 72% were bilateral cases and 28% were unilateral (Gelfand & Silman, 1993). Some possible reasons to explain why bilateral functional losses might be more common are (1) an underlying organic loss is more likely to be experienced in both ears, (2) it is easier to respond the same way for both ears, and (3) the belief that "real" hearing losses "should be" bilateral. On the other hand, sensing a difference between the ears might influence the patient to exaggerate the impairment in only one ear. A loss might be exaggerated in the poorer ear to maximize the benefits that can be derived from the loss in that ear. Alternatively, the patient might feign a loss in the good (or "better") ear because he (1) believes that hearing losses "should be" bilateral, or (2) envisions greater benefits from an impairment in both ears instead of just one.

Nonorganic Hearing Loss in Adults: Motivating Factors

Because functional losses do not have an organic basis they must be due to either **psychogenic** causes or to **malingering** or **feigning**. The psychogenic explanation says the hearing loss is the result of unconscious psychodynamics, and includes such phenomena as hysterical and conversion reaction deafness. It implies the patient actually experiences impaired hearing and he truly believes the hearing loss is real. Malingering means the patient is faking a hearing loss he does not have, or is falsely exaggerating whatever amount of loss he actually does have. Malingering may be motivated by financial or other benefits that the patient associates with a hearing loss. Financial gain is often an issue with injury-related lawsuits, and with veterans' and workers' compensation claims. Here, worse hearing translates into larger legal settlements, pensions, and/or compensation payments. The other real or perceived benefits to be derived from an exaggerated hearing loss may be summarized as the desire for real or perceived special attention, preferential treatment, considerations, and support in a host of social and occupational life situations.

Goldstein (1966) argued that exaggerated hearing losses are due to malingering because they cannot meet the criteria for a psychogenic disorder, which must include alleviation of the nonorganic hearing loss when the underlying psychiatric disorder is resolved. Others argued that we cannot ascribe a patient's functional loss to malingering (unless he admits feigning) because we really do not know why his responses are exaggerated, which may well include a psychogenic cause (Hopkinson, 1967, 1973; Chaiklin & Ventry, 1963; Ventry, 1968). This is one of the reasons for using nonjudgmental, descriptive terms such as "functional hearing loss." Nobel (1978, 1987) has challenged the concept of "functional *hearing loss*" as a clinical entity and the appropriateness of the term itself to describe the exaggeration of thresholds during compensation evaluations. He argued that we are dealing with faking that is related to a process that is legalistic and adversarial rather than clinical, and that is often itself unfair. This point of view makes sense, but it does not explain why patients should have exaggerated losses when monetary issues are not involved.

Reported cases of psychogenic hearing loss are noticeably sparse. For example, Ventry (1968) presented only one case to make his point, and Coles (1982) reported that he *might* have seen three cases, but was not certain. The author came across only one reasonably convincing case of psychogenic hearing loss among all the patients seen in a Veterans Administration audiology program over about 15 years. This patient had psychiatric diagnoses that included an infantile personality and conversion reactions. He had various somatic disorders that responded to placebo treatments, among which was a functional hearing loss that he insisted was helped by a hearing aid. The intangible nature of other people's motivations and the desire to be fair minded makes it hard to conclude with absolute certainty that psychogenic cases of nonorganic hearing loss do not exist. However, it appears that these cases are few and far between.

Even in the absence of a deeply rooted psychogenic cause, it is still reasonable to ask what psychological factors are associated with nonorganic hearing loss. Most of what we know about the personality and other psychosocial characteristics of individuals with nonorganic hearing loss is based on a fairly small number of studies reported during the 1940s through the 1960s. These culminated with the authoritative and well-known study by Trier and Levy (1965), who compared adult male veterans with functional losses and those with organic hearing impairments. The subjects with nonorganic hearing loss had an average intelligence quotient (IQ) of 98.7, which was slightly but significantly lower than an average IQ of 106.8 in the organic group. Compared to those with organic losses, the functional group was found to exhibit more emotional disturbances, nervousness and submissiveness, hypochondria and preoccupation with their hearing problems, tinnitus, tendencies to exploit their physical symptoms, and variability in the manifestation of the effects of their hearing losses. In addition, the individuals in the functional group earned $1300 less per year than their organic loss counterparts, and their mean family incomes were $2000 per year lower. This reflects a major economic difference between the two groups because the median regional family income at that time was about $7000. Trier and Levy hypothesized that the patients with nonorganic hearing loss experienced general feelings of inadequacy, which included the belief that they were incapable wage earners. These beliefs led to exaggeration of their impairments for monetary compensation to help provide for their families, and doing so caused them to suffer a loss of self-esteem.

Nonorganic Hearing Loss in Children

Nonorganic hearing losses in children have been described by many investigators (Dixon & Newby, 1959; Barr, 1963; Rintelmann & Harford, 1963; Ross, 1964; Berger, 1965; Lumio, Jauhiainen, & Gelhar, 1969; McCanna & DeLupa, 1981; Veniar & Salston, 1983; Aplin & Rowson, 1986, 1990; Bowdler & Rogers, 1989). These studies have shown that nonorganic hearing loss tends to occur in children

who fail hearing screening tests at school. Many of these children do not show any evidence of hearing impairment except for the failed screening tests and functional losses on subsequent audiological evaluations, and for the most part their nonorganic hearing losses are usually resolved over time. Different samples of children with nonorganic hearing loss have been described as having normal intelligence and academic performance (e.g., Dixon & Newby, 1959); normal intelligence but poor educational achievement (e.g., Barr, 1963); and widely ranging (and below-average mean) intelligence with a substantial rate of poor academic achievement (e.g., Aplin & Rowson, 1990). These observations suggest that children with nonorganic hearing loss can vary widely in terms of their intellectual abilities and academic performance.

Financial rewards are clearly not the motivation for nonorganic hearing loss in children. Instead, children with pseudohypacusis are usually motivated by the secondary gains of having a hearing impairment. For example, a hearing loss can serve as a justification for underachievement at school, and to lighten the academic demands made upon him by teachers and parents, and can also provide a means to obtain needed attention and emotional support at home or school (Lumio, Jauhiainen, & Gelhar, 1969; Aplin & Rowson, 1986). These gains become apparent to the child who has failed a routine hearing screening test. Ross (1964) recommended that actual hearing losses should be identified as soon as possible, preferably during the screening process before referrals are made, to avoid undue attention and concern that could precipitate pseudohypacusis in children who are actually normal. The majority of children with nonorganic hearing loss do not appear to have significant emotional problems, but this certainly does occur. There is also evidence of psychodynamic origins in at least some cases of childhood nonorganic hearing loss (e.g., Hallewell, Goetzinger, Allen, & Proud, 1966; Lumio, Jauhiainen, & Gelhar, 1969; Broad, 1980).

Several modified testing methods can help obtain improved thresholds from children with nonorganic losses. Ross (1964) modified an earlier method used by Dixon and Newby (1959) to arrive at the **Variable Intensity Pulse Count Method**. The child's task is to count the number of tones that are heard. Groups of tones are then presented, composed of various numbers of tones at different levels. Testing begins above the child's admitted threshold. Once she is responding properly, the tone levels are manipulated until finding the lowest level at which the child is able to respond appropriately three times in a row. The success of this procedure depends on presenting it to the child as a test of *counting*

rather than hearing. In the **Yes-No Method** (Miller, Fox, & Chan, 1968; Frank, 1976) the child is told to immediately say "yes" whenever she hears a tone and "no" whenever she does not hear one. The tones are then presented using an ascending technique. Any response associated with the presentation of a tone indicates that the child heard the tone, regardless of whether she says "yes" or a "no." This technique depends on the immaturity of the child's logic, which allows her to say "no" in response to a supposedly inaudible tone without realizing that any response demonstrates that the tone was actually heard.

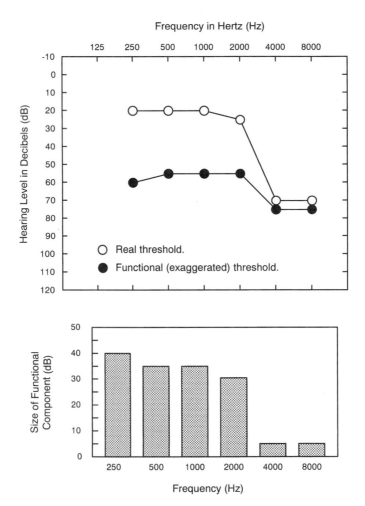

FIGURE 14–1   Example of how the configuration of functional components is related to the configuration of the underlying sensorineural hearing loss sloping precipitously at 4000 Hz.

Relation to Organic Hearing Thresholds

Patients with nonorganic hearing loss have functional components that are related to the configuration of the underlying, organic thresholds (Coles & Mason, 1984; Gelfand & Silman, 1985, 1993; Gelfand, 1993). This relationship is seen most clearly in patients who actually have precipitously sloping sensorineural losses, as illustrated in Figure 14–1. Notice how the functional components are relatively large for the frequencies up to 2000 Hz, where the organic thresholds are relatively low, and become abruptly smaller

beginning at 4000 Hz, where the organic thresholds get abruptly worse. Similarly, functional patients who really have sloping losses tend to have nonorganic components that become progressively smaller as their real thresholds become progressively worse (Figure 14–2). However, functional components and underlying organic thresholds are not related in patients who actually have normal hearing and mild losses.

Patients with functional loss seem to use an internalized reference level or "anchor" that has a certain loudness level, which we will call the "target." It appears that they will not respond to a test stimulus until its loudness

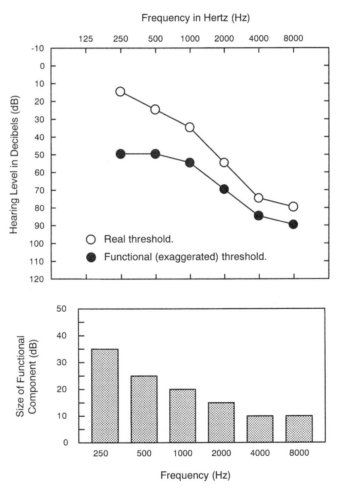

FIGURE 14–2 Example of how the configuration of functional components is related to the configuration of the underlying sloping sensorineural hearing loss.

level reaches the target (Gelfand & Silman, 1985, 1993; Gelfand, 1993). The inverse relationship between the degree of organic loss and the size of the functional component at each frequency appears to be produced by the following mechanism: Because of loudness recruitment, test tones reach the target at lower sensation levels (SLs) for frequencies where the underlying organic thresholds are higher (worse), and at higher SLs where the underlying thresholds are lower (better), within the same ear. This occurs because loudness recruitment is related to the amount of sensorineural loss (Chapter 10). Larger functional components are more common at lower frequencies and smaller ones are more common at higher frequencies because most sensorineural losses tend to worsen with increasing frequency. These relationships cause the exaggerated audiograms of patients with underlying high-frequency losses to appear relatively flattened (Coles & Mason, 1984). Functional components tend not to be systematically related to the underlying organic thresholds in patients who really have normal and mildly impaired hearing because these patients do not experience substantial loudness level differences between test frequencies.

Even though the configurations of functional components are consistently related to the configurations of the underlying losses, patients vary widely in terms of the absolute sizes of their functional components. This variability is probably influenced by differences between patients with respect to (1) the loudness level used as the target, (2) the range between the organic threshold and the highest stimulus level the patient is willing tolerate, and (3) the amount of recruitment.

Clinical Signs and Manifestations of Nonorganic Hearing Loss

Presenting and Behavioral Manifestations of Nonorganic Hearing Loss

The first factors that raise the index of suspicion for a possible nonorganic hearing loss involve real-world considerations about who referred the patient and why the evaluation is being done, rather than his clinical behavior or complaints. These include referrals made by attorneys, insurance companies, or compensation boards. Also included are referrals that are in any way related to legal issues, accidents, employment and/or work environment issues, or any form of claim that deals with any kind of pension or compensation.

The characteristics of patients with functional hearing loss are well established in the audiologic literature (Chaiklin & Ventry, 1963; Hopkinson, 1973; Coles, 1982). Many of these patients exaggerate the behaviors and complaints that they associate with people who have real hearing problems. Examples include leaning forward, turning the head to favor the "better side," cupping a hand over one ear to make sounds louder, and obviously gazing at the talker's mouth to demonstrate a reliance on lipreading. Some patients talk loudly in an exaggerated effort to hear their own voices. Many functional patients fail to have the speech and voice aberrations associated with long-standing hearing losses, but the same behavior also occurs in many patients with organic impairments. Functional patients may also constantly ask for repetition and clarification, or even insist on having things written for them. Vague complaints about hearing problems, excessive needs to rely on lipreading, and a lack of knowledge about the use of hearing aids by a patient who "used to own one" also raise the index of suspicion for pseudohypacusis. One might observe the patient conversing effortlessly with others in the waiting room even though his audiometric thresholds would make this impossible. Few adult feigners make this mistake when the clinician is present unless they are caught off guard. However, it is not uncommon for children with nonorganic hearing loss to carry on a conversation in an informal setting but not in a test situation.

Two caveats should be mentioned about the behavioral manifestations of nonorganic hearing loss. First, even though many patients are caricature-like in their portrayal of these behaviors, there are many others whose deportment typifies any patient with a real hearing impairment, or who play the part with practiced subtlety. Subtlety should not be surprising because, after all, patients do talk to other patients and are perfectly capable of reading an audiology textbook. Second, the diagnosis of pseudohypacusis depends on *test results*. Behavioral signs of exaggeration raise the index of suspicion for a nonorganic hearing loss and also provide support for any test findings that are obtained, but they do not indicate a functional loss themselves.

Indicators of Nonorganic Hearing Loss in the Routine Evaluation

Several signs of nonorganic hearing loss are obtained during the routine audiological evaluation that is administered to almost every patient. The fact that functional impairments can be revealed by routine testing is important because the clinician does not have to suspect a patient of exaggerating his hearing loss before she is able to test for it. Acoustic reflex tests are covered later along with other physiological measures, even though they are most certainly part of the routine evaluation battery.

LACK OF FALSE ALARM RESPONSES

Almost all patients who have normal hearing and organically based hearing losses will occasionally respond even though no tone has been presented. These responses that are made during the silent periods between tone presentations are called **false-positive responses** or **false alarms**. False alarms can be disturbing to the audiologist because they make it more difficult to establish the patient's threshold; however, they do demonstrate that the patient is highly motivated to hear every possible signal, no matter how faint it might be. Patients with functional losses obviously do not share this desire and often fail to elicit any false alarms. For example, Chaiklin and Ventry (1965b) found that false alarms were elicited by 86% of patients with real hearing losses compared to only 22% for those with pseudohypacusis. They recommended that pure-tone testing should

include one-minute "silent periods," during which no stimuli are presented, as a check for false alarms. One should consider the possibility of nonorganic hearing loss if the patient does not produce any false alarms, especially during these rather long silent intervals.

THRESHOLD VARIABILITY

Pure-tone thresholds are usually repeatable within a range of ± 5 dB, and test-retest reliability is certainly expected to be within ± 10 dB. Thresholds that vary by 15 dB or more from test to retest are associated with a nonorganic hearing loss (Chaiklin & Ventry, 1965b). On the other hand, good test-retest does not rule out a nonorganic hearing loss because many functional patients are able to produce thresholds that are quite reliable (Berger, 1965; Shepherd, 1965).

ABSENCE OF A SHADOW CURVE

Recall that cross-hearing means that the test signal is actually heard by the opposite ear instead of by the ear being tested. With this in mind, consider the audiogram in Figure 14–3a, which is from a patient who is unilaterally deaf in the left ear and has normal hearing in the right ear. The unmasked thresholds for the left ear are actually due to cross-hearing in the right ear, and are known as a shadow curve. The hearing levels of the shadow audiogram are in the 50 to 65 dB HL range because they depend on interaural attenuation and the bone-conduction thresholds of the better ear. In this case, the right ear has bone-conduction thresholds of 0 dB HL and interaural attenuation is in the 50 to 65 dB range. Hence, the right cochlea is able to hear the tones presented to the left ear by air-conduction at 50 to 65 dB HL. The shadow curve disappears when the deaf left ear is retested with masking noise in the opposite ear.[1] Figure 14–3b shows the unmasked audiogram of a patient with *nonorganic* unilateral deafness

---

[1] If these points are not clear, the student should review the material on cross over, cross hearing, interaural attenuation, and masking in Chapters 5 and 9.

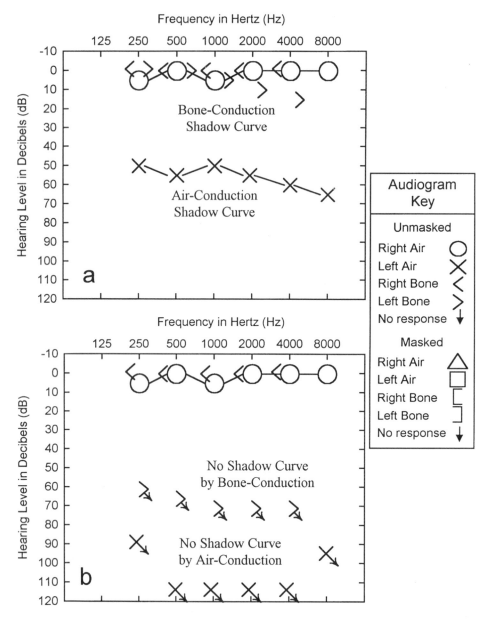

FIGURE 14–3 (a) Shadow curves occur for air-conduction and bone-conduction in the unmasked audiogram of a patient who is completely deaf in the left ear and normal in the right ear. (b) Shadow curves are missing in the unmasked audiogram of a patient who is feigning unilateral deafness in the left ear.

in the left ear and normal hearing in the right ear. There is *no shadow curve* because the patient refuses to respond to any sound being presented to the left ear, no matter how intense it might be. He is unaware that the normal right ear would have started hearing these tones by the time they reached about 50 to 60 dB HL in a genuinely deaf left ear, and it is the absence of the shadow curve that reveals the nonorganic origin of the loss. Similarly, a real unilateral loss has a shadow curve for bone-conduction. However, the "no response" symbols for bone-conduction show that this functional patient would not respond when the bone vibrator was on the left side of his head, in spite of the fact that little interaural attenuation occurs for bone-conduction.

The absence of a shadow curve for air-conduction is a strong indicator of nonorganic hearing loss when there is a unilateral (or asymmetrical) hearing loss so large that it must result in cross-hearing of the signals being presented to the poorer ear. In addition, because there is little interaural attenuation for bone-conduction, the absence of a shadow curve for bone-conduction is a very strong sign of pseudohypacusis. However, we must be mindful of several considerations and caveats in this context: (1) *Unmasked* air- and bone-conduction thresholds from the poorer side are needed to tell whether shadow curves are present or absent. (2) Instead of thinking in terms of specific hearing levels where shadow curves "must be," it is wiser to consider whether the signal being directed to the poorer is likely to reach the bone-conduction threshold of the better ear. (3) Although the prior consideration is similar to the "Do I need to mask?" question, there is one important distinction: The masking decision uses the smallest reasonable amount of interaural attenuation because it is better to mask when it was not necessary rather than to misdiagnose the hearing loss. However, when dealing with a nonorganic hearing loss, we must think in terms of the *largest* amount of interaural attenuation that is reasonably possible because we do not want to classify a loss as exaggerated without good cause. (4) We must be sure that the absence of a bone-conduction shadow curve is not due to problems with the placement of the bone vibrator on the "bad" side.

ATYPICAL SPEECH AUDIOMETRY RESPONSES

Functional patients often give a variety of atypical responses to spondee words during speech recognition threshold (SRT) testing (Chaiklin & Ventry, 1965b). They often miss spondee words previously repeated correctly at lower hearing levels. For example, a patient might not repeat "farewell" at 55 dB HL even though she could repeat that word at 45 dB HL earlier during the same test. They also give many half-word responses to the spondee words (e.g., "cow" for "cowboy," or "well" for "farewell"), and even monosyllabic word responses that are unrelated to the spondee that was presented (e.g., "ball" for "armchair").

Functional patients may also obtain higher than expected speech recognition scores when tested at low sensation levels (SLs) relative to their admitted thresholds (Gold, Lubinsky, & Shahar, 1981). This suggests a nonorganic hearing loss because high speech recognition scores are not expected until the presentation level reaches about 30 dB SL or even higher (Chapter 8). For example, suppose a patient whose SRT is 50 dB HL is able to score 92% correct for words presented at 60 dB HL, which is only 10 dB SL (re: SRT). Such high scores rarely occur at only 10 dB SL. This implies that 60 dB HL is more than just 10 dB above the SRT, and for this to be true the patient's real SRT must be lower (better) than 50 dB HL.

SRT-PTA DISCREPANCY

The pure-tone average (PTA) of the 500-, 1000-, and 2000-Hz thresholds and the SRT normally agree within reasonable limits. In contrast to the agreement between the SRT and PTA in patients with real hearing losses, Carhart (1952) observed that the SRT is often better (lower) than the PTA in patients with functional losses. An **SRT-PTA discrepancy** (or PTA-SRT discrepancy) of 12 dB or more is considered to indicate a nonorganic hearing loss (Chaiklin & Ventry, 1965b). For example, if a patient has a PTA of 47 dB HL and an SRT of 30 dB HL, he would be considered to have a nonorganic hearing loss because his SRT is better than his PTA by ≥ 12 dB. A significant SRT-PTA discrepancy has been shown to be the best audiometric indicator of functional losses (Ventry & Chaiklin, 1965).

One must be mindful of the shape of the audiogram when making the SRT-PTA comparison. Suppose a patient has an SRT of 20 dB HL and the following pure-tone thresholds:

Frequency (Hz):	250	500	1000	2000	4000	8000
Threshold (dB HL):	15	20	30	65	70	80

The 2000-Hz threshold is clearly out of line with the thresholds at 500 and 1000 Hz. Hence, the SRT should be compared to the two-frequency PTA of 500 and 1000 Hz, which is $(20 + 30)/2 = 25$ dB HL. The SRT-PTA discrepancy is only 5 dB, which is perfectly acceptable. In contrast, the three-frequency PTA is $(20 + 30 + 65)/3 = 38$ dB HL. This results in an 18 dB SRT-PTA discrepancy, giving the false impression of a nonorganic hearing loss. This example shows that the two-frequency PTA should also be considered before labeling a patient as functional. In fact, it is even occasionally appropriate to compare the SRT to the single frequency that has the best tonal threshold, which is usually 500 Hz but can be 250 Hz (Gelfand & Silman, 1985, 1993; Silman & Silverman, 1991).

The size of the SRT-PTA discrepancy also appears to be affected by how the SRT and pure-tone thresholds are tested. Exaggerated losses are more clearly identified (i.e., the discrepancy is bigger) when the SRT is obtained with an ascending testing method compared to a descending method (Conn, Ventry, & Woods, 1972; Schlauch, Arnce, Olson, Sanchez, & Doyle 1996). This difference can be seen by comparing the first two bars in Figure 14–4. Schlauch et al (1996) also demonstrated that the SRT-PTA discrepancy can be enhanced considerably by using a descending method for pure tones with an ascending method for the SRT (third bar in Fig. 14–4); and they recommended this approach as a screening test for functional loss. The descending pure-tone procedure involves (1) presenting the first tone at each frequency at high level (90 dB HL), (2) working downward in 10-dB steps, and (3) then following the ASHA (1978) method to arrive at a threshold (see Chapter 5).

AUDIOGRAM CONFIGURATION

The classical literature described nonorganic hearing loss as "saucer-shaped" or "flat," but it has been shown that no particular audiometric configurations are characteristic of functional losses (Chaiklin, Ventry, Barrett, & Skalbeck, 1959; Chaiklin & Ventry, 1965a). On the other hand, the *functional components* of exaggerated audiograms are related to configuration of the *underlying, organic thresholds* (Coles & Mason, 1984; Gelfand & Silman, 1985, 1993; Gelfand, 1993). This relationship

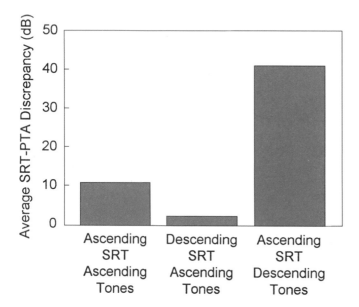

FIGURE 14–4 The size of the discrepancy between the speech recognition threshold (SRT) and pure-tone average (PTA) depends on whether ascending or descending methods were used to arrive at the SRT and the pure-tone thresholds. Based on data of Schlauch, Arnce, Olson, Sanchez, Doyle (1996).

is seen most clearly in patients who actually have precipitously sloping sensorineural losses, as illustrated in Figure 14–1. Notice how the functional components are relatively large for the frequencies up to 2000 Hz, where the underlying thresholds are relatively good, and become abruptly smaller beginning at 4000 Hz, where the organic thresholds get abruptly worse. Similarly, functional patients who really have sloping losses tend to have nonorganic components that become progressively smaller as their real thresholds worsen with increasing frequency (Figure 14–2). In general, the functional components are (1) bigger at the lower frequencies where the organic thresholds are better, and (2) smaller at the higher frequencies where the organic thresholds are worse.

As explained earlier, this appears to happen because patients with functional impairments use an internalized reference level or "anchor" that has a certain loudness level; they will not respond to a test tone (or other test stimulus) until its loudness level reaches that of the anchor (Gelfand & Silman, 1985, 1993; Gelfand, 1993). Within an ear, functional components are smaller at the frequencies where the actual losses are worse and larger at the frequencies where the real thresholds are better because loudness recruitment is related to the degree of hearing loss (Chapter 10). As a result, the majority of functional components tend to be wider at lower frequencies and narrower at higher frequencies simply because high-frequency losses are so common.

Tests for Nonorganic Hearing Loss

Many tests for nonorganic hearing loss have been developed over the years. Most of them identify the presence of an exaggerated hearing loss, but some of these tests can be used to make an estimate of the patient's actual organic hearing levels.

Behavioral Tests

ASCENDING-DESCENDING GAP TESTS

Recall that an unusual amount of threshold variability is often but not always found among functional patients. One way to help identify patients with functional losses is to use techniques that cause their exaggerated thresholds to be even more variable. This can be done by testing the threshold for the same tone separately with an ascending approach and with a descending approach (Harris, 1958; Hood, Campbell, & Hutton, 1964; Kerr, Gillespie, & Easton, 1975). The difference between these two thresholds is usually called the **ascending-descending gap**, and the testing itself can be done by either manual or Bekesy audiometry. When Bekesy audiometry is used, the method is known as the **Bekesy Ascending-Descending Gap Evaluation (BADGE)** (Hood, Campbell, & Hutton, 1964). The common feature of these methods is that one threshold is obtained by starting at a low hearing level and increasing the intensity, whereas the other threshold is obtained by starting at a high hearing level and decreasing the intensity. As illustrated in Figure 14–5, the ascending-descending gap is narrow for real thresholds and wide for exaggerated hearing losses. Functional patients have wide ascending-descending gaps because it is hard to maintain the same frame of reference for the exaggerated threshold "target" when it is being approached from below as when it is being approached from above.

Bekesy Audiometry

Type V Bekesy Pattern In the four conventional Bekesy audiogram patterns, the continuous and pulsed tone tracings are either interleaved, or the continuous tracings are tracked below the pulsed tone tracings (Chapter 10). These configurations occur because (1) continuous tone thresholds may be either the same as or worse than the pulsed tone thresholds, and (2) higher (poorer) thresholds are plotted downward on the audiogram. In contrast, patients with nonorganic hearing loss have the opposite arrangement—*their pulsed tracings are tracked below the continuous tracings*, which is known as the **type V Bekesy** pattern (Jerger & Herer, 1961). A typical example of a type V Bekesy audiogram is shown in Figure 14–6. Sweep-frequency tracings are preferred over the

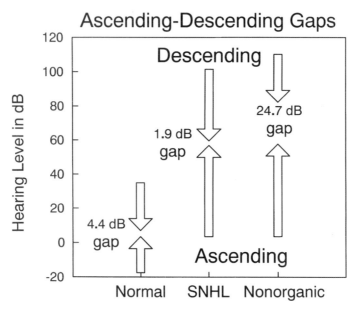

FIGURE 14–5   Conceptual illustration of the ascending-descending gaps associated with real thresholds (normal and sensorineural hearing loss) and exaggerated hearing losses. Values based on data reported by Cherry and Ventry (1976).

fixed-frequency method when conventional Bekesy audiometry is being used to identify nonorganic hearing loss (Rintelmann & Harford, 1967).

Why does the pulsed tracing fall below the continuous one on the type V Bekesy audio-

gram? It appears that this pattern is due to the effects of loudness memory as the functional patient attempts to keep the continuous and pulsed tones at a targeted loudness above his real thresholds. This notion is based on findings by Rintelmann and Carhart (1964). Their

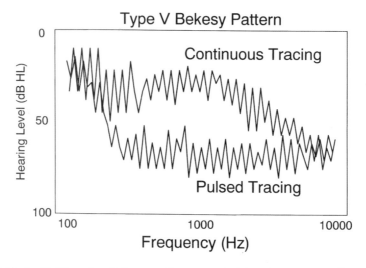

FIGURE 14–6   Unlike other Bekesy audiograms, the Type V pattern is distinguished by a pulsed tracing that falls below the continuous tracing.

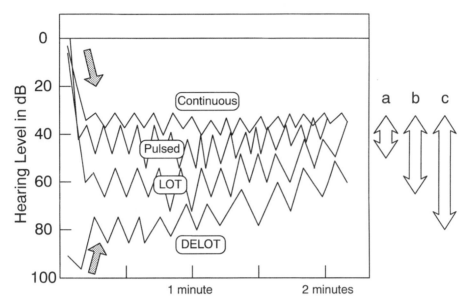

FIGURE 14–7 Type V fixed-frequency Bekesy tracings using a standard pulsed tone, lengthened off-time (LOT), and descending lengthened off-time (DELOT). Notice how the separation between the continuous and pulsed tracings for the conventional Bekesy **(a)** gets wider for the LOT **(b)** and even wider for the DELOT **(c)**.

subjects heard a 1000-Hz "target" tone at a certain level immediately before doing a sweep-frequency Bekesy tracing. The task was to keep the sweep-frequency tone at the same loudness that was recalled for the target tone. To do this, more intensity was needed when the sweep-frequency tone was pulsed and less intensity was needed when it was continuous. In other words, the pulsed tone needed more intensity than the continuous tone to reach the same recalled loudness. Consequently, the pulsed tracing was tracked below the continuous tracing (recall again that "more intensity" is "lower down" on the audiogram).

Lengthened Off-Time (LOT) Test Conventional Bekesy audiometry uses pulsed tones that are *on* and *off* for equal amounts of time (200-msec *on* and 200-msec *off*). The **Lengthened Off-Time (LOT) test** (Hattler, 1968, 1970, 1971) is a test for nonorganic hearing loss that uses Bekesy audiometry in which the pulsed tones have an *off-time* that is length-

ened from 200 ms to 800 ms.[2] In addition, the LOT test uses fixed-frequency rather than sweep-frequency tracings. Procedurally, the LOT test is just like standard fixed-frequency Bekesy audiometry except that the continuous tracing is compared to a pulsed tracing that is obtained with a tone that pulses at a rate of 200-msec *on* and 800-msec *off*. The LOT test increases the degree to which the pulsed tracing falls below the continuous tracing in functional patients, thereby improving the identification of functional impairments with the type V Bekesy pattern. This can be seen by comparing the conventional pulsed and LOT tracings in Figure 14–7.

---

[2] The *ratio* of the *on–time* to the *on–time plus off–time*, is often called the **duty cycle**. In these terms, conventional Bekesy pulsed tones have a duty cycle of $200/(200 + 200) = 200/400 = 0.5$, or 50%, and the duty cycle for the LOT Bekesy is $200/(200 + 800) = 200/1000 = 0.2$, or 20%.

DELOT Test   The **Descending-LOT (DELOT) test** (Chaiklin, 1990) combines the LOT with the BADGE. Recall that the BADGE (Hood, Campbell, & Hutton, 1964) is an ascending-descending gap test that uses Bekesy audiometry. The DELOT test begins with the same ascending continuous and 200-msec *on*/800-msec *off* pulsed tracings that are used in the LOT test. It then adds a *third* 200-msec *on*/800-msec *off* pulsed tracing that begins 25 dB above the worst (highest) threshold found on the LOT test. This will be a descending tracing because it starts from above the patient's apparent threshold. Functional patients tend to produce DELOT tracings that fall below the LOT tracing on the Bekesy audiogram (i.e., at higher hearing levels). This widens the gap between the continuous and pulsed tracings, making the type V pattern even clearer, as can be seen in Figure 14–7. Chaiklin (1990) recommended screening for nonorganic hearing loss with the DELOT at 500 Hz, which is supported by what we know about the configuration of functional components (Coles & Mason, 1984; Gelfand & Silman, 1985, 1993; Gelfand, 1993).

Stenger Test

A tone presented from the right earphone is heard in the right ear, and a tone presented from the left earphone is heard in the left ear. However, a tone presented from both earphones is heard as a single, fused image that seems to be located somewhere in the head. This phenomenon is called **binaural fusion**. The image is heard in the middle of the head if the tone has the same sensation level in both ears. This is a midline lateralization. Small differences in the SLs at the two ears will cause the tone to be perceived toward the side with the higher sensation level, that is, it will be lateralized to the right or to the left. Consider the following example, which is broken down into three parts:

1. A 1000-Hz tone presented *only* to the *right* ear at *10 dB SL* is heard in the *right* ear.
2. A 1000-Hz tone presented *only* to the *left* ear at *20 dB SL* is heard in the *left* ear.

3. If *both* of these tones are presented *simultaneously*, then the listener hears *one tone* in her *left* ear.

The third part of this example illustrates the lateralization of the fused image to the (left) ear where the SL is higher. We could also say that the sound is *audible* in both ears, but that the patient is only *aware* of it in the left ear (where the SL is higher), in which case the situation is called the **Stenger phenomenon (effect)**. More formally, the Stenger effect states that when a sound is presented to both ears, the listener is aware of its presence only in the ear where it has a higher sensation level (or more loosely, where it is "louder").

The **Stenger test** makes use of the Stenger effect in a clinical test for *unilateral* functional hearing loss. It was first described by Stenger in 1900 as a tuning-fork procedure and is now performed audiometrically in a variety of ways (Watson & Tolan, 1949; Altshuler, 1970). The Stenger test can be used to identify a unilateral nonorganic hearing loss, and to also estimate the patient's real thresholds in that ear. It is called the **pure-tone Stenger test** when testing is done with pure tones and the **speech Stenger test** when spondee words are used as the stimuli. There must be a unilateral or asymmetrical hearing loss in which the two ears differ by at least 30 dB (preferably ≥ 40 dB) at each frequency where the pure-tone Stenger test is performed. The speech Stenger test requires a similar difference between the two SRTs.

The Stenger can be administered immediately after finding the voluntary thresholds for both ears. As far as the patient is concerned, the Stenger is part of the pure-tone threshold test, during which she is to respond whenever a tone is heard. In fact, the patient should not even be aware a special test is being administered. The question is whether she will or will not respond to various tones presented slightly above and/or below the voluntary thresholds of the two ears, either alone or in combination. The easiest way to learn the Stenger test is to work through the procedure itself. We will do this for two patients who have voluntary

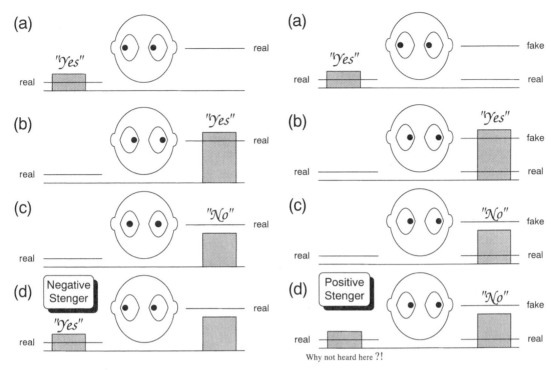

FIGURE 14–8 Negative Stenger test results for a patient with a real unilateral hearing loss. "Real" represents a true, organically based threshold. (See text.)

FIGURE 14–9 Positive Stenger test results for a patient with a nonorganic unilateral hearing loss. "Real" represents a true, organically based threshold; "fake" indicates the exaggerated voluntary threshold. (See text.)

thresholds of 0 dB HL in the right ear and 50 dB HL in the left ear. The unilateral hearing loss in the left ear will be real in the first example and functional in the second example. Even though the Stenger test has numerous variations, most experts agree that test tones should be presented at 5 to 10 dB HL above and/or below the voluntary thresholds. We will use 10 dB.

Figure 14–8 illustrates the results of a Stenger test for a patient with a *real* unilateral hearing loss in her left ear. Her thresholds are represented by the reference lines on each side of the head. The patient responds ("yes") when a 10-dB tone is presented to her right ear because it is above her threshold (Fig. 14–8a). She also responds ("yes") when a 60 dB HL tone is presented to her left ear because it too is above her threshold (Fig. 14–8b). In Figure 14–8c, she does not respond ("no") when a 40 dB HL tone is presented to

her left ear because it is 10 dB below her threshold (i.e., she does not respond because she really cannot hear it). Two tones are presented simultaneously in Figure 14–8d. One of them is 10 dB *above* the better ear's threshold, just like Figure 14–8a, and the other one is 10 dB *below* the poor ear's threshold, just like Figure 14–8c. The patient responds ("yes") because she can hear the tone in her better right ear. She is not influenced by the below-threshold 40-dB tone in her left ear because she cannot hear it. This is called a *negative Stenger test result* and suggests the threshold in the poorer ear is real.

Now let us see what happens when the same Stenger test is given to a patient who has a *nonorganic* unilateral loss, as illustrated in Figure 14–9. Here, the left ear's 50 dB HL threshold is represented by a line labeled "fake" because it is exaggerated. His real thresholds are 0 dB HL in both ears, and these are represented by the lines labeled "real." The patient responds ("yes") to a 10 dB HL tone in his right ear because it is above his threshold (Fig. 14–9a). He also responds ("yes") when a 60 dB HL tone is presented to his left ear because it is loud enough to be higher than his exaggerated threshold (Fig. 14–9b). The 40 dB HL tone in Figure 14–9c is well above his real threshold, but he fails to respond ("no") because the tone is lower than his exaggerated threshold (i.e., he denies hearing the tone even though he really can hear it). The stimulus combination in Figure 14–9d is the same as it was in Figure 14–8d: two tones are presented simultaneously; one *is 10 dB above the better ear's threshold*, just like Figure 14–9a, and the other one is *10 dB below the poor ear's threshold*, just like Figure 14–9c. A patient with a real loss would not hear the below–threshold tone in the left ear, and would thus respond to the above-threshold tone in the right ear. However, even though 40 dB HL is 10 dB below the exaggerated threshold, it is also 40 dB *above the real threshold* (0 dB HL). Here comes the Stenger effect: A 1000-Hz tone is in the right ear at 10 dB SL and also in the left ear at 40 dB SL. The fused image of these two tones is heard only in the left ear. Hence, all the patient knows about is the 40 dB HL tone in the left ear, which is lower than his exaggerated loss. He therefore refuses to respond ("no"). This is a *positive Stenger test result*, indicating a functional loss in the poorer ear. Why? Because if the hearing loss in his left ear were real, he still would hear the above-threshold tone in the right ear! The only thing that could prevent him from hearing the 10 dB SL tone in the right ear would be a tone that is heard at an even higher sensation level in the left ear.

The speech Stenger test is done in the same way as the pure-tone Stenger, except spondee words are used instead of pure-tone tones, and the test is done at sensation levels relative to the SRTs of the two ears.

When it is performed as just described, the Stenger test only shows that a unilateral nonorganic hearing loss is present. The Stenger test can also be used to approximate the organic thresholds of the poorer ear. Threshold determination with the Stenger test goes well beyond our current scope, but the basic idea is to vary the level of the tone presented to the "bad" ear until the Stenger test result changes from positive to negative. The **Fusion Inferred Threshold (FIT) test** (Bergman, 1964) is another advanced technique that relies on binaural fusion to estimate organic thresholds in patients with functional hearing loss.

DELAYED AUDITORY FEEDBACK TESTS

DAF Speech Test People expect to hear what they are saying simultaneously as they are talking. If a person speaks into a microphone and hears himself through earphones, then it is possible to insert a time delay between when he says something and when he hears it. This phenomenon is called **delayed auditory feedback (DAF)** or **delayed side-tone for speech**, and it causes disruptions of the talker's speech production in terms of such characteristics as rate, fluency, intensity, and vocal quality. It is a simple matter to apply DAF for speech as a test for nonorganic hearing loss (Tiffany & Hanley, 1952; Hanley & Tiffany, 1954): The patient is asked to read a passage. His speech is picked up by a microphone, subjected to a time delay of about 180 ms, and then directed to his earphones. Pseudohypacusis is indicated if the patient's speech production can be disrupted by DAF at hearing levels below the patient's SRT.

Delayed Feedback Audiometry A more effective application of DAF for the assessment of functional loss is **delayed feedback audiometry (DFA)** (Ruhm & Cooper, 1964; Cooper, Stokinger, & Billings, 1976), which might also be called the **tonal DAF tapping test**. The patient is asked to tap out a simple rhythmic pattern on a key or button. The tapping pattern is "4 taps-pause-2 taps," and is repeated over and over again:

❑❑❑❑ ❑❑, ❑❑❑❑ ❑❑, ❑❑❑❑ ❑❑, ❑❑❑❑ ❑❑…

The button controls a test tone so that the tapping pattern produces a pattern of tones.

These tones are subjected to a 200-msec time delay, and are then directed into one of the patient's earphones. If the patient is able to hear these delayed auditory feedback tones, then his tapping pattern will be disrupted. The tone key is also connected to a chart recorder. The basic procedure is to have the patient keep tapping the required pattern while increasing the hearing level of the DAF tones. At the same time, the audiologist watches the chart recorder for any aberrations in the tapping pattern. The presence of a nonorganic hearing loss is indicated if the tapping pattern is disrupted by DAF tones at levels lower (better) than the patient's admitted thresholds. The main advantage of DFA is that tapping patterns tend to be disrupted by DAF tones that are within 5 to 10 dB of a person's real threshold, which makes it possible to estimate a functional patient's organic hearing levels. However, it is sometimes necessary for the DAF tone to reach a much higher sensation level before it interferes with the tapping pattern (Alberti, 1970). The main limitation of DFA is that the patient must be able and willing to produce the tapping pattern and to maintain it over time.

LOMBARD REFLEX TEST

The **Lombard reflex** or **effect** is the elevation of vocal effort that occurs when talking in the presence of noise (Lombard, 1911). In addition to "talking louder," the Lombard effect also involves several vocal and articulatory changes associated with the increased vocal effort while the noise is present (Junqua, 1993). We have all experienced this effect when we try to continue speaking even though a loud airplane or train is passing by. The Lombard reflex may be used as a test for nonorganic hearing loss on the following basis: A Lombard effect can only be caused by a noise that can be heard. If a noise that is below her voluntary thresholds can induce a patient to raise her speaking level, then her hearing must actually be better than admitted. The **Lombard test** can be accomplished in a variety of ways, but the basic procedure may be described as follows: The patient is asked to read a passage, during which the clinician monitors the level of the patient's speech on the VU meter of the audiometer. Noise is introduced into both of the patient's earphones and its intensity is raised while the audiologist watches the VU meter (and listens) for changes in the patient's vocal level. An exaggerated hearing loss is suspected if the patient's speech level is raised by a noise that is lower than the patient's admitted thresholds.

DOERFLER-STEWART TEST

The Doerfler-Stewart (1946) test is based on the notions that a masking noise will cause functional patients to stop repeating spondee words even though the noise level is below the speech level, and interferes with the patient's ability to use a target loudness as a frame of reference for consistent responses. It was originally described as a binaural test that employed saw-tooth noise, but has also been used as a monaural test and with other noises (e.g., speech noise). The procedure involves several SRTs, a noise detection threshold, determining how much noise is needed to interfere with the patient's repetition of spondee words at various levels relative to the SRTs, and calculations among the various measures to decide whether a functional loss is present. Because it relies on this cumbersome procedure just to identify a nonorganic hearing loss as present (which is done more efficiently with many other tests), it is not surprising that the **Doerfler-Stewart test** is rarely if ever used any more. Those who are interested in this test can find a detailed description and normative information in Hopkinson (1978).

SWITCHING SPEECH TEST

The **switching speech (or story) test** is an uncommon method for detecting unilateral functional losses. Various descriptions are available (e.g., Watson & Tolan, 1949; Calearo, 1957), but the basic idea is as follows: A passage, or a series of questions, is presented to the patient with the speech being switched back and forth between the patient's right and left earphones, so each ear gets only part of the information. The presentation levels are above the threshold of the "good" ear and below the admitted threshold of the "bad" ear. A functional loss is revealed by the ensuing confusion and/or how the patient recounts the story or answers the questions. Tests of this type are not recommended because they rely on a very cumbersome approach just to identify a unilateral nonorganic hearing loss, and it is not surprising that they are rarely if ever used.

Physiological Tests

The physiological changes that occur in response to the reception of a sound stimulus reflect the patient's organically based hearing because they occur regardless of whether the patient chooses to volunteer a behavioral response. For this reason, physiological tests are particularly attractive as tests for nonorganic hearing loss. Although physiological tests are said to be objective, one should realize that this objectivity does not extend to the clinician who can be subject to biases in her interpretation of the physiological results. We will go over only the major physiological approaches to nonorganic hearing loss, but most physiological measurements that have been used to test hearing have also been tried with functional hearing loss.

ELECTRODERMAL (PSYCHOGALVANIC SKIN RESPONSE) AUDIOMETRY

Electrodermal audiometry (EDA) is the measurement of hearing with the **electrodermal** or **psychogalvanic skin response (PGSR)**, and was employed to confirm the veracity of voluntary thresholds and assess patients with nonorganic hearing loss until the mid-1970s. The PGSR is a change in electrical resistance of the skin that occurs in response to some stimulus. In EDA, electrodes on the fingertips were used to monitor skin resistance changes in response to hearing a test tone (or speech). Even though sounds can be used to obtain PGSR results, noxious stimuli such as mild electrical shocks are much more effective and reliable.

For this reason, the usual EDA procedure involved presenting mild shocks along with tones above the patient's voluntary threshold. These shock-tone pairings enabled the tone itself to reliably elicit a PGSR as a result of classical conditioning. This is the same kind of classical conditioning we all learned about in Psych 101, which caused Pavlov's dogs to salivate whenever they heard a bell that was previously paired with food. The PGSR instrument registered the patient's electrodermal responses on a strip-chart recording. Organic hearing thresholds could then be approximated by finding the lowest tone (or speech) levels that resulted in a measurable skin resistance change. In spite of its effectiveness as a tool in the evaluation of nonorganic hearing loss, electrical safety considerations have relegated EDA to the history books. A detailed discussion of this approach may be found in Ventry (1975).

ACOUSTIC REFLEX

Acoustic reflex thresholds (ARTs) have been used as a physiological test for functional hearing loss since the 1960s (Feldman, 1963; Lamb & Peterson, 1967; Alberti, 1970). This is not surprising because most audiological evaluations include acoustic reflex testing as a matter of routine, so that applying ARTs to the assessment of functional impairment comes almost without cost. The other physiological tests mentioned in this chapter do not enjoy this advantage.

A functional impairment is suspected when an ART occurs at or below the patient's hearing threshold, or at an atypically low level even though it exceeds the hearing threshold. How high must an ART be? Recall from Chapter 7 that ARTs depend on the hearing threshold in normal and cochlear-impaired patients, and that there is a range of ARTs that occurs for any given amount of loss. In that chapter we considered ARTs to be atypically high if they exceeded the 90th percentiles. Now we are concerned with atypically low ARTs, and we will use the 10th percentiles as the lower cutoff values for the degree of apparent hearing loss (Gelfand & Piper, 1984; Gelfand, Schwander, & Silman,

1990; Gelfand, 1994). However, the 10th percentiles may be used to identify functional losses only when the voluntary thresholds are *at least 60 dB HL* at the frequency where the ART is tested (Gelfand, 1994). Real and feigned losses up to 55 dB HL cannot be distinguished by ARTs because tonal ARTs are essentially the same for hearing thresholds up to roughly 50 to 60 dB HL. Table 14–1 shows the 10th percentile lower cutoff values for hearing losses ≥ 60 dB HL due to real cochlear impairments at 500, 1000, and 2000 Hz (Gelfand, Schwander, & Silman, 1990).

The modified bivariate method, which uses the ARTs for both broadband noise (BBN) and tones to identify hearing loss (Chapter 7), has also been proposed as a test for functional impairment (Silman, Gelfand, Piper, Silverman, & VanFrank, 1984; Silman, 1988). This technique reveals the existence of nonorganic hearing losses in young adults who actually have normal hearing (Silman, 1988). However, the modified bivariate cannot be expected to identify functional losses in patients who have a significant degree of underlying organic hearing loss, or those who are ≥ 45 years old. This limitation occurs because the bivariate method depends on the broadband noise ART, which is affected by sensorineural losses and aging.

Gelfand (1994) suggested the following guidelines for interpreting acoustic reflex tests with regard to functional losses. It is assumed that the patient's voluntary thresholds show some degree of significant hearing loss.

1. Reflex thresholds at or below the voluntary threshold for the same tones suggest functional impairments.
2. Modified bivariate results falling within the "normal area" of the bivariate graph (Chapter 7) strongly suggest a nonorganic hearing loss and also that the organic hearing thresholds are more or less within the normal range.
3. Tenth percentiles are appropriate when the voluntary thresholds are at least 60 dB HL at the frequencies used for reflex testing. In this case, a functional loss may be suspected if ARTs fall (a) below the 10th percentiles, and/or (b) up to 5 dB above a voluntary threshold that is ≥ 90 dB HL.
4. Just because the modified bivariate results fall in the "impaired area" of the bivariate graph and the ARTs are at or above the 10th percentiles does not rule out an exaggerated loss.

AUDITORY EVOKED POTENTIALS

Several investigators have reported that the auditory brainstem response (ABR) can be used to identify patients with nonorganic hearing loss, as well as to estimate organic hearing sensitivity in many if not all cases (Alberti, 1970; Sanders & Lazenby, 1983). The

TABLE 14–1   Tenth percentile cutoff values in dB HL for acoustic reflex thresholds (ARTs) for hearing losses ≥60 dB HL at 500, 1000, and 2000 Hz

Hearing Threshold *(dB HL)*	*Frequency*		
	500 Hz	*1000 Hz*	*2000 Hz*
60	85	85	85
65	90	90	90
70	95	95	90
75	95	95	95
80	100	100	100
85	100	100	110
≥90	(10 dB above the hearing threshold)[a]		

[a] An ART that is no more than 5 dB above the hearing threshold is considered to be atypically low for hearing losses ≥90 dB HL. This criterion places the lower cutoff value at 10 dB above the hearing threshold assuming that testing is done in 5-dB steps.

Based on Gelfand, Schwander, Silman (1990).

major limitations of the ABR in functional hearing loss are due to its reliance on wide band stimuli such as clicks. The affect of high-frequency hearing losses on the ABR can be a complicating factor when assessing nonorganic hearing loss in adults, because they usually have at least some degree of underlying organic hearing loss, particularly in the higher frequencies. Cortical auditory evoked potentials are also useful in the assessment of functional hearing loss (Alberti, 1970; Coles & Mason, 1984). A major advantage of cortical potentials is that they make it possible to screen for exaggerated losses and to estimate organic thresholds on a frequency-by-frequency basis. Coles and Mason (1984) suggested that a functional loss is indicated if there is a discrepancy between voluntary thresholds and cortical response findings averaging more than 7.5 dB for three frequencies, or more than 15 for a single frequency.

OTOACOUSTIC EMISSIONS

Otoacoustic emissions (OAEs) have great potential as a test for at least some patients with nonorganic hearing loss because they are obliterated by many sensorineural losses. Functional losses have been identified by transient-evoked OAEs (Robinette, 1992; Musiek, Bornstein, & Rintelmann, 1995; Kvaerner, Engdahl, Aursnes, Arnesen, & Mair, 1996; Durrant, Kesterson, & Kamerer, 1997), as well as by distortion-product OAEs (Lonsbury-Martin, Martin, & Telischi, 1999). It is clear that OAEs will be a very useful tool for identifying exaggerated losses in patients whose hearing is really normal or near normal. However, it is not likely that OAEs will become a "definitive" test for nonorganic hearing loss because the majority of adults with functional impairments also have some degree of underlying organic hearing loss.

Some Comments About Counseling in Cases of Nonorganic Hearing Loss

Counseling a patient with a nonorganic hearing loss is a tricky matter. The main goal is to get the patient to elicit valid and reliable responses, if at all possible. In the overwhelming majority of cases, one should *avoid being adversarial, judgmental, or accusatory, and also avoid the use of labels* when counseling a patient who has a nonorganic overlay. Let us be tersely candid to drive home the point: Using words such as "malingering" and "feigning" is like calling the patient a liar or worse, and many patients translate clinical-sounding words such as "functional," "nonorganic," and "psychogenic" into "crazy liar." Offending the patient is almost always counterproductive. Instead of being confrontational, give the patient as much emotional room as possible so he has the option of changing his responses without losing face. A good initial approach is to simply reinstruct the patient about the tasks, subtly emphasizing the importance of responding no matter how soft the tones are, etc. If a reason is needed, allude to benign miscommunication that was not the patient's fault. The strategic placement of a physiological test sometimes motivates the patient to consider a change in response behavior, especially if the right "spin" is put on the test description ("This test helps us make a diagnosis because it directly tests your hearing nerve"). If all fails (as it often does), the next approach is generally to point out that there are "discrepancies" that make a diagnosis impossible at this time, and to schedule another appointment.

Prudence and discretion are equally important when counseling children with functional losses and their parents. The issue of secondary gain was discussed earlier. It is generally agreed that a normal-hearing child with a nonorganic hearing loss should not be confronted with the issue of his exaggerated thresholds (Veniar & Salston, 1983; Bowdler & Rogers, 1989; Rintelmann & Schwan, 1999). On the contrary, the wise course of action is usually to advise the child that his hearing is normal and to treat him as a normal-hearing child. Supportive psychotherapy has been found beneficial in some children with functional hearing losses (e.g., Veniar & Salston, 1983; Bowdler & Rogers, 1989; Andaz, Heyworth, & Rowe, 1995), although the clinician should be alert to the possibility of more significant emotional problems (e.g., Aplin & Rowson, 1986; Brooks & Geoghegan, 1992). Hence, psychological referrals should be made when these are appropriate.

Perhaps the most important point to be made in this context is that counseling by a student is not appropriate when nonorganic hearing loss is an issue. New clinicians are equally well advised to involve or at least consult an experienced supervisor whenever these situations arise.

REFERENCES

Alberti PWRM. 1970. New tools for old tricks. *Ann Otol Rhinol Laryngol* 79, 800–807.

Altshuler MW. 1970. The Stenger phenomenon. *J Commun Dis* 3, 89–105.

American Speech and Hearing Association, Committee on Audiometric Evaluation (ASHA). 1978. Guidelines for manual pure-tone threshold audiometry. *ASHA* 20, 297–301.

Andaz C, Heyworth T, Rowe S. 1995. Nonorganic hearing loss in children—a 2-year study. *J Oto-Rhino-Laryngol & Its Related Specialties* 57, 33–35.

Aplin DY, Rowson VJ. 1986. Personality and functional hearing loss in children. *Br J Clin Psychol* 25, 313–314.

Aplin DY, Rowson VJ. 1990. Psychological characteristics of children with functional hearing loss. *Br J Audiol* 24, 77–87.

Baran JA, Musiek FE. 1994. Evaluation of the adults with hearing complaints and normal audiograms. *Hearing Today* 6, 9–11.

Barr B. 1963. Psychogenic deafness in school children. *Int Audiol* 2, 125–128.

Berger K. 1965. Nonorganic hearing loss in children. *Laryngoscope* 75, 447–457.

Bergman M. 1964. The FIT test. *Arch Otolaryngol* 80, 440–449.

Bowdler DA, Rogers J. 1989. The management of pseudohypacusis in school-age children. *Clin Otolaryngol* 15, 211–215.

Broad RD. 1980. Developmental and psychodynamic issues related to cases of childhood functional hearing loss. *Child Psychiatry Hum Dev* 11, 49–58.

Brooks DN, Geoghegan PN. 1992. Nonorganic hearing loss in young persons: Transient episode or deep-seated difficulty. *Br J Audiol* 26, 347–350.

Calearo C. 1957. Detection of malingering by periodically switched speech. *Laryngoscope* 67, 130–136.

Carhart R. 1952. Speech audiometry in clinical evaluation. *Acta Otolaryngol* 41, 18–42.

Chaiklin J. 1990. A descending LOT-Bekesy screening test for functional hearing loss. *J Speech Hear Dis* 55, 67–74.

Chaiklin J, Ventry IM. 1963. Functional hearing loss. In Jerger J (Ed.): *Modern Developments in Audiology.* New York: Academic Press, 76–125.

Chaiklin J, Ventry IM. 1965a. Evaluation of pure-tone audiogram configurations used in identifying adults with functional loss. *J Audiol Res* 5, 212–218.

Chaiklin J, Ventry IM. 1965b. Patient errors during spondee and pure-tone threshold measurement. *J Audiol Res* 5, 219–230.

Chaiklin J, Ventry IM, Barrett LS, Skalbeck GS. 1959. Pure-tone threshold patterns observed in functional hearing loss. *Laryngoscope* 69, 1165–1179.

Cherry R, Ventry IM. 1976. The ascending-descending gap: A tool for identifying a suprathreshold response. *J Audiol Res* 16, 281–287.

Coles RRA. 1982. Non-organic hearing loss. In Gibb AG, Smith MFW (Eds.): *Butterworth's International Medical Reviews.* London: Butterworth, 150–176.

Coles RRA, Mason SM. 1984. The results of cortical electric response audiometry in medico-legal investigations. *Br J Audiol* 18, 71–78.

Coles RRA, Priede VM. 1971. Non-organic overlay in noise-induced hearing loss. *Proc R Soc Med* 64, 41–63.

Conn M, Ventry IM, Woods RW. 1972. Pure-tone average and spondee threshold relationships in simulated hearing loss. *J Aud Res* 12, 234–239.

Cooper WA Jr, Stokinger TE, Billings BL. 1976. Pure-tone delayed auditory feedback: Development of criteria of performance deterioration. *J Am Auditory Soc 1*, 192–196.

Dixon RF, Newby HA. 1959. Children with nonorganic hearing problems. *Arch Otolaryngol* 70, 619–623.

Doerfler LG, Stewart KC. 1946. Malingering and psychogenic deafness. *J Speech Dis* 11, 181–186

Durrant JD, Kesterson RK, Kamerer DB. 1997. Evaluation of the nonorganic hearing loss suspect. *Am J Otol* 18, 361–367.

Feldman AS. 1963. Impedance measurements at the eardrum as an aid to diagnosis. *J Speech Hear Res* 6, 315–327.

Frank T. 1976. Yes-no test for nonorganic hearing loss. *Arch Otolaryngol* 102, 162–165.

Gelfand SA. 1993. Organic thresholds and functional components in experimentally simulated exaggerated hearing loss. *Br J Audiol* 27, 35–40.

Gelfand SA. 1994. Acoustic reflex threshold tenth percentiles and functional hearing impairment. *J Am Acad Audiol* 5, 10–16.

Gelfand SA, Piper N. 1984. Acoustic reflex thresholds: Variability and distribution effects. *Ear Hear* 5, 228–234.

Gelfand SA, Schwander T, Silman S. 1990. Acoustic reflex thresholds in normal and cochlear-impaired ears: Effects of no-response rates on 90th percentiles in a large sample. *J Speech Hear Dis* 55, 198–205.

Gelfand SA, Silman S. 1985. Functional hearing loss and its relationship to resolved hearing levels. *Ear Hear* 6, 151–158.

Gelfand SA, Silman S. 1993. Functional components and resolved thresholds in patients with unilateral nonorganic hearing loss. *Br J Audiol* 27, 29–34.

Gold S, Lubinsky R, Shahar A. 1981. Speech discrimination scores at low sensation levels as possible index of malingering. *J Aud Res* 21, 137–141.

Goldstein R. 1966. Pseudohypacusis. *J Speech Hear Dis* 31, 341–352.

Hallewell JD, Goetzinger CP, Allen ML, Proud GO. 1966. The use of hypnosis in audiologic assessment. *Acta Otolaryngol* 61, 205–208.

Hanley CN, Tiffany W. 1954. An investigation into the use of electro-mechanically delayed side tone in auditory testing. *J Speech Hear Dis* 19, 367–374.

Harris DA. 1958. A rapid and simple technique for the detection of non-organic hearing loss. *Arch Otolaryngol* 68, 758–760.

Hattler KW. 1968. The type V Bekesy pattern: The effects of loudness memory. *J Speech Hear Res* 11, 567–575.

Hattler KW. 1970. Lengthened off-time: A self-recording screening device for nonorganicity. *J Speech Hear Dis* 35, 113–122.

Hattler KW. 1971. The development of the LOT-Bekesy test for nonorganic hearing loss. *J Speech Hear Res* 14, 605–617

Hood WH, Campbell RA, Hutton CL. 1964. An evaluation of the Bekesy ascending-descending gap. *J Speech Hear Res* 7, 123–132.

Hopkinson NT. 1967. Comment on "Pseudohypacusis." *J Speech Hear Dis* 32, 293–294.

Hopkinson NT. 1973. Functional hearing loss. In Jerger J (Ed.): *Modern Developments in Audiology*, 2nd ed. New York: Academic Press, 175–210.

Hopkinson NT. 1978. Speech tests for pseudohypacusis. In Katz J (Ed.): *Handbook of Clinical Audiology*, 2nd ed. Baltimore: Williams & Wilkins, 291–303.

Jerger J, Herer G. 1961. Unexpected dividend in Bekesy audiometry. *J Speech Hear Dis* 26, 390–391.

Junqua JC. 1993. The Lombard reflex and its role on human listeners and automatic speech recognizers. *J Acoust Soc Am* 93, 510–524.

Kerr AG, Gillespie WG, Easton JM. 1975. A simple test for malingering. *Br J Audiol* 9, 24–26.

Kvaerner KJ, Engdahl B, Aursnes J, Arnesen AR, Mair IWS. 1996. Transient-evoked otoacoustic emissions—helpful tool in the detection of pseudohypacusis. *Scand Audiol* 25, 173–177.

Lamb LE, Peterson JL. 1967. Middle ear reflex measurements in pseudohypacusis. *J Speech Hear Dis* 32, 46–51.

Lombard E. 1911. Le signe de l'elévation de la voix. *Ann Maladiers Oreill Laryngx Nes Pharynx* 37, 101–119.

Lonsbury-Martin BL, Martin GK, Telischi FF. 1999. Otoacoustic emissions in clinical practice. In Musiek FE, Rintelmann WF (Eds.): *Contemporary Perspectives in Hearing Assessment*. Boston: Allyn & Bacon, 167–196.

Lumio JS, Jauhiainen J, Gelhar K. 1969. Three case of functional deafness in the same family. *J Laryngol* 83, 299–304.

McCanna DL, DeLupa G. 1981. A clinical study of twenty-seven children exhibiting functional hearing loss. *Lang Speech Hear Serv Schools* 12, 26–35.

Miller AL, Fox MS, Chan G. 1968. Pure-tone assessments as an aid in detecting suspected non-organic hearing disorders in children. *Laryngoscope* 78, 2170–2176.

Musiek FE, Bornstein SP, Rintelmann WF. 1995. Transient evoked otoacoustic emissions and pseudohypacusis. *J Am Acad Audiol* 6, 293–301.

Nobel W. 1978. *Assessment of Impaired Hearing*. New York: Academic Press.

Nobel W. 1987. The conceptual problem of "functional hearing loss." *Br J Audiol* 21, 1–3.

Rintelmann WF, Carhart R. 1964. Loudness tracking by normal hearers via Bekesy audiometer. *J Speech Hear Res* 7, 79–93.

Rintelmann WF, Harford E. 1963. The detection and assessment of pseudohypoacousis among school-age children. *J Speech Hear Dis* 28, 141–152.

Rintelmann WF, Harford E. 1967. The type V Bekesy pattern: Interpretation and clinical utility. *J Speech Hear Res* 10, 733–744.

Rintelmann WF, Schwan SA. 1999. Pseudohypacusis. In Musiek FE, Rintelmann WF (Eds.): *Contemporary Perspectives in Hearing Assessment*. Boston: Allyn & Bacon, 415–435.

Robinette MS 1992. Clinical observations with transient evoked otoacoustic emissions with adults. *Semin Hear* 13, 23–36.

Ross M. 1964. The variable intensity pulse count method (VIPCM) for the detection and measurement of the pure-tone thresholds of children with functional hearing losses. *J Speech Hear Dis* 29, 477–482.

Ruhm HB, Cooper WA Jr. 1964. Delayed feedback audiometry. *J Speech Hear Dis* 29, 448–455.

Sanders JW, Lazenby BB. 1983. Auditory brain stem response measurements in the assessment of pseudohypacusis. *Am J Otol* 4, 292–299.

Saunders GH, Haggard MP. 1989. The clinical assessment of obscure auditory dysfunction—1. Auditory and psychological factors. *Ear Hear* 10, 200–208.

Schlauch RS, Arnce KD, Olson LM, Sanchez S, Doyle TN. 1996. Identification of pseudohypacusis using speech recognition thresholds. *Ear Hear* 17, 229–236.

Shepherd DC 1965. Non-organic hearing loss and the consistency of behavioral responses. *J Speech Hear Res* 8, 149–163.

Silman S. 1988. The applicability of the modified bivariate plotting procedure to subjects with functional hearing loss. *Scand Audiol* 17, 125–127.

Silman S, Gelfand SA, Piper N, Silverman CA, VanFrank L. 1984. Prediction of hearing loss from the acoustic-reflex threshold. In Silman S (Ed.): *The Acoustic Reflex: Basic Principles and Clinical Applications*. Orlando: Academic Press, 187–223.

Silman S, Silverman CA. 1991. *Auditory Diagnosis: Principles and Applications*. San Diego: Academic Press.

Tiffany W, Hanley CN. 1952. Delayed speech feedback as a test for auditory malingering. *Science* 115, 59–60.

Trier TR, Levy R. 1965. Social and psychological characteristics of veterans with functional hearing loss. *J Aud Res* 5, 241–256.

Veniar FA, Salston RS. 1983. An approach to the treatment of pseudohypacusis in children. *Am J Dis Child* 137, 34–36.

Ventry IM. 1968. A case for psychogenic hearing loss. *J Speech Hear Dis* 33, 89–92.

Ventry IM. 1975. Conditioned galvanic skin response audiometry. In Bradford LJ (Ed.): *Physiological Measures of the Audio-Vestibular System*. New York: Academic Press, 215–247.

Ventry IM, Chaiklin J. 1965. The efficiency of audiometric measured used to identify functional loss. *J Aud Res* 5, 196–211.

Watson LA, Tolan T. 1949. *Hearing Tests and Hearing Instruments*. Baltimore: Williams & Wilkins.

15

Audiological Management of the Hearing Impaired

In the grand sense, the terms **audiological (re)habilitation** and **aural (re)habilitation** refer to a wide range of modalities employed by the audiologist to maximize the hearing-impaired patient's ability to live and communicate in a world of sound. Many clinicians use the term **rehabilitation** when working with someone who has an impairment of an already-developed skill, such as an adult with an adventitious hearing loss, and **habilitation** when dealing with an individual who has not yet developed a skill, such as a child with prelingual hearing loss. The modalities of audiological intervention include the use of physical instruments such as hearing aids, group amplification systems, cochlear implants, tactile aids, and assistive devices, as well as therapeutic approaches like patient and family counseling, developing effective communication strategies, and auditory-visual training. To this list must be added referrals to and interactions with other professionals who are involved with the patient's management, such as speech-language pathologists, physicians, psychologists, teachers, etc.

Hearing Aids

It almost goes without saying that the first order of business in the audiological management of a hearing-impaired person must be to increase the intensities of sounds so they become audible. **Hearing aids** are devices that boost sound levels so the patient can hear them. This process is called **amplification**.

Most simply, a hearing aid amplifies sounds just like a megaphone, except the amplified sound is directed right into the listener's ear. It is easiest to think of a hearing aid in terms of its major parts, as shown in Figure 15–1. The hearing aid's **microphone** picks up sounds and converts them into an electrical signal. A device that transforms energy from one form to another is called a **transducer**. Thus, the microphone is an acoustic-to-electrical transducer. Once the sound has been changed into an electrical signal it can be manipulated by electronic circuits. Obviously, the principal manipulation is to boost its intensity, that is, to **amplify** it. This is done by the **amplifier**. The amplified electrical

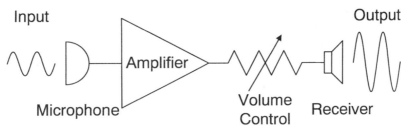

FIGURE 15–1 A simplified hearing aid diagram showing the microphone, amplifier, and receiver. Notice how the output from the receiver is larger than the input into the microphone. The battery is not shown for simplicity.

443

signal is then converted back into sound by an electrical-to-acoustic transducer or loudspeaker. The hearing aid's loudspeaker is called the **receiver**. The amplified sound from the receiver is directed into the patient's ear. Two other components of all hearing aids should be mentioned at this time. One is the **battery**, which provides the power to accomplish all of the hearing aid's functions. The other is the **earmold**, which is the object actually inserted into the patient's ear. In fact, the majority of modern hearing aids are completely contained within the earmold itself. Earmolds are almost always custom-made from an impression taken of the ear.

The sounds picked up by the microphone are called the **input** to the hearing aid and the sounds produced by the receiver are called the **output**. The patient hears the output from the hearing aid. The amount of amplification is called **gain**. Suppose the input is speech at 60 dB SPL and the output is the same speech signal that has been amplified to 95 dB SPL. How much amplification has occurred? The obvious answer is 35 dB because the signal coming out of the instrument is 35 dB higher than the signal that went in. Thus, gain is simply the difference in decibels between the intensity coming out of a hearing aid and the intensity that went in. Numerically, gain (in dB) equals output (in dB SPL) minus input (in dB SPL). Ten decibels of gain means the output is 10 dB higher than the input, and 0 dB of gain means the input and output are the same. Notice that input and output are given in SPL, but gain is not expressed in SPL. The reason is that the input and output are physical magnitudes, whereas gain refers to the *difference* between them. In fact, 10 decibels of gain is simply referred to as "10 dB gain." (The quantitatively oriented student should note that gain is actually the ratio of the intensity of the output to the intensity of the input.) Any hearing aid has a range of gains that it can generate, and the patient has some degree of control over this gain by using a **volume control** (more technically called a **gain control**), just like the volume control of a radio.

The intensity of a hearing aid's output cannot be limitless. The greatest sound magnitude that can be produced by a hearing aid is quite descriptively called its **maximum power output (MPO)** or **output sound pressure level (OSPL)**. We will see later that OSPL is more completely called OSPL90, which means how much is coming out of the hearing aid ("O") in decibels of sound pressure level ("SPL") when the input to the hearing aid is a 90 dB SPL signal ("90"). In order to understand what we mean by OSPL, suppose you set a hearing aid to its *highest gain* by turning its volume control all the way up and you also *keep increasing the input*. The output will get bigger and bigger as the input rises, but the output will eventually reach a maximum. Here, the output cannot get any higher no matter how much you raise the input (remember that the volume control is already turned all the way up). At this point we say the hearing aid is **saturated**. This is analogous to what happens when you keep pouring more and more water into a sponge. It will soak up all the water until some maximum amount is absorbed. At that point we say that the sponge is saturated, meaning that it cannot hold any more water no matter how much more water you pour into it.

These notions are shown by the **input-output function** in Figure 15–2a. The diagonal line shows how output increases with input up to a maximum value, where the line becomes horizontal because output no longer rises with increasing input. Thereafter, the horizontal line shows that the output stays at this level. For example, an OSPL of 124 dB means that 124 dB SPL is the strongest sound the hearing aid is capable of producing. In other words, OSPL refers to the output of the hearing aid in dB SPL when the hearing aid is saturated. In fact, OSPL used to be called **saturation sound pressure level (SSPL)**.

Once the hearing aid's maximum power output is reached, its output cannot become any greater than this ceiling no matter how much more the input might increase or the volume control might be turned up. When this happens, the parts of the amplified sound that would have exceeded the ceiling

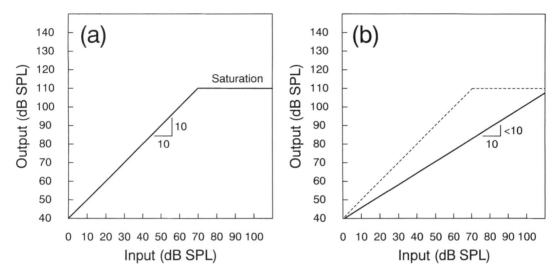

FIGURE 15–2 (a) With linear amplification, each 10-dB increase of input (on the x-axis) results in a 10-dB increase in the output (on the y-axis) until saturation is reached, where output no longer increases with input. (b) With compression amplification, 10-dB increases of input result in less than 10-dB increases in output, so the output does not become uncomfortably loud or reach saturation. The linear amplification function from frame *a* is shown as a dotted line for comparison.

are clipped off, resulting in a distortion of the amplified signal descriptively known as **peak clipping**. Many hearing aids employ special **compression** or **automatic gain control (AGC)**[1] circuits that slow down the rate of amplification for louder sounds so the clipping level is never reached, as illustrated in Figure 15–2b. Compression has other uses as well, such as preventing loud sounds from becoming uncomfortably loud, which is often desirable for patients who have trouble with loudness recruitment.

Two more commonly encountered hearing aid components are worthy of mention. One of these is the **tone control**. It adds flexibility to the instrument by adjusting the relative levels of the higher and lower frequencies much like the bass and treble on a stereo set.

The **telecoil** is a circuit that allows the hearing aid to pick up magnetic signals generated by many telephone receivers instead of using the microphone. Telecoils are associated with a switch labeled "M/T" or "M/T/MT," allowing the patient to select between using

the hearing aid's microphone (**M**) in the normal manner, the telecoil (**T**) while bypassing the microphone, or in some cases to use the microphone and telecoil simultaneously (**MT**). The telecoil allows the patient to hear the telephone signal without interference from noises in the room, and/or to attend to a telephone conversation that would not be possible using the microphone. The MT position might be selected when the patient desires to hear the phone clearly but also needs to hear what is going on around her, or when she needs her hearing aid to monitor her own voice while speaking on the phone.

Types of Hearing Aids

Hearing aids are most broadly classified in terms of whether they are body or ear-level devices, and among the latter, whether they are worn behind the ear, in the ear, or built into eyeglass frames. Figure 15–3 shows several examples. Originally, the larger body aids were the most common devices, but smaller and less conspicuous devices now dominate the market (e.g., Strom, 2000). One

---

[1] Sometimes called **automatic volume control (AVC)**.

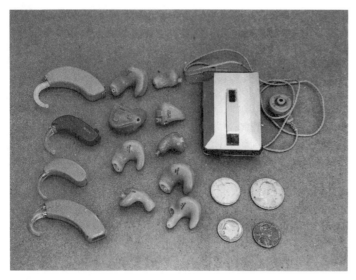

FIGURE 15-3 Examples of various types of hearing aids. Behind-the-ear instruments are on the left, in-the-ear instruments are in the middle, and a body hearing aid is on the right. Several coins are shown for size comparison.

is tempted to the conclude that this simply reflects the ability of technological advances to meet patients' desires for hearing aids that are cosmetically acceptable. While the cosmetic issue is real and highly relevant, it is by no means the only reason for the preponderance of small instruments. Technological advances have not only made it possible for modern hearing aids to be smaller, but more importantly modern hearing aids are capable of being genuine high-fidelity devices (Killion, 1993). In addition, having a device in the patient's ear means the microphone is picking up sounds as they appear at the patient's ear. This permits the listener to receive a more realistic representation of his acoustic environment, and maximizes the ability to take advantage of binaural cues.

Body Hearing Aids

Body hearing aids contain all of their components and controls (except for the receiver and earmold) in a case about the size of a small pocket calculator. A wire leads from the case to the receiver and earmold at the patient's ear. The case is usually worn somewhere on the chest. Typical locations are in a chest-level pocket, clipped to a shirt, jacket, or undergarment, or in a specially made harness. Body instruments now account for less

than 1% of the hearing aids dispensed in the United States.

Body instruments have always been the most powerful hearing aids, and this continues to be true. Thus, body aids are primarily used for the most severe hearing losses. However, considerable amounts of gain are also available in modern ear-level instruments, so high power is no longer the exclusive domain of the body instrument. Because of their size, body aids have controls and batteries that are larger, more accessible, and easier to manipulate than other types of hearing instruments. This is advantageous for patients with arthritis and other handicapping conditions, as well as for some elderly patients and younger children. An unfortunate dilemma exists because economic considerations make it practical for body aids to be manufactured only as powerful (high gain) instruments. This is a problem for individuals who need both large controls due to manual dexterity or other limitations, and low to moderate amounts of gain.

In addition to being big enough to accommodate larger components and batteries, another reason body aids can provide the greatest amounts of gain involves the problem of **acoustic feedback**. This is the whistle or whine produced when the output from the receiver is picked up by the microphone; feedback is a bigger problem when the microphone and receiver are closer together than when they are further apart. The wide separation between the microphone (on the chest) and receiver (at the ear) with body aids makes feedback less of a problem than it is for ear-level instruments, where the two transducers are very close together.

Body instruments have many limitations, as well. The most obvious problem is cosmetic undesirability, but it is not the only one. Many of the problems are due to the location of the microphone on the torso instead of at ear level. Noise is picked up by the microphone when clothing brushes across the case. The amount and thickness of clothing covering the case can reduce the sound reaching the microphone. (Consider how different one's aided hearing would be with the microphone covered by a sweater and overcoat.) The body itself can adversely affect the intensity and spectrum of the sounds reaching the microphone. These effects are known as the "body shadow" and the "body baffle." Finally, body aids cause sounds to be picked up as though the ears were located on the chest instead of on the sides of the head. This distorts the perception of auditory space and detracts from the perceptual advantages afforded by binaural hearing even if two hearing aids are being used.

EAR-LEVEL HEARING AIDS

Ear-level instruments have all of their components in a small package worn in or near the ear, and comprise 98 to 99% of all hearing aids now being dispensed in the United States. They include behind-the-ear, in-the-ear, in-the canal, and eyeglass instruments. A hearing aid is an ear-level instrument as long as the microphone and receiver are at the patient's ear. This includes currently available or future ear-level units that use a radio signal (or wire) to communicate with signal processing circuits contained in a case that might be kept in one's shirt pocket. In general, the smaller ear-level instruments provide less gain and flexibility than the larger ones, but there is extensive overlap among instrument types. Moreover, the ongoing development of programmable and signal processing hearing aids (see below) continues to cloud the traditional distinctions. The acoustic feedback issue discussed above as a benefit for body aids is of course a limiting factor for ear-level devices.

Behind-the-ear (BTE) instruments have their components contained in a crescent-shaped plastic case that fits behind the auricle. For this reason, BTE instruments are also called **post-auricular** hearing aids. The sound from the receiver is transmitted through a plastic tube to an earmold in the patient's ear. The more powerful models of BTE instruments rival the amounts of gain that could only be provided by body aids in the past, although many patients with very severe and profound losses still require body instruments. Slightly less than 20% of the hearing aids dispensed in the United States in 1999 were BTE instruments.

Eyeglass hearing aids have their components built into the temple piece of the patient's glasses. Similar to BTEs, the receiver output goes through a plastic tube to an earmold in the patient's ear. These devices afford some apparent cosmetic advantage over BTE instruments. They have also been used in CROS-type hearing aids (see below) that use a wire to connect components on the two sides of the head. They have been almost completely replaced with the successful advent of in-the-ear hearing aids. Even their use to hide the wires of CROS-type instruments has been superseded by radio connections between in-the-ear units in the two ears. Further, these instruments have various practical problems because they are part of and inseparable from the patient's eyeglasses. It is thus not surprising that they now represent less than 1% of all hearing aids dispensed.

In-the-ear (ITE) hearing aids have all of their components built into the earmold, and are now the most commonly used hearing aids. In spite of their small size, the technology has progressed to the point that a majority of patients can now be fitted with ITE-type instruments. In-the-ear hearing aids vary widely in size. The largest ones fill the whole concha and extend into the ear canal. Smaller size units take up less and less of the concha, and the smallest ones fit completely into the ear canal. The latter group is now recognized as a distinct category of instruments called **completely-in-the-canal (CIC)** hearing aids (Chasin, 1994; Gudmundsen, 1994; Mueller, 1994). To be considered a CIC instrument, the outermost part of the device must be at least 1 to 2 mm inside of the ear canal entrance. In addition, most CICs are also **deep canal fittings**, which means the device extends into the bony part of the canal, so its receiver end is within about 5 mm of the eardrum. (Actually a deep canal fitting can be achieved with any kind of hearing aid as long as its earmold extends this deep into the external auditory meatus.) In addition to their obvious cosmetic advantage, CIC hearing aids also offer several acoustic benefits. For example: (1) locating the microphone inside the meatus entrance makes it possible to take advantage of pinna and concha effects; (2) compared to shallower ones, deep canal fittings provide more gain and output because the sound is directed into a smaller volume; and (3) they are less likely to make the wearer's own speech sound as if he is talking inside a barrel because the *occlusion effect* is minimized in the bony section of the canal.

DIRECTIONAL HEARING AIDS

Hearing aids with directional microphones are called **directional** hearing aids. **Directional microphones** are designed to be more sensitive to sounds coming from certain directions and less sensitive to sounds coming from other directions. This is in contrast to the more common type of microphone, which is more or less equally sensitive to sounds coming from all directions, or **omnidirectional**. In the directional mode, the hearing aid provides more amplification for sounds coming from the front compared to sounds coming from behind the patient. As a result, the directional hearing aid provides the patient with an improved signal-to-noise ratio in situations where the desired signal is coming from the front and noise is coming mainly from behind. For an informative review of directional hearing aids, see the tutorial by Ricketts and Mueller (1999).

STATE-OF-THE-ART INSTRUMENTS

Hearing aids are considered to be **adaptive** hearing aids when some characteristic of the amplification process is affected by changes in the input signal, that is, when the hearing aid automatically reacts or adapts to the signal. These adaptations may be the activation of circuits that use special filters to reduce noise, or that adjust the amount of gain produced when the level of the input sound changes, either across the board for all frequencies or only within certain bandwidths. Terms such as **automatic signal processing** are often associated with these types of instruments. These kinds of instruments may use traditional electronic (analog) circuits, digital technology, or a combination of the two. In **digital** or **digital signal processing (DSP)** hearing aids, the signal entering the microphone is first transformed into digital form (i.e., a code in which binary numbers represent the sound signal) by an *analog-to-digital (A/D) converter*. Then, all aspects of the amplification process are accomplished digitally, in the same way a personal computer handles the activities involved in word processing. After digital processing, the signal is transformed back into analog form by a *digital-to-analog (D/A) converter*, and transduced into amplified sound by a receiver.

Programmable hearing aids are instruments that can be programmed to provide several different kinds of amplification characteristics for use under different kinds of circumstances, such as speech communication in quiet and in the presence of competing noises, listening to music, etc. The wearer can select among the different settings using a switch on the hearing aid itself or with a small remote control device that can be kept in a pocket or handbag. It is interesting to note that approximately 39% of United States hearing aid sales in 1999 were programmable or DSP instruments.

BONE-CONDUCTION HEARING AIDS

The hearing aids described so far have been *air-conduction* instruments in which the sound is directed into the ear from a miniature loudspeaker (the receiver) via the normal air-conduction route. **Bone-conduction hearing aids** present amplified sound to the patient using a **bone-conduction vibrator** just like the ones used in bone-conduction audiometry (Chapter 5). The vibrator is typically held in place with a spring headband or built into the temple portion of eyeglasses. Bone-conduction instruments are used only when air-conduction hearing aids are ruled out because of *atresia of the ear canal* or *certain conductive pathologies* like active drainage from the ear, or in situations in which ear disease is activated when an earmold is used.

SURGICALLY IMPLANTED HEARING AIDS

It is sometimes warranted to consider the use of surgically implanted hearing aids in some patients who have permanent conductive hearing losses, particularly if they cannot use regular hearing aids because of medical considerations such as those just mentioned for bone-conduction instruments (e.g., Johnson, Meikle & Vernon, 1988; Weber & Roush, 1991; Mylanus, Snik, Jorritsma, & Cremers, 1994; Weber & Fredrickson, 2000). These devices have some advantages over conventional bone-conduction hearing aids, such as the elimination of feedback, headband pressure, and the instability of vibrator positioning, as well as some improvement in high-frequency response and reduced distortion. On the other hand, implantable devices cannot be used when surgery is contraindicated, and involve all the risks associated with surgery and anesthesia.

Hearing Aid Configurations

Hearing aids can be worn in one or both ears. **Monaural amplification** means that one hearing aid is being used in one ear, and is illustrated in Figure 15–4a. **Binaural amplification** refers to the use of two separate hearing aids, one in each ear (Fig. 15–4b), and provides patients with the benefits of binaural hearing. The hallmark of binaural amplification is the use of two independent instruments, which preserves the acoustical differences between signals picked up separately by the two ears, technically known as **dichotic** inputs.

It is also possible to connect the single output of one hearing aid—almost always a body instrument—to both ears with a wire that is split so it can connect to two receivers, as in Figure 15–4c. This configuration is called a **Y-cord** fitting due to the shape of the wire. Here, the two ears are receiving identical (**diotic**) signals instead of the dichotic stimulation that occurs with two independent instruments. For this reason, Y-cord arrangements constitute **pseudobinaural** (as opposed to true binaural) amplification, and their use is discouraged.

Figure 15–4 also illustrates two kinds of hearing aid configurations that can be used when the patient must rely on just one ear to hear sounds from both sides of the head. The criteria for these configurations are discussed later, but for now let us assume that one ear is completely deaf. In cases like this, sounds coming from the deaf side reach the good ear at a reduced level due to the acoustical shadow cast by the head. This **head shadow effect** is substantial, especially for the frequencies above 1000 Hz where it grows with increasing frequency and reaches a size of about 15 to 20 dB (Shaw, 1974). The **CROS (contralateral routing of signals)** hearing aid (Harford & Barry, 1965) picks up sounds with a microphone placed at one ear and transmits the signal around the head via a wire or a radio signal to a second instrument at the *opposite ear*, which receives the amplified sound (Fig. 15–4d). For example, sounds picked up by a microphone at the right ear would be delivered via a receiver in the left ear. This arrangement overcomes the head shadow, allowing the left ear to hear sounds originating from the deaf right side. In addition to hearing sound from the impaired side via the hearing aid, the good ear hears other sounds naturally through a large opening in the earmold. Figure 15–4e shows a variation

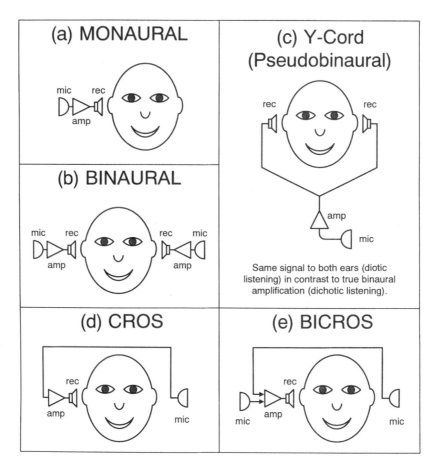

FIGURE 15–4   Typical hearing aid configurations: (a) monaural, (b) binaural, (c) Y-cord or pseudobinaural, (d) CROS, (e) BICROS.

of the CROS hearing aid called **BICROS (bilateral CROS)** (Harford, 1966). Here, sounds from both sides are picked up by microphones that are located at both ears, and the amplified signals are directed to a single receiver located in just one ear.

Electroacoustics Characteristics of Hearing Aids

Precise terminology is important when dealing with sophisticated devices such as hearing aids. The manner in which hearing aid characteristics are specified is defined in the ANSI S3.22 (1996) standard. In addition to defining terms, the standard also specifies how hearing aid characteristics are to be tested, and gives allowable **tolerances** that tell how closely a given hearing aid must adhere to the specifications provided by the manufacturer. As a result, we all use the same language, test hearing aids the same way, and know when a hearing aid is operating properly. In addition to audiologists, speech-language pathologists, teachers of the deaf, and others who work with the hearing impaired often need to read hearing aid specifications to understand the functioning (and malfunctioning) of their patients' hearing aids, and must often "translate" this material for others. Parts of this section are a bit technical, but the student will probably find that having some details about the most commonly encountered measurements in an introductory text will serve as a convenient ready reference, if not right away then surely some time in the future.

The definitions of a hearing aid's characteristics are closely related to how they are measured. For example, we already know that **gain** refers to the amount of amplification or "boost" provided by a hearing aid, defined as the difference between the output level (from the receiver) and the input level (that enters the microphone). Let us see how this is actually done. Figure 15–5 shows a conceptualized block diagram of a **hearing aid test system**, and Figure 15–6 shows a picture of a commercial system. The hearing aid being tested is located inside a sound-treated test box to minimize the effects of noise in the surrounding room, as shown in Figure 15–7. The test box also contains a loudspeaker that produces test sounds that are picked up by the hearing aid's microphone. The hearing aid's receiver is connected to a **2-cc coupler**, which is a metal cavity with a volume of 2 cc that is designed for testing hearing aids (technically called an **HA1** or **HA2 coupler**, depending on the type being used). There is a measuring microphone at the other end of the coupler, which monitors the output of the hearing aid. This arrangement is somewhat reminiscent of that described for earphone calibration in Chapter 4. The measuring microphone leads to instrumentation that analyzes the sounds produced by the hearing aid. In other words, (1) the loudspeaker produces sounds that become the input to the

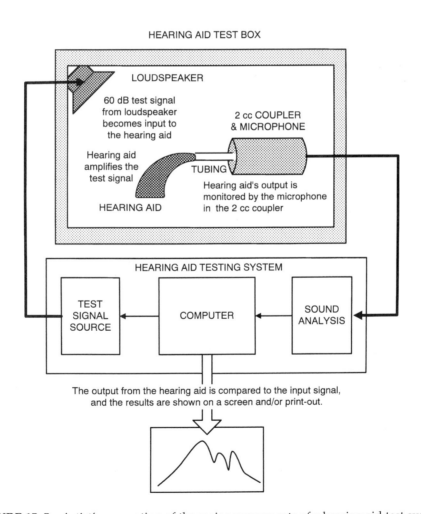

FIGURE 15–5 Artist's conception of the major components of a hearing aid test system.

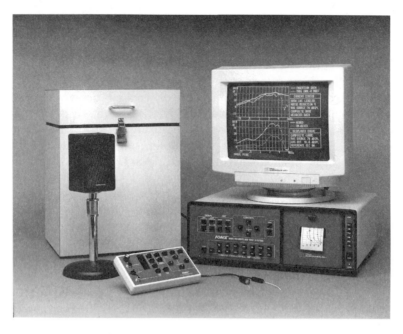

FIGURE 15–6 A typical hearing aid test system. Photograph courtesy of Frye Electronics, Inc., Tigard, OR.

hearing aid, (2) the hearing aid amplifies those sounds and its receiver broadcasts its output into the coupler, and (3) the measuring microphone picks up the hearing aid's output in the coupler. The test instrumenta-

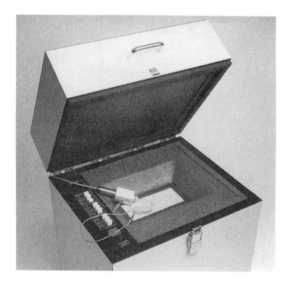

FIGURE 15–7 A hearing aid in the test box. Photograph courtesy of Frye Electronics, Inc., Tigard, OR.

tion is able to determine what the hearing aid has done to the signal because it controls the loudspeaker (hearing aid input) and also receives the hearing aid's output via the measuring microphone. These measurements can then be viewed on a screen or printed out, usually in the form of a graph. We will review several of the measurements that are made using this kind of a testing system.

Full-on gain means the amount of gain provided by a hearing aid when (1) its volume control is turned up to its highest (hence, full-on) position, and (2) the input signal is 60 dB SPL (or 50 dB SPL for a compression hearing aid).[2] As for most measurements done according to this standard, the test range must include the frequencies between at least as low as 200 Hz up to at least 5000 Hz. The hearing aid's output is then measured as a function of frequency over this range.

---

[2] Technically, full-on gain must be based on a 50-dB input if the spread between the full-on gain curve and the OSPL90 curve (described below) is less than 4 dB at any frequency from 200 to 5000 Hz.

A convenient summary value called the **high-frequency average (HFA)** is used for most ANSI S.3.22 measurements. The HFA is obtained by simply averaging the results obtained at 1000, 1600, and 2500 Hz. The HFA is often provided automatically by commercial hearing aid test systems to make the testing process more convenient and efficient. The HFA full-on gain is simply the average of the amounts of full-on gain obtained at *1000 Hz, 1600 Hz, and 2500 Hz*. For example, if the full-on gains are 30 dB at 1000 Hz, 34 dB at 1600 Hz, and 36 dB at 2500 Hz, then the HFA full-on gain would be 33 dB. The tolerance for **HFA full-on gain** is ± 5 dB, meaning that a hearing aid's actual HFA full-on gain must be within 5 dB of the value indicated in the manufacturer's specifications. The use of a high-frequency average is sometimes inappropriate, such as when a hearing aid is designed to amplify mainly in the low frequencies. In those cases, the manufacturer may replace the HFA with a **special purpose average (SPA)** composed of three other frequencies that are appropriate for the hearing aid in question.

Recall that the output sound pressure level represents the maximum output of a hearing aid in dB SPL. Output sound pressure level is determined by turning the hearing aid's volume control to the full-on position and presenting a 90 dB SPL signal from the loudspeaker. This value is called **OSPL90** because we are measuring the OSPL that results from a 90-dB input. Remember that the "90" refers to the 90-dB input, and that the amount of the OSPL90 is the level coming out of the hearing aid (its output). For example, if the 90 dB SPL input causes a hearing aid to produce an output of 129 dB SPL, then the OSPL90 is 129 dB. As for full-on gain, OSPL90 is measured from 200 to 5000 Hz, resulting in an **OSPL90 curve** like the one shown in Figure 15–8. The highest point on the OSPL90 curve is called **maximum OSPL90**, and must be no more than 3 dB higher than the amount shown on the manufacturer's specifications. The **HFA-OSPL90** of a hearing aid is obtained by averaging the values of OSPL90 at 1000, 1600, and 2500 Hz. For the OSPL90 curve in the figure, HFA-OSPL90 would be (134 + 128 + 128)/3 = 130 dB SPL. The tolerance for HFA-OSPL90 is ±4 dB.

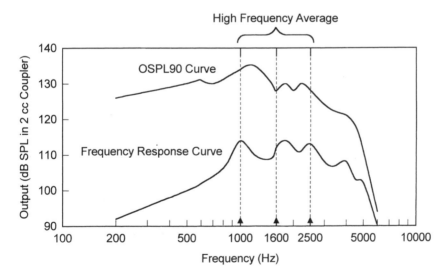

FIGURE 15–8 Examples of an OSPL90 curve (above) and a frequency response curve (below) based on ANSI S3.22-1996. The highest point on the OSPL90 curve is called maximum OSPL90. The decibel values of the 1000-, 1600-, and 2500-Hz points on the OSPL90 curve are averaged to find HFA-OSPL90. The average of the three corresponding points on the frequency response curve is 17 dB below HFA-OSPL90 at the reference test position. OSPL90 used to be called SSPL90, and will often be encountered using that terminology.

The two measures described so far are made with the volume control in the full-on position; however, hearing aids are actually used with the volume control set to some intermediate position. In other words, although OSPL90 and full-on gain tell us the maximum amounts of power and gain, we are especially concerned with how the hearing aid functions at the lower volume control setting actually used by the patient for conversational speech purposes. The amount of gain provided at the volume control position actually selected by the patient is termed "use gain." Of course, we have no way of knowing where a particular patient will set the volume control. For this reason, we need to test the hearing aid with a volume control setting that makes sense and is clearly defined so the measurements are meaningful and consistent. The volume control setting used for testing purposes is called the **reference test position**. The underlying concept is to find the volume control position that would just prevent the peaks of speech from exceeding OSPL90. In other words, we do not want the loudest aspects of conversational speech to saturate the hearing aid. Speech peaks are about 12 dB above the average level of speech. Hence, the volume control setting has to be set so that the average speech level is 12 dB below OSPL90. Now, the hearing aid will actually be tested with 60 dB SPL tones, which are 5 dB lower than the average conversational speech level of 65 dB SPL (at one meter from the talker). As a result, we want to set back the volume control by the equivalent of an additional 5 dB, so the amplified tones are 17 dB below OSPL90. Our summary figure is always the high-frequency average, so we want to set the volume control so that the amplified HFA of the tones is 17 dB below HFA-OSPL90. (The volume control is kept at the full-on setting for aids that do not provide enough amplification to make this adjustment possible and also for AGC instruments.)

How is the reference test position found? Remember that we have already found HFA-OSPL90; this was 130 dB SPL in the above example. Hence, we are looking for the volume control setting that causes an HFA output of $130 - 17 = 113$ dB SPL. We now turn down the hearing aid volume control by some "guestimated" amount, close the test box, and push the button that causes the loudspeaker to present 60 dB SPL test tones. Commercial testing systems will present the three needed tones (1000, 1600, and 2500 Hz) and even calculate the resulting HFA output from the hearing aid. We compare this value to the desired amount (113 dB in our example). If we are off by more than 1 dB, then we open the test box, readjust the hearing aid volume control a bit in the right direction (down if the output was too high, up if it was too low), close the box, and press the button to repeat the test. This process continues until we find the volume control setting that gives the desired value (17 dB below HFA-OSPL90 within ±1 dB). This setting is the reference test position, which is used for the remainder of the tests.

The amount of gain provided by a hearing aid in the reference test position is called its **reference test gain (RTG)**. The RTG is found by subtracting 77 dB from the HFA-OSPL90. In our example, this is $130 - 77 = 53$ dB. Why? Because (1) the output in the reference test position is 17 dB below OSPL90, (2) gain is output minus input, and (3) the input is 60 dB. Using our example, the "long way" is to find the output in the reference test position by subtracting 17 dB from OSPL90, or $130 - 17 = 113$ dB, and then to find the reference test gain by subtracting the 60 dB input, or $113 - 60 = 53$ dB. It is quicker and easier to combine the 17 dB and the 60 dB into 77 dB, and to find the RTG in one step by subtracting 77 from the OSPL90, or $130 - 77 = 53$ dB. No tolerances are specified for the RTG because the standard considers it to be given for information purposes.

The lower curve in Figure 15–8 is the hearing aid's **frequency response curve**, and is obtained by measuring the output as a function of frequency from 200 to 5000 Hz with a 60 dB SPL input (or 50 dB for AGC aids) and the volume control in the reference test position. Before we can address tolerances for the frequency response curve, an intermediate step is needed so that they will be meaningful. The **frequency range** is determined from the frequency response curve as shown in Figure 15–9 by (1) calculating an HFA from the 1000, 1600, and 2500 Hz points on the frequency response curve; (2) measuring down to a point 20 dB below this HFA; and (3) drawing a horizontal line. This horizontal line will intersect the frequency response curve at two points, called the *low-frequency cutoff* (f_1) *and the high-frequency cutoff* (f_2). The frequency range is the distance between these two points (from f_1 to f_2), and no tolerances apply to it. The tolerances are different for the lower- and higher-frequency parts (bands) of the curve: (1) ±4 dB for the lower band, which includes the frequencies from $1.25f_1$ (or 200 Hz, whichever is higher) up to 2000 Hz; and (2) ±6 dB for the higher band, which includes the frequencies from 2000 Hz up to $0.8f_2$ (or 4000 Hz, whichever is lower).

Although not part of the hearing aid standard per se, a gain curve obtained at the reference test position can be shown by plotting the frequency response curve in terms of *decibels of gain* rather than in dB SPL. This kind of a graph is shown in Figure 15–10, and is generally known as a **reference test gain curve**. It is usually provided by the hearing aid test system at the touch of a button, and is very useful because it directly

shows the amount of amplification provided by the hearing aid (in the 2-cc coupler) on a frequency-by-frequency basis.

The quality of amplification is adversely affected by **distortion** or **noise** produced by the hearing aid. **Harmonic distortion** occurs when the output contains spurious signals at multiples (harmonics) of the input signal. Suppose the input is a 500-Hz tone and the output includes 500, 1000, and 1500 Hz. The 500-Hz signal is the fundamental frequency or first harmonic, and would be the only frequency present in a "perfectly clean" output. The output at 1000 Hz is second harmonic distortion (a spurious signal generated at twice the fundamental, 2 × 500 Hz) and 1500 Hz is third harmonic distortion (3 × 500 Hz). The **percentage of total harmonic distortion (%THD)** is measured while the hearing aid is at its reference test setting. These measurements are done at 500 Hz and 800 Hz using 70 dB SBL input signals, and at 1600 Hz using a 65 dB SPL input. For special purpose hearing aids, harmonic distortion is measured using tones that are one-half the frequencies used for the SPA. Two methods are available for measuring a hearing aid's harmonic distortion, and are shown in Table 15–1 for the convenience of the mathematically oriented student. Regardless of which

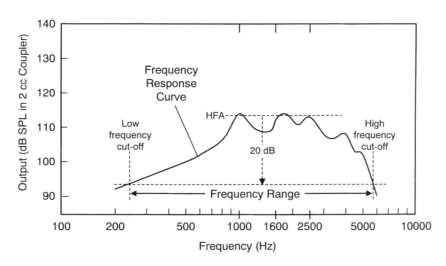

FIGURE 15–9 The frequency range is obtained from the frequency response curve, as shown.

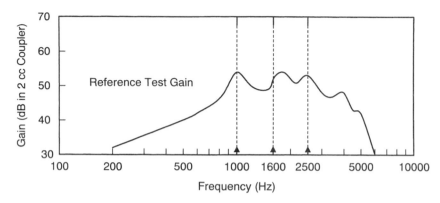

FIGURE 15–10   The reference test gain curve shows the frequency response in decibels of gain instead of dB SPL, and represents the amount of amplification provided by the hearing aid (in a 2-cc coupler) on a frequency-by-frequency basis.

method is used, the total harmonic distortion of a hearing aid may not exceed the manufacturer's specifications by more than 3%.

A special rule applies when the hearing aid amplifies the frequency corresponding to the second harmonic considerably more than the frequency being used to test for harmonic distortion: Harmonic distortion does not have to be tested for a given frequency if the frequency response curve rises to the extent that the level of the second harmonic is 612 dB stronger than at the test frequency. For example, if the frequency response curve shows a level of 92 dB at 500 Hz and 104 dB or more at 1000 Hz (the second harmonic of 500 Hz), then it is not necessary to measure harmonic distortion for 500 Hz. This rule avoids exaggerating the percentage of total harmonic distortion.

Equivalent input noise is a measure of the noise generated by the hearing aid at the reference test setting based on a comparison of the outputs when there is an input signal and when there is no input signal. The math-minded will find the formulas for equivalent input noise in Table 15–2. A hearing aid may not exceed the manufacturer's specifications for equivalent input noise by more than 3 dB.

Several special tests are required for AGC hearing aids. Recall that the input-output function shows how the output of a hearing aid increases as the input level is raised (as in Fig. 15–2). With the volume control set to the reference test position, input-output curves are measured for input levels from 50 to 90 dB SPL in 5-dB steps at one or more frequencies (250, 500, 1000, 2000, and/or 4000 Hz). The hearing aid's **input-output function** is compared to the curve in the manufacturer's specifications by lining them up at the point corresponding to the 70 dB input. The output values for the hearing aid must be within ±5 dB of those in the specifications.

TABLE 15–1   Methods and formulas for determining percent total harmonic distortion (%THD) for hearing aids[a]

		Where:
Method A	$\%THD = 100 \times \sqrt{\dfrac{p_2^2 + p_3^2 + p_4^2 + \ldots}{p_1^2}}$	p_1 = pressure of 1st harmonic (fundamental); p_2 = pressure of 2nd harmonic; p_3 = pressure of 3rd harmonic; etc
Method B	$\%THD = 100 \times \sqrt{\dfrac{p_2^2 + p_3^2 + p_4^2 + \ldots}{p_1^2 + p_2^2 + p_3^2 + \ldots}}$	

[a] Method A should be used when %THD exceeds 30%.

TABLE 15–2   Determining the equivalent input noise of a hearing aid

Regular hearing aids	$L_n = L_2 - (L_{av} - 60)$ dB	Where:
		L_n = equivalent input noise
		L_{av} = average output with 60 dB inputs at 1000,
AGC hearing aids	$L_n = L_2 - (L_{av} - 50)$ dB	1600, and 2500 Hz
		L_2 = output with no input, representing inherent
		noise of hearing aid

Level changes occur all the time in the real world, such as when a talker suddenly raises his voice to emphasize a point, when a loud drum beat occurs during a musical piece, or when a truck backfires. Instead of acting instantaneously when the input level rises, there will be a delay before the hearing aid's AGC circuit actually reduces the gain in response to the higher level, called **attack time**. Similarly, there will be also be a delay before the gain returns to its original amount after the louder input ends, called **release time**. Attack time is measured by abruptly increasing the input signal from 55 to 90 dB SPL, and measuring how long it takes for the output to stabilize at the level associated with the 90 dB input (± 3 dB). Release time is measured by abruptly decreasing the input signal from 90 to 55 dB SPL, and measuring how long it takes for the output to stabilize at the level associated with the 55 dB input (± 4 dB). Attack and release times must be within $\pm 50\%$ or ± 5 msec (whichever is larger) of the manufacturer's specifications.

Telecoil performance is tested by measuring the hearing aid's output in response to a magnetic signal instead of sound. To do this, the hearing aid is switched to the telecoil (T) setting and the volume control is placed in the reference test position. The hearing aid is placed on a **telephone magnetic field simulator (TMFS)**, which produces the magnetic test signal, and a frequency response curve is obtained. This curve is called a **SPLITS curve** because it shows the sound pressure level (SPL) as a function of frequency produced by the hearing aid when it is activated by an induction telephone simulator (ITS). Averaging the values at 1000, 1600, and 2500 Hz gives us the **HFA-SPLITS** for the hearing aid, which must be within ± 6 dB of the manufacturer's

specifications. (As with the microphone measurements, a special frequency average may be used, if appropriate.) Finally, the hearing aid's **simulated telephone sensitivity (STS)** is determined by subtracting reference test gain plus 60 dB (already known from previous measurements) from the HFA-SPLITS. The STS gives us an idea of how the hearing aid's gain using the telecoil compares to its normal gain.

Two-cc coupler measurements are excellent for their intended purposes, which involve the reliable determination of hearing aid operating characteristics. However, 2-cc couplers do not replicate the acoustics of the human ear, and the arrangement in the test box certainly does not replicate how sounds are affected by the human head and body. These characteristics are closely replicated by using another kind of coupler called the **Zwislocki ear simulator** (Zwislocki, 1971) that is mounted in the ear of a dummy that acoustically mimics the human head and torso, like the **Knowles Electronics Manikin for Acoustic Research (KEMAR)** (Burkhard & Sachs, 1975). This type of system is shown in Figure 15–11, and is very useful when it is necessary to make electroacoustic measurements that simulate real-world conditions (ANSI S3.35-1997).

REAL-EAR (PROBE-TUBE) MEASUREMENTS

The measurements described so far tell us how the hearing aid is working as an electroacoustic instrument. But how do we determine whether the hearing aid is actually providing the prescribed amplification performance to a specific, real patient? To do this, actual hearing aid performance must be determined with the hearing aid on the patient herself.

(a)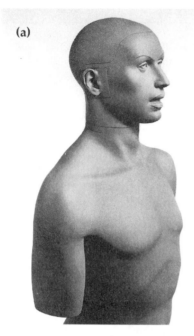

(b)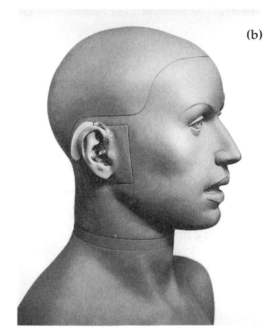

FIGURE 15–11   (a) The KEMAR manikin. (b) A hearing aid being tested on KEMAR. Photographs courtesy of Knowles Electronics, Inc.

The major aspects of a typical real-ear measurement system are shown in Figure 15–12. An example of a commercially available system is shown in Figure 15–13. A soundfield loudspeaker is used to present the stimulus sounds,[3] which are picked up by specially placed measurement microphones, to be described momentarily. The core of the system is a computer that controls the loudspeaker and analyzes the sounds monitored by the microphones. The results are displayed on a screen, and can be printed out as desired. Many commercially available systems are programmed to provide a variety of prescription formulas, making it very easy to compare actual hearing aid performance with the prescribed targets.

The key aspect of the real-ear system involves the use of two microphones mounted on the head. One is called the **reference microphone,** which picks up sounds outside

the ear, very close to the hearing aid's microphone just before they enter the hearing aid. The other microphone is the **probe microphone**. Even though this microphone is physically located outside the ear, it is connected to a fine pliable **probe-tube** that is inserted into the ear canal, with its tip within a few millimeters of the eardrum. The probe-tube and microphone (hereafter called the probe-tube) therefore monitor the sound as it is actually received by the eardrum.

Two different kinds of measurements are made with the probe-tube system just described. The first measurement is made *without* the hearing aid. The stimulus from the loudspeaker is picked up by both the reference microphone and the probe-tube. The reference microphone monitors the signal before it enters the ear canal and the probe tube monitors the signal at the eardrum. The signal will usually be about 12 to 17 dB stronger in the 2700- to 5000-Hz range at the eardrum (probe-tube) compared with outside the ear (reference microphone). This boost at the eardrum is due to the **ear canal resonance effect** explained in Chapter 2. The first measurement is called the

[3] The student should be aware that important issues must be considered when making soundfield measurements even though the details are too advanced for an introductory text. For a clear and detailed tutorial, see ASHA (1991).

Probe-tube system with unoccluded ear canal.

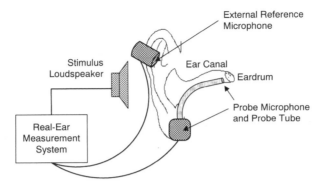

Probe-tube system with a hearing aid in place.

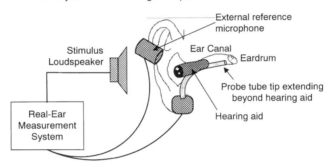

FIGURE 15–12 Conceptual representation of real-ear measurements.

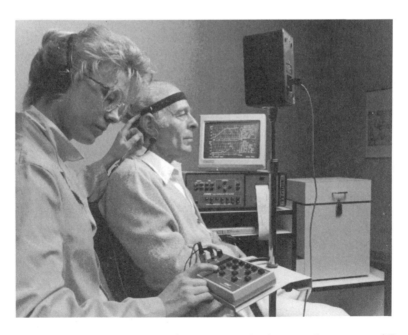

FIGURE 15–13 Real-ear assessment of a hearing aid. Photograph courtesy of Frye Electronics, Inc., Tigard, OR.

459

real-ear unaided response (REUR), and is retained in the memory of the analysis system.

The second measurement is made *with* the hearing aid in the ear. The real-ear system assembly is left in place and the hearing aid is inserted into the patient's ear, being careful not to crimp or displace the probe-tube. The probe-tube now extends beyond the inside (receiver) end of the hearing aid, so that it monitors the output of the hearing aid that is actually being received by the patient's eardrum. The stimulus signal is then presented from the loudspeaker. The reference microphone monitors the input to the hearing aid and the probe-tube monitors the output of the in-place hearing aid at the eardrum. The difference between them is automatically calculated by the analysis system, and is called the **real-ear aided response (REAR)**.

It would seem that the REAR represents the actual gain provided by the hearing aid. However, let us not forget that a certain amount of gain is provided by the ear canal resonance *without* the hearing aid, represented by the REUR that was previously measured and is being kept in the system's memory. Hence, in order to arrive at the true gain being provided by the hearing aid, the real-ear system must subtract the unaided response from the aided response. The resulting *true gain* is called the **insertion gain** or **real-ear insertion gain (REIG)**, and the curve showing insertion gain as a function of frequency is the **real-ear insertion response (REIR)**.

We verify whether a hearing aid is providing the patient with the intended amount of amplification by comparing the real-ear insertion gain to the prescribed insertion gain target values based on the prescription method being used. Real-ear measurements are not limited to gain. For example, probe-tube measurements also allow us to determine the OSPL90 at the patient's eardrum, which is shown as a function of frequency by the **real-ear saturation response (RESR)**. The phrase "saturation response" here reflects the influence of the term "saturation sound pressure level (SSPL)," which was used before the term was changed to OSPL in the ANSI S3.22 (1996) standard. Just as the REIR is

compared to prescribed insertion gain target values, the RESR is compared to prescribed target values for OSPL90 at the eardrum. Notice that the patient does not have to do anything except quietly sit still while the measurements are being made. In other words, the real-ear approach provides extensive and detailed information about what the hearing aid is actually delivering to the patient's eardrum without the need for tedious and time-consuming behavioral measurements. A concomitant major advantage is that we can almost instantly view the results of any number of hearing aid adjustments on the patient. This is a priceless capability when verifying, fine-tuning, or modifying a hearing aid fitting.

FUNCTIONAL GAIN MEASUREMENTS

The actual amount of amplification provided by a hearing aid can also be tested behaviorally by the **functional gain method**, although it lacks many of the advantages just described for probe-tube measurements. This approach involves obtaining soundfield thresholds under two conditions: (1) without the hearing aid (unaided thresholds), and (2) while wearing the hearing aid (aided thresholds). The amount of functional gain is determined by finding the difference between the two thresholds at each frequency of interest. In other words, functional gain (dB) equals unaided threshold (dB HL) minus aided threshold (dB HL). For example, if an unaided threshold is 55 dB HL and the aided threshold is 30 dB HL, then the functional gain is $55 - 30 = 25$ dB. Functional gain is then compared to the target gain at each frequency to verify that the hearing aid provides the prescribed amplification. If we assume the target gain is 27 dB in the current example, then the 25 dB of functional gain would be compared to the 27 dB target gain.

It is more convenient to work in terms of aided thresholds instead of functional gain values during behavioral testing. Under these circumstances, *aided threshold targets* may be established by subtracting the prescribed target gain from the patient's unaided threshold at each frequency. In the prior example, where the unaided threshold was 55 dB HL and the prescribed target gain was 27 dB, the prescribed target aided threshold would be $55 - 27 = 28$ dB HL. The 30 dB HL aided threshold would then be compared to the 28 dB HL target aided threshold. Converting insertion gain into aided thresholds is also useful when explaining amplification to the patient.

Candidacy for Amplification

The primary step in the audiological management of hearing-impaired patients involves providing them with amplification, or at least making decisions about it. However, as important as amplification is, we must be forever mindful of the fact that the hearing aid is *part* of the aural rehabilitation process and not an end unto itself.

Who is a candidate for amplification? The consensus of current opinion is that any patient complaining of auditory difficulties in communicative situations should be viewed as a potential candidate for audiological intervention, such as hearing aids or other kinds of assistive devices (Hawkins Beck, Bratt, Fabry, Mueller, & Stelmachowicz, 1991). Clearly, the patient must have some degree of hearing loss, and the need for amplification unquestionably rises as the degree of hearing loss worsens. Hence, it is easy to say that a patient with a pure-tone average (PTA) or speech recognition threshold (SRT) of 50 dB HL in both ears needs a hearing aid. But let us see what happens when we play the "countdown" game: Is a hearing aid needed at 45 dB? Absolutely. At 40 dB? Yes. At 35 dB? Of course. At 30 dB? Sure. How about 25 dB or 20 dB? Well, uh . . . Notice how we quickly reach a range of losses where we cannot definitively say "yes" or "no." (The same frustrating game can be played counting up from a threshold of 0 dB HL.) One of the reasons for hedging on the answer is that the overall degree of hearing loss is only one of the many variables to be considered. For example, hearing losses typically increase with frequency, so a patient can have quite a nasty hearing impairment even though the PTA and/or SRT may be just 10 dB (or even zero). Then, of course, there is the issue of unilateral and asymmetrical impairments: Does Mrs. Jones need a hearing aid if her right ear has a 50-dB loss but her left ear is normal? What about Mr. Smith who also has a 60-dB loss in the right ear and a 30-dB loss in the left?

We must also deal with the special case of infants and small children. Here, even relatively small amounts of hearing loss can have numerous adverse effects (e.g., Bess, Dodd-Murphy, & Parker, 1998), and *early identification* linked with *early intervention*—including amplification—produces impressive benefits (e.g., Yoshinaga-Itano, Sedey, Coulter, & Mehl, 1998; Yoshinaga-Itano, 1999). Thus, amplification should be introduced as early as possible once there has been a diagnosis of a hearing loss capable of having an impact on speech and language development (e.g., PWG, 1996).

Complicating matters is the distinction between the *need for amplification* due to the extent and impact of the auditory deficit versus how much *benefit the patient experiences* from the hearing aid. When the hearing loss is moderate to severe, unaided speech communication is belabored or impossible (*need*) and this situation improves appreciably albeit not totally when hearing aids are worn (*benefit*). What's more, the improvement is readily appreciated by the patient and by others. However, the need for amplification can be ambiguous in cases considered to be marginal because of a mild, high-frequency, or unilateral loss. Here the degree to which the hearing loss affects speech communication is often subtle, inconsistent, and situational, depending on such factors as speaking level, whether there are background or competing noises, and the communicative demands of the patient's occupational and social interactions.

The benefits of amplification can be similarly subtle and inconsistent in patients with marginal impairments, so that a patient may need a hearing aid but perceive little or no benefit from it. However, little perceived benefit does not mean no benefit. The subtle benefits of amplification often become apparent when the patient forgets to bring his hearing aid to an important meeting or must do without the instrument while it is being repaired. At the opposite extreme, patients with profound losses have the greatest need for hearing aids, but they often receive relatively little benefit in terms of auditory speech reception because their residual auditory capability is often minimal. Again, however, remember that limited benefit for the purpose of hearing speech is not the same as no benefit at all. On the contrary, patients with profound losses benefit considerably from their hearing aids in terms of the ability to hear for alerting, warning, and emergency signals, and as an aid to lipreading.

Clearly, hearing aid candidacy depends on more than auditory status alone, and is particularly affected by the patient's communicative requirements and the need to rely on auditory information. Other motivational factors interact with the hearing loss to induce the patient to see an audiologist, and then to follow the recommendation to obtain hearing aids and to use them. Some of the major factors that appear to motivate patients to obtain a hearing aid for the first time include communication problems at home, in noisy listening situations, social situations, and at work, as well as encouragement by the spouse (Bender & Mueller, 1984). Acceptance of the hearing impairment itself and of the need for clinical assistance to deal with it also weighs heavily in the patient's decision to obtain amplification. A patient in one of the "marginal" categories is often not willing to accept himself as hearing impaired, let alone so much so that amplification is needed. This is particularly true when the loss has developed slowly and insidiously over a long period of time.

Several other issues often result in delaying the decision to use hearing aids. These factors include whether the patient's primary care physician refers her to an audiologist or at least actively encourages her to do so, the relatively high cost of the instruments, cosmetic considerations, and the related issue of concern about the stigma still attached to hearing aid use. Because of the implications of all these factors, it is often helpful to use **self-assessment scales** (discussed below) that address the auditory, social/occupational, and emotional impact of hearing impairment in the assessment of hearing aid candidacy, as well as other aspects of audiological practice (e.g., ASHA, 1998).

Monaural versus Binaural Amplification

It is desirable to provide the hearing-impaired listener with usable binaural hearing whenever possible. For practical purposes, this means binaural amplification is preferred over a monaural hearing aid for most patients with bilateral hearing losses, and many patients with unilateral hearing losses should benefit from the use of a hearing aid in the impaired ear. The desirability of binaural amplification reflects several advantages of binaural hearing compared to monaural hearing (Valente, 1982; deJong, 1994; Gelfand, 1998): Binaural summation results in an advantage over monaural listening corresponding to about 3 dB at threshold and approximately 6 dB at suprathreshold levels. Binaural difference limens for both frequency and intensity are smaller (better) than the corresponding values for monaural hearing. Binaural hearing maximizes directional hearing ability (e.g., sound localization) and alleviates the head shadow effect. In addition, binaural listening reduces the adverse effects of noise and reverberation on speech intelligibility in real-world listening conditions (sometimes called binaural "squelch").

There is also a compelling negative reason to choose binaural amplification whenever possible. Silman, Gelfand, and Silverman (1984) demonstrated that adults with bilateral sensorineural hearing losses who use monaural hearing aids can develop an **auditory deprivation effect** in which speech recognition scores deteriorate over time in their *unaided* ears even though intelligibility scores remain unchanged in their aided ears. In contrast, binaural hearing aid users do not experience a speech recognition deficit in either ear. This phenomenon has been corroborated by numerous studies (e.g., Gelfand, Silman & Ross, 1987; Stubblefield & Nye, 1989; Silverman & Silman, 1990; Silman,

Silverman, Emmer, & Gelfand, 1992; Hurley, 1993, 1999; Gelfand, 1995). The auditory deprivation effect is not limited to adults. Gelfand and Silman (1993) demonstrated that it also occurs in children with bilateral losses who use monaural amplification, but not in children who use binaural hearing aids.

Once a patient has developed an auditory deprivation effect, adding a second hearing aid to the previously unfitted ear may reduce or alleviate the problem in some but not all cases (Silverman & Silman, 1990; Silman, Silverman, Emmer, & Gelfand, 1992; Hurley, 1993; Gelfand, 1995). At least three patterns of auditory deprivation development and recovery or no recovery have been identified (Gelfand, 1995): (1) Speech recognition deteriorates within about two years of monaural amplification and *recovers completely* within about two years after binaural hearing aids are introduced. (2) The largest group experiences a *significant but incomplete amount of recovery* from auditory deprivation after switching to binaural amplification, although the time frames vary widely for both the development of deterioration with one aid and recovery with two aids. (3) An auditory deprivation effect takes several years to develop and there is *no recovery* with a second hearing aid, even after several years of binaural amplification. In addition, some patients actually reject a second hearing aid even though the auditory deprivation effect has been reduced or eliminated by its use (e.g., Hurley, 1993).

The foregoing discussion demonstrates that binaural hearing aids should be the first consideration for patients with bilateral hearing losses. This conclusion agrees with the consensus of opinion in the field (e.g., Hawkins et al, 1991; PWG, 1996). However, it must be kept in mind that binaural amplification is not always the best overall choice for every patient. For example, it has been shown that some patients actually experience a **binaural interference effect**, in which the participation of the more impaired ear (as with binaural hearing aids) results in a deterioration of performance rather than an improvement (Jerger et al, 1993). In addition, binaural hearing aids may be rejected by the patient due to any number of reasons that might be perceptual, behavioral, physical, cognitive, emotional, and/or financial.

Candidacy for binaural hearing aids becomes controversial when patients have asymmetrical losses, that is, bilateral impairments that are significantly different between the two ears. In terms of the "common wisdom," enthusiasm for binaural hearing aids begins to wane when the two ears have pure-tone averages that differ by more than 15 dB and/or speech recognition scores that differ by more than 8%; and binaural amplification is considered progressively less desirable as the inter-ear difference gets wider. It is reasonable to anticipate that patients with large inter-ear differences probably will not have the same chances of success with binaural hearing aids as their counterparts with more symmetric losses. However, there is no compelling reason to rule out binaural amplification without even a try simply because there is an audiometric difference between the ears, especially with criteria as small as the ones just mentioned (Courtois, Johansen, Larsen, et al, 1988; Sandlin, 1994). One should be alert to the possibility of the binaural interference phenomenon when binaural hearing aids are rejected or when binaural performance is poorer than that of the better ear alone.

CROS-Type Fittings

It is not uncommon to find patients in whom one ear is normal and the other has a unilateral hearing loss that is unaidable. The impaired ear might be unaidable because it is totally deaf or due to a medical condition that precludes the use of a hearing aid, such as chronic drainage. Even an ear with a reasonable amount of residual hearing sensitivity sometimes proves to be unaidable due to for example, an extremely low speech recognition score. These patients must rely on one ear, which means that sounds originating from the impaired side will be received at a reduced level due to the head shadow. Depending on the communicative and other demands of their work and social environments, some individuals in this situation can function with little or no difficulty by relying on the remaining normal ear, but others experience a considerable disadvantage and need assistance to hear sounds originating from the impaired side. Imagine, for example, the disadvantage experienced by an executive who cannot hear the comments made by people sitting to her left at a business meeting, or the impact of a deaf right ear on a taxi driver who cannot hear what his passengers are saying. The CROS hearing aid was introduced for patients of this type, who have one normal ear and one substantially impaired ear that is not aidable (Harford & Barry, 1965).

The "good ear" does not have to be completely normal for CROS to be used. Instead, the *open earmold* used in CROS amplification can also be beneficial when there is a high-frequency hearing loss in the better ear (Harford & Dodds, 1966). This arrangement works for two reasons. First, the open earmold facilitates high-frequency amplification without amplifying the lows. Second, having the microphone and receiver in separate ears avoids the acoustic feedback problem that is likely to occur when the microphone and receiver are able to communicate via an open earmold in the same ear. Feedback is minimized with CROS because the distance between the microphone and receiver minimizes the feedback with CROS, and this separation is enhanced by the head shadow. The use of open earmolds to remove the lows in a regular (one ear) hearing aid is known as an **IROS** ("I" for ipsilateral) fitting on analogy to CROS, even though the term is a misnomer. *Vents* are more commonly drilled through the earmold for the same purpose.

The BICROS arrangement is considered when the patient has an unaidable poorer ear for any of the above-mentioned reasons, as well as a hearing loss that can benefit from a hearing aid in the better ear (Harford, 1966). It is easiest to think of this arrangement as a regular hearing aid in the better ear, with its own microphone, receiver, and the appropriate kind of earmold (instead of an open CROS-type earmold), plus an additional "offside" microphone that is located at the unaidable poorer ear on the other side of the head.

Hearing Aid Selection and Fitting

Prefitting Considerations

The first steps in the process of providing the patient with amplification include patient assessment (see Candidacy for Amplification, above), obtaining medical clearance, and providing the patient with initial counseling. The purpose of the medical clearance is to meet legal and regulatory requirements and to be sure no medical problems exist that would contraindicate a hearing aid or would create the need for special considerations. Otologic and related pathologies are discussed in Chapter 6. Initial counseling should address such issues as the reasons for amplification and other aural rehabilitation services that might be indicated; the kinds of instrument(s) that are appropriate; the reasons for preferring binaural amplification, if appropriate; and realistic goals and expectations regarding what hearing aids can and cannot do. Other issues often discussed at this point revolve around such practical matters as the costs involved, where the instrument can be purchased, the 30-day trial period, batteries, instrument warrantees, and insurance, etc. The patient and his family[4] should have a clear and realistic understanding of these issues so they can be active participants in the aural rehabilitation process, of which the hearing aids are one part (ASHA, 1998). Earmold impressions might be taken at this point or at a subsequent time, depending on the kind of instruments being considered and who will be dispensing them. These issues are included in the *assessment* and *treatment planning* stages shown in Table 15–3.

Instrument Selection/Evaluation/Fitting

The process of providing the patient with amplification has been described by various terms over the years, such as *hearing aid evaluation, hearing aid consultation, hearing aid*

---

[4] As well as other pertinent individuals (caregivers, etc.) depending on the patient's particular circumstances.

TABLE 15–3   Summary of the ASHA (1998) hearing aid fitting guidelines for adults

Assessment stage	Determine nature and magnitude of hearing loss. Assess hearing aid/rehabilitation candidacy based on audiometric data, self-assessment protocols, etc. Consider patient's unique circumstances (e.g., physical status, mental status, attitude, motivation, sociological status, communication status).
Treatment planning stage	Audiologist, patient, and family/caregivers review findings to identify needs, arrive at rehabilitative goals, plan intervention strategies, understand treatment benefits/limitations/costs and how outcomes are assessed.
Selection stage	Hearing aid(s) selected in terms of electroacoustic (e.g., frequency-gain, OSPL90, input-output function) and other (monaural/binaural; style and size, etc.) characteristics.
Verification stage	ANSI S3.22 measurements (hearing aid electroacoustics) and real-ear measurements (e.g., prescriptive targets, performance on patient). Physical and listening checks for physical fit, intermittencies, noisiness, etc. Determine whether audibility, comfort, and tolerance expectations are achieved.
Orientation stage	Counseling on hearing aid use and care, realistic expectations, etc.; and explore the candidacy for assistive devices, audiologic rehabilitation assessment, and further intervention.
Validation stage	Assess intervention outcomes, reduction of disability, goals addressed using such measures as self-assessment tools, objective or subjects measures of speech perception, other means.

selection, and *hearing aid fitting*. The nature of the fitting process has evolved over the years and continues to do so, and no one method is applicable in all cases, let alone universally accepted. Contemporary approaches implicitly accept a concept that has traditionally been called *selective amplification*. This term originally meant that the amount of gain at each frequency should depend on the degree and configuration of the patient's hearing loss. A more modern definition would say that the hearing aid's electroacoustic characteristics should be chosen or adjusted so that they are most appropriate for the nature of the patient's hearing loss. The selective amplification concept is so ingrained in modern clinical philosophy that the term itself is rarely used anymore. However, the student should be aware that this was not always the case. For example, the influential Harvard (Davis, Stevens, Nichols, Hudgins, Marquis, Peterson, & Ross, 1947) and MedResCo (1947) reports concluded that most patients could be optimally fitted with a hearing aid that has a flat or slightly rising frequency response, so that an individualized selection process would be superfluous in all but un-

usual cases. The ensuing controversy lasted for decades.[5] As already indicated, individualized hearing aid selection has proven to be the accepted approach, although numerous different methods have been proposed to accomplish this. These methods can be categorized into two broad groups, which we will call the comparative and prescriptive approaches.

COMPARATIVE HEARING AID EVALUATIONS

The traditional hearing aid evaluation (HAE) involves preselecting a number of hearing aids that appear to be appropriate for the patient on the basis of their electroacoustic specifications, and then comparing the patient's performance with each of these instruments using a variety of speech tests presented from loudspeakers. The procedures involved in the comparative hearing aid evaluation originally described by Carhart (1946) began with

---

[5] These and other classical papers have been reproduced with informative commentaries by Levitt, Pickett, and Houde (1980).

unaided measurements of SRT, the tolerance limit for loud speech, and a speech recognition score for PB-50 words presented at 25 dB HL, after which the patient took a series of tests with each of the hearing aids being compared. These tests began by finding the volume control setting where the patient judged speech presented at 40 dB HL to be comfortably loud. This was followed by (1) SRTs at the comfort and full-on gain settings; (2) tolerance limits at the comfort and full-on gain settings; (3) determining the signal-to-noise (S/N) ratio for speech, that is, finding the level of noise that rendered speech at 50 dB HL to be barely audible; and (4) speech recognition scores for words presented at 25 dB SL.

The extensive testing of the **original Carhart method** quickly led to the use of all kinds of abbreviated variations, generically known as **comparative hearing aid evaluations** or **modified Carhart methods**. In a typical evaluation of this type, the patient would be tested with each hearing aid to obtain an SRT and speech recognition scores for words presented in quiet and/or against a background of noise. Other methods compared hearing aids on the basis of judgments of the quality and/or intelligibility of amplified speech using various selection strategies that involve paired comparisons (e.g., Punch & Beck, 1980; Punch & Parker, 1981; Neuman, Levitt, Mills, & Schwander, 1987; Cox & McDaniel, 1989; Surr & Fabry, 1991; Kuk, 1994). In effect, the hearing aid with the best speech recognition score (or judgment rating) was considered the best choice for the patient. These procedures were often followed by a short trial period with the hearing aid. Once a particular instrument was selected, the patient would be given a recommendation to purchase an instrument of the same make and model, and would subsequently return to the clinic for verification of adequate performance with the purchased instrument.

The comparative HAE approach has largely been abandoned in favor of prescriptive approaches. The principal reason for this has been the inability of currently employed speech recognition tests to distinguish among hearing aids adequately and reliably. For example, in their classic study, Walden, Schwartz, Williams, Holum-Hardangon, and Crowley (1983) found that the mean difference in speech recognition scores for words presented in noise was only 4.3% among acoustically similar hearing aids. In addition, only 4.5% of the speech recognition score differences were large enough to be significant on an individual patient basis. Why is this a problem if the hearing aids were acoustically similar? The reason is that this is the same situation involved in a real-world comparative HAE, where the audiologist starts by preselecting several apparently appropriate (hence fairly similar) instruments to compare behaviorally on the patient. Walden et al also found that the mean speech recognition score difference was only 14.2% even for acoustically dissimilar hearing aids. In other words, speech recognition scores were able to distinguish only among instruments so different that an experienced audiologist would never have preselected them for comparison on the same patient to begin with. What's more, fewer than half (48.1%) of the speech recognition score differences were large enough to be significant on an individual patient basis even though the instruments were so dissimilar acoustically. In addition, just because a hearing aid had the highest speech recognition score did not mean it would also be the one judged best by a patient after a trial period of actual use, except for the subgroup where the scores were significantly different to begin with.

The traditional comparative HAE also faces at least two practical limitations. First, the majority of modern fittings use ITEs and canal aids, which do not lend themselves to comparative assessments because they are custom-ordered. The second pragmatic limitation is related to the nature of programmable instruments. The comparative HAE was originally developed to compare hearing aids with only one frequency response and perhaps a second tone control setting. A simple two-position tone control switch could effectively double the number of comparisons. Modern programmable instruments have a variety of different settings used by the same patient under different listening conditions and are, in effect, several hearing aids packaged as one. There are so many permutations that comparative assessments are simply unrealistic.

PRESCRIPTIVE HEARING AID FITTING

Contemporary hearing aid fitting approaches involve prescriptive methods (e.g., ASHA, 1998; Table 15–3). Fundamentally, **prescriptive methods** use a "formula" to prescribe the amplification characteristics considered to be most appropriate for a patient. The very idea of using formulas to prescribe gain might seem strange. After all, we know from common experience that eyeglasses often restore "20-20" visual acuity. Consequently, it would seem that the amount of gain should be equal to the amount of hearing loss because this would restore 0 dB HL thresholds. This notion would be a great idea except for the fact that it is wrong. Equating gain with the amount of loss invariably results in too much amplification, subjecting the patient to excessive amounts of loudness and distortion, and placing the patient at risk for developing a noise-induced hearing loss. In fact, if we try to give patients too much gain, they often negate the intent by turning down the volume control, and may even reject amplification altogether. If the goal of amplification is not to restore normal hearing, then, alas, what is the goal? The answer is to provide the amount and configuration of gain that maximizes the audibility of conversational speech without making the amplified signal uncomfortably loud. Skinner (1988) described this gain configuration as the one that provides the patient with the best compromise between maximum speech intelligibility and acceptable sound quality.

Hearing aid prescription formulas are really explicitly described sets of rules used to determine the amounts and configurations of gain and output sound pressure level[6] that are most desirable for the patient (the *selection stage* in Table 15–3). Depending on which prescriptive method is used, the formula might use the patient's thresholds, comfortable listening levels, and/or loudness discomfort levels as a function of frequency. This information might come from the patient's audiogram, specially administered tests, or a combination of both. Reviews of this topic and summaries of prescriptive formulas for adults and children are available in several sources (e.g., Skinner, 1988; Mueller, Hawkins, & Northern, 1992; Valente, 1994; PWG, 1996; Traynor, 1997). The student should keep in mind that prescriptive approaches are in a state of evolutionary development, so that modifications and new methods are frequently encountered, and that different prescriptive methods can recommend different gain configurations for the same patient.

Prescriptive formulas or methods for hearing aid characteristics can be classified as either threshold-based or suprathreshold-based approaches. **Threshold-based methods** determine the prescription from the patient's unaided thresholds. The prototype method is Lybarger's (1944) **half-gain rule**, which essentially states that the amount of gain should be 50% of the threshold hearing level at each frequency except 500 Hz, where 30% gain is recommended. Many threshold-based methods have been proposed that prescribe different amounts and configurations of gain, as well as addressing severe-to-profound hearing losses and considerations involved in the fitting of sophisticated state-of-the-art instruments (e.g., McCandless & Lyregaard, 1983; Byrne & Dillon, 1986; Libby, 1986; Schwartz, Lyregaard, & Lundh, 1988; Berger, Hagberg & Rane, 1988; Byrne, Parkinson, & Newal, 1990; Killion, 1996; Seewald, Cornelisse, Ramji, Sinclair, Moodie, & Jamieson, 1997; Dillon, 1999a,b).

The **suprathreshold-based methods** employ one or more above-threshold measures to arrive at the prescription, such as most comfortable listening levels (MCLs), loudness discomfort levels (LDLs), or loudness judgments for narrow bands of noise or warble tones as a function of frequency. Some of these methods attempt to prescribe the gain configuration needed to place the *long-term average speech spectrum* at the listener's MCL

---

[6] Many of these procedures refer to saturation sound pressure level (SSPL), which was the former terminology for OSPL.

or approximately midway between the patient's thresholds and loudness discomfort levels (e.g., Watson & Knudsen, 1940; Shapiro, 1976, 1980; Bragg, 1977; Cox, 1988; Skinner, 1988). An approach by Levitt, Sullivan, Neuman, and Rubin-Spitz (1987) amplifies the speech signal to levels 10 dB below the patient's LDLs for most frequencies. Another protocol uses thresholds and loudness judgments, and attempts to enable the patient to experience soft sound levels as audible and soft, average sound levels as comfortable, and high sound levels as loud but not uncomfortably loud (Cox, 1995; Valente & Van Vliet, 1997).

In addition to the desired amount of gain as a function of frequency, it is also important to prescribe OSPL90 values that do not exceed the patient's loudness discomfort levels. Output sound pressure levels can be prescribed based on loudness discomfort level measurements (using, e.g., narrow-band noises or warble tones) or employing various estimating procedures (e.g., Cox, 1983, 1985; Hawkins, Walden, Montgomery, & Prosek, 1987; PWG, 1996; Cox, Alexander, Taylor, & Gray, 1997; ASHA, 1998; Dillon & Storey, 1998; Storey, Dillon, Yeend, & Wigney, 1998; Dillon, 1999a).

The prescription may also be viewed in terms of **targets**. For example, the targeted frequency response expresses the amount of gain that we want delivered to the patient's eardrum at each frequency. Similarly, maximum output is also prescribed in terms of target values for OSPL90 at the patient's eardrum. The ideal hearing aid would be the one that actually provides these targeted values. To achieve this goal with BTE and body hearing aids, the clinician selects a stock instrument based on the information provided in the manufacturer's specifications book. For ITE and canal aids, the audiologist places a customized order with the manufacturer, who then fabricates an instrument using electronic and acoustical methods that should provide the prescribed characteristics.

Once the hearing aid is obtained, we must confirm that it is working without problems (e.g., noisiness or intermittencies), that it fits

properly and comfortably, and that it actually provides the intended amplification characteristics (the *verification stage* in Table 15–3). That the instrument actually meets the intended electroacoustic characteristics selected by the audiologist is **verified** by testing the instrument in a hearing aid test box using the measurements described in the ANSI S3.22 (1996) standard. These are essential measurements about the hearing aid itself, but they do not tell us what the instrument is doing for the patient. Hence, we must also test the hearing aid *on the patient* to verify that it is actually providing her with the intended performance. The *preferred method* for verifying hearing aid performance with respect to the patient involves **real-ear (or probe-tube) measurements**, although some of the information can also be determined behaviorally with **functional gain measurements** (PWG, 1996; ASHA, 1998). It is often necessary for the audiologist to "fine-tune" the hearing aid's characteristics to bring them as close as possible to the targeted values. This is done by adjusting the hearing aid's internal controls (known as trim pots) or with program adjustments for state-of-the-art programmable hearing aids.

In addition to verifying the adequacy of the fitting in terms of consistency with the prescribed characteristics, it is also desirable to validate the benefits afforded to the patient using formal and/or informal techniques (Hawkins et al, 1991; ASHA, 1998), corresponding to the validation stage in Table 15–3. **Validation** may be accomplished in a variety of ways that might employ, for example, speech intelligibility tests, quality and/or intelligibility judgments, or other assessment tools. Notice that speech intelligibility assessment is now used as one of several ways to validate the adequacy of a hearing aid fitting, whereas it was the criterion measure for selecting among instruments in the traditional HAE approach.

Postfitting Considerations

There is almost always a 30-day trial period during which the patient may elect to return the hearing aid. Although one should not lose sight of the consumer protection aspects of the trial period, it is probably more important for the audiologist and patient to consider it at the time when the *orientation stage* (Table 15–3) of the hearing aid fitting process takes place. Consequently, the patient should be urged to return for consultation several times during this period, not just at the end. Schedule the first follow-up appointment before the patient leaves.

Once the hearing aid fitting has been judged acceptable, the patient and any significant others (family, parents, etc., depending on the specific circumstances) should be instructed about all aspects of the use and care of the instruments. The patient should know how to insert and remove the instrument, use its controls, clean and maintain it, replace batteries, etc. She should understand the goals of amplification, realistic expectations for what hearing aids can and cannot do, and the nature of effective listening strategies. These initial clinical counseling activities should also include the consideration of assistive devices and other aural rehabilitation services.

A word about batteries is in order before proceeding. The patient and others who handle the instruments should also be made aware that hearing aid batteries are to be treated as a dangerous poison. This is not an overstatement. Batteries should be inaccessible to children and pets; even adult patients should be reminded never to use their lips as an extra set of hands while changing batteries. Special attention should be given to battery safety with pediatric patients and others who require special supervision.

Group and Classroom Amplification Systems

Effects of Noise and Room Acoustics

In spite of the benefits provided by their personal hearing aids, hearing-impaired children still have considerable problems communicating in classrooms because of **noise** and **reverberation**. **Group** or **classroom amplification systems** are used to minimize

these effects, and thereby present an optimal signal to each hearing-impaired child (or adult) in the room. The term *auditory trainer* is sometimes encountered when these kinds of systems are used in therapy. Personal amplification systems are also available for individual use. Even though we are focusing on the hearing-impaired child who is trying to listen to the teacher in a classroom, one should realize that the same issues apply to *all* hearing-impaired persons in *all* noisy and/or reverberant environments, such as theaters, houses of worship, and auditoriums.

Room acoustics have a considerable impact on the effectiveness and quality of communication, and the importance of hearing in all facets of education makes classroom acoustics in particular an area of major concern (e.g., ASHA, 1995; Crandell, Smaldino, Flexer, 1997; Palmer, 1997; Federal Register, 1998; Rosenberg, Blake-Rahter, Heavner, Allen, Redmond, Phillips, & Stigers, 1999; Crandell & Smaldino, 2000). Recommended acoustical criteria for classrooms include (1) a maximum unoccupied noise level of 30 dBA, (2) a signal-to-noise ratio of at least +15 dB at the child's ear, and (3) a maximum reverberation time of 0.4 seconds (ASHA, 1995).

Classroom noise comes from a variety of sources inside and outside the room, with which we are all familiar from common experience. Ambient noise levels vary among classrooms, but are typically about 60 dB or more (Ross & Giolas, 1971; Crandell, Smaldino, & Flexer, 1997; Rosenberg et al, 1999; Crandell & Smaldino, 2000). In contrast, Hodgson, Rempel, and Kennedy (1999) found that university classrooms and lecture halls have an average noise level of 44.4 dBA.

Particularly important for speech understanding is the relationship between the levels of the teacher's speech and the noise at the child's ears (or the microphones of her hearing aids). Recall that this relationship is a **signal-to-noise (S/N) ratio or SNR**. [The SNR is often called the **message-to-competition ratio (MCR)** when the noise is a competing speech signal, or the **speech-to-babble (S/B) ratio** when the noise is a babble composed of several voices.] Positive SNRs mean that the level of the signal (the speech) is greater than that of the noise, and negative SNRs indicate that the noise is stronger than the speech. For example, a +6 dB SNR means the signal is 6 dB greater than the noise, and a −6 dB SNR means the noise is 6 dB higher than the speech. A 0 dB SNR means the levels of the signal and noise are the same. Figure 15–14 illustrates these relationships as well as the manner in which SNR deteriorates with distance from the talker. Notice that the SNR falls from +18 dB immediately in front of the teacher's lips (1 foot) to 0 dB at a distance of just 8 feet, and to −6 dB when the child is 16 feet away. These are not uncommon distances in typical classrooms. Hearing-impaired persons need higher SNRs than normal individuals to achieve similar levels of performance while listening to speech in noise (Dubno, Dirks, & Morgan, 1984; Gelfand, Ross, & Miller, 1988). Hearing-impaired children require SNRs of at least +10 to +20 dB for effective classroom performance (Gengel, 1971; Finitzo-Hieber & Tillman, 1978), and ASHA (1995) recommends a minimum SNR of +15 dB at the child's ears. Yet, typical schoolroom SNRs are often only +1 to +6 dB

(Finitzo, 1988). In fact, even children who have minimal amounts of sensorineural hearing loss (with pure-tone averages between 15 and 30 dB HL) have significantly poorer speech recognition than their normal hearing counterparts, and the disadvantage becomes greater as the SNR decreases (Crandell, 1993), as illustrated in Figure 15–15.

Reverberation is the term used to describe the reflections of sounds from the walls, floors, ceilings, and other hard surfaces in the room. This multiplicity of reflections is perceived as a prolongation of the duration of a sound in a room. It can be heard by sharply clapping one's hands once in a classroom, and noticing that the resulting sound lingers after the initial sound. Reverberation is measured in terms of **reverberation time**, which is the duration of the reflections. Specifically, reverberation time is how long it takes for the reflected sounds to fall to a level that is 60 dB less than the original sound. Typical classroom reverberation times range from about 0.4 to 1.2 seconds (ASHA, 1995; Crandell & Smaldino, 2000). Speech recognition is adversely affected by reverberation because the reflections mask the direct sound

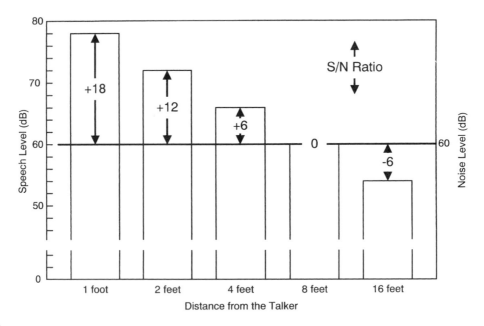

FIGURE 15–14   Speech level and signal-to-noise (S/N) ratio at various distances from the talker's lips (idealized).

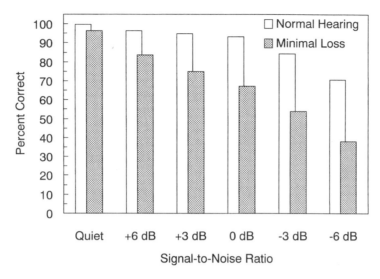

FIGURE 15–15 Percent correct speech recognition ability on BKB sentences for children with normal hearing and minimal sensorineural hearing losses (pure-tone average 15 to 30 dB HL). Based on data by Crandell (1993).

and also because some speech cues are distorted by their prolongation (Nabelek & Robinette, 1978; Gelfand & Silman, 1979; Gelfand, 1998). Speech perception worsens as reverberation time gets longer and when reverberation is mixed with noise, and the effect is greater for people with hearing loss than it is for those with normal hearing (Gelfand & Hochberg, 1976; Finitzo-Hieber & Tillman, 1978; Nabelek & Robinette, 1978; Yacullo & Hawkins, 1987; Crandell & Smaldino, 2000).

The effects of noise and reverberation depend a lot on the distance between the teacher and the child. Let's see why: Under the simplest conditions, sound pressure level drops by 6 dB whenever the distance from the sound source doubles. Suppose the teacher's overall speech level is 78 dB at one foot in front of her lips. The speech level will be 72 dB (i.e., 6 dB less) when the distance doubles to 2 feet, then it will drop to 66 dB at 4 feet, 60 dB at 8 feet, and 54 dB at 16 feet. Thus, if the noise level is 60 dB, then the SNR will be 0 dB at a distance of 8 feet and −6 dB at 16 feet from the teacher. The effects of reverberation are also smaller near the teacher's lips and become greater with distance. This is so because the intensity of the original sound is relatively greater than that of the reflections close to the source, whereas the reflections are dominant at some distance away from the source.

We can now appreciate why a hearing-impaired child experiences so much difficulty listening through her hearing aids in a classroom. Hearing aids pick up all sounds present at their microphones, which are located on the child who is sitting in a noisy and reverberant classroom. Thus, the hearing aid delivers a noisy and reverberant signal to the child. The workable solution is to place a microphone close to the teacher's lips where her speech is least affected by the acoustics of the room. The signal from this optimally placed microphone can then be amplified and sent directly to receivers in the child's ears. This simple strategy is the basis for many of the group amplification systems about to be described.

Types of Group Amplification Systems

The basic components of almost all group amplification systems involve a microphone placed close to the teacher's mouth, an amplifier with its controls, and some type of receiver to direct the amplified sound into the child's ears. The principal difference among the various types of systems has to do with how the signal picked up by the teacher's microphone is transmitted to the receivers at the children's ears. To keep the hands free, most systems use *lapel microphones, lavaliere microphones* that hang from a cord around the neck, or *boom microphones* connected to a headset like the ones used by telephone operations. It is important that the microphone be placed so that it properly picks up the talker's speech and also does not interfere with speech reading (Medwetsky & Boothroyd, 1991; Lewis, 1994a,b). Some systems also include microphones for each child, typically called **environmental microphones**. Environmental microphones permit the children to hear each other, and also allow each child to monitor her own speech.

HARD-WIRED SYSTEMS

The oldest and technologically simplest classroom amplification systems involved components that were physically connected by wires. The teacher's microphone was wired to a console containing an amplifier and controls, from which wires went to control boxes and headsets at each of the children's desks. Hardwired systems can provide high sound levels with good fidelity. They are also relatively low in cost and easy to repair. However, the teacher and students can move no further than the lengths of the cables allow, making them physically restrictive and inflexible. In addition, these systems typically lack environmental microphones, so that student participation and self-monitoring are limited at best.

INDUCTION-LOOP SYSTEMS

Induction-loop classroom amplification systems use a *magnetic signal* to transmit the teacher's speech to the children in the room. The teacher's microphone connects to an amplifier and then to a wire (**induction-loop**) that encircles the classroom, as in Figure 15–16. The induction-loop sends a magnetic signal into the room, which is then received by the telecoil of each child's hearing aid. Thus, the child's hearing aid becomes the final amplification device and receiver in induction-loop systems (although special induction receivers are also available). This is made possible by switching the hearing aid to its "T" position to receive the signal from the induction-loop, or to the "MT" position to hear the teacher via the telecoil and to hear other students and monitor his own speech through the microphone. The benefits and limitations of induction-loop systems are listed in Table 15–4.

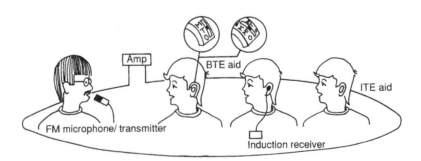

FIGURE 15–16 Induction-loop systems transmit a magnetic signal to the telecoils of a student's own hearing aids, or to a special induction receiver. In the modem induction-loop system shown here, the teacher uses a wireless microphone/transmitter that sends an FM radio signal to the induction-loop amplifier. From Lewis (1994a), with permission of American Speech-Language-Hearing Association.

TABLE 15–4   Some advantages and limitations of various group amplification systems[a]

Induction-loop systems
  Advantages
    Usable with a wide range of hearing losses
    Relative freedom of movement within the room
    Takes advantage of individual hearing aids as receivers for system
    Relatively low cost to school
  Limitations
    Hearing aids must have telecoils
    Hearing aids function differently via telecoil compared to microphone
    Broken hearing aid denies child access to group system
    Signal varies with location in the room
    Signal varies with how telecoil is oriented with respect to the loop
    Interference from loops in other rooms (cross-talk)
    Interference from other electromagnetic signals
    Cannot be used outside of room with induction loop (not portable)
FM systems
  Advantages
    Usable with a wide range of hearing losses
    No cross-talk between rooms because any FM channels available
    Environmental microphones for class participation and self-monitoring
    Usable outside of building (portable)
    Personal hearing aids not needed with self-contained FM system
  Limitations
    Child must wear FM receiver unit
    Interference from other FM sources
    Personal hearing aids and coupling needed with personal FM systems
    More complicated maintenance and troubleshooting
    Relatively higher relative cost
Infrared systems
  Advantages
    Convenient for use in theaters, houses of worship, other public forums
    No cross-talk between rooms
    Do not require personal hearing aid
  Limitations
    Output levels generally more limited than FM and induction loop system
    Signals blocked by obstructions between transmitter and receiver
    Interference from sunlight prevents outside use (not portable)
    No environmental microphones
Soundfield amplification systems
  Advantages
    Advantageous for a wide range of groups
    Receiving device not needed
    Provides improved signal for everyone in room
    Does not stigmatize individuals
    Reduces teacher's vocal stress
    Easily maintained
    Relatively lower cost
  Limitations
    If used all by itself, useful only with relatively milder hearing losses.
    Loudspeakers must be properly placed and oriented.
    Cannot be used outside of room where installed (not portable).

[a] Gilmore and Lederman (1989); Leavitt (1991); Flexer (1992, 1994); Beck et al (1993); Lewis (1994a,b); Crandell, Smaldino, & Flexer (1995); Compton (2000).

FM SYSTEMS

Most modern classroom amplification systems are **FM (frequency modulation) systems**, and a great deal of attention has been given to their use in a wide variety of applications (Ross, 1992; ASHA, 2000; Lewis, 1994a,b). In an FM system, the teacher's voice is picked up by a portable microphone/transmitter and is sent by an FM radio signal to receivers worn by each child (Fig. 15–17). The Federal Communications Commission has designated two bandwidths (72–76 mHz and 216–217 mHz) for use with FM amplification systems, which are each broken down into 10 wide-band channels and/or as many as 40 narrow-band channels. The FM receiver can deliver the signal to the child directly through a variety of transducers, or it can be connected to the child's own hearing aid. **Personal FM receivers** usually connect to the child's own hearing aid(s), whereas **self-contained FM receivers** contain circuits and controls that enable them to replace the child's hearing aids while in the classroom. Various combinations are shown in Figure 15-18. A third type of available FM receiver is either built into a behind-the-ear hearing aid or snaps onto the bottom of the hearing aid. Class participation and self-monitoring are made possible by environmental microphones on each receiver. Clinical guidelines for the fitting and monitoring of FM systems are provided by ASHA (2000). Some of the principal advantages and disadvantages of FM systems are outlined in Table 15–4.

The FM receiver can be connected (coupled) to the child's hearing aids by direct audio input or induction (Fig. 15–18). **Direct audio input** involves a wire that plugs into both the FM receiver and the hearing aid, and requires the hearing aid to be equipped with a direct audio input jack. With **induction coupling**, the FM receiver sends a magnetic signal to the hearing aid's telecoil by way of a personally worn inductor, which comes in two general styles. **Neck-loop inductors** are induction loops worn around the child's neck. **Silhouette inductors** house the inductor in a flat case that has the same shape as the hearing aid, and are worn next to the hearing aid itself. One should be aware the hearing aid's output can be different when it is coupled to an FM system compared to when it is used alone (Hawkins & Schum, 1985).

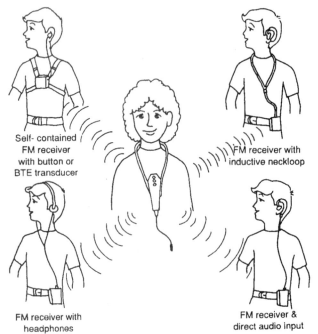

Self- contained FM receiver with button or BTE transducer

FM receiver with inductive neckloop

FM receiver with headphones

FM receiver & direct audio input

FIGURE 15–17 An FM amplification systems showing various receiver options. From Lewis (1994a), with permission of American Speech-Language-Hearing Association.

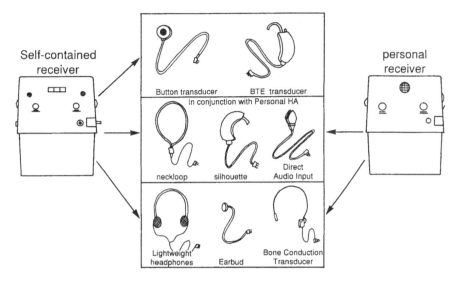

FIGURE 15–18 Options available for delivering the signal from the FM receiver to the wearer's ear(s). From Lewis (1994a), with permission of American Speech-Language-Hearing Association.

INFRARED SYSTEMS

With an **infrared system**, the signal from the talker's microphone is sent by an infrared light transmitter to individually worn receivers in the room. The infrared receivers convert the light signal back to sound, which is directed into the wearer's ears. A typical infrared device is shown in Figure 15–19. These systems are rarely used in regular classrooms, but are widely used as assistive devices by hearing-impaired persons in theaters, houses of worship, auditoriums, and other public forums. The system shown in the figure includes a transmitter for personal use, such as improving the hearing-impaired person's ability to hear television programs. Some of their advantages and limitations are listed in Table 15–4.

SOUNDFIELD AMPLIFICATION SYSTEMS

Soundfield (or **soundfield FM**) **amplification systems** (Crandell & Smaldino, 1992; Crandell, Smaldino, & Flexer, 1995, 1997) differ from the other approaches described because they transmit amplified sound directly into the room (a soundfield) rather than to individually worn receivers. Specifically, the signal from the talker's microphone is sent by an FM transmitter to an amplifier, and is then directed to several loudspeakers placed

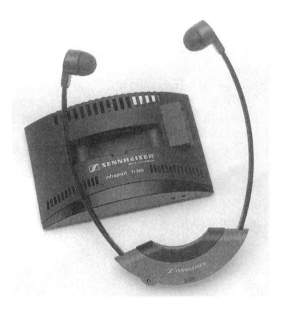

FIGURE 15–19 An infrared system transmitter and receiver. Photography courtesy of Sennheiser Electronic Corp.

around the room. The idea is to keep the level of the talker's speech about 10 dB higher than the ambient noise level all through the room, so that everyone present is provided with an improved signal. Although implementing a soundfield amplification system is beyond our scope (see, e.g., Crandell, Smaldino, & Flexer, 1995, 1997), it should be noted that the proper acoustical analyses need to be done, and that the system cannot be a haphazard modification of a public address (PA) system with a few loudspeakers. For example, soundfield amplification is not appropriate in highly reverberant rooms, and improper loudspeaker arrangements may result in an amplified signal that is inferior to the original one (Leavitt, 1991; Flexer, 1992, 1994; Crandell, Smaldino, & Flexer, 1995; Rosenberg et al, 1999).

Soundfield amplification produces several kinds of benefits for a wide range of individuals (see, e.g., Flexer, 1992, 1994; Crandell, Smaldino, & Flexer, 1995): Among the advantageous outcomes are improved speech recognition performance, attending skills and academic performance for students, as well as reduced vocal (and other) stress for teachers. Those who appear to benefit from soundfield amplification include

- children under about 15 years old;
- children with all kinds of hearing disorders (conductive, sensorineural, minimal, unilateral, fluctuating);
- children with language, articulation, learning and attention disorders, and developmental delays; and
- children who are not native speakers of English.

Several of the benefits and limitations of soundfield amplification systems are enumerated in Table 15–4.

Cochlear Implants

Some hearing losses are so extensive that there is little if any residual hearing, and the patient is unable to derive any appreciable benefit from even the most powerful hearing aids. Other types of sensory aids are needed for these patients. **Cochlear implants** attempt to provide the patient with information about sound by converting it into an electrical current, and then using this electrical signal to directly stimulate any remaining auditory nerve fibers the patient might still have.

Cochlear implants are composed of both internal components that are surgically installed and external devices worn outside the body (Figs. 15–20 to 15–23). The **external components** include (1) a **microphone** that picks up sound and converts it into an electrical signal; (2) the **speech processor** that analyzes the sound and converts it into a code representing various aspects of the sound; (3) a **transmitter** that sends the encoded information to the implanted device via an electromagnetic or radio frequency (RF) signal. The **surgically implanted components** include (1) a **receiver** that picks up the signal from the external transmitter, and (2) the **electrical stimulator** with its **electrodes** that are inserted into the cochlea (Fig. 15–23). The electrodes send the encoded information to the remaining fibers of the auditory nerve in the form of an electrical signal. In addition, a ground electrode is placed somewhere outside the cochlea, such as in the middle ear. Speech processor units are available in both body-worn and ear-level styles, as shown in the figures.

Cochlear implants are generally categorized as either single-channel or multiple-channel devices. Early cochlear implants were **single-channel** devices, exemplified by the 3M/House single-electrode system. This implant treats the sound entering the microphone as a whole, and delivers an electrical signal to the remaining auditory nerve fibers via an electrode inserted approximately 6 mm into the scale tympani through the round window. To do this, the sound picked up by the microphone is used to modulate a carrier signal, which in turn becomes the electrical code conveyed by the electrode. The 3M/House device was discontinued in 1987, and all modern cochlear implants are multiple-channel units.

Multiple-channel cochlear implants use several electrodes laid out along the cochlea, as illustrated in Figure 15–23. Cochlear Corporation's *Nucleus 22* and *24* systems have

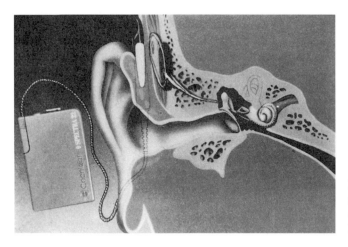

FIGURE 15–20 Representation of a cochlear implant in a patient, showing external and implanted components. Picture courtesy of Cochlear Corp.

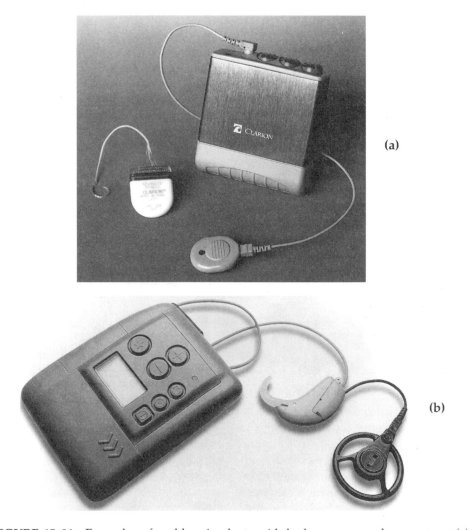

(a)

(b)

FIGURE 15–21 Examples of cochlear implants with body worn speech processors. (a) Clarion system showing speech processing (above), headpiece containing the microphone and external transmitter (below) and implanted electrical stimulator and electrodes (left). Photograph courtesy of Advanced Bionics Corp. (b) Nucleus 24 system showing speech processor left, ear-level microphone (center), and external transmitter (right). The implanted components are shown in Figure 15-22. Photograph courtesy of Cochlear Corp.

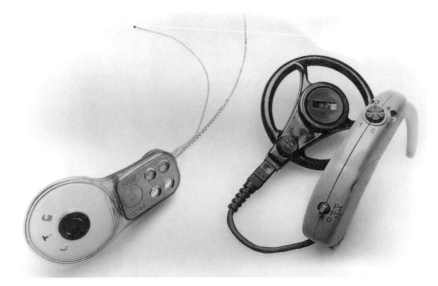

FIGURE 15–22   Example of a cochlear implant with an ear-level speech processor (Nucleus 24). Left: implanted electrical stimulator and electrodes. Right: Ear-level speech processor and microphone unit along with the external transmitting coil. Photograph courtesy of Cochlear Corp.

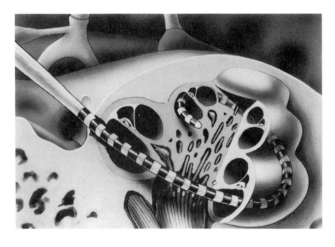

FIGURE 15–23 Illustration of the electrodes of a multiple-channel cochlear implant inserted into the cochlea. Electrodes representing higher frequencies are toward the base of the cochlea and those representing lower frequencies are toward the apex. Picture courtesy of Cochlear Corp.

22 evenly spaced electrodes, Advanced Bionics' *Clarion* systems employ 16 electrodes in eight pairs, and the Med-EL *CIS Pro+* and *TEMPO+* systems have 24 electrodes arranged in 12 pairs. In each case, the electrodes closer to the base of the cochlea represent higher frequencies and those toward the apex represent lower frequencies. In other words, the electrode layout follows the pattern of how frequencies are arranged by place along the cochlea. The cochlear implant's microprocessor analyzes the incoming sound in terms of various parameters, which are coded into combinations of tiny currents delivered to the electrodes laid out in the cochlea. Various coding strategies are used to represent the speech signal. For example, the patterns of stimulation from the array of electrodes might represent the spectral peaks of the incoming sound, speech features like formants and fricative noises, or the waveform of the incoming signal. Some approaches activate one electrode at a time in rapid succession, whereas other systems activate sev-

eral electrodes simultaneously. Information about the intensity of a sound is provided by the strength of the current coming from the electrodes. Some cochlear implants use just one program and other systems can store several programs in the processor's memory.

Cochlear implants are in a stage of rapid, ongoing development, and this evolutionary process will continue well into the future. This is true of the technology itself and every aspect of its experimental and clinical use. For example, there are ongoing changes in the instrumentation and processing strategies, who is considered a candidate for implantation, in how and when performance is tested, and in the content and duration of training. It is thus difficult to describe the benefits provided by cochlear implants in unequivocal terms. The situation is further complicated when the patients are children because the effects of developmental factors come into play.

In spite of differences in subjects, implant devices, processing strategies, testing methods, and a host of other variations among studies, we are still able to delineate many important generalities about the benefits and limitations of cochlear implants (e.g., Staller, Dowell, Beiter, & Brimacombe, 1991; Geers & Moog, 1994; Nicholas, 1994; Waltzman, Cohen, Gomolin, et al, 1994; NIH, 1995; Waltzman, Fisher, Niparko, et al, 1995; Nevins & Chute, 1996; Osberger, Robbins, Todd, Riley, Kirk, & Carney, 1996; Clark, Cowan, & Dowell, 1997; Staller, Menapace, Domico, et al, 1997; Tyler, Parkinson, Fryauf-Bertchy, et al, 1997; Sehgal, Kirk, Suirsky, & Miyamoto, 1998; Beiter & Brimacombe, 2000; Chute & Nevins, 2000; Waltzman & Shapiro, 2000). Cochlear implants provide several types of auditory perceptions, such as (1) general sound awareness; (2) temporal parameters (e.g., beginning and ending of a sound, duration, temporal patterns); (3) intensity discrimination; (4) pitch discrimination (which was limited to below about 300 Hz in the single-channel devices); (5) environmental sound recognition; and (6) widely variable speech recognition. Above and beyond auditory perception, per se, enhancement of

speechreading performance is an especially important benefit of cochlear implantation. In addition, it has been established that:

- Performance varies very widely among cochlear implant users.
- Performance is appreciably better with multiple-channel implants than it is for single-channel units. For example, single-channel implant users get some speech recognition on closed-set (multiple-choice) tests but essentially no speech understanding on open-set (fill-in) tests, whereas at least some degree of open-set speech recognition ability is enjoyed by most multiple-channel cochlear implant users.
- Multiple-channel devices yield open-set speech recognition scores ranging from 0% to 100%, depending on the individual, device, processor, conditions, and test used.
- Cochlear implantation results in enhancement of speech and language development in deaf children.
- Performance with cochlear implants improves over time (with increased duration of implantation).
- Speech perception skills improve when implants are "upgraded" from older processing approaches to more sophisticated processing strategies.

Finally, it has been found that the chances of success with cochlear implants are improved when (1) the onset of the hearing impairment is postlingual rather than prelingual, (2) the duration of deafness is shorter rather than longer, and (3) implantation occurs sooner rather than later.

It should be apparent that cochlear implants provide considerable benefits compared to no usable hearing, but in absolute terms, these advantages may not compare favorably with those typically obtained by even severely hearing-impaired patients who are able to use hearing aids. Even though current cochlear implants do not provide the typical listener with a means to use audition as an independent vehicle for communication, they serve as a valuable aid to speechreading and as a supplement to other communicative intervention strategies.

The Food and Drug Administration (FDA) has approved cochlear implants for clinical use with both adults and children. Certainly, this does not mean that every child and adult is an appropriate candidate for an implant. This is so because only limited benefits can be expected from a cochlear implant, and its installation requires that the patient undergo surgery and general anesthesia. Therefore, it is imperative that the patient be audiologically and medically suited for a cochlear implant.

The original conception of an audiologically appropriate candidate for cochlear implantation was a patient with a bilateral, profound sensorineural hearing loss who did not receive any significant benefits from hearing aids. The requirement for no significant benefits from hearing aids is rather straightforward among adults, who can be formally tested and also have a known history of unsuccessful hearing aid experience. However, this can be a tricky issue in young children. A trial period with hearing aids and/or tactile aids is usually in order before the viability of a cochlear implant is assessed. This period should be combined with a pretraining program especially for young children (e.g., Beiter, Staller, & Dowell, 1991; NIH, 1995).

Implantation criteria are changing rather rapidly as more information and experience are accumulated. The original requirement that patients be postlingually deafened adults slowly evolved to include postlingually deafened children, and then prelingually deaf children. The 1995 National Institutes of Health consensus statement on cochlear implants (NIH, 1995) recommended considering implantation for (1) adults with severe to profound losses and best aided open-set sentence recognition scores of ≤30%; and (2) children as young as 2 years old with bilateral profound losses ≥ 90 dB HL and only minimal speech perception performance under the best amplified conditions after a trial period that includes intensive auditory training. However, current thinking is to consider implantation in marginal or borderline cases, with criteria like sentence recognition scores of (1) ≤40% (≤50% in some clinical trials) and ≤20% for consonant–vowel nucleus–consonant

(CNC) word recognition for adults, and (2) ≤20% on the Lexical Neighborhood Test or the Modified Lexical Neighborhood Test for children. Moreover, the FDA now approves cochlear implantation for children as young as 18 months (12 months in some clinical trials).

Several medical and surgical criteria must be met for cochlear implantation (e.g., Pyman, Brown, Dowell, & Clark, 1990; Gray, 1991; NIH, 1995; Chute & Nevins, 2000; Waltzman & Shapiro, 2000). There must be working auditory nerve fibers that can be stimulated by the implant and the existence of the relevant cochlear anatomy. These criteria are met by using high-resolution computerized tomography (CT scans) to rule out such structural abnormalities as cochlear agenesis or dysplagia, or the absence of an auditory nerve. The viability of the remaining auditory nerve fibers can be tested by seeing if an auditory sensation is produced by electrical stimulation of the promontory. This procedure involves inserting a needle electrode through the tympanic membrane. (Another test site is the round window niche.) The integrity of the existing auditory nerve fibers can also be demonstrated by the presence of low-frequency audiometric thresholds providing they are actually heard as opposed to being tactile responses. In addition to these factors, the patient's general health must be good enough to undergo surgery and general anesthesia.

Realistic expectations play an especially important role in cochlear implant candidacy. This issue cannot be taken lightly because patients and their parents can develop the faulty belief that cochlear implants are an overnight cure for deafness. This misconception is fostered by the mystique associated with surgery and is nurtured by unrealistic media coverage that is occasionally given to high-tech innovations. The patient and/or parents need to know what the implant can and cannot do, the variability of the results, and the importance of a strong commitment to training after the device is installed. Moreover, even though cochlear implant surgery has a relatively low incidence of major complications, they can and do occur, and these issues should be discussed with the patient and/or parents.

After the surgery is completed and healing has occurred, the next step is to program the device for optimal use by the individual patient. The **programming** process is also called **mapping**. Programming involves adjusting the electrical currents produced by the electrodes to yield appropriate thresholds and comfortable listening levels, and allocating frequency bandwidths to the various electrodes. Children often require a period of preprogramming training to teach them the tasks involved in programming the cochlear implant. A period of auditory training is needed after the implant has been installed and programmed. This can last anywhere from a month or so for adults with adventitious deafness to a comprehensive, long-term intervention program for children with prelingual deafness.

Tactile Aids

Tactile aids are another class of sensory aids for the deaf that use tactile sensations to *substitute* for auditory ones. Tactile aids are similar to cochlear implants in the sense that sounds picked up by a microphone are analyzed and encoded by a single- or multiple-channel processor. However, instead of converting sound into an electrical signal that is transmitted to the auditory nerve and perceived auditorily, tactile aids transmit a stimulus to the skin that is perceived tactually. Either a **vibrator (vibrotactile stimulator)** or an **electrical (electrotactile or electrocutaneous) stimulator** can be used to produce the tactile responses. The stimulators have been worn at various sites, such as the wrist, arm, chest, abdomen, waist, and thighs. (Even though some of the best performance has been obtained when vibrators are worn on the fingertips, this location is not practical because it interferes with manual tasks.) Tactile aids are not the only kind of sensory substitution method that have been used. For example, various kinds of visual displays have also been designed and studied; however, this approach has not achieved clinical acceptance.

Single-channel tactile devices often used the incoming speech signal to modulate the vibration, and represent sound amplitude as the strength of the vibration. This approach is analogous to what was described for single-channel cochlear implants. **Multiple-channel** tactile aids use an array of vibrators laid out on the skin. Multiple-channel tactile aids like the one shown in Figure 15–24 have stimulators arranged in a line. Here, frequency information is represented by which vibrators are active, and intensity is coded as the strength of the vibration. This is analogous to the arrangement of electrodes in a cochlear implant. More complicated representations use a matrix of stimulators in columns and rows, so that the vibratory pattern represents the spectrum of an incoming sound as a graph "drawn" on the skin.

Tactile aids have been studied in some detail (e.g., Sherrick, 1984; ASHA, 1986; Hnath-Chisolm & Kishon-Rabin, 1988; Cowan, Blamey, Galvin, Sarant, Alcantara, & Clark, 1990; Carney, Osberger, Carney, Robbins, Rehshaw, & Miyamoto, 1993; Osberger, Maso, & Sam, 1993; Seffens, Eilers, Fishman, Oller,

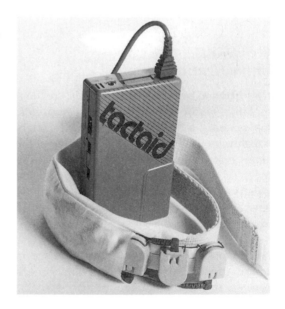

FIGURE 15–24 An example of a currently available multiple-channel tactile aid (Tactaid 7), showing its array of seven vibrators. Photograph courtesy of Audiological Engineering Corp.

& Urbano, 1994; Weisenberger & Percy, 1995; Kishon-Rabin, Boothroyd, & Hanin, 1996; Ertmer, Kirk, Sehgal, Riley, & Osberger, 1997; Sehgal, Kirk, Svirsky, Ertmer, & Osberger, 1998; Galvin, Mavrias, Moore, Cowan, Blamey, & Clark, 1999; Plant, Gnosspelius, & Levitt, 2000). Although tactile aids are much cheaper than cochlear implants and also do not involve surgery, considerable training and practice are needed to make optimal use of the tactual signals. Many of the benefits provided by multiple-channel cochlear implants, including the important benefit of enhancing lipreading, have also been reported for multiple-channel tactile aids. However, cochlear implant results are considerably more impressive. In addition, cochlear implants provide at least some degree of open set word recognition for auditory-only stimulation but tactile aids do not appear to do this for tactual-only stimulation. Nevertheless, it is important to remember that tactile aids are desirable instruments for many patients, such as those who are not candidates for cochlear implants or choose not to have one, and are also beneficial during the period prior to receiving an implant, for preimplantation training, etc.

Assistive Devices for the Hearing Impaired

In addition to personal hearing aids, cochlear implants, tactile aids, and group amplification systems, a diverse and growing variety of technologies are available to help meet the communicative requirements of the hearing impaired and deaf. These are often called **assistive listening devices**, but the more general term **assistive devices** is preferred because not all approaches involve the auditory channel (Compton, 2000). Some devices must be used alone, while others are used in combination with one's hearing aids, speech reading, and sign language interpreters.

Telephone Devices

Hearing aid compatibility has been required for most new telephones since 1991. The simplest systems are telephones that provide amplified signals, often with a volume control. The use of special telephone amplifiers is facilitated by the common use of modular telephone connectors, which are available as special replacement handsets or as in-line amplifiers installed between the telephone and the handset. One should be sure to check for electronic compatibility with the telephone when using replacement handsets and in-line amplifiers. Several telephones specially designed for use by the hearing impaired are also available, as are various portable amplifiers. Portable amplifiers and other instruments can pick up either acoustic or magnetic signals from telephones, or are connected by direct audio input.

Telecommunication devices for the deaf (TDDs) or **text telephones (TTs)** as well as personal computers (PCs) provide telephone access for those who cannot hear amplified speech from the telephone. The TDD is basically a portable terminal that sends and receives typed messages via the telephone. The TDD and telephone are often connected using an acoustic coupler. Communication between people using voice telephones and TDDs (or a computer) is made possible by dual-party relay systems, which telephone companies must provide under Public Law 101-336 (the Americans with Disabilities Act). Communication between TDDs and PCs has been somewhat of a problem because TDDs have traditionally used a system called **Baudot code**, whereas PCs use **ASCII code** and also operate at much faster transmission rates. As one might expect, TDDs are now available that can use both formats.

Television and Related Devices

Closed captioning is probably the most well-known assistive approach in current use. It involves providing subtitles on a television monitor or movie screen giving the gist of what is being said from moment to moment. Although closed captioning previously necessitated the use of a decoder box, Public Law 101-431 (the Television Decoder Circuitry Act of 1990) mandates that closed caption decoders be built into all new television sets with screens 13 inches in size and larger. **Real-time captioning** involves providing the detailed text of what is being said, and is often desirable for lectures and similar situations.

Alerting and Safety Devices

Many hearing-impaired individuals cannot rely upon the auditory channel to know when the doorbell is ringing, the alarm clock sounds, or when emergency signals like smoke or burglar alarms go off. For this reason, sound signals like bells, tones, buzzers, and sirens are supplemented or replaced with flashing lights and/or vibrators on all kinds of common devices. In addition, special purpose devices are also available, such as lights or vibrators that indicate when a call is coming in on a telecommunication device, or when the baby is crying. We should not forget that hearing ear dogs can often supplement electronic alerting devices, and can serve as portable alerting devices as well as companions to their severely hearing impaired or deaf owners.

Intervention Approaches

Auditory and Visual Training

One of our principal goals is to maximize the amount and quality of speech information that the hearing-impaired patient can obtain. This involves (1) providing an optimum acoustical signal with hearing aids or other devices, and (2) training the patient to derive the most information about the spoken message from what he hears and sees by using the acoustical and visual representations of speech to the fullest, and taking advantage of various forms of contextual and linguistic cues. Even though we will be considering some aspects of speechreading and auditory training separately, the student should know from the outset that combined auditory-visual training is usually the preferred treatment mode. Also, virtually all practice exercises can be done in the auditory, visual, or combined audiovisual modes. In fact, it is not uncommon to present exercises in all three modes to demonstrate to the patient the benefits of using all possible communication channels, and to give him practice in doing so. In addition, most techniques are successfully used in both individual and group therapy.

Analytical and Synthetic Approaches

Therapy methods are traditionally divided into analytical and synthetic approaches. **Analytical** exercises concentrate on the recognition of individual sounds and words, and might be thought of as the "micro" approach. In contrast, **synthetic** methods can be conceived of as the "macro" approach because they concentrate upon deriving the meaning of what is being said rather than trying to catch every sound or word. These alternative approaches trace their origins to the classical schools of thought in lipreading instruction. The classical analytical schools were the Mueller-Walle (Bruhn, 1920) and Jena (Bunger, 1932) methods, and the traditional synthetic schools of thought were described by Nitchie (1912) and by Kinzie and Kinzie (1931), and are mentioned for historical perspective. Strict adherence to one approach is a thing of the past, and even the traditional schools actually used both analytical and synthetic activities. The terms *analytical* and *synthetic* continue to be employed to describe the two different classes of activities that are used.

Analytic exercises are the most formal. Typical syllable discrimination exercises might involve presenting the patient with two syllables (e.g., "ba–da," or "da–da") and having him indicate whether they are the same or different, or having the patient choose which one of three syllables is different from the other two (e.g., "se–sa–sha"). The same tasks can also be done with words. Recognition drills might involve having the patient identify the presented syllable or word by repeating it, or by choosing it from among a number of choices. The syllables or words selected depend on the focus of the exercise. In addition, the patient is usually given feedback after each response.

There is an almost unlimited variety of synthetic techniques. These include counseling about effective communicative strategies and group discussion as well as practice exercises, per se. One type of exercise involves practice in receiving the main ideas of a sentence, paragraph, or passage-length material. For example, one might first give the patient the key words and/or the general topic of a passage, which is then presented to him. Responses can include anything from answering specific questions to having the patient retell the passage, or to incorporate the main ideas of the passage into a subsequent discussion. Another type of synthetic exercise involves having the patient fill in the gaps in a passage. A useful group therapy exercise involves videotaping a group discussion among several hearing-impaired patients, which is subsequently shown to them. The group can then discuss the communicative styles and strategies used, dealing with such topics as taking advantage of context, listening for main ideas rather than trying to catch every word, the importance of asking for clarification when needed, etc.

Continuous-Discourse Tracking

DeFilipo and Scott (1978) described a technique known as **continuous-discourse tracking**, which is popular both as a therapy approach and as a testing procedure. In speech tracking, the clinician orally presents a passage to the patient, who must in turn repeat it back verbatim and on an ongoing basis. Thus, the patient literally tracks what the clinician is saying: the clinician says a phrase, the patient repeats it word-for-word, the clinician presents the next phrase, the patient says it back exactly, etc. This continues until the patient makes an error. Then the clinician provides the patient with a variety of clues and prompts to help her get the correct word(s). The prompts might include repeating the misperceived word, paraphrasing it, using fill-ins, or any of a host of other tactics to help the patient get the correct word. Tracking performance is assessed in terms of the number of words per minute that can be repeated by the patient.

Effectiveness of Formal Training Exercises

There is no question that formal training procedures are essential and beneficial for hearing-impaired children. On the other hand, the ability of formal auditory training and lipreading instruction to improve the speech recognition ability of adults with adventitious hearing losses is another issue. Several carefully carried-out studies have shown various kinds of improvements from both lipreading instruction and auditory training (Walden, Prosek, Montgomery, Scherr, & Jones, 1977; Walden, Erdman, Montgomery, Schwartz, & Prosek, 1981; Montgomery, Walden, Schwartz, & Prosek, 1984; Rubinstein & Boothroyd, 1987). However, there are inconsistencies among at least some of the findings, and information about the long-term effectiveness of formal auditory-visual training is lacking. A compelling result in this context was reported by Rubinstein and Boothroyd (1987). They found that the only speech recognition measure showing a significant improvement after either analytical or synthetic auditory training regimens was the probability-high SPIN test (Kalikow, Stevens, & Elliot, 1977), which reflects the listener's ability to take advantage of the context of the test word. We will find that although formal auditory-visual training exercises are used, these are only one part of modern aural rehabilitation approaches for adults, which concentrate on the patient's overall communicative situation.

Adult Auditory-Training Approaches

The traditional approach to auditory training for adults was outlined by Carhart (1960). The goal was to train the patient "to take full advantage of the auditory cues that are still available to him" (p. 381). This involved counseling about the nature of the hearing disorder and listening strategies, reporting on various listening assignments, and formal analytic listening drills. Practice exercises were initially done in quiet, and then under more difficult listening conditions, such as in the presence of noise or reverberation.

Garstecki (1981) described a systematic auditory-visual training paradigm that manipulates the redundancy of the communicative situation in terms of (1) message type, (2) noise type, (3) signal-to-noise ratio, and (4) situational cues. Message type has to do with the content of the speech material, going from low message content materials like syllables or individual words to high content materials like paragraphs or stories. Noise type refers to the kind of acoustical background that is present during the speech. This may be quiet, white noise, one or more competing talkers, etc. The signal-to-noise (S/N) ratio refers to the intensity relationship between the speech signal and the noise being used. It can range from speech that is 12 dB greater than the noise (+12 dB SNR) down to noise levels that are 6 dB higher than the speech (−6 dB SNR). Situational cues involve the visual or auditory context of the speech material. The types of cues used may be *related* to the message versus *distracting*, or may be *omitted* altogether. Pretests are used to determine the combination of these parameters where the patient is able to achieve a certain percent correct level of performance (the "criterion level"). This becomes the starting point for training. Individual and group practice exercises are designed to help him to perform at successively lower levels of redundancy. Communication strategies such as making predictions from situational and nonverbal cues and optimizing listening situations are also provided.

Speechreading (Lipreading) Considerations

Lipreading or **speechreading** involves deriving meaning about what is being said by watching the talker. Although we will use the two terms interchangeably, "speechreading" is usually considered to be the preferred term because information is obtained from the visible movements of the articulators, facial expressions, gestures, etc., and not just the lips. Speechreading involves the visual channel of speech communication. It is a natural means of communication that we all use to supplement hearing, especially when listening conditions become difficult. It should thus come as no surprise that all people with hearing impairments must rely on speechreading to a greater or lesser extent. In fact, one of the most elegant distinctions between "hearing impairment" and "deafness" is that the primary channel of speech perception is audition for the former and vision for the latter (Ross, Brackett, & Maxon, 1982).

Speechreading skills vary widely among individuals. We can use lipreading tests to gain some insight into a given patient's speechreading ability, but it is difficult to predict how much a given patient will benefit from lipreading training. Typical reasons for testing speechreading skills are to (1) determine her basic speechreading ability, (2) help decide what kinds of training programs

TABLE 15–5   The Utley Lipreading Test, Form A (Utley, 1946)

1. All right.	17. What did you want?
2. Where have you been?	18. How much do you weigh?
3. I have forgotten.	19. I cannot stand him.
4. I have nothing.	20. She was home last week.
5. That is right.	21. Keep your eye on the ball.
6. Look you.	22. I cannot remember.
7. How have you been?	23. Of course.
8. I don't know if I can.	24. I flew to Washington.
9. How tall are you?	25. You look well.
10. It is awfully cold.	26. The train runs every hour.
11. My folks are home.	27. You had better go slow.
12. How much was it?	28. It says that in the book.
13. Good night.	29. We got home at six o'clock.
14. Where are you going?	30. We drove to the country.
15. Excuse me.	31. How much rain fell?
16. Did you have good time?	

TABLE 15–6   The Denver Quick Test of Lipreading Ability

1. Good morning,	11. May I help you?
2. How old are you?	12. I feel fine.
3. I live in (state of residence).	13. It is time for dinner.
4. I have only one dollar.	14. Turn right at the corner.
5. There is somebody at the door.	15. Are you ready to order?
6. Is that all?	16. Is this charge or cash?
7. Where are you going?	17. What time is it?
8. Let's have a coffee break.	18. I have a headache.
9. Park your car in the lot.	19. How about going out tonight?
10. What is your address?	20. Please lend me 50 cents.

From Alpiner, J.G. 1987. Evaluation of adult communication function. In J.G. Alpiner & P.A. McCarthy (eds.). Rehabilitative Audiology: Children and Adults. Baltimore: Williams & Wilkins, 44–114. Used with permission.

are most appropriate for her needs (e.g., by skill level), (3) help decide how to place her in a speechreading program (e.g., with new versus experienced lipreaders), and (4) ascertain the effects of the lesson (O'Neil & Oyer, 1981). A large variety of speechreading tests are available, and two of the more commonly used test lists are shown in Tables 15–5 and 15–6. These are the sentence part of the **Utley Lipreading Test** (Utley, 1946), which requires the patient to repeat what has been said; and the **Denver Quick Test of Lipreading Ability** (Alpiner, 1987), which requires the patient to identify the main idea expressed in each sentence.

One should be aware of the factors that affect speechreading because this becomes the basis for counseling patients about effective listening strategies and for many practice exercises. Optimal speechreading requires adequate illumination of the talker's face, and the lipreader should try to orient himself so light falls on the talker's face instead of in his own eyes. Other factors that affect speechreading to a greater or lesser extent include the distance between the talker and lipreader, viewing angle, familiarity with the speaker, articulation, speaking rate, facial expressions and gestures, age, feedback between the talker and speechreader; distracting behaviors (e.g., chewing and random gestures), as well as environmental distractions. Unfortunately, our understanding about how some of these factors influence lipreading has been clouded by inconsistent findings across studies. A number of these issues are being reex-

amined using more modern approaches. Speaking rate and viewing angle are two examples. Ijsseldijk (1992) found that different speaking rates and facial views (full face, two-thirds profile, and lips only) did not affect the speechreading performance of 8- to 16-year-olds who had profound hearing losses. Performance was improved by repetition of the material.

Speechreading is also affected by context, situational cues, knowledge of the topic, linguistic factors (e.g., sentence structure and word familiarity), and the redundancy of the message. As one might expect, the speechreader's visual acuity affects lipreading ability, but contrary to common wisdom, lipreading performance is not related to his personality attributes and intelligence (as long as it is not impaired).

Homophonous Sounds and Words

Certain speech sounds look the same "on the lips," such as /p/, /b/, and /m/, and therefore cannot be distinguished from one another on the basis of speechreading alone. Such sounds are called **homophonous sounds** or **homophemes**. Similarly, words that look the same are called **homophonous words** (e.g., "pat," "bat," and "mat"). Therefore, the speechreader can only distinguish among sounds that belong to *different* homophonous groups, but cannot be expected to distinguish between sounds *within* the same group. Such visually distinguishable groups of sounds are also called **visemes** (Fisher, 1968). Owens and Blazek (1985) found sets of homophonous sound groups that were in good agreement with visually identifiable articulatory movements described by Jeffers and Barley (1971). These are shown in Table 15–7. The existence of homophonous sounds and words brings home the point that lipreading cannot independently serve as a replacement for hearing, and one must learn to make use of linguistic and contextual constraints as well as the redundancy of the message.

Auditory-Visual Speech Perception

Speech perception is improved by the use of hearing plus speechreading, compared to either audition or vision alone (Walden, Prosek & Worthington, 1974; Erber, 1975; MacLeod & Summerfield, 1987). It is easy to understand why this occurs. It is not always possible to determine what is being said from either audition or vision alone because (1) speechreading does not give enough information for adequate speech understanding all by itself, and (2) sound cues may be inaudible or distorted due to adverse listening conditions or a hearing impairment. Combined hearing and speechreading provides the person with complementary cues, so that the total amount of information becomes sufficient to perceive what is being said. For example, place of articulation cues (e.g., "pile" vs. "tile") that might be misheard because of a hearing loss can be filled-in by speechreading, and voicing distinctions (e.g., "bad" vs. "pad") that are not visible can often be filled-in by hearing.

TABLE 15–7   Visemes (Owens and Blazek, 1985) and their associated articulatory movements (Jeffers and Barley, 1971)

Visemes	Articulatory movements
p, b, m	Lips together
f, v	Lower lip to upper teeth
θ, ð	Tongue between teeth
w, r	Puckered lips
tʃ, ʤ, ʃ, ʒ	Lips forward
t, d, s, k, n, g, l	Teeth approximated

It is clear we want hearing-impaired patients to use both hearing and lipreading whenever possible, but many people think of lipreading as an "alternative" to hearing, or are reluctant for whatever reason to both look and listen. It is therefore important to make the patient aware that almost everybody benefits from the *combined* use of speechreading and audition, including those with profound hearing losses who must use powerful hearing aids or cochlear implants to receive even a modicum of auditory input. Telling this to the patient is often not enough. A simple and effective demonstration involves giving the patient a speech recognition "test" by hearing alone (with your mouth covered), speechreading alone (with no sound), and then by hearing plus speechreading. The speech level used should be reasonably difficult for the patient, so that there is room to show how the scores improve when audition and vision are combined. This exercise can usually be done sitting face-to-face in a regular room (unless it is done as part of a formal assessment) with whatever kind of speech material is appropriate to demonstrate the intended effect. It is often useful for this type of exercise to be worked into individual and group practice sessions

Framework for Intervention with Adults

A useful framework for understanding modern approaches to aural rehabilitation for adults is provided by a model described by Goldstein and Stephens (1981). It includes both evaluation and remediation phases that address the communicative needs of the hearing-impaired patient in a rather holistic manner. A particularly inviting aspect of this approach is that it is easily applied to a broad range of patients of all ages.

Goldstein and Stephens' *evaluation phase* explores several phases of the patient's communicative situation as well as interrelated factors: (1) *Communication status* is assessed in terms of all components, such as auditory, visual, language and manual/gesture skills. (2) *Associated variables* (e.g., psychological, sociological, vocational, and educational) are explored to determine their interactions with the hearing disorder and the need for coordinated efforts with other professionals. (3) *Related conditions* such as the patient's overall mobility, manual dexterity, visual disorders, and the existence of ear pathologies might affect the intervention plan, and are therefore assessed. The student should consider how factors such as these would change with aging: the differences in approach and supportive counseling that would be appropriate for those who need various degrees of assistance to accomplish their daily activities, and for those who are in nursing facilities. (4) Finally, the patient's *attitude* toward the rehabilitation process is assessed, and will actually be one of the first issues handled during the remediation phase.

The *treatment phase* also addresses several broad areas of remediation: (1) *Psychosocial counseling* is provided, dealing with such factors as explaining the nature of the hearing loss, helping the patient and her family understand its ramifications, and dealing with the patient's attitudes regarding aural rehabilitation. Of course, audiological counseling should not meander into the realm of psychotherapy, the need for which should be handled by appropriate referrals. (2) *Amplification* and other instruments are a major component of the intervention process. These instruments include hearing aids, group amplification devices, and other assistive listening and warning devices. The instruments must be selected and fitted, and must also be adjusted over time. The audiologist also orients and instructs the patient (and often others as well) regarding the use and care of each device, its use in various situations, and in coordination with other devices, etc. (3) *Communication training* involves learning strategies to improve communicative situations and listening effectiveness, as well as developing skills through auditory-visual training, and other activities. (4) The *overall coordination* phase of the program deals with making use of other professionals and resources that are appropriate in a given

case, such as vocational rehabilitation, social work, psychology, medicine, etc.

Self-Assessment Scales

Self-assessment scales and questionnaires are valuable tools for identifying the nature and scope of a patient's communicative and related problems. In addition to describing the direct communicative impact of the hearing loss, many self-assessment scales also provide insights about its psychological, social, and vocational impact upon the patient. Most self-assessment instruments present statements or questions for which the patient must reply along a scale describing how common or true a situation is, how much difficulty or benefit is experienced, or how much he agrees or disagrees with what it says. For example, he might reply on a scale of 1 to 5 (or 1 to 3, 1 to 7, etc.) from "always" to "never," "very little" to "very much," or "completely agree" to "completely disagree."

The information derived from self-assessment scales helps define the kinds of rehabilitative efforts needed by isolating specific problems and difficult environmental situations; it also provides us with a basis for counseling the patient and significant persons in her life. In addition, the outcome of a hearing aid fitting or other aspects of the rehabilitation process can be validated by comparing self-assessment scales administered before and after intervention, as well as over the course of the management program. Some scales ask the patient to indicate several areas of concern or special relevance to his own situation, which become the basis for assessing intervention outcomes. Self-assessment scales are also used in hearing screening programs (Chapter 13). Table 15–8 shows several representative self-assessment scales and the topics they address. The questionnaires in their entirety may be found in the original papers cited and in several current aural rehabilitation texts (e.g., Sanders, 1993; Schow & Nerbonne, 1996; Alpiner & McCarthy, 2000; see also Chapter 13).

TABLE 15-8 Characteristics of several self-assessment scales

Reference	Scale	Characteristics
Alpiner, Chevrette, Glascoe, Metz, and Olsen, 1974	Denver Scale of Communicative Function	Family, self, social-vocational, communication
Giolas, Owens, Lamb, and Schubert, 1979	Hearing Performance Inventory (HPI)	Speech understanding, sound intensity, response to auditory failure, social, personal, occupational
Schow and Nerbonne, 1980	Nursing Home Hearing Handicap Index (NHHI)	Communication, self, social; both self-administered and staff-administered versions
Schow and Nerbonne, 1980	Quantified Denver Scale (QDS)	Modification of Denver Scale
McCarthy and Alpiner, 1980, 1983	McCarthy-Alpiner Scale of Hearing Handicap (M-A Scale)	Psychological, social, vocational
Schow and Nerbonne, 1982	Self-Assessment of Communication (SAC), Significant Other Assessment of Communication (SOAC)	Communication situations, feelings, opinions about others' views. SOAC completed by familiar other
Ventry and Weinstein, 1982	Hearing Handicap Inventory for Elderly (HHIE)	Social-situational, emotional
Demorest and Erdman, 1986	Communication Profile for the Hearing Impaired (CPHI)	Twenty-five scales addressing communicative performance, importance, environment, strategies; personal adjustment; response biases
Cox, Gilmore, and Alexander, 1991	Profile of Hearing Aid Performance (PHAB)	Ratings given with and without hearing for situations involving familiar talkers, ease of communication, reverberation, reduced cues, background noise, aversiveness of sounds, distortion of sounds
Newman, Weinstein, Jacobson, and Hug, 1991	Hearing Handicap Inventory for Adults (HHIA)	Modification of HHIE for use with nonelderly adults
Cox and Alexander, 1995	Abbreviated Profile of Hearing Aid Performance (APHAB)	Abbreviated version of PHAB addressing ease of communication, reverberation, background noise, aversiveness of sounds
Kaplan, Bally, Brandt, Busacco, and Pray, 1997	Communication Scale for Older Adults (CSOA)	Communication strategies; communication attitudes; for use with noninstitutionalized elderly adults
Dillon, James, and Ginis, 1997	Client Oriented Scale of Improvement (COSI)	Patient nominates up to five specific situations of concern in order of importance, before treatment, each situation rated according to (a) how much better/worse, and (b) ease of communication, after treatment
Anderson and Smaldino, 1998	Listening Inventories for Education (LIFE)	(a) Student appraisal and (b) teacher appraisal of the classroom listening environment; and (c) teacher appraisal of impact of intervention methods in the classroom.
Cox and Alexander, 1999	Satisfaction with Amplification in Daily Live (SADL)	Global (overall) satisfaction with hearing aid, positive effects, service and cost, positive image, negative features
Gatehouse, 1999	Glasgow Hearing Aid Benefit Profile (GHABP)	Addresses initial disability, handicap, hearing aid usage, hearing aid benefit, residual disability, and satisfaction for each of four situations plus four additional situations nominated by the patient

Speech Production Management

Speech conservation efforts are sometimes needed because speech production occasionally deteriorates in adults who develop hearing losses. Aberrations of final consonants, sibilants, and vocal loudness or quality are among the reported speech production problems of these patients (Calvert & Silverman, 1975). The incidence of these problems is exceedingly variable, and it is affected by the degree and configuration of the hearing loss, among other less clear factors. In fact, significant amounts of speech deterioration in cases of adult-onset deafness have been reported to occur by some (Cowie & Douglas-Cowie, 1983) but not by others (Goehl & Kaufman, 1984). In addition, speech deterioration effects due to adult-onset hearing losses tend to develop gradually over time. Cases of clinically significant speech deterioration have been rare (but not absent) in the author's experience, and the dearth of coverage on this topic in current aural rehabilitation textbooks seems to confirm this. Jackson (1982) has provided one of the few available discussions of the topic, and includes clinically applicable material. Even though these effects are relatively uncommon, we must be alert to their development so that the appropriate intervention can be undertaken.

Intervention Considerations for Children

Recall that early identification linked to early intervention is a primary goal in the audiological management of the hearing-impaired child. The importance of early intervention is highlighted by the finding that language performance is significantly better in children whose hearing losses are identified before six months of age compared to those identified after six months old (Yoshinaga-Itano et al, 1998). Our goal from the very beginning of the intervention process is to integrate the development of auditory skills into the child's overall speech-language and educational program. This process of audiological rehabilitation for the very young hearing-impaired child begins at home, and most if not all of the earliest activities are carried out by parents or other caregivers. The intervention environment expands as the child enters preschool, elementary, and then higher grades, where the direct provision of services is taken on by professionals.

One of the most well-known approaches to auditory training for children was described by Carhart (1960). This approach stresses the development of (1) sound awareness, (2) gross sound discriminations, and then (3) discrimination among speech sounds. The first goal is to make the child aware that sounds exist, that she should attend to them, and that sounds are associated with objects and activities in her environment. This involves surrounding the child with the sounds of everyday life and associating them with the objects and activities that produce them. Work on sound discrimination begins with gross distinctions between sounds that are very different, and then proceeds to finer distinctions. Typical noise-makers used for these activities include drums, horns, toys, or other objects that produce reasonably distinctive sounds that are within the child's aided audible range. Work on speech sound discriminations also follows the general path of starting with more gross discriminations (e.g., between vowels and consonants) and then moving on to finer ones (e.g., place differences between consonants).

A more current approach to the kinds of skills that need to be addressed in auditory training for hearing-impaired infants and young children is employed in the **SKI-HI program** (Clark & Watkins, 1985; Watkins & Clark, 1993). Here, activities are designed to address a series of 11 major classes of auditory/speech/language skills that are arranged into four overlapping developmental phases. Phase I includes (1) attending to sound, and (2) early vocalization skills. Phase II involves (3) recognizing sounds, (4) locating sound sources, and (5) vocalizing with inflections. The skills in Phase III include (6) locating sounds that are at some distance as well as at levels above and below the child, and (7) the production of several vowels and consonants. Phase IV is concerned with the discrimination and comprehension of (8) environmental sounds, (9) vocal sounds, words, and phrases, and (10) distinct speech sounds; as well as (11) the imitation and/or meaningful production of speech. The SKI-HI program itself is a well-known example of early intervention approaches in which the professional clinician guides parents, family members, and other caregivers so that they can provide the child with a comprehensive at-home program of auditory, speech, and language stimulation.

Erber (1982) stresses that auditory training should be incorporated into the child's overall communicative activities and school program. In his auditory training approach, the child's auditory skills are viewed in terms of a model that takes into account both the speech stimulus and the response task. The *speech stimulus* involves the characteristics and complexity of the speech material that the child must perceive, and may involve any of six levels: (1) *speech elements*, (2) *syllables*, (3) *words*, (4) *phrases*, (5) *sentences*, and (6) *connected discourse*. The *response task* involves the kind of perceptual activity that in involved in responding to the speech signal. These include four general categories: (1) *detection*, (2) *discrimination*, (3) *identification*, and (4) *comprehension*.

Auditory activities can be viewed in terms of any combination of these six speech materials and four response tasks. The child's auditory skills are assessed in terms of Erber's model with the **Glendonald Auditory Screening Procedure (GASP)**. The GASP includes three combinations of these stimuli and response tasks: (1) detection of speech elements, (2) word identification, and (3) sentence comprehension.

Auditory training activities in Erber's approach may involve any of three general styles, including (1) practice on specific tasks, (2) a moderately structured method, and (3) a natural conversational method. Practice on specific tasks is the most structured approach. It focuses on a specific listening skill, and involves structured activities in which the teacher determines the speech stimuli, and the range of responses to be used by the child. A moderately structured activity might use material selected from recent classwork

in a multiple-choice identification task, followed by comprehension tasks or basic speech development activities, procedures, and comprehension tasks. The natural conversational approach is the most flexible method, in which auditory training activities are integrated into the context of the current classroom activity. The approach is *adaptive* in the sense that the nature of the child's responses for one activity influences the nature of the subsequent activity.

The **Developmental Approach to Successful Listening II (DASL-II)** program developed by Stout and Windle (1992) also uses a sequential approach to auditory training in which a child's auditory capabilities are addressed in terms of sound awareness, phonetic listening, and auditory comprehension. Similar to the program described by Erber, DASL-II employs an auditory skills test to determine the child's level of auditory performance so that she can be placed properly in the intervention program.

Sanders (1993) presents a comprehensive intervention approach for hearing-impaired children. Several of its aspects are mentioned to give the student a flavor for the approach, although these points do not even begin to the scratch the surface. Sanders' intervention procedures for younger preschool children are directed toward the development of auditory behavior in the child, and are analogous to but more comprehensive than what Carhart (1960) described as developing sound awareness and discriminations. The major areas of concentration include (1) parent/caregiver education, (2) stimulating the use of hearing, (3) optimization of the child's auditory environment, and (4) developing auditory discrimination and recognition.

Intervention approaches for older preschool children realize the place of the preschool educational environment as a supplement to at-home activities, and highlight the importance of learning through active experiences. Structured communication training is introduced. This includes the use of (1) language that is appropriate for the child's developmental level, (2) maximizing redundancy in order to optimize the child's understanding of relationships and the ability to make accurate predictions about what is being said, and (3) techniques to encourage the development of auditory/visual perceptions.

The intervention process for the hearing-impaired school-age child is multifaceted. A major issue to be faced is the choice of the type of school placement, which is discussed below. Several of the audiologist's responsibilities at this level include providing information to the classroom teacher about issues such as the manner in which hearing loss affects communication, the use and care of hearing aids and other amplification and assistive devices, preferential seating to optimize the hearing-impaired child's auditory-visual reception of classroom activities, etc. Auditory-visual training and language enrichment are integrated into the overall academic program.

Speech Production Assessment and Training

The speech production characteristics of children with hearing impairments have been described for those who have mild-to-moderate losses (Markides, 1970, 1983; Elfenbein, Hardin-Jones, & Davis, 1994) and severe hearing impairments (McDermott & Jones, 1984), as well as for those with profound losses who are typically described as deaf (Hudgins & Numbers, 1942; Smith, 1975). Speech production problems are observed among children with all levels of loss; however, speech does not generally become significantly unintelligible until the loss is worse than roughly 70 dB HL (Jensema, Karchmer, & Trybus, 1978), beyond which it becomes more unintelligible as the person's hearing loss and speech reception capabilities become worse (Boothroyd, 1984, 1985). It is therefore not surprising that speech production considerations are a major issue in the habilitation and education of hearing-impaired and deaf children. Details of speech production evaluation and training for hearing-impaired and deaf children are not outlined here because they are well beyond the scope of an introductory audiology text, and are generally within the province of speech-language pathologists and deaf educators. However, the interested student will find excellent coverage in several well-known texts on the subject (Vorce, 1974; Calvert & Silverman, 1975; Ling, 1976; Hochberg, Levitt, & Osberger, 1983).

Educational Options and Approaches

The legal requirement for providing comprehensive educational and related services to hearing-impaired and deaf children is well established. Children with hearing impairments are included among those with a wide range of handicaps covered under the Individuals with Disabilities Education Act of 1975, better known as Public Law (PL) 92-142. For our purposes, PL 94-142 (along with its extensions under PL 99-457) mandates (1) the least restrictive, individually appropriate free public education for hearing-impaired children from 3 to 21 years old, (2) the provision of the full range of intervention modalities involved in aural rehabilitation, and (3) empowers parents with significant input into the child's educational plan.

EDUCATIONAL PLACEMENT OPTIONS

Potential educational placements for hearing-impaired children fall along a continuum from attending conventional classes in a regular school (mainstreaming) to being enrolled in a residential school for the deaf. Complete mainstreaming is considered to be the least restrictive environment and the residential school represents the most restrictive one. The options between these extremes (going from less to more restrictive) include mainstreaming with various modifications of the environment (e.g., an FM system) and/or some adjustments in the requirements (e.g., modified assignments or tests), or with a modified curriculum; attending regular classes but spending part of the time getting individualized assistance in a resource room or with an itinerant specialist teacher or therapist; being enrolled in special classes for the hearing impaired inside the regular school building; and attending a day school for the deaf. There is good evidence to suggest that overall academic performance is best when high-quality services are provided in less restrictive settings (Ross, Brackett, & Maxon, 1982).

What constitutes the optimal educational placement for a given hearing-impaired child can be a vexing question. The factors to be considered go beyond the degree of hearing loss, and include such issues as the kinds of special services needed by the child, the presence of other handicaps, maximization of the child's psychosocial development, family considerations, geographical limitations, and viewpoints about educational approaches for the hearing impaired.

COMMUNICATIVE APPROACHES

Several communication approaches and techniques are available for use by the hearing impaired and deaf. Because the means of communication cannot be separated from the overall habilitation and education of this population, the choice of which communication method will be used is a central issue in the education of the hearing impaired and deaf. Audiologists have a responsibility to inform parents about the approaches available for their children. However, we must remember that we share this responsibility with other professionals such as educators of the deaf and speech-language pathologists, and that the final placement decision rests with the child's parents.

Oral/Aural Method   Candidly stated, there is no question that spoken language is the means of communication naturally developed by normal individuals, and is employed by the overwhelming preponderance of people throughout the world. These points provide the basic argument for teaching the hearing impaired to employ spoken language as their principal means of communication, as well. This viewpoint has been implied throughout the current discussion. Educational approaches that use spoken language as the primary and often exclusive means of communication are said to employ the **oral/aural method**.

It is unlikely that anyone would disagree with this point of view *provided* we are discussing children whose residual auditory capabilities are sufficient for hearing to be the principal channel for receiving language. However, the oral/aural method becomes an issue of heated controversy when we are dealing with children whose hearing is so impaired that the visual channel effectively becomes their natural, primary channel for receiving linguistic information. This group generally includes those with profound hearing losses, whom we operationally define as being deaf. The fundamental arguments against using the oral/aural method are (1) that these children learn visually oriented or manual systems as their natural, primary means of communication, and (2) that the manual method is the preferred system within the deaf community. This line of reasoning leads to the use of the manual and total communication methods in the education of deaf children.

Manual Systems   **American Sign Language (ASL)** has developed as the manual language of the deaf community. It is not a "translation" of the English language into a set of equivalent signs, but is rather a language unto itself with its own lexicon and grammatical rules. This concept can be difficult for hearing individuals to understand even if they have learned to speak a foreign language like Spanish or German, all of which are spoken languages. In contrast to *spoken* languages, which are suited to transmission via sound (acoustic spectra that change with time), ASL is a manual system suited to the visual channel. Thus, ASL uses *spatial* dimensions (hand shakes, movements, and locations and orientations relative to the signer's body) over time. Signed English (Bornstein, 1974) is similar in many ways to ASL with modifications intended for use by younger children, such as the addition of signed pronouns, helping verbs, and syntactic markers. A variety of other signing systems have been developed over the years, which have attempted to represent the spoken language manually; however, these have not received the wide acceptance enjoyed by ASL.

Fingerspelling involves hand positions and motions corresponding to the conventional 26 letter alphabet. Words are spelled out in order. Fingerspelling is employed by users of both oral/aural and manual systems.

Cued speech (Cornet, 1967) is a visual system used to supplement lipreading. It uses a total of 12 hand postures and positions produced by the talker while speaking to help the speechreader distinguish between homophonous sounds.

Total Communication Total communication encourages the combined use of both speech and/or sign language in whatever combination fosters the child's best language development (Jordan, Gustason, & Rosen, 1979). This approach has replaced oralism as the principal means of communication in most educational institutions for the hearing impaired.

The relative advantages of oral versus total communication programs for the speech communication abilities of profoundly hearing-impaired children has always been controversial. Studies comparing the effects of these two types of settings have yielded conflicting results. One reason for the inconsistencies involves comparisons among elementary school children whose communicative skills are still being developed. Geers and Moog (1992) improved our understanding of this issue by comparing two large, well-matched groups of teenagers with profound hearing impairments who were educated in either oral versus total communication programs since they were in preschool. They found that speech perception, speech production, and oral communication skills were significantly better for the subjects who were educated in oral programs.

Todoma Todoma is a manual system employed by individuals who are both deaf and blind. In the Todoma method, the "listener" feels the talker's face and neck. Reed, Rabinowitz, Durlach, Braida, Conway-Fithian, and Schultz (1985) found that speech reception

by Todoma relies principally on the feel of lip and jaw movements, laryngeal vibration, and oral air flow, and secondarily on the feel of muscle tension and nasal air flow.

REFERENCES

Alpiner JG. 1987. Evaluation of adult communication function. In Alpiner JG, McCarthy PA (Eds.): *Rehabilitative Audiology: Children and Adults*. Baltimore: Williams & Wilkins, 44–114.

Alpiner JG, Chevrette W, Glascoe G, Metz M, Olsen B. 1974. The Denver Scale of Communicative Function. Unpublished, University of Denver.

Alpiner JG, McCarthy PA (Eds.). 2000. *Rehabilitative Audiology: Children and Adults*, 3rd ed. Baltimore: Lippincott Williams & Wilkins.

American National Standards Institute (ANSI). 1996. ANSI S3.22-1996. *American National Standard Specification of Hearing Aid Characteristics*. New York: ANSI.

American National Standards Institute (ANSI). 1997. ANSI S3.35-1985 (R1997). *American National Standard Method of Measurement of Performance Characteristics of Hearing Aids Under In Situ Working Conditions*. New York: ANSI.

American Speech-Language-Hearing Association (ASHA). 1986. Report of the ad hoc committee on cochlear implants. *ASHA* 28, 29–52.

American Speech-Language-Hearing Association (ASHA). 1991. Sound field measurement tutorial. *ASHA* 33 (suppl 3), 25–37.

American Speech-Language-Hearing Association (ASHA). 1995. Position statement and guidelines for acoustics in educational settings. *ASHA* 37 (suppl 14), 15–19.

American Speech-Language-Hearing Association (ASHA). 1998. Guidelines for hearing aid fitting for adults. *Am J Audiol* 7(1), 5–13.

American Speech-Language-Hearing Association (ASHA). 2000. Guidelines for fitting and monitoring FM systems (in press).

Anderson K, Smaldino JJ. 1998. *Listening Inventories for Education (L.I.F.E.)*. Tampa: Educational Audiology Association.

Beck L, Compton C, Gilmore R, Hanna W, Lederman N, Marshall B, O'Brien J, Preves D, Stone R, Teder H, Wilber L. 1993. Telecoils: Past, present and future. *Hear Instr* 44, 22–27, 40.

Beiter AL, Brimacombe JA. 2000. Cochlear implants. In Alpiner JG, & McCarthy PA (Eds.): *Rehabilitative Audiology: Children and Adults*, 3rd ed. Baltimore: Lippincott Williams & Wilkins, 473–500.

Beiter AL, Staller SJ, Dowell RC. 1991. Evaluation and device programming in children. *Ear Hear* 12 (suppl), 25S–33S.

Bender D, Mueller HG. 1984. Factors influencing the decision to obtain amplification. Paper presented at American Speech-Language-Hearing Association Convention. San Francisco.

Berger KW, Hagberg EN, Rane RL. 1988. *Prescription of Hearing Aids: Rationale, Procedure, and Results*. Kent, OH: Herald.

Bess FH, Dodd-Murphy J, Parker RA. 1998. Children with minimal sensorineural hearing loss: Prevalence, educational performance, and functional status. *Ear Hear* 19, 339–354.

Boothroyd A. 1984. Auditory perception of speech contrasts by subjects with sensorineural hearing loss. *J Speech Hear Res* 27, 134–144.

Boothroyd A. 1985. Residual hearing and the problem of carry-over in the speech of the deaf. *ASHA report no. 15*, 8–14.

Bornstein H. 1974. Signed English: A manual approach to English language development. *J Speech Hear Dis* 39, 330–343.

Bragg VC. 1977. Toward a more objective hearing aid fitting procedure. *Hear Instr* 28, 6–9.

Bruhn, M. 1920. *The Mueller-Walle Method of Lipreading for the Deaf*. Lynn, MA: Nichols.

Bunger A. 1932. *Speech Reading—Jena Method*. Danville: Interstate.

Burkhard M, Sachs R. 1975. Anthropomorphic manikin for acoustic research. *J Acoust Soc Am* 58, 214–222.

Byrne D, Dillon H. 1986. The National Acoustic Laboratories' (NAL) new procedure for selecting the gain and frequency response of a hearing aid. *Ear Hear* 7, 257–265.

Byrne D, Parkinson A, Newall P. 1990. Hearing aid gain and frequency response requirements for the severely/profoundly hearing impaired. *Ear Hear* 11, 40–49.

Calvert DR, Silverman SR. 1975. *Speech and Deafness*. Washington, DC: Alexander Graham Bell Association for the Deaf.

Carhart R. 1946. Tests for selection of hearing aids. *Laryngoscope* 56, 780–794.

Carhart R. 1960. Auditory training. In Davis H, Silverman SR (Eds.): *Hearing and Deafness*. New York: Holt, Rinehart & Winston, 368–386.

Carney AE, Osberger MJ, Carney E, Robbins AM, Rehshaw J, Miyamoto RT. 1993. A comparison of speech discrimination with cochlear implants and tactile aids. *J Acoust Soc Am* 94, 2036–2049.

Chasin M. 1994. The acoustic advantages of CIC hearing aids. *Hear J* 47, 13–17.

Chute PM, Nevins ME. 2000. Cochlear implants in children. In Roeser RJ, Valente M, Hosford-Dunn H (Eds.): *Audiology: Treatment*. New York: Thieme, 511–535.

Clark GM, Cowan RSC, Dowell RC (eds.). 1997. *Cochlear Implantation for Infants and Children*. San Diego: Singular.

Clark T, Watkins S. 1985. *Programming for Hearing Impaired Infants Through Amplification and Home Visits*, 4th ed. Logan: Utah State University.

Compton CL. 2000. Assistive technology for the enhancement of receptive communication. In Alpiner JG, McCarthy PA (Eds.): *Rehabilitative Audiology: Children and Adults*, 3rd ed. Baltimore: Lippincott Williams & Wilkins, 501–555.

Cornet R. 1967. Cued speech. *Am Anals Deaf* 112, 3–13.

Courtois J, Johansen PA, Larsen BV, et al. 1988. Hearing aid fitting in asymmetrical hearing loss. In Jensen JH (Ed.): *Hearing Aid Fitting: Theoretical and Practical Views* (13th Danavox Symposium). Copenhagen: Stougaard Jenson, 243–255.

Cowan RCS, Blamey PJ, Galvin KL, Sarant JZ, Alcantara JL, Clark GM. 1990. Perception of sentences, words, and speech features by profoundly hearing-impaired children using a multichannel electrotactile processor. *J Acoust Soc Am* 88, 1374–1384.

Cowie R, Douglas-Cowie E. 1983. Speech production in profound post-lingual hearing deafened adults. *J Laryngol Otol* 96, 101–112.

Cox RM. 1983. Using ULCL measures to find frequency-gain and SSPL90. *Hear Instr* 34, 17–21, 39.

Cox RM. 1985. A structured approach to hearing aid selection. *Ear Hear* 6, 226–239.

Cox RM. 1988. The MSUv3 hearing instrument prescription procedure. *Hear Instr* 39, 6–10.

Cox RM. 1995. Using loudness data for hearing aid selection: The IHAFF approach. *Hear J* 47, 2, 10, 39–42.

Cox RM, Alexander GC. 1995. The abbreviated profile of hearing aid benefit. *Ear Hear* 16, 176–186.

Cox RM, Alexander GC. 1999. Measuring satisfaction with amplification in daily life: The SADL scale. *Ear Hear* 20, 306–320.

Cox RM, Alexander GC, Taylor IM, Gray GA. 1997. The Contour Test of loudness perception. *Ear Hear* 18, 388–400.

Cox RM, Gilmore C, Alexander GC. 1991. Comparison of two questionnaires for patient-assessed hearing aid benefit. *J Am Acad Audiol* 2, 134–145

Cox RM, McDaniel DM. 1989. Development of the Speech Intelligibility Rating (SIR) Test for hearing aid comparisons. *J Speech Hear Res* 32, 347–352.

Crandell CC. 1993. Speech recognition in noise by children with minimal degrees of sensorineural hearing loss. *Ear Hear* 14, 210–216.

Crandell CC, Smaldino JJ. 1992. Sound-field amplification in the classroom. *Am J Audiol* 1, 16–18.

Crandell CC, Smaldino JJ. 1994. An update on classroom acoustics for children with hearing impairment. *Volta Rev* 96, 291–306.

Crandell CC, Smaldino JJ. 2000. Room acoustics for listeners with normal-hearing and hearing impairment. In RJ Roeser, M Valente, H Hosford-Dunn (Eds.): *Audiology: Treatment*. New York: Thieme, 601–637.

Crandell CC, Smaldino JJ, Flexer C. 1995. *Sound-Field FM Amplification: Theory and Practical Applications*. San Diego: Singular.

Crandell CC, Smaldino JJ, Flexer C. 1997. A suggested protocol for implementing sound-field FM technology in the educational setting. *J Educ Audiol* 5, 13–21.

Davis H, Stevens SS, Nichols RH, et al. 1947. *Hearing Aids: An Experimental Study of Design Objectives*. Cambridge: Harvard University Press.

DeFilipo CL, Scott BL. 1978. A method for training and evaluating the recognition of ongoing speech. *J Acoust Soc Am* 63, 1186–1192.

deJong R. 1994. Selecting and verifying hearing aid fittings for symmetrical hearing loss. In Valente M (Ed.): *Strategies for Selecting and Verifying Hearing Aid Fittings*. New York: Thieme, 180–206.

Demorest ME, Erdman SA. 1986. Scale composition and analysis of the communication profile for the hearing impaired. *J Speech Hear Res* 29, 515–535.

Dillon H. 1999a. NAL-NL1: A new procedure for fitting non-linear hearing aids. *Hear Instr* 52, 10–16.

Dillon H. 1999b. Using the NAL-NL1 prescriptive procedure with advanced hearing instruments. *Hear Rev* 6, 8–20.

Dillon H, James A, Ginis J. 1997. Client Oriented Scale of Improvement (COSI) and its relationship to several other measures of benefit and satisfaction provided by hearing aids. *J Am Acad Audiol* 8, 27–43.

Dillon H, Storey L. 1998. The National Acoustics Laboratories' procedure for selecting the saturation sound pressure level of hearing aids: Theoretical derivation. *Ear Hear* 19, 255–266.

Dubno J, Dirks DD, Morgan DE. 1984. Effects of age and mild hearing loss on speech recognition in noise. *J Acoust Soc Am* 76, 87–96.

Elfenbein JL, Hardin-Jones MA, Davis JM. 1994. Oral communication skills of children who are hard of hearing. *J Speech Hear Res* 37, 216–226.

Erber NP. 1975. Auditory-visual perception of speech. *J Speech Hear Dis* 40, 481–492.

Erber NP. 1982. *Auditory Training.* Washington, DC: AG Bell Association for the Deaf.

Ertmer DJ, Kirk KI, Sehgal ST, Riley AI, Osberger MJ. 1997. Comparison of vowel production by children with multichannel cochlear implants or tactile aids: Perceptual evidence. *Ear Hear* 18, 307–315.

Federal Register. 1998. Architectural and Transportation Compliance Board. Petition for rulemaking: Request for information on acoustics. *Federal Register* 63:104: 29679–29686.

Finitzo T. 1988. Classroom acoustics. In Roeser RJ, Downs MP (Eds.): *Auditory Disorders in School Children,* 2nd ed. New York: Thieme, 221–233.

Finitzo-Hieber T, Tillman T. 1978. Room acoustics effects on monosyllabic word discrimination ability for normal and hearing impaired children. *J Speech Hear Res* 21, 440–458.

Fisher CG. 1968. Confusions among visually perceived consonants. *J Speech Hear Res* 11, 796–804.

Flexer C. 1992. FM classroom public address systems. In Ross M (Ed.): *FM Auditory Training Systems: Characteristics, Selection and Use.* Timonium, MD: York Press, 189–210.

Flexer C. 1994. *Facilitating Hearing and Listening in Young Children.* San Diego: Singular.

Galvin KL, Mavrias G, Moore A, Cowan, RSC, Blamey PJ, Clark GM. 1999. A comparison of Tactaid II+ and Tactaid 7 use by adults with profound hearing impairment. *Ear Hear* 20, 471–482.

Garstecki DC. 1981. Auditory-visual training program for hearing-impaired adults. *J Acad Rehabil Audiol* 14, 223–238.

Gatehouse S. 1999. Glasgow hearing aid benefit profile: Derivation and validation of a client-centered outcome measure for hearing aid services. *J Am Acad Audiol* 10, 80–103.

Geers AE, Moog JS. 1992. Speech perception and production skills of students with impaired hearing from oral and total communication settings. *J Speech Hear Res* 35, 1384–1393.

Geers A, Moog J. 1994. Spoken language results: Vocabulary, syntax and communication. *Volta Rev* 96, 97–108.

Gelfand SA. 1995. Long-term recovery and no recovery from the auditory deprivation effect with binaural amplification: Six cases. *J Am Acad Audiol* 6, 141–149.

Gelfand SA. 1998. *Hearing: An Introduction to Psychological and Physiological Acoustics,* 3rd ed. New York: Marcel Dekker.

Gelfand SA, Hochberg H. 1976. Binaural and monaural speech discrimination under reverberation. *Audiology* 15, 72–84.

Gelfand SA, Ross L, Miller S. 1988. Sentence reception in noise from one versus two sources: Effects of aging and hearing loss. *J Acoust Soc Am* 83, 248–256.

Gelfand SA, Silman S. 1979. Effects of small room reverberation upon the recognition of some consonant features. *J Acoust Soc Am* 66, 22–29.

Gelfand SA, Silman S. 1993. Apparent auditory deprivation in children: Implications of monaural versus binaural hearing. *J Am Acad Audiol* 4, 313–318.

Gelfand SA, Silman S, Ross L. 1987. Long-term effects of monaural, binaural and no amplification in subjects with bilateral hearing loss. *Scand Audiol* 16, 201–207.

Gengel R. 1971. Acceptable speech-to-noise ratios for aided speech discrimination by the hearing impaired. *J Aud Res* 11, 219–222.

Gilmore R, Lederman N. 1989. Induction loop assistive listening systems: Back to the future? *Hear Instr* 40, 14–20.

Giolas TG, Owens E, Lamb SH, Schubert ED. 1979. Hearing performance inventory. *J Speech Hear Dis* 44, 169–195.

Goehl M, Kaufman DK. 1984. Do the effects of adventitious deafness include disordered speech? *J Speech Hear Dis* 49, 58–64.

Goldstein DP, Stephens SDG. 1981. Aural rehabilitation: Management model I. *Audiology* 20, 432–452.

Gray RF. 1991. Cochlear implants: The medical criteria for patient selection. In Cooper H (Ed.): *Cochlear Implants: A Practical Guide.* London: Whurr, 146–154.

Gudmundsen GI. 1994. Fitting CIC hearing aids—some practical pointers. *Hear J* 47, 10, 45–47.

Harford E. 1966. Bilateral CROS: Two-sided listening with one hearing aid. *Arch Otolaryngol* 84, 426–432.

Harford E, Barry J. 1965. A rehabilitative approach to the problem of unilateral hearing impairment: The contralateral routing of signals (CROS). *J Speech Hear Dis* 30, 121–138.

Harford E, Dodds E. 1966. The clinical application of CROS: A hearing aid for unilateral deafness. *Arch Otolaryngol* 83, 455–464.

Hawkins DB, Beck LB, Bratt GW, Fabry DA, Mueller HC, Stelmachowicz PB. 1991. The Vanderbilt/Department of Veterans Affairs 1990 conference consensus statement: Recommended components of a hearing aid selection procedure for adults. *Audiol Today* 3, 16–18

Hawkins DB, Schum D. 1985. Some effects of FM-system coupling on hearing aid characteristics. *J Speech Hear Dis* 50, 132–141.

Hawkins DB, Walden BE, Montgomery A, Prosek RA. 1987. Description and validation of an LDL procedure to select SSPL90. *Ear Hear* 8, 162–169.

Hnath-Chisolm T, Kishon-Rabin L. 1988. Tactile presentation of voice fundamental frequency as an aid to the reception of speech pattern contrasts. *Ear Hear* 9, 329–334.

Hochberg I, Levitt H, Osberger MJ. 1983. *Speech of the Hearing Impaired: Research, Training, and Personal Preparation.* Baltimore: University Park Press.

Hodgson M, Rempel R, Kennedy S. 1999. Measurement and prediction of typical speech and background noise levels in university classrooms during lectures. *J Acoust Soc Am* 105, 226–233.

Hudgins CF, Numbers F. 1942. An investigation of the intelligibility of the speech of the deaf. *Genetic Psych Monogr* 25, 289–392.

Hurley RM. 1993. Monaural hearing aid effect. *J Am Acad Audiol* 4, 285–294.

Hurley RM. 1999. Onset of auditory deprivation. *J Am Acad Audiol* 10, 529–534.

Ijsseldijk FJ. 1992. Speechreading performance under different conditions of video image, repetition, and speech rate. *J Speech Hear Res* 35, 466–471.

Jackson PL. 1982. Techniques for speech conservation. In Hull R (Ed.): *Rehabilitative Audiology*. New York: Grune & Stratton, 129–152.

Jeffers J, Barley M. 1971. *Speechreading*. Springfield, IL: CC Thomas.

Jensema CJ, Karchmer MA, Trybus R. 1978. *The Rated Intelligibility of Hearing-Impaired Children: Basic Relationships*. Washington, DC: Gallaudet College.

Jerger J, Silman S, Lew HL, Chmiel R. 1993. Case studies in binaural interference: Converging evidence from behavioral and electrophysiological measures. *J Am Acad Audiol* 4, 122–131.

Johnson R, Meikle M, Vernon J. 1988. An implantable bone-conduction hearing device. *Am J Otol* 9, 93–100.

Jordan I, Gustason G, Rosen R. 1979. An update on communication trends in programs for the deaf. *Am Ann Deaf* 125, 350–357.

Kalikow DN, Stevens DN, Elliot LL. 1977. Development of a test of speech intelligibility in noise using sentence materials with controlled word predictability. *J Acoust Soc Am* 61, 1337–1351.

Kaplan H, Bally S, Brandt F, Busacco D, Pray J. 1997. Communication scale for older adults (CSOA). *J Am Acad Audiol* 8, 203–217.

Killion MC. 1993. The K-amp hearing aid: An attempt to present high fidelity for persons with impaired hearing. *Am J Audiol* 2, 52–74.

Killion MC. 1996. Talking hair cells: What they have to say about hearing aids. In Berlin CI (Ed.): *Hair Cells and Hearing Aids*. San Diego: Singular.

Kinzie C, Kinzie R. 1931. *Lipreading for the Deafened Adult*. Chicago: Winston.

Kishon-Rabin L, Boothroyd A, Hanin L. 1996. Speechreading enhancement: A comparison of spatial-tactile display of voice fundamental frequency (F_o) with auditory F_o. *J Acoust Soc Am* 100, 593–602.

Kishon-Rabin L, Haras N, Bergman M. 1997. Multisensory speech perception of young children with profound hearing loss. *J Speech Lang Hear Res* 40, 1135–1150.

Kuk F. 1994. A screening procedure for modified simplex in frequency-gain response selection. *Ear Hear* 15, 62–70.

Leavitt R. 1991. Group amplification systems for students with hearing impairment. *Semin Hear* 12, 380–387.

Levitt H, Pickett JM, Houde RA. 1980. *Sensory Aids for the Hearing Impaired*. New York: IEEE Press.

Levitt H, Sullivan JA, Neuman AC, Rubin-Spitz JA. 1987. Experiments with a programmable master hearing aid. *J Rehabil Res Dev* 24, 29–54.

Lewis DE. 1994a. Assistive devices for classroom listening. *Am J Audiol* 3, 58–69.

Lewis DE. 1994b. Assistive devices for classroom listening: FM systems. *Am J Audiol* 3, 70–83.

Libby E. 1986. The 1/3–2/3 insertion gain hearing aid selection guide. *Hear Instr* 37, 27–28.

Ling D. 1976. *Speech and the Hearing-Impaired Child: Theory and Practice*. Washington, DC: Alexander Graham Bell Association for the Deaf.

Lybarger SF. 1944. U.S. Patent application SN 543, 278.

MacLeod, A, Summerfield, Q. 1987. Quantifying the contribution of vision to speech perception in noise. *Br J Audiol* 21, 131–141.

Markides A. 1970. The speech of deaf and partially-hearing children with special reference to factors affecting intelligibility. *Br J Commun Dis* 5, 126–140.

Markides A. 1983. *The Speech of Hearing-Impaired Children*. Dover, NH: Manchester University Press.

McCandless GA, Lyregaard PE. 1983. Prescription of gain/output (POGO) for hearing aids. *Hear Instr* 34, 16–21.

McCarthy PA, Alpiner JG. 1980. An assessment scale of hearing handicap for use in family counseling. *J Acad Rehabil Audiol* 16, 256–270.

McCarthy PA, Alpiner JG. 1983. McCarthy-Alpiner Scale of Hearing Handicap. Unpublished.

McDermott R, Jones T. 1984. Articulation characteristics and listeners? Judgments of the speech of children with severe hearing loss. *Lang Speech Hear Services Schools* 15, 110–126.

Medical Research Council (MedResCo). 1947. *Hearing Aids and Audiometers*. Report of the Committee on Electro-Acoustics. Special Report 261. London: His Majesty's Stationery Office.

Medwetsky L, Boothroyd A. 1991. Effect of microphone placement on the spectral distribution of speech. Paper presented at American Speech-Language-Hearing Association Convention. Atlanta, GA.

Montgomery AA, Walden BE, Schwartz DM, Prosek RA. 1984. Training auditory-visual speech reception in adults with moderate sensorineural hearing loss. *Ear Hear* 5, 30–36.

Mueller HG. 1994. Small can be good too! *Hear J* 47, 11.

Mueller HG, Hawkins DB, Northern JL. 1992. *Probe Microphone Measurements: Hearing Aid Selection and Assessment*. San Diego: Singular.

Mylanus EAM, Snik AFM, Jorritsma FF, Cremers CWRJ. 1994. Audiologic results for the bone-anchored hearing aid HC220. *Ear Hear* 15, 87–92.

Nabelek A, Robinette L. 1978. Reverberation as a parameter in clinical testing. *Audiology* 17, 239–259.

National Institutes of Health (NIH). 1995. *NIH Consensus Statement: Cochlear Implants in Adults and Children*. 13, 1–30.

Neuman AC, Levitt H, Mills R, Schwander T. 1987. An evaluation of three adaptive hearing aid selection strategies. *J Acoust Soc Am* 82, 1967–1976.

Nevins ME, Chute PM. 1996. *Children with Cochlear Implants in Educational Settings*. San Diego: Singular.

Newman CW, Weinstein BE, Jacobson GP, Hug GA. 1991. Test-retest reliability of the Hearing Handicap Inventory for Adults. *Ear Hear* 12, 355–357.

Nicholas JG. 1994. Sensory aid use and the development of communicative function. *Volta Rev* 96, 181–198.

Nitchie E. 1912. *Lipreading: Principles and Practice*. New York: Stokes.

O'Neil JJ, Oyer HJ. 1981. *Visual Communication for the Hard of Hearing*. Englewood Cliffs, NJ: Prentice-Hall.

Osberger MJ, Maso M, Sam LK. 1993. Speech intelligibility of children with cochlear implants, tactile aids, or hearing aids. *J Speech Hear Res* 36, 186–203.

Osberger MJ, Miyamoto RT, Zimmerman-Philips S, Kemink JL, Stroer BS, Firszt JB, Novack MA. 1991. Independent evaluation of the speech perception abilities of children with the Nucleus 22-channel cochlear implant system. *Ear Hear* 12 (suppl), 66S–80S.

Osberger MJ, Robbins A, Todd S, Riley A, Kirk KI, Carney A. 1996. Cochlear implants and tactile aids for children with profound hearing impairment. In Bess F, Gravel J, Tharpe AM (Eds.): *Amplification for Children with Auditory Deficits.* Nashville: Bill Wilkerson Center Press, 283–308.

Owens E, Blazek B. 1985. Visemes observed by hearing-impaired and normal-hearing adult viewers. *J Speech Hear Res* 28, 381–393.

Palmer CV. 1997. Hearing and listening in a typical classroom. *Lang Speech Hear Services Schools* 28, 213–218.

Pediatric Working Group of the Conference on Amplification for Children with Auditory Deficits (PWG). 1996. Amplification for infants and children with hearing loss. *Am J Audiol* 5, 53–68.

Plant G, Gnosspelius J, Levitt H. 2000. The use of tactile supplements in lipreading Swedish and English: A single-subject study. *J Speech Lang Hear Res* 43, 172–183.

Pollack MC. 1988. *Amplification for the Hearing-Impaired,* 3rd ed. New York: Grune & Stratton.

Punch JL, Beck EL. 1980. Low-frequency response of hearing aids and judgments of aided speech quality. *J Speech Hear Dis* 45, 325–335.

Punch JL, Parker CA. 1981. Pairwise listener preferences in hearing aid evaluation. *J Speech Hear Res* 24, 366–374.

Pyman BC, Brown AM, Dowell RC, Clark GM. 1990. Preoperative evaluation and selection of adults. In Clark GM, Tong YC, Patrick JF (Eds.): *Cochlear Prostheses.* Edinburgh: Churchill Livingstone, 125–134.

Reed CM, Rabinowitz WM, Durlach NI, Braida LD, Conway-Fithian S, Schultz MC. 1985. Research on the Todoma method of speech communication. *J Acoust Soc Am* 77, 247–257.

Ricketts T, Mueller HG. 1999. Making sense of directional microphone hearing aids. *Am J Audiol* 8, 117–127.

Rosenberg GG, Blake-Rahter P, Heavner J, Allen L, Redmond BM, Phillips J, Stigers K. 1999. Improving classroom acoustics (ICA): A three-year FM sound-field classroom amplification study. *J Educ Audiol* 7, 8–28.

Ross M (Ed.). 1992. *FM Auditory Training Systems: Characteristics, Selection and Use.* Timonium, MD: York Press.

Ross M, Brackett D, Maxon AM. 1982. *Hard of Hearing Children in Regular Schools.* Englewood Cliffs, NJ: Prentice-Hall.

Ross M, Giolas T. 1971. Three classroom listening conditions on speech intelligibility. *Am Ann Deaf* 116, 580–584.

Rubinstein A, Boothroyd A. 1987. Effect of two approaches to auditory training on speech recognition by hearing-impaired adults. *J Speech Hear Res* 30, 153–160.

Sanders DA. 1993. *Management of Hearing Handicap: Infants to Elderly.* Englewood Cliffs, NJ: Prentice-Hall.

Sandlin RE. 1994. Fitting binaural amplification to asymmetrical hearing loss. In Valente M. (Ed.): *Strategies for Selecting and Verifying Hearing Aid Fittings.* New York: Thieme, 207–227.

Schow RL, Nerbonne MA. 1980. Hearing handicap and Denver scales: Applications, categories, interpretation. *J Acad Rehabil Audiol* 13, 66–77.

Schow RL, Nerbonne MA. 1982. Communication screening profile: Use with elderly clients. *Ear Hear* 3, 135–147.

Schow RL, Nerbonne MA. 1996. *Introduction to Aural Rehabilitation,* 3rd ed. Boston: Allyn & Bacon.

Schwartz D, Lyregaard PE, Lundh P. 1988. Hearing aid selection for severe-to-profound hearing losses. *Hear J* 4, 13–17.

Seewald RC, Cornelisse LE, Ramji KV, Sinclair ST, Moodie KS, Jamieson DG. 1997. *DSL 4.1 for Windows: Software Implementation of the Desired Sensation Level [DSL(i/o)] Method for Fitting Linear Gain and Wide Dynamic Range Compression Hearing Instruments.* London, Ontario: University of Western Ontario.

Seffens ML, Eilers RE, Fishman L, Oller DK, Urbano RC. 1994. Early vocal development in tactually aided children with severe-profound hearing loss. *J Speech Hear Res* 37, 700–711.

Sehgal ST, Kirk KI, Svirsky M, Ertmer DJ, Osberger MJ. 1998. Imitative consonant feature production by children with multichannel sensory aids. *Ear Hear* 19, 72–84.

Sehgal ST, Kirk KI, Svirsky M, Miyamoto RT. 1998. The effects of processor strategy on the speech perception performance of pediatric Nucleus multichannel cochlear implant users. *Ear Hear* 19, 149–161.

Shapiro I. 1976. Hearing aid fitting by prescription. *Audiology* 15, 163–173.

Shapiro I. 1980. Comparison of three hearing aid prescription procedures. *Ear Hear* 1, 211–214.

Shaw E. 1974. Ear canal pressure generated by a free sound field. *J Acoust Soc Am* 56, 1848–1861.

Sherrick CE. 1984. Basic and applied research in tactile aids for deaf people: Progress and prospects. *J Acoust Soc Am* 75, 1325–1342.

Silman S, Gelfand SA, Silverman CA. 1984. Late-onset auditory deprivation: Effects of monaural versus binaural hearing aids. *J Acoust Soc Am* 76, 1357–1361.

Silman S, Silverman CA, Emmer M, Gelfand SA. 1992. Adult-onset auditory deprivation. *J Am Acad Audiol* 3, 390–396.

Silverman CA, Silman S. 1990. Apparent auditory deprivation from monaural amplification and recovery with binaural amplification: Two case studies. *J Am Acad Audiol* 1, 175–180.

Skinner MW. 1988. *Hearing Aid Evaluation.* Englewood Cliffs, NJ: Prentice-Hall.

Smith C. 1975. Residual hearing and speech production in deaf children. *J Speech Hear Dis* 18, 795–811.

Staller SJ, Dowell RC, Beiter AL, Brimacombe JA. 1991. Perceptual abilities of children with the Nucleus 22-channel cochlear implant. *Ear Hear* 12 (suppl), 34S–47S.

Staller SJ, Menapace C, Domico E, et al. 1997. Speech perception abilities of adult and pediatric Nucleus implant recipients using the spectral peak (SPEAK) strategy. *Otol Laryngol Head Neck Surg* 117, 236–242.

Storey L, Dillon H, Yeend I, Wigney D. 1998. The National Acoustics Laboratories' procedure for selecting the saturation sound pressure level of hearing aids: Experimental validation. *Ear Hear* 19, 267–279.

Stout G, Windle J. 1992. *Developmental Approach to Successful Listening II*. Englewood, CO: Resource Point.

Strom KE. 2000. The hearing care market at the turn of the 21st century. *Hear Rev* 7, 8–22, 100.

Stubblefield J, Nye C. 1989. Aided and unaided time-related differences in word discrimination. *Hear Instr* 40, 38–45.

Surr RK, Fabry DA. 1991. Comparison of three hearing aid fittings using the speech intelligibility rating (SIR) test. Ear Hear 12, 32–38.

Traynor RM. 1997. Prescriptive procedures. In H Tobin (Ed.): *Practical Hearing Aid Selection and Fitting*. Washington, DC: U.S. Department of Veterans Affairs, 59–74.

Tyler R, Parkinson AJ, Fryauf-Bertchy H, et al. 1997. Speech perception by prelingually deaf children and postlingually deaf adults with cochlear implant. *Scand Audiol* 26 (suppl 46), 65–71.

Utley J. 1946. A test of lipreading ability. *J Speech Dis* 11, 109–116.

Valente M. 1982. Binaural amplification. *Audiol J Cont Ed* 7, 79–93.

Valente M (Ed.) 1994. *Strategies for Selecting and Verifying Hearing Aid Fittings*. New York: Thieme.

Valente M, Van Vliet D. 1997. The Independent Hearing Aid Fitting Forum (IHAFF) protocol. *Trends in Amplification* 2, 6–35.

Ventry IM, Weinstein BE. 1982. Identification of elderly people with hearing problems. *Ear Hear* 3, 128–134.

Vorce E. 1974. *Teaching Speech to Deaf Children*. Washington, DC: Alexander Graham Bell Association for the Deaf.

Walden BE, Erdman SA, Montgomery AA, Schwartz DM, Prosek RA. 1981. Some effects of training on speech recognition of hearing-impaired adults. *J Speech Hear Res* 24, 207–216.

Walden BE, Prosek RA, Montgomery AA, Scherr CK, Jones CJ. 1977. Effects of training on the visual recognition of consonants. *J Speech Hear Res* 20, 130–145.

Walden BE, Prosek RA, Worthington DW. 1974. Predicting audiovisual consonant recognition performance of hearing-impaired adults. J Speech Hear Res 17, 270–278.

Walden BE, Schwartz DM, Williams DL, Holum-Hardengen LL, Crowley JM. 1983. Test of the assumptions underlying comparative hearing aid evaluations. *J Speech Hear Dis* 48, 264–273.

Waltzman SB, Cohen NL, Gomolin RH, et al. 1994. Long-term results of early cochlear implantation in congenitally and prelingually deafened children. *Am J Otol* 15 (suppl 2), 9–13.

Waltzman SB, Fisher SG, Niparko JK, et al. 1995. Predictors of postoperative performance with cochlear implants. *Ann Otol Rhinol Laryngol* 104 (suppl 165), 15–18.

Waltzman SB, Shapiro WH. 2000. Cochlear implants in adults. In Roeser RJ, Valente M, Hosford-Dunn H (Eds.): *Audiology: Treatment*. New York: Thieme, 537–546.

Watkins S, Clark T. 1993. *SKI-HI Resource Manual: Family-Centered Home-Based Programming for Infants, Toddlers, and Pre-School Aged Children with Hearing Impairment*. Logan: Hope.

Watson NA, Knudsen VO. 1940. Selective amplification in hearing aids. *J Acoust Soc Am* 11, 406–419.

Weber BA, Roush J. 1991. Implantable bone-conduction hearing device: Practical considerations. *J Am Acad Audiol* 2, 123–127.

Weber DA, Fredrickson JM. 2000. Implantable hearing aids. In Roeser RJ, Valente M, Hosford-Dunn H (Eds.): *Audiology: Treatment*. New York: Thieme, 489–520.

Weisenberger JM, Percy ME. 1995. The transmission of phoneme-level information by multichannel tactile speech perception aids. *Ear Hear* 16, 392–406.

Yacullo WS, Hawkins DB. 1987. Speech recognition in noise and reverberation by school-age children. *Audiology* 26, 235–246.

Yoshinaga-Itano C. 1999. Early identification: An opportunity and challenge for audiology. *Semin Hear* 20, 317–331.

Yoshinaga-Itano C, Sedey AL, Coulter DK, Mehl AL. 1998. Language of early- and later-identified children with hearing loss. *Pediatrics* 102, 1161–1171.

Zwislocki J. 1971. *An Ear-Like Coupler for Earphone Calibration*. Lab of Sensory Communication Report LSC-S-9. New York: Syracuse University.

16

The Effects of Noise and Industrial Audiology

This chapter is concerned with the branch of audiology that deals with the effects and ramifications of excessive sound exposure. Terms like *noise exposure* and *sound exposure* will be used interchangeably in this context because we are dealing with issues involving too much sound. The topics that will be addressed here include the effects of noise on hearing ability and speech communication, its nonauditory effects, occupational noise exposure and industrial hearing conservation, and the related issue of workers' compensation for noise-induced hearing losses. We will begin by expanding on several concepts about how noises are described and measured, which is often part of audiological practice and is also prerequisite to understanding the effects of noise exposure.

Noise Levels and Their Measurement

We are already familiar with the concepts involved in describing the magnitude and spectral content of a sound in terms of its overall sound pressure level (SPL), octave-band levels, and weighted (A, B, C) sound levels. It is also important to characterize noise exposures in terms of their *temporal characteristics* (Hamernik & Hsueh, 1991; Ward, 1991). Noise exposures are considered **continuous** if they remain above the level of "effective quiet" (the level below which a noise is too soft to cause a threshold shift). Noises that are not continuous may be considered (1) **interrupted** if they are on for relatively long periods of time (hours) above the level of effective quiet; (2) **intermittent** if the noise exposure is broken up by short breaks (e.g., a few seconds to an hour) of quiet or effective quiet; or (3) **time-varying** if the noise stays above effective quiet but its level varies over time. **Transient noises** produced by the sudden release of energy (e.g., gun shots) are called **impulse** noises, and often exceed 140 dB SPL. On the other hand, **impact** noises are transients caused by impacts between objects (e.g., hammering on metal), and are usually less than 140 dB SPL. Special sound level meters with extremely fast response characteristics are needed to measure transient noises accurately.

Most noise events last for some period of time, from a few seconds to many hours. Also, the levels of the noise will usually vary during this period, often considerably. It is desirable to integrate these noise levels into a single number that summarizes the overall level of the exposure "averaged" over its duration, called its **equivalent level (L_{eq})**. However, it is important to remember that decibels are logarithmic values, so that combining a series of sound level measurements into L_{eq} cannot be done by using their simple arithmetic average. Instead, L_{eq} is obtained using a method analogous to the one described in Chapter 1 for combining octave-band levels into overall SPL or dBA. The curious student will find the appropriate formulas and descriptions of their use in Berger, Ward, Morrill, and Royster (1986). In practice, L_{eq} values are often obtained directly using an integrating sound level meter or a dosimeter (described below). Special types of L_{eq} are used for compliance with occupational hearing conservation regulations (e.g., OSHA, 1983). The equivalent level for a

24-hour period of exposure is often expressed as $L_{eq}(24)$. When annoyance is an issue, the **day-night level** (DNL or L_{dn}) is used to describe the equivalent noise level for a 24-hour period in a way that assigns a penalty to nighttime noises because these are considered more objectionable. This is done by adding 10 dB to all noise levels that occur between the hours of 10 P.M. and 7 A.M. **Community noise equivalent level** (CNEL) is a variation of the DNL concept that adds a 5-dB penalty for evening noises and a 10-dB penalty for nighttime noises. All-day equivalent levels do not adequately represent objectionable single noise events like aircraft fly-overs, so a supplemental measurement is often necessary to characterize them. These single incidents can be expressed in terms of an equivalent one-second exposure called **sound exposure level** (SEL). There are also other approaches to identify the interference or annoyance capability of noises. For example, the spectrum of a noise can be compared to **noise criterion** (NC) **curves**, including the **balanced noise criterion** (NCB) **curves** that also consider the effects of vibration and audible rattles (Beranek, 1957, 1989).

Noise Level Surveys

Noise surveys (or **sound surveys**) are systematic measurements of the sound levels in an industrial setting, or in other environments like the neighborhoods in the vicinity of an airport. Noise surveys are done for several reasons: (1) To identify locations where individuals (typically employees) are exposed to noise levels that exceed a certain criterion. This criterion is usually a **time-weighted average** (TWA) of ≥85 dBA because this value is the level specified by federal occupational hearing conservation regulations (OSHA, 1983). The time-weighted average is a special kind of equivalent level normalized to an eight-hour workday. (2) To identify which employees are being exposed to noise levels of ≥85 dBA TWA or some other level of interest. (3) To ascertain which noise sources may require engineering controls, and to provide

engineers with the information they need to determine what kinds of noise control methods are best suited to the problem at hand. (4) To determine how much attenuation must be provided by the hearing protection devices (e.g., earplugs and earmuffs) used by noise-exposed employees. (5) In addition, the information provided by noise surveys can also be used to identify and help alleviate problems pertaining to the audibility of emergency warning signals and the effectiveness of speech communication in the workplace. Levels in dBA are usually needed for determining employee noise exposures. Octave-band levels are needed to evaluate the nature of the noise in detail, and for engineering purposes such as determining appropriate noise control techniques, and for assessing hearing protectors. Noise levels in dBC are also needed for assessing hearing protectors, especially when octave-band levels are not available. Environmental noise surveys often use other measurements to concentrate on annoyance factors around airports, major highways, and other nonoccupational noise sources.

The noise level measurements obtained in various locations can be used to develop **noise level maps**. Noise maps are diagrams that depict noise levels as contour lines superimposed on the floor plan of the area that was surveyed. The contours on a noise map show which areas have similar noise levels, like contours on a geographical map show regions with similar elevations above sea level. An example of a noise level contour map is shown in Figure 16–1. Maps of this type make it easier to identify noise sources and employees who are being exposed to unacceptable noise levels, and to communicate this information to others. In addition to area measurements, it is usually necessary to measure representative personal exposures (1) because noise levels often vary with location; (2) because many employees move around among work locations that have different noise levels, and/or in and out of noise exposure areas; and (3) to account for times when employees may be away from high-noise locations, such as lunch and rest breaks. Simi-

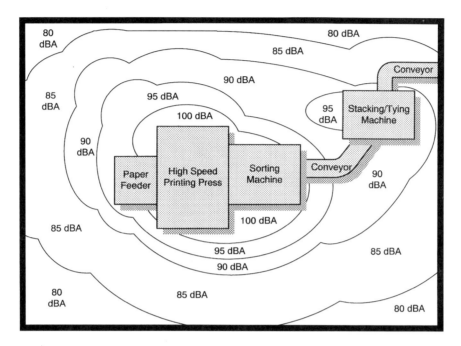

FIGURE 16–1   A typical noise contour map.

lar noise contour maps are made around air-ports and other environmental noise sources.

Sound Level Meters   The principal noise measurement tools are sound level meters and noise dosimeters. Recall from Chapter 1 that the **sound level meter (SLM)** is the basic instrument for measuring the magnitude of sound. The SLM can be used to measure over-all sound pressure level at its linear setting, weighted sound levels in dBA, dBB, and dBC, as well as octave- and third-octave-band levels with the appropriate filters. The character-istics of the A-, B- and C-weightings and the octave-band were summarized in Figure 1–21 and Table 1–2 of Chapter 1. In this section we will expand on some of the fundamental aspects of sound measurement, and apply this information to noise measurement.

Sound level meters are classified as types 0, 1, 2, and S (ANSI-S1.4, 1983, R1997). The most precise sound level meters with the most restricted tolerances are **Type 0** or **lab-oratory standard** models. These instruments have the most exacting tolerances, which

requires them to be correct within ±0.7 dB from 100 to 4000 Hz. Type 0 SLMs are used for exacting calibration and reference pur-poses under laboratory conditions, but are not required for noise level analyses. **Type 1** or **precision** SLMs are intended for precise sound level measurements in the laboratory and in the field, and have tolerances of ±1 dB from 50 to 4000 Hz. **General purpose** or **type 2** SLMs are field measurement instru-ments with tolerances as narrow as ±1.5 dB from 100 to 1250 Hz, and are the ones required to meet the noise level compliance standards of the Occupational Safety and Health Administration (OSHA) and other regulatory agencies. The student can get an appreciation for the tolerance differences among the three classes of SLMs from the samples listed in Table 16–1. One can also find "survey" (formerly type 3) SLMs, but they are not appropriate for our use. **Special purpose (type S)** SLMs have a limited num-ber of selected functions intended for a par-ticular application rather than all of the features of the type 0, 1, and 2 meters.

TABLE 16–1   Tolerance limits (maximum allowable measurement errors) at selected frequencies for type 0, 1, and 2 sound level meters (ANSI-S1.4, 1983, R1997)

Frequency (Hz)	Tolerances in dB for		
	Type 0	Type 1	Type 2
31.5	±1	±1.5	±3
63	±1	±1	±2
125	±0.7	±1	±1.5
250	±0.7	±1	±1.5
500	±0.7	±1	±1.5
1000	±0.7	±1	±1.5
2000	±0.7	±1	±2
3150	±0.7	±1	±2.5
4000	±0.7	±1	±3
6300	−1.5 to +1	−2 to +1.5	±4.5
8000	−2 to +1	−3 to +1.5	±5

It takes a certain amount of time for a meter to respond to an abrupt increase in sound level. Response time is expressed as a **time constant**, which is how long it takes the meter to reach 63% of its eventual maximum reading. Sound level meters have "slow" and "fast" response speeds that date back to the early days of their development, and are specified for use in many noise measurements by various federal and state laws and regulations. In particular, OSHA requires most noise measurements to be made at the slow speed. The **slow** speed has a time constant of 1 second. This sluggish response has the effect of averaging out sound level fluctuations, making the meter easier to read; but it also makes the slow speed inappropriate for estimating sound level variability over time. With a time constant of 0.125 seconds, the **fast** speed is better suited for assessing the variability of a sound, but the fluctuating meter readings make it more difficult to determine an overall level. However, even the fast response is far too slow for measuring transient noises like impulses and impacts. A **true peak** or **instantaneous** response setting is needed to measure these kinds of sounds. At their true peak settings, type 0 SLMs must be able to respond to pulses as short as 50 *micro*seconds, and type 1 and 2 meters must be able to respond to 100-

microsecond pulses. It is important to be aware that the **impulse** setting on SLMs, which has a 35 *milli*second rising time constant and a 1.5 second decay time, is not appropriate for measuring impulse sounds, in spite of its name.

Dosimeters   **Noise dosimeters** are sound measurement devices that are used to record the amount of sound exposure that accumulates over the course of an entire workday. An example is shown in Figure 16–2. A dosimeter may be thought of as a sound level meter that has been modified to simplify and automate the process of making noise exposure measurements over a period of time, making noise exposure monitoring a very practical activity. **Personal** noise exposure measurements are obtained by having an employee wear the dosimeter over the course of the workday. In this case, the dosimeter is typically carried on the employee's belt with its microphone located on top of his shoulder. **Area** sound exposure measurements may be obtained by placing the dosimeter at an appropriate location in the work environment. Most dosimeters have a very large dynamic range, which means they are able to integrate a wide range of intensity levels into the exposure measurements. To comply with federal regulations (OSHA, 1983), dosi-

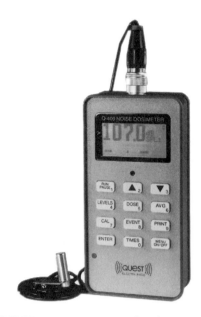

FIGURE 16–2   An example of a noise dosimeter commonly used for industrial noise exposure measurements. Courtesy of Quest Technologies, Inc.

meters usually include all sound levels ≥80 dB in the noise measurements, whereas those below this *floor* or lower threshold are omitted. (Other floors are also available, but are not appropriate for compliance with noise exposure regulations.) The overall, accumulated noise exposure for the workday is generally given in terms of a noise dose (analogous to a radiation dose), and/or the equivalent time-weighted average in dBA for an 8-hour exposure. In addition, modern dosimeters can make measurements in both dBA and dBC using all kinds of meter responses (slow, fast, instantaneous, etc.), provide various kinds of accumulated exposure levels, and provide a profile showing a detailed noise exposure history for the period that was monitored. This information may be printed out or transferred to a computer.

The Noise Spectrum   Spectral information is not provided by the overall noise level measurements obtained with the linear setting of an SLM, or with its A, B, and C weighting

networks. However, a general idea about the spectral content of a noise can sometimes be obtained by comparing the sound levels measured with the linear and A-weighted settings of the sound level meter. This is possible because the overall SPL provided by the linear setting treats all frequencies equally, whereas the low frequencies are de-emphasized by the A-weighting network. In effect, a noise level reading in dB SPL includes the lows, whereas dBA "ignores" the lows. For this reason, a difference between the two levels implies that the noise contains low-frequency energy "seen" by the dB SPL reading but "ignored" by the dBA reading. On the other hand, similar levels in dB SPL and dBA imply that the noise does not have much energy in the low frequencies. This kind of comparison can also be made between noise levels in dBA and dBC because the C-weighting network largely approximates the linear response.

The spectrum of a noise can be determined by **octave-band analysis**, and an even finer picture of the spectrum of a noise from a **third-octave-band analysis**. These measurements can be done with a sound level meter that has octave- or third-octave filters, or with a self-contained instrument often called an octave-band analyzer (or third-octave band analyzer). Figure 16–3 shows an example of an octave-band analysis using the noise present in a hypothetical industrial environment. Notice that the amplitude of this noise is generally greater in the lower frequencies, except for a pronounced peak in the 2000 Hz octave-band. This peak happens to be associated with the operation of a particular machine in the plant. These spectral characteristics cannot be ascertained from the overall noise level measurements, which were 90 dBA and 91 dB SPL. The dBA and dB SPL values are very close because of the dominance of the peak in the 2000 Hz octave-band. Another approach is to use a **spectrum analyzer** that determines the spectrum by performing a Fourier analysis on the sound electronically using a process called **fast Fourier transformation (FFT)**.

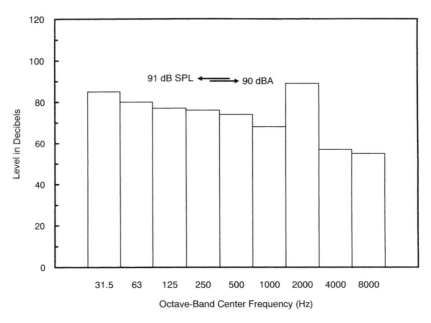

FIGURE 16–3   Octave-band levels of the noise in a hypothetical industrial environment with an overall noise level corresponding to 91 dB SPL and 90 dBA. Notice the noise has a low-frequency emphasis as well as the dominant 89-dB peak in the 2000-Hz octave-band.

Effects of Noise

Effects of Noise on Hearing

NOISE-INDUCED HEARING LOSS

The effect of noise exposure on hearing sensitivity is expressed in terms of threshold shift. A **temporary threshold shift (TTS)** is a temporary change in hearing sensitivity that occurs following an exposure to high sound levels, and is a phenomenon that we have all experienced. The basic concept of a TTS is very simple. Suppose someone's threshold is 5 dB HL, and she is exposed to a relatively intense noise for a period of time. Retesting her hearing after the noise stops reveals her threshold has changed (shifted) to 21 dB HL, and retesting a few hours later shows her threshold has eventually returned to 5 dB HL. Her threshold shift soon after the noise ended is 21 − 5 = 16 dB (the difference between the pre- and postexposure thresholds), and it is a temporary threshold shift because her threshold eventually returned to

its preexposure value. If her threshold never returned to its preexposure value, then it would have been a **permanent threshold shift (PTS)**, also known as a **noise-induced permanent threshold shift (NIPTS)** or a **noise-induced hearing loss (NIHL)**.

Temporary and permanent threshold shifts have been studied in great detail and involve many factors (Miller, 1974; Clark, 1991a; Hamernik, Ahroon, & Hsueh, 1991; Melnick, 1991; Ward, 1991). The nature of noise-induced damage to the auditory system was discussed in Chapter 6. In general, higher-frequency noise exposures cause larger threshold shifts than do equally intense lower-frequency exposures. In addition, the greatest amount of TTS tends to occur at a frequency that is about one-half octave higher than the offending band of noise. However, not all sounds affect hearing sensitivity. The term **equivalent quiet** (or **effective quiet**) describes the intensity below which sound exposures do not cause a TTS. The weakest sound pressure levels that cause a TTS are about 75 to 80 dB for broadband noise, and decrease with frequency from 77 dB for the 250-Hz octave-band to 65 dB for the 4000-Hz octave-band. Thus, we are interested in the duration and intensity of exposures that are above equivalent quiet. In any case, it is stressed that noise-induced threshold shifts are very *variable* across individuals.

Temporary threshold shift is usually measured 2 minutes after a noise is turned off because its value is unstable before that point, and is thus called **TTS$_2$**. The three functions in Figure 16–4 illustrate how TTS$_2$ is affected by the duration and intensity of a noise exposure. We will assume that all three exposures are above equivalent quiet, and that the TTS$_2$ is being measured at the frequency most affected by our hypothetical band of noise. All three functions show that TTS$_2$ increases as the duration of the exposure gets progressively longer. As we would expect, more TTS$_2$ is produced by higher noise levels than by softer ones for any par-

ticular exposure duration. The rate at which TTS$_2$ grows with duration is essentially linear when plotted on a logarithmic scale. However, TTS$_2$ grows faster as the intensity of the noise increases, that is, the lines get steeper going from 80 dB to 90 dB to 100 dB. The linear increase continues for durations up to about 8 to 16 hours. The functions then level off to become asymptotic (shown by the horizontal line segments), indicating that TTS$_2$ does not increase any more no matter how much longer the noise is kept on. In other words, the horizontal lines show the biggest TTS$_2$ that a particular noise is capable of producing regardless of its duration. This maximum amount of TTS$_2$ is called the **asymptotic threshold shift (ATS)**.

The threshold shift produced by a noise exposure is largest when it is first measured (i.e., TTS$_2$), and then decreases with the passage of time since the noise ended. This process is called recovery, and is illustrated in Figure 16–5. Notice that the time scale is

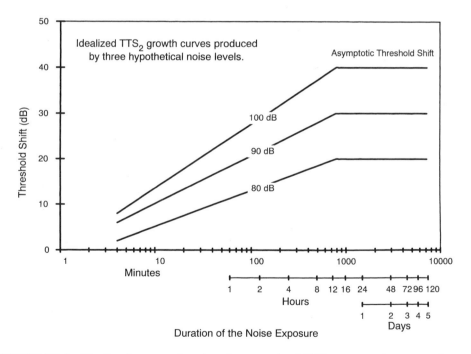

FIGURE 16–4 Idealized curves showing the growth of TTS$_2$ at some frequency due to increasing durations of exposure to a narrow band noise at three different hypothetical levels above equivalent quiet (80, 90, and 100 dB). Duration is shown on a logarithmic scale. A maximum amount of ATS (asymptotic threshold shift) is eventually reached for each noise level.

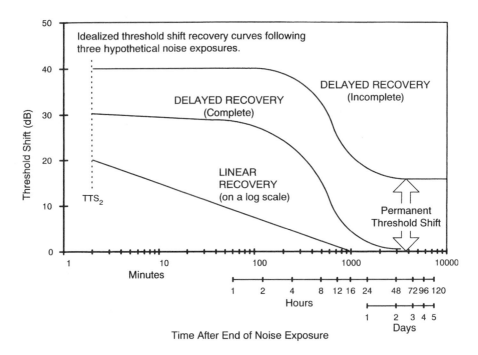

FIGURE 16–5 Idealized recovery from noise-induced threshold shift with time after the exposure has ended. Duration on a logarithmic scale. Notice the largest threshold shift never recovered completely, leaving a permanent threshold shift.

logarithmic, as it was in the prior figure. As a rule, *complete* linear recovery is expected to occur within about 16 hours after the noise ends, providing the TTS_2 is less than roughly 40 dB *and* it was caused by a continuous noise exposure lasting no more than 8 to 12 hours (shown by the lowest function in the figure). Otherwise, the recovery will be *delayed* (e.g., if the noise was intermittent, more than 8 to 12 hours in duration, and/or there is more TTS_2). The middle curve in the figure is an example of delayed recovery that eventually becomes complete after 2 days. However, once the amount of TTS_2 gets into the vicinity of about 40 dB, there is a likelihood that recovery may be *incomplete* as well as delayed. The top curve in the figure shows an example. Here, what started out as a 40-dB TTS ends up as a 15-dB PTS—an irreversible noise-induced hearing loss.

Even though the PTS is usually smaller than the original size of the TTS, it is possible for the PTS to be as large as the TTS. However, it cannot be any larger. Recall that TTS increases with the duration of a noise until the

asymptotic threshold shift is reached. This means that there is a maximum amount of TTS (i.e., ATS) that can be caused by a particular noise at a given intensity, no matter how long it lasts. Consequently, the biggest PTS that can be caused by that noise is limited to the ATS. Keep in mind, however, that the TTS caused by a noise exposure is often superimposed upon a preexisting sensorineural loss. For example, a TTS of 15 dB experienced by a patient who started out with a loss of 30 dB HL would bring his threshold to 45 dB HL.

Occupational Noise Exposure The early use of terms like *boilermakers' disease* to describe deafness among industrial workers highlights the fact that occupational noise exposure has been recognized as a major cause of hearing loss for a very long time. Industrial noises vary widely in intensity, spectrum, and time course. We can get a sense of the intensities involved from the partial list in Table 16–2, based on studies analyzed by Passchier-Vermeer (1974) and Rösler (1994). Overall, somewhere between 36 and 71% of manufacturing employ-

TABLE 16–2   Some examples of various occupational noise level intensities

Noise Type	Example(s) of Reported Levels
Miscellaneous industrial	88–104 dB SPL; 80–103 dBA
Weaving machines	102 dB SPL
Boiler shop	91 dBA
Riveting	113 dB SPL
Shipyard caulking	111.5 dB SPL
Drop forging	
Background	109 dB SPL
Drop hammer	126.5 peakSPL
Mining industry trucks	102–120 dB SPL
Mining equipment	96–114 dB SPL
Military weapons	168–188 peakSPL

Derived from Passchier-Vermeer (1974) and Rösler (1994).

ees have daily workplace exposures of 90 dBA or more (Royster & Royster, 1990b).

Numerous studies have reported the noise-induced hearing losses experienced by workers in many industries. Based on an analysis of eight well-documented studies, Passchier-Vermeer (1974) reported that (1) occupational NIHL at 4000 Hz increases rapidly for about 10 years, at which time it is similar to the amount of TTS associated with an 8-hour exposure to a similar noise, and (2) the con-

tinued development of NIPTS at 4000 Hz slows down or plateaus thereafter. On the other hand, NIHL at 2000 Hz develops slowly for the first 10 years, after which the loss at 2000 Hz increases progressively with time. The general pattern of development of occupational NIHL is illustrated in Figure 16–6. Here, we see the median NIHLs of female workers who were exposed to noise levels of 99 to 102 dB SPL for durations of 1 to 52 years in the jute weaving industry (Taylor, Pearson, & Mair, 1965). As a group, their hearing losses started as a 4000-Hz notch, and became deeper and wider as they were exposed to more years of noise exposure. It is important to remember that these are median audiograms, and that Taylor et al (1965) reported a great deal of variability among individuals.

Rösler (1994) compared the long-term development of NIHL in 11 studies representing a wide variety of different kinds and levels of occupationally related noises. Figure 16–7 summarizes the mean (or median) audiograms after (a) 5 to 10 and (b) (25 years of exposure, and shows presbycusis curves for comparison. Notice the similarity among the configurations after (25 years of exposure in spite of the widely variant kinds of noises. The "outliers" in Figure 16–7b are the two

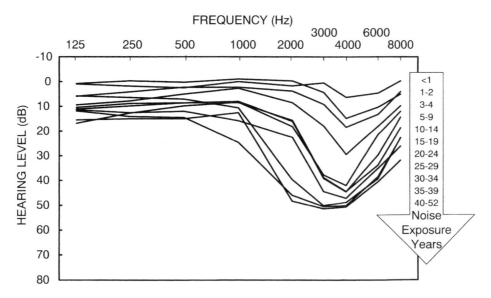

FIGURE 16–6   Median audiograms of female weavers exposed to 99-102 dB SPL noises for 1 to 52 work years. Based on Taylor, Pearson, and Mair (1965).

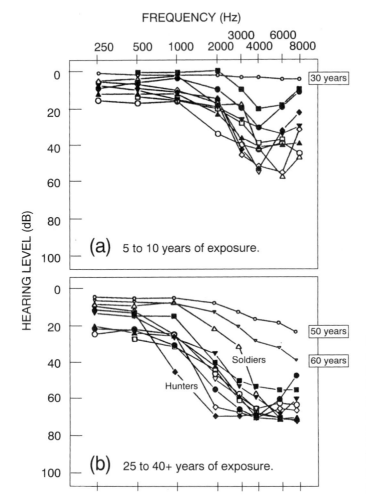

FREQUENCY (Hz)

(a) 5 to 10 years of exposure.

(b) 25 to 40+ years of exposure.

FIGURE 16–7 Mean (or median) audiograms after (a) 5 to 10 years and (b) 25 to 40+ years from 11 studies involving different kinds of occupational noises. For reference and comparison purposes, the open circles labeled 30 years in (a) and 50 and 60 years in (b) are due to age alone, based on ISO-1999 (1990). Adapted from Rösler (1994) with permission of *Scandinavian Audiology*.

groups of firearms users. Finnish regular army personnel developed their maximum average losses within the first 5 to 10 years, and are the least affected in Figure 16–7b. On the other hand, Eskimos who hunted without hearing protectors at least weekly since childhood had thresholds that continued to deteriorate throughout a period of about 45 years, and are the most affected in Figure 16–7b.

Nonoccupational Noise Exposure Industrial noise exposures are not the only origin of NIHL. Hearing loss is also caused by *environmental* and other *nonoccupational* noise exposures, and is sometimes called **sociocusis**. This is not surprising when we realize that many sounds encountered in daily life and leisure activities produce noise levels

that approach and often far exceed 90 dBA. Some examples are shown in Figure 16–8. Recreational impulse noises produce peak SPLs of 160 to 170+ dB for rifles and shotguns (Odess, 1972; Davis, Fortnum, Coles, Haggard, & Lutman, 1985), and 140 dB for toy cap pistols (Suter, 1992a). Rock music averages 103.4 dBA (Clark, 1991b), and car stereo systems have been "clocked" at 140 dB SPL (Suter, 1992a).[1] Rifles and shotguns often cause an asymmetrical loss that is poorer in the left ear, which usually faces the muzzle.

---

[1] Interestingly, Florentine, Hunter, Robinson, Ballou, and Buus (1998) found that about 9% of the subjects they studied had maladaptive patterns of listening to loud music suggestive of those associated with substance abuse.

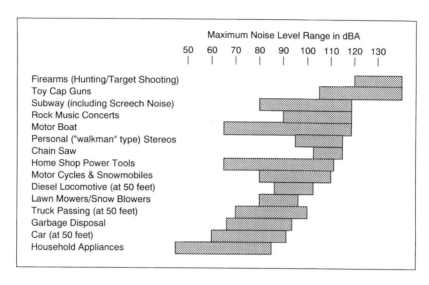

FIGURE 16–8 Typical sources of environmental noise and their approximate maximum levels in dBA, based on data reported by the EPA (1974) and Clark and Bohne (1984).

Individual Susceptibility and Interactions with Other Factors Individual susceptibility to NIHL varies widely and is affected by several factors (Boettcher, Henderson, Gratton, Danielson, & Byrne, 1987; Henderson, Subramaniam, & Boettcher, 1993). At first glance, it would seem wise to use *temporary threshold shifts* as the test for susceptibility to NIHL because they precede permanent threshold shifts, and the amount of TTS after an 8-hour workday seems to be similar to the amount of PTS after 10 years of occupational exposure on a group basis. However, the correlation between TTS and PTS is too ambiguous for TTS results to be used as a test of one's susceptibility to NIHL, especially when intermittent exposures and impulse noises are involved. The use of TTS testing is also unattractive because of litigation fears.

The effect of noise exposure is exacerbated by *vibration*, but vibration alone does not produce a hearing loss. Susceptibility is also affected by the effectiveness of the *acoustic reflex* and possibly by the *efferent auditory system*. Susceptibility is also affected by *noise exposure history*: repeated intermittent noise exposures produced progressively smaller hearing losses in laboratory animals over time (Clark, Bohne, & Boettcher, 1987; Subra-

maniam, Campo, & Henderson, 1991a,b). Does a prior noise exposure affect susceptibility to future exposures? This question has been addressed by measuring threshold shifts in lab animals that were subjected to (1) a *prior* (initial) noise exposure, (2) followed by a *recovery period*, and (3) then subjected to a *subsequent* noise exposure (Canlon, Borg, & Flock, 1988; Campo, Subramaniam, & Henderson, 1991; Subramaniam, Henderson, Campo, & Spongr, 1992). Subsequent low-frequency exposures produced smaller threshold shifts after a low-frequency prior exposure; but susceptibility to a subsequent high-frequency noise was made worse by prior exposures (with low- or high-frequency noises).

Susceptibility to NIHL is increased by *nonauditory factors*, as well, including *ototoxic drugs* (aminoglycocides and Cis-platinum, possibly and less so for salicilates) and *industrial and environmental toxins* (e.g., solvents, carbon monoxide). Other nonauditory factors have been identified, but they account for a very small part of the variability, often with inconclusive or equivocal results. These include the following, with the more susceptible groups identified in parentheses: *age* (very young and the elderly); *gender* (males); *eye color* (blue); and *smoking* (smokers).

DAMAGE RISK CRITERIA AND NOISE EXPOSURE STANDARDS

There are probably two closely related key questions that concern people about noise exposure and hearing loss: First, what are the chances of getting a hearing loss from being exposed to some noise for some period of time? Second, how much noise exposure is acceptable before it becomes damaging to hearing? These questions are addressed by **damage risk criteria (DRC)**, which are standards or guidelines that pertain to the hazards of noise exposure. However, this apparently straightforward issue actually involves many interrelated questions, the answers to which are complicated, not necessarily understood, and often controversial. Some questions deal with the noise and predicting its effects: How should noise be quantified for the purpose of assessing damage risk, and how should we handle different kinds of noises (continuous, impulsive, intermittent, and time varying)? Are there valid and reliable "predictors" of NIHL, and if so, what are they and how are they related to hearing loss? Other questions deal with the amount of NIHL and how many people are affected: How much hearing loss is acceptable or at least tolerable, and at which frequency(ies)? Since people vary in susceptibility, what is the acceptable/tolerable percentage of the population that should be "allowed" to develop more than the acceptable/tolerable amount of NIHL? Still other questions pertain to distinguishing between different sources of hearing impairment: Can we separate NIPTS from other sources of hearing impairment (e.g., pure presbycusis and disease), and if so, how? Can we distinguish between the effects of *occupational* noise exposure and *nonoccupational* causes of hearing loss, including nonoccupational noise exposures? The latter is an important issue because we are usually concerned with industrial exposures. For this reason, we often use the term *industrial noise-induced permanent threshold shift* to refer to the part of a hearing loss actually attributable to industrial (or other occupational) noise exposures. These questions should be kept in mind when dealing with the effects of noise exposure in general, and particularly when dealing with hearing conservation programs and assessing hearing handicap for compensation purposes.

One approach to damage risk criteria is to protect just about everybody from just about any degree of NIHL. This notion is illustrated by the "Levels Document" issued by the Environmental Protection Agency (EPA, 1974), which suggested that NIPTS could be limited to less than 5 dB at 4000 Hz in 96% of the population by limiting noise exposures to 75 dB $L_{eq(8)}$ or 70 dB $L_{eq(24)}$ over a 40-year period. Changing the criterion to 77 dB $L_{eq(24)}$ would protect 50% of the population.

The Committee on Hearing and Bioacoustics and Biomechanics (CHABA) published damage risk criteria intended to limit the amount of industrial NIPTS to 10 dB at ≤1000 Hz, 15 dB at 2000 Hz, and 20 dB at ≥3000 Hz among 50% of workers who are exposed to steady or intermittent noises for 10 years (Kryter, Ward, Miller, & Eldredge, 1966). The CHABA DRC was based on the amount of TTS_2 that occurs after an 8-hour noise exposure, and relied on the notion that this value seems to correspond to the amount of NIPTS after 10 years of occupational exposure. However, it has never been proven that TTS validly predicts NIPTS, and this notion has several serious problems (e.g., Melnick, 1991; Ward, 1991). Damage risk criteria for impulsive noises using similar criteria were introduced by Coles, Garinther, Rice, and Hodge (1968). The CHABA damage risk criteria required noises to be measured in third-octave- or octave-bands, and expressed maximum exposure levels for durations up to 8 hours per day. The maximum allowable octave-band levels for an 8-hour exposure were about 85 dB for frequencies ≥1000 Hz but were higher for lower frequencies, because they cause smaller threshold shifts than do equally intense higher frequency exposures. The allowable noise levels also became higher as the duration of the exposure decreased below 8 hours, because the amount of threshold shift is related to exposure duration. Botsford (1967) developed equivalent values that make it possible to apply the CHABA damage risk criteria to noises measured in dBA instead of octave-band levels.

Several well-known approaches and estimates of the risks for developing a hearing loss due to occupational noise exposure have been developed over the years (e.g., NIOSH, 1972, 1998; EPA, 1973; ISO, 1990, ANSI, 1996; Prince, Stayner, Smith, & Gilbert, 1997). The NIOSH (1972) risk criteria were based on linear fit to the data collected in the 1968–1972 NIOSH Occupational Noise and Hearing Survey (Lempert & Henderson, 1973), which was reanalyzed using a best-fitting nonlinear model by Prince et al (1997), also known as the NIOSH-1997 model. (The 1968–1972 survey provides valuable data that are still used today because it pre-dated regulations requiring the use of hearing protectors [see below], the use of which makes it hard to determine actual exposure levels from modern noise surveys.) The criteria for material impairment used by Prince et al (1997) involved an average hearing loss in both ears of more than 25 dB for certain combinations of frequencies: (a) 500, 1000, and 2000 Hz; (b) 1000, 2000, and 3000 Hz; and (c) 1000, 2000, 3000, and 4000 Hz. The latter is similar to the criterion recommended by ASHA (1981), discussed later in this chapter.[2] In addition, the National Institute for Occupational Safety and Health (NIOSH, 1998) has adopted a binaural average loss exceeding 25 dB HL for the 1000–4000 Hz average as its criterion for material hearing impairment.

The International Standards Organization *ISO 1999* standard (1990) considers the hearing loss of noised-exposed people to be due to the combination of an age-related component and NIPTS, which are almost additive.[3] Formulas are used to predict the effects of noise exposure levels (from 85 to 100 dBA) and durations (up to 40 years) at each frequency for different percentiles of the population (e.g., the 10% with the most loss, the 10% with the least loss, medians, etc.). This approach has been adopted by the American National Standards Institute in *ANSI Standard S3.44* (1996). In effect, NIPTS is determined by comparing the thresholds of a noise-exposed group to a comparable unexposed group of the same age. These standards provide two sets of age-related hearing level distributions. One is based on a population *highly screened* to be free of ear disease and noise exposure (representing more-or-less "pure" presbycusis), and the other is from an essentially *unscreened general population*. It is important to remember that the estimated risk of NIHL will be affected by which noise-free sample is used.

To estimate the risks to hearing attributable to a certain amount of occupational noise exposure, we need to compare the percentage of people exposed to that noise who get material amounts of hearing impairment to the percentage of unexposed people of the same age who also get a material hearing impairment. Obviously, the risk estimate will depend on the *criterion* used to determine when a *material hearing impairment* begins. In other words, **excess risk** for occupational hearing impairment is simply the percentage of exposed people with material impairments minus the percentage of unexposed people with material impairments. Figure 16–9 shows the amount of excess risk of hearing impairment due to 40 years of occupational noise exposures of 80, 85, and 90 dBA (8 hours TWA) estimated by several of the methods just described. It is clear that excess risk becomes readily apparent by the time occupational noise exposure levels reaches 85 dBA even though the actual percentages estimated by the various methods and pure tone combinations differ. The only "outlier" among the methods seems to be ISO-1990, which appears to underestimate the amount of excess risk compared to the other methods. It is interesting to note in this context that excess risk estimates based on the ANSI (1996) method agreed with the NIOSH-1997

---

[2] Prince et al (1997) weighted the 1000–4000 Hz average based on the based on the articulation index (see below) as opposed to ASHA's (1981) simple 1000–4000 Hz average; however, both variations yield similar risk estimate outcomes.

[3] Specifically, the total hearing loss in dB due to age and NIPTS combined (TOTAL) is related to the hearing loss due to age (AGE) and the NIPTS according to the formula: TOTAL = AGE + NIPTS − (AGE × NIPTS)/120. Subtracting the term (AGE x NIPTS)/120 prevents the total loss from becoming impossibly large and also causes the combined effects of age and noise to be somewhat less than additive.

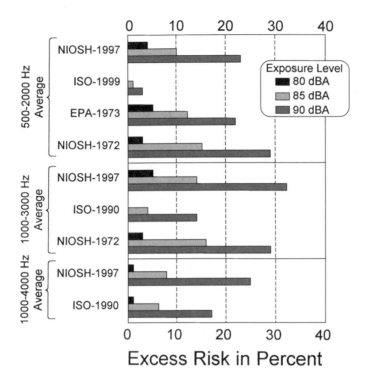

FIGURE 16–9 Excess risk of material hearing impairment (binaural average >25 dB HL) using various approaches and pure tone averages expected to result from 40 years of occupational noise exposures of 80, 85, and 90 dBA (8 hours TWA) among 60-year-old workers. The approach labeled NIOSH-1997 refers to Prince et al. (1997). Based on NIOSH (1998).

estimates for 65-year-old workers, but ANSI (1996) underestimated excess risk encountered for 45-year-olds (Prince et al, 1997).

OSHA Noise Exposure Criteria Noise exposure standards are particularly effectual when they carry the weight of law. Numerous examples are found in state and local ordinances and in military regulations, but the most influential are federal labor regulations found in the Walsh-Healey noise standard and OSHA Hearing Conservation Amendment (HCA) (DOL, 1969; OSHA, 1983). These noise exposure limits are shown in Table 16–3 (first and second columns), where we see that the maximum noise exposure limit is 90 dBA for 8 hours. In addition, impulse or impact noises are not supposed to exceed 140 dB peak SPL. If the noise level exceeds 90 dBA, then the exposure duration must be reduced by one-half for each 5-dB increase. In other words, the maximum exposures are 8 hours at 90 dBA, 4 hours at 95 dBA, 2 hours at 100

dBA, down to 1/4-hour at 115 dBA. However, the noise level is not permitted to exceed 115 dBA even for durations shorter than 1/4-hour. This trade-off of 5 dB per doubling of time is called the **5-dB trading rule** or **exchange rate**, and is based on the premise that sounds that produce equal amounts of TTS are equally hazardous. This is the same **equal-TTS** principle discussed previously for the CHABA damage risk criteria. The major alternative approach is to reduce the intensity by 3 dB for each doubling of duration (the **3-dB trading rule** or **exchange rate**), which is employed by the military, the EPA, and many foreign countries. The 3-dB trading rule is based on the **equal-energy** concept that considers equal amounts of noise energy to be equally hazardous, and is more strongly supported by scientific evidence than the 5-dB rule (e.g., Suter, 1992b; NIOSH, 1998).

The maximum allowable noise exposure is known as the **permissible exposure level (PEL)**, and is considered to be one full dose

TABLE 16–3 Maximum permissible noise exposures according to the OSHA (1983) regulations using and NIOSH (1998) recommendations

Maximum Exposure Level in dBA	Maximum Exposure Durations	
	OSHA HCA (1983) Regulations[a]	NIOSH (1998) Recommendations
85[b]		8 hours
88		4 hours
90[c]	8 hours	2 hours, 31 minutes
92	6 hours	1 hour, 35 minutes
95	4 hours	47 minutes, 37 seconds
97	3 hours	30 minutes
100	2 hours	15 minutes
102	1 hour, 30 minutes	9 minutes, 27 seconds
105	1 hour	4 minutes, 43 seconds
110	30 minutes	1 minute, 29 seconds
115	15 minutes or less	28 seconds

[a]From Table G-16, OSHA (1983), which also indicates: "When the daily noise exposure is composed of two or more periods of noise exposure of different levels, their combined effect should be considered, rather than the individual effect of each. If the sum of the following fractions: $C_1/T_1 + C_2/T_2 \ldots C_n/T_n$ exceeds unity [i.e., 1], then the mixed exposure should be considered to exceed the limit value. C_n indicates the total time of exposure at a specified noise level, and T_n indicates the total time of exposure permitted at that level."

[b]OSHA (1983) PEL for an 8-hour TWA exposure.

[c]NIOSH (1998) REL for an 8-hour TWA exposure.

of noise. Using the OSHA (1983) criteria, a person has received **one dose** (or a **100% dose**) of noise regardless of whether he was exposed to 90 dBA for 8 hours or 105 dBA for 1 hour. This is the same kind of terminology that is used for exposures to radiation or noxious chemicals—a full day's dose is a full dose whether it accumulates over 8 hours or just a few minutes. Because of the 85-dB PEL and the 5-dB trading rule, an 8-hour exposure to 85 dBA would be a 1/2-dose (50% dose) and an 8-hour exposure to 80 dBA would be a 1/4-dose (25% dose). Similarly, an 8-hour exposure to 95 dBA would be a 200% dose or two doses. Hence, we can also express a noise exposure in terms of an *equivalent 8-hour exposure*, that is its 8-hour TWA. Equivalent values of noise level exposures in terms of TWA and dosage are shown in Figure 16–10.[4] Using the plot labeled "OSHA

(1983)," we see that the following are examples of equivalent noise exposures:

90 dBA TWA and 1 dose and a 100% dose (the PEL);
95 dBA TWA and 2 doses and a 200% dose;
100 dBA TWA and 4 doses and a 400% dose;
105 dBA TWA and 8 doses and an 800% dose;
120 dBA TWA and 70 doses and a 6000% dose.

Noises that have been measured in terms of octave-band levels need to be converted into 0 dBA so that allowable exposures can be determined for them. The methods used to convert octave-band levels into overall level in dBA were described in Chapter 1. However, a simplified approach for compliance with the OSHA noise standard can be achieved by using the conversion chart shown in Figure 16–11. The procedure involves plotting the octave-band levels of the noise on the chart, and then comparing them to the conversion curves. The highest curve that is crossed by any part of the noise spectrum constitutes the *equivalent* noise level in dBA. This value in dBA can then be used to assign noise exposure limits according to the first and second columns of Table 16–3 for OSHA purposes.

---

[4] For reference purposes, the relationship between TWA in dBA and noise dose in percent (D) can be calculated as follows: TWA=16.61 × log (D/100) + 90 for OSHA (1983) purposes, and TWA = 10 × log (D/100) + 85 according to the NIOSH (1998) criteria.

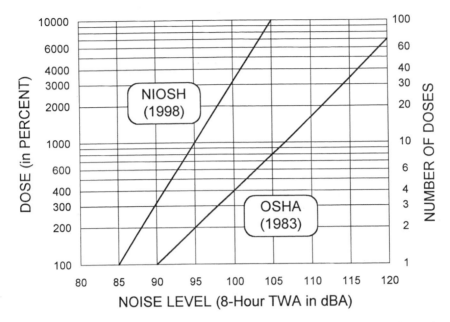

FIGURE 16–10   Noise exposure in terms of 8-hour TWA in dBA and noise dose (shown in percent on the left axis and as the number of doses on the right axis) according to OSHA (1983) regulations and NIOSH (1998) recommended criteria (see text).

NIOSH Noise Exposure Criteria   We are very interested in the OSHA HCA because it continues to be the dominant force in occupational hearing conservation in most indus-

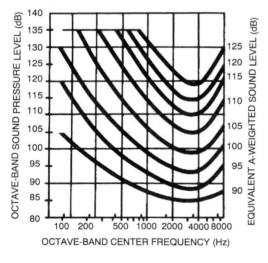

FIGURE 16–11   Curves for converting octave-band levels into equivalent A-weighted sound level (based on Figure G-9, OSHA, 1983). Octave-band sound levels measured for a noise are plotted on this graph (using the left axis). The highest contour penetrated by the noise spectrum constitutes the equivalent noise level in dBA (using the right axis).

tries[5] as the legally enforceable federal regulation. However, the National Institute of Occupational Safety and Health (NIOSH, 1998) developed revised criteria and recommendations for occupational hearing conservation programs that have considerable efficacy because they reflect the preponderance of scientific evidence. With regard to noise exposure limits, NIOSH called for (1) replacing the PEL of 90 dBA TWA with a **recommended exposure level (REL)** of 85 dBA TWA (2) changing the exchange rate from the 5-dB rule to the 3-dB (equal energy) rule, and (3) setting a ceiling exposure of 140 dBA regardless of the type of the noise.

The 85-dBA REL and 3-dB exchange rate used by NIOSH result in different and more protective exposure values than those used by OSHA, which is seen clearly by comparing the two sets of maximum exposure durations in Table 16–3. For example, notice that

---

[5] The Mine Safety and Health Administration (MSHA) has jurisdiction over the mining industry, and proposed a set of regulations in 1996, although these are not in effect as of this writing.

a 90-dBA exposure is permissible for 8 hours by OSHA but for only 2½ hours by NIOSH, and that OSHA permits a 1-hour exposure to 100 dBA compared to only 15 minutes according to the NIOSH recommendations. Noise exposure dosages are also considerably different according to the two sets of criteria. Referring to the plot labeled "NIOSH (1998)" in Figure 16–10, we see that a TWA of 85 dBA corresponds to one dose or a 100% dose according to NIOSH; OSHA's 90-dBA PEL is considered to be two doses or a 200% dose, and 105 dBA constitutes 100 doses or a 10,000% dose. Although the graph only goes up to a 10,000 dose, a 120-dBA TWA exposure would correspond to about a 316,000% dose (roughly 316 doses).

Other Effects of Noise

The effects of noise exposure are not limited to hearing impairment. We often experience many of the noises that we encounter as being disturbing in a way that goes beyond being too loud. Traffic and construction noise, airplane fly-overs, sirens, squeaky floor boards, the screech of fingernails drawn across a blackboard, and a neighbor's loud music are but a few examples. These sounds may be unwanted for one or more reasons. For example, sounds might be unwanted because they interfere with one's work, leisure activities, rest, or sleep; interfere with speech communication; are distracting or startling; or convey a disturbing meaning.

NOISINESS AND ANNOYANCE

Kryter (1985) distinguishes between two types of unwanted sounds, described as perceived noisiness and annoyance. **Perceived noisiness** (or just **noisiness**) is the "unwantedness" of a sound that is not unexpected or surprising, does not cause pain or provoke fear, and has nothing to do with the meaning of the sound. The same physical factors that make a sound louder also make it noisier, but noisiness is also affected by the time course of a sound. For example, increasing the duration of a sound beyond a second does not

make it louder but does make it noisier. Also, a sound that builds up over time is noisier than a sound that dies down over the same amount of time (e.g., an approaching train is noisier than a departing train). The magnitude of perceived noisiness can be quantified in **noys** (analogous to loudness in sones), and equally objectionable sounds can be expressed in units of **PNdB (perceived noise decibels)** (analogous to loudness level in phons). If one sound is twice as noisy as another, then it will be 10 PNdB higher and it will have double the number of noys.

In contrast to perceived noisiness, **annoyance** is the objectionability of a sound that involves the novelty, meaning, or emotional implications of the sound, as well as its physical characteristics. It has been suggested that noise levels would have to be ≤45 dB DNL in homes, hospital, and schools, and ≤55 dB outdoors to meet the goal of avoiding all interference and annoyance by noise (EPA, 1974). The amount of annoyance increases with increasing noise levels (e.g., Kryter, 1985), and also appears to be related to the source of the noise. For example, Miedema and Vos (1998) found that annoyance due to transportation noises is related to the mode of transportation, with the percentage of highly annoyed individuals being the greatest for aircraft noise, followed by road traffic noise, and then by railroad noise.

Fields (1993) found that residential noise annoyance is affected by the amount of isolation from noise at home, fear of danger from the noise sources, beliefs about noise prevention, general noise sensitivity, concern about the non-noise consequences of the noise source, and beliefs about the importance of the noise source. However, annoyance was not substantially affected by ambient noise levels, the number of hours spent at home, or a variety of demographic variables (e.g., age, sex, socioeconomic status). Fields (1998) also found the annoyance resulting from a particular noise source (e.g., aircraft) is little if at all affected by the amount of ambient noise produced by other noise sources (e.g., road traffic noises). Miedema and Vos (1999) found that fears relating to the noise source and self-assessed noise sensitivity had a large effect on transportation noise annoyance, but that most demographic factors had small effects on annoyance. They also found that younger and older adults were less annoyed by transportation noise than were those in the roughly 30- to 50-year-old range.[6] Miedema and Vos pointed out that the lessening of noise annoyance among older persons may be part of a more general aging-related development because the amount of annoyance caused by environmental odors also decreases among older individuals (Miedema, 1992).

SPEECH COMMUNICATION INTERFERENCE

Interference with speech communication is one of the most important and pervasive problems caused by noise. The adverse effects of noise on speech communication are experienced in many ways: masking of the speech signal may render it completely inaudible, or it may be audible but limited in intelligibility; speaker effort must be increased; listening becomes laborious and stressful; there is an increased need for repetition, clarification, and confirmation of the message; reliance on visual cues becomes increasingly important; message content may have to be adjusted or limited; distances between the talker and listener must be reduced; and errors and confusion abound.

How does a particular noise affect speech communication in a given environment? The most direct answer comes from giving subjects speech intelligibility tests for various kinds of materials (words, sentences, etc.) in each situation, but this approach is unrealistic. The practical solution is to make acoustical measurements of the noise, and then to predict how it should affect communication based on known relationships between noise

and speech intelligibility. We will briefly outline the principal methods.

Articulation Index   The **articulation index (AI)** is a method for predicting speech intelligibility from the audibility of speech signals, which was originated by French and Steinberg (1947). Audibility depends on how well the speech signal can be heard above the listener's threshold and any noise that is present.

Some background information is needed to understand the AI. French and Steinberg measured speech intelligibility when subjects were provided with only part of the frequency range. One set of experiments involved **high-pass filtering**, which means that the frequencies above a certain cutoff frequency were "passed" and the frequencies below the cutoff were "rejected" or not passed. For example, if the cutoff frequency is 800 Hz, then the subjects could hear the frequencies above 800 Hz (the "pass band") but could not hear the frequencies below 800 Hz (the "reject band"). This was done for many different cutoff frequencies, and the results are shown by the curve marked "high pass" in Figure 16–12. Intelligibility is close to 100% when the high-pass cutoff is 200 Hz, at point **a**, because the subjects can hear all of the frequencies above 200 Hz and are only denied the small range below it. Performance falls as the cutoff moves upward in frequency, and is only about 5% at point **b**, where the high-frequency cutoff is 5000 Hz. This happens because high-pass filtering at 5000 Hz is the same as removing the wide range of important frequencies below 5000 Hz. The same measurements were done with **low-pass filtering**, and these results are shown by the curve marked "low pass." Notice that intelligibility is very good (about 95%) for low-pass filtering at 5000 Hz, at point **c**, because the subjects can hear all of the frequencies up to 5000 Hz. However, intelligibility drops to near zero for the 200 Hz cutoff, at point **d**, because the subjects can hear only the frequencies up to 200 Hz but cannot hear anything higher than 200 Hz (because passing the lows is the same as

---

[6] The curvilinear (rising then falling) relationship between age and annoyance found by Miedema and Vos (1999) does not really disagree with Fields' (1993) analysis, which fundamentally found that there was not a linear (straight-line) relationship between age and annoyance.

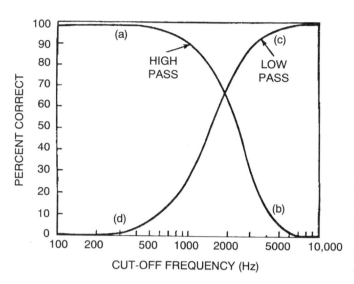

FIGURE 16–12 Correct identification of syllables as a function of high- and low-pass filtering. Points labeled **a, b, c,** and **d** refer to the text. Adapted from French and Steinberg (1947), with permission of the *Journal of the Acoustical Society of America.*

rejecting the highs). Notice that the two curves *intersect* at about 1900 Hz (where the score happens to be 68%). This means that the frequencies above 1900 Hz provide as much information about speech intelligibility as the frequencies below 1900 Hz. The frequency range of speech has been divided into two ranges or bandwidths (≤1900 Hz and ≥1900 Hz), each of which makes the same contribution to speech intelligibility. If the frequencies above and below 1900 Hz contribute equally, why do they intersect at 68% instead of at 50%? The answer is the speech signal contains **redundant** information. Incidentally, 1900 Hz and 68% are not magical values; the curves will intersect at different locations depending on the nature of the speech material being tested.

It is also possible to divide the frequency range into 20 bands, each of which makes an equal contribution to speech intelligibility. French and Steinberg (1947) did this very thing to develop the original version of the articulation index. Specifically, the AI is composed of 20 contiguous bands found to be equally important for speech understanding. Hence, each band contributes 5% to intelligibility (20 bands × 5% = 100%). The AI is expressed as a decimal value between 0 and 1.0, where 1.0 is the same as 100% (20 bands × 0.05 = 1.0). Each band is counted according to

the audibility of the speech signal it contains. We are concerned with the effects of noise on speech communication, so we will assume that the sounds are well above threshold, and concentrate on the signal-to-noise ratio (S/N) in each band. (Recall that S/N ratio is the number of decibels for the signal minus the number of decibels for the noise.) A 30-dB range of S/N ratio is considered, where an S/N ratio of +18 dB gets "full credit" for the band (0.05) down to −12 dB, which gets no credit for that band (0.0). In effect, each decibel of S/N ratio counts for 1/30 of the band's 0.05 value. This S/N ratio is used to determine how much of the band's 0.05 value will be counted. The resulting 20 values (one from each band) are added to arrive at the AI, which will range from 0 to 1.0. The original AI has been modified to use standard third-octave and octave-bands, adjustments in the importance attached to each band, etc., which is leading to the development of a new standard for a **speech intelligibility index (SII)**, as well as for use with the hearing impaired (e.g., Kryter, 1962; ANSI-S3.5, 1986; ANSI-S3.5, 1997; Pavlovic, Studebaker, & Sherbecoe, 1986; Pavlovic, 1987, 1991).

The AI can be used to predict the intelligibility of various kinds of speech material, some examples of which are illustrated in Figure 16–13. For example, an AI of 0.5

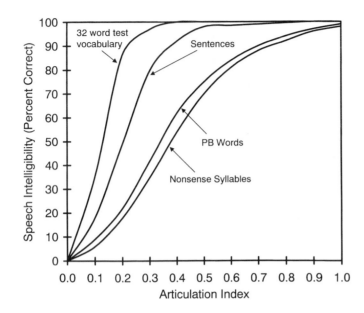

FIGURE 16–13 Relationship between the articulation index and speech intelligibility for various materials. Based on Kryter (1962, 1985) and ANSI-S3.5 (1969, R1986).

corresponds to intelligibility scores of roughly 70% for nonsense syllables, 75% for monosyllabic (PB) words, 97% for sentences, and 100% when the test vocabulary is limited to only 32 words. As a rule of thumb, the conditions for speech communication are (1) probably satisfactory when the AI is above 0.6, (2) unsatisfactory when the AI is under 0.3, and (3) sufficiently suspicious to warrant intelligibility testing (if possible) when the AI is between 0.3 and 0.6 (Beranek, 1954/1986). Notice in Figure 16–13 that an AI of 0.3 corresponds to word intelligibility of roughly 45% and sentence scores of about 80%, whereas performance reaches approximately 85% for words and about 98% for sentences when the AI is 0.6.

Speech Interference Level   The **speech interference level (SIL)** (Beranek, 1954/1986) is a simplified variation of the articulation index that identifies how much noise will just permit communication to take place. The SIL is provided for various distances between the talker and listener, and for different amounts of vocal effort from normal conversational speech to shouting. Figure 16–14 shows SIL values developed by Beranek (1954/1986). It shows, for example, that (1) normal conversational speech can just take place at a distance of 12 feet providing the noise (i.e., the SIL) is

43 dB, but at no more than 4 feet if the SIL is 53 dB; (2) an SIL of 61 dB will allow communication to take place for raised speech level at 3 feet, very loud speech at 6 feet, and when shouting at 12 feet; and (3) an SIL of 71 dB limits the distance to 4 feet when shouting, 2 feet for very loud speech, 1 foot for raised speech, and just 6 inches for normal speech.

The SIL itself is obtained by simply averaging the noise levels in three or four bands. The original SIL used the 600 to 1200 Hz, 1200 to 2400 Hz, and 2400 to 4800 Hz bands, and included the 300 to 600 Hz band in the average if its level was >10 dB more than in the 600 to 1200 Hz band. Many modifications of the SIL have been developed using the *preferred* octave-bands centered at 500, 1000, 2000, and 4000 Hz (called **PSIL** for this reason), as well as measurements in dBA and dBC (e.g., Webster, 1969, 1978; ANSI S3.14-1977, R1997; Lazarus, 1987). The current version of the SIL uses the 500, 1000, 2000, and 4000 Hz bands (ANSI-S3.14, 1977, R1997).

Speech Transmission Index   The **speech transmission index (STI)** (Steeneken & Houtgast, 1983; Anderson & Kalb, 1987) is another method for estimating speech communication efficiency from acoustical measurements. It extends the AI concept to account for the effects of all kinds of distortions,

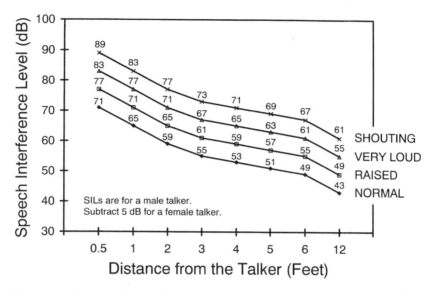

FIGURE 16–14 The speech interference levels (SILs) at which word intelligibility is barely reliable at distances of 1/2 foot to 12 feet away from the talker in an environment without reflections, for various levels of vocal effort (normal, raised, very loud, shouting). Subtract 5 dB for female talker. Add 5 dB for sentences or if a limited vocabulary is used. Based on data by Beranek (1954/1986).

including those that occur over time, like reverberation. **Reverberation** refers to multiple echoes from reflective surfaces in a room that continue for a period of time after the original sound has ended. Some degree of reverberation adds "liveness" to a room, but substantial reverberation is a very common problem that causes speech intelligibility to deteriorate. The STI uses a sophisticated method of physical analysis called the **modulation transfer function (MTF)** to determine how a test signal is affected by noise and distortion in the octave-bands from 125 to 8000 Hz. The MTF results are converted to a transmission index for each band. The bands are weighted according to their importance for speech communication (as for the AI), and are then combined to produce the STI, which ranges from 0 to 100% (or 0 to 1.0). The higher the STI, the better are the conditions for speech communication. The curves in Figure 16–15 show how speech recognition is related to the STI.

A simple and efficient method for making STI measurements is provided by the **rapid speech transmission index (RASTI)** (IEC, 1987), which can be accomplished using

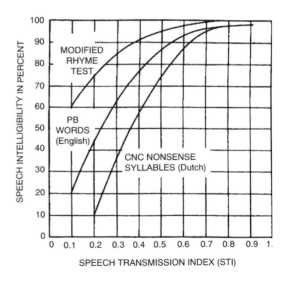

FIGURE 16–15 The relationship between the speech transmission index and speech recognition scores for PB-50 words (English), the Modified Rhyme Test (MRT; estimated), and Dutch CVC nonsense syllables. Adapted from Anderson and Kalb (1987) with permission of the *Journal of the Acoustical Society of America*.

instrumentation made for this purpose (e.g., Bruel & Kjaer, 1985). The equipment includes a loudspeaker placed in the location of a talker and a microphone placed where the listener would be. The loudspeaker presents a test signal into the room being evaluated, and the sound picked up by the microphone reflects how the original test signal has been affected by the noise and other acoustical characteristics in the room. The results are expressed as RASTI values from 0 to 1.0, which can be used to indicate relative speech intelligibility; for example, ≤0.29, bad; 0.3 to 0.44, poor; 0.45 to 0.59, fair; 0.6 to 0.74, good; ≥0.75, excellent (Orfield, 1987).

NONAUDITORY EFFECTS OF NOISE

Exposure to noise can have wide-reaching negative effects on many aspects of physical and mental health and performance. Many of these are mentioned here so the student will have a general idea of how noise can affect other aspects of life besides hearing and speech communication. These include: (1) interference with sleep; (2) stress and anxiety reactions; (3) startle responses and reflexive muscle reactions; (4) changes in heart rate, breathing pattern, gastrointestinal motility, pupillary size, and digestive secretions; (5) nervous system arousal, revealed by changes in electroencephalogram (EEG) activity and reduced galvanic skin resistance; (6) constriction and flow reduction in peripheral blood vessels; (7) vestibular disturbances with very intense sounds; (8) negative impact on the performance of cognitive and sensorimotor tasks due to arousal, distraction, startle responses, and increased fatigue after completion of tasks; (9) increased incidences of cardiovascular, vestibular, and ear-nose-throat disorders; (10) a slight effect on prematurity and reduced birth weight; and (11) evidence of relatively poorer school performance (Cohen, 1977; Miller, 1974; Cohen & Weinstein, 1981; Kryter, 1985; Suter, 1992a).

Occupational Hearing Conservation

The requirements of occupational hearing conservation programs are largely defined by compliance with federal regulations known as the **Hearing Conservation Amendment (HCA)** (OSHA, 1983). The current HCA is the culmination of a series of laws and regulations beginning with noise exposure regulations instituted in 1969 under the authority of the Walsh-Healey Public Contracts Act of 1935 (DOL, 1969). Subsequently, the Williams-Steiger Occupational Safety and Health Act of 1970 established OSHA under the Department of Labor. In turn, OSHA amended the Walsh-Healey noise standard by developing the original version of the HCA in 1971. After a long and bumpy evolution (see, e.g., Suter, 1984; Suter & vonGierke, 1987), the final form of the HCA was published in the Federal Register on March 8, 1983 (OSHA, 1983).

The HCA requires that a **hearing conservation program** must be implemented for all employees who are exposed to noise levels of 85 dBA TWA, or a 50% dose (recall that the PEL is 90 dBA TWA or a 100% dose). A time-weighted average of 85 dBA (or a 50% dose) is often called the **action level** for this reason, although we will see that some aspects of the program are triggered when exposures achieve 90 dBA TWA. In contrast, NIOSH (1998) called for all components of the hearing conservation program to be triggered at 85 dBA TWA. The OSHA-mandated hearing conservation program involves five major components: monitoring of noise levels; audiometric testing; hearing protectors (ear plugs or muffs that reduce the sound levels reaching the eardrum); a training program; and record keeping. Invaluable information and guidance pertaining to the details of hearing conservation programs may be found in several readily available sources (e.g., Miller & Silverman, 1984; Gasway, 1985; Berger et al, 1986; Lipscomb, 1988; NIOSH, 1990, 1996, 1998; Royster & Royster, 1990a; Suter, 1993).

MONITORING OF NOISE LEVELS

The Hearing Conservation Amendment requires noise level monitoring to be done whenever there is information suggesting that employees might be exposed to noise levels

≥85 dBA TWA. All continuous, intermittent, and impulsive noises between 80 and 130 dB are integrated into the noise exposure measurements. Representative personal noise exposure sampling is done when area-wide monitoring is not appropriate, such as when the employees move around a lot, or when there are variations in sound level within the area in question. All affected employees must be notified that they are being exposed to noise levels ≥85 dBA TWA. Noise level monitoring must be repeated whenever changes occur that might cause (1) additional employees to be exposed to ≥85 dBA TWA, or (2) the employees' hearing protectors no longer to be providing adequate attenuation.

AUDIOMETRIC TESTING

The audiometric testing component of the program includes a baseline audiogram, annual audiograms, certain retests, and referrals. Air-conduction audiograms are done for each ear for at least *500, 1000, 2000, 3000, 4000, and 6000 Hz*, using a manual, self-recording, or microprocessor-controlled (computerized) audiometer. These tests may be performed by an audiologist, a physician, or a technician who is certified by the Council of Accreditation in Occupational Hearing Conservation (CAOHC) or who has demonstrated satisfactory competence. Technicians who operate microprocessor-based audiometers do not have to be certified. All technicians must be responsible to an audiologist or a physician. The term "physician" is used here even though the HCA actually says "an otolaryngologist or physician" because all otolaryngologists are physicians. Confusing wording is also found in the HCA with regard to technicians who may operate manual versus microprocessor-controlled audiometers. The fact that technicians can be certified by CAOHC or have "satisfactorily demonstrated competence" effectively negates any distinction between a certified or uncertified technician.

Employees must have a **baseline audiogram** within the first 6 months of exposure to noise levels ≥85 dBA TWA. Future audiograms will be compared to the baseline audiogram to determine if there has been any deterioration of hearing that may have been caused by occupational noise exposure. To minimize the effects of TTS on the baseline audiogram, employees must be without workplace noise exposure for at least 14 hours before testing, and must be advised to avoid nonoccupational noise exposures during this period, as well. However, hearing protectors may be used as a substitute for being away from workplace noise during the 14 hours before testing. A special exception to the 6-month time limit for baseline audiograms is allowed if the audiometric services are provided by a mobile testing van that comes to the workplace. Mobile testing vans are often used when on-site testing facilities are not available. In these cases, the time limit for the baseline audiogram is extended to a full year, but hearing protectors must be used after the first 6 months.

Annual monitoring audiograms are done for each employee exposed to noise levels ≥85 dBA TWA. The annual audiogram is compared to the baseline audiogram to determine if there has been a **standard threshold shift** in either or both ears. A standard threshold shift is simply a change for the worse in threshold with an *average of 10 dB or more at 2000, 3000, and 4000 Hz*. An **age correction** may be made when determining if there has been a standard threshold shift, which essentially reduces the size of the threshold shift by an amount that is attributed to presbycusis. Table 16–4 shows the age correction values that may be used for this purpose, and illustrates the procedure prescribed by the HCA. A retest may be done within 30 days if there has been a standard threshold shift, in which case the retest may be used as the annual audiogram. Comparisons between annual and baseline audiograms may be done by a technician. However, problem cases are reviewed by an audiologist or a physician, who also determines if there is a need for further evaluation.

NIOSH (1998) recommended the replacement of OSHA's standard threshold shift (which averages across frequencies) with a **significant threshold shift**, defined as change for the worse of ≥15 dB at any of the required test

TABLE 16–4   Age correction values for males and females (according to Tables F-1 and F-2, OSHA, 1983)

Frequency (Hz):	Males					Females				
	1000	2000	3000	4000	6000	1000	2000	3000	4000	6000
Age (years)										
20 or younger	5	3	4	5	8	7	4	3	3	6
21	5	3	4	5	8	7	4	4	3	6
22	5	3	4	5	8	7	4	4	4	6
23	5	3	4	6	9	7	5	4	4	7
24	5	3	5	6	9	7	5	4	4	7
25	5	3	5	7	10	8	5	4	4	7
26	5	4	5	7	10	8	5	5	4	8
27	5	4	6	7	11	8	5	5	5	8
28	6	4	6	8	11	8	5	5	5	8
29	6	4	6	8	12	8	5	5	5	9
30	6	4	6	9	12	8	6	5	5	9
31	6	4	7	9	13	8	6	6	5	9
32	6	5	7	10	14	9	6	6	6	10
33	6	5	7	10	14	9	6	6	6	10
34	6	5	8	11	15	9	6	6	6	10
35	7	5	8	11	15	9	6	7	7	11
36	7	5	9	12	16	9	7	7	7	11
37	7	6	9	12	17	9	7	7	7	12
38	7	6	9	13	17	10	7	7	7	12
39	7	6	10	14	18	10	7	8	8	12
40	7	6	10	14	19	10	7	8	8	13
41	7	6	10	14	20	10	8	8	8	13
42	8	7	11	16	20	10	8	9	9	13
43	8	7	12	16	21	11	8	9	9	14
44	8	7	12	17	22	11	8	9	9	14
45	8	7	13	18	23	11	8	10	10	15
46	8	8	13	19	24	11	9	10	10	15
47	8	8	14	19	24	11	9	10	11	16
48	9	8	14	20	25	12	9	11	11	16
49	9	9	15	21	26	12	9	11	11	16
50	9	9	16	22	27	12	10	11	12	17
51	9	9	16	23	28	12	10	12	12	17
52	9	10	17	24	29	12	10	12	13	18
53	9	10	18	25	30	13	10	13	13	18
54	10	10	18	26	31	13	11	13	14	19
55	10	11	19	27	32	13	11	14	14	19
56	10	11	20	28	34	13	11	14	15	20
57	10	11	21	29	35	13	11	15	15	20
58	10	12	22	31	36	14	12	15	16	21
59	11	12	22	32	37	14	12	16	16	21
60 or older	11	13	23	33	38	14	12	16	17	22

Example of how to use age correction values: Using 4000 Hz as an example, suppose the threshold on the annual audiogram is 20 dB at age 32, and the threshold on the baseline audiogram was 5 dB at age 20. The uncorrected threshold shift would be

$$20 \text{ dB (annual)} - 5 \text{ dB (baseline)} = 15 \text{ dB (threshold shift)}$$

Now, find the age correction values that apply to the baseline and annual audiogram. Find the difference between these age correction values. For males at 4000 Hz, these values are 14 dB at age 32 and 11 dB at age 20, and the difference between them is

$$14 \text{ dB (at age 32)} - 11 \text{ dB (at age 20)} = 3 \text{ dB (age correction)}$$

This difference becomes the age correction. It is subtracted from the uncorrected threshold shift to find the age corrected threshold shift. In our example, this is

$$15 \text{ dB (uncorrected)} - 3 \text{ dB (correction)} = 12 \text{ dB (age-corrected)}$$

The age-corrected threshold shift is then used to find the (now age-corrected) standard threshold shift.

frequencies (500, 1000, 2000, 3000, 4000, or 6000 Hz) in either ear. It also recommended abandoning the practice of using age corrections in the threshold shift calculations. Some of the other substantial changes to OSHA's audiometric testing rules included the following: Testing should include 8000 Hz—albeit optionally—to improve the diagnostic usefulness of the results. An immediate retest should be done when the monitoring audiogram shows significant threshold shift before scheduling the employee to return for a confirmation test (which is used to establish the persistence of the threshold shift). An **exit audiogram** should be obtained when an employee is no longer exposed to potentially hazardous noise levels or leaves the employer. In addition, employees should be away from noise exposures of ≥85 dBA for 12 hours before the baseline and exit audiograms, and hearing protectors should not be used as a substitute for the noise-free period.

FOLLOW-UP AND REFERRAL PROCEDURES

An employee who has sustained a standard threshold shift must be advised of this within 21 days. Unless a physician determines that the standard threshold shift was unrelated to occupational noise exposure, the employee must be provided with hearing protectors and be *required* to use them, or be refitted with new ones that provide greater attenuation if he is already using hearing protectors. *Referrals* for audiological and/or otological evaluations are made if more testing is needed or if there is suspicion of ear pathology related to the use of hearing protectors. Employees must also be *informed* about any suspicion of ear diseases that are not related to hearing protector use. Just as an employee must be told about the presence of a standard threshold shift, he must also be informed if subsequent tests show that the standard threshold shift is not consistent. In that case, he may choose to stop using hearing protectors providing his noise exposures are less than 90 dBA TWA. The annual audiogram becomes a **revised baseline audiogram** for future comparisons if the audiologist or

physician judges that (1) there is a persistent standard threshold shift, or (2) the thresholds on the annual audiogram are better (lower) than those on the baseline.

AUDIOMETER CALIBRATION AND TESTING ENVIRONMENT

Audiometers used in the occupational hearing conservation program are required to be calibrated to ANSI S3.6 (1969, R1989) specifications (see Table 4-1 in Chapter 4) for at least the frequencies between 500 and 6000 Hz. A *biological calibration* using a person who has known thresholds as well as a listening check for distortion and spurious noises must be accomplished daily before any testing is done. An *acoustical calibration* is required at least annually, and an *exhaustive calibration* must be done at least once every 2 years. In addition, the HCA calls for an acoustical calibration to be done whenever the biological calibration is off by ≥10 dB, and for an exhaustive calibration whenever there is a deviation of ≥15 dB on an acoustical calibration.

The HCA permits the audiometric test room to have ambient noise octave-band levels that are substantially higher than the maximum ambient noise levels specified by the ANSI S3.1-1991 standard for audiometric environments, as shown in Table 16–5. The serious implication of this discrepancy is that a test room can meet the HCA requirements for audiometric testing without really being quiet enough for thresholds to be obtained down to 0 dB HL. This can be a source of error and variability that should be avoided by using test rooms that come as close as possible to meeting the ANSI (1991a) standard for audiometric test environments whenever feasible. Testing in rooms meeting the ANSI (1991a) standard is recommended by NIOSH (1998).

HEARING PROTECTORS

The employer must *provide* a reasonable choice of adequate hearing protectors free of charge to all employees who are exposed to noise levels of ≥85 dBA TWA, and replace

TABLE 16–5   Comparison between the octave-band levels (in dB) of ambient noise in an audiometric test room allowed by the Hearing Conservation Amendment (OSHA, 1983) and those specified by ANSI standards (ANSI S3.1-1991a)

Center Frequency (Hz)	HCA (1983) (dB)	ANSI-S3.1 (1991) (dB)	Discrepancy (dB)
500	40	19.5	20.5
1000	40	26.5	13.5
2000	47	28	19
4000	57	34.5	22.5
8000	62	43.5	18.5

them as necessary. The employer is also responsible for the proper initial fitting of hearing protectors, providing employees with training in their use and care, and supervising their correct use. There are three classes of employees who not only must be provided with ear protectors but also are required to actually use them. They include all employees exposed to levels exceeding the PEL of 90 dBA TWA, and employees exposed at ≥85 dBA TWA who (1) are waiting longer than 6 months for a baseline audiogram under the exception for mobile test vans, or (2) have experienced a standard threshold shift. Here, again, the onus for compliance is upon the employer. Hearing protectors are discussed in more detail below.

Efforts to reduce noise exposure have concentrated on the use of hearing protectors. However, the Walsh-Healey regulation actually states that when employees are exposed to noise levels above the PEL "feasible *administrative or engineering controls shall be utilized.*" If engineering and/or administrative controls fail to reduce sound levels within the levels of Table G-16 [i.e., the PELs identified in the first and second columns of Table 16–3], then "personal protective equipment shall be provided and used to reduce sound levels within the levels of the table" (OSHA, 1983, 29 CFR 1910.95 (b)(1), emphasis added). It is important to be aware that the HCA did *not* supersede or replace these requirements of the original regulations.

TRAINING PROGRAM

Employers are responsible for providing an annual training program for employees

exposed to ≥85 dBA TWA and ensure they participate in the program. The training program is required to address at least three topics: (1) the effects of noise on hearing; (2) hearing protectors, including their purpose, advantages and disadvantages of different types, and their selection, fitting, use, and care; and (3) the purposes of and procedures involved in audiometric testing.

Although annual training sessions are required, it would be foolish to believe that the effectiveness of any hearing conservation program can be maintained by a passively supported meeting once a year, no matter how impressive the talker, demonstrations, and videotapes might be. Several sessions spread over the year can be helpful, especially if they are interactive and relatively short. All kinds of educational and training materials are available, including motivational posters that not only prompt employees to wear their hearing protectors, but also remind them how to do so properly. Motivational approaches run the gamut from simple praise to innovative reward systems, but also include disciplinary personnel actions. The importance of active support by management, including supervisors and foremen, cannot be over-stressed, so that employees are aware that the hearing conservation program is treated as a mutually beneficial commitment that is enthusiastically encouraged and actively enforced.

RECORD KEEPING

Employers are required to keep records on noise exposure measurements, audiometric tests, and the background levels in the test rooms. In addition to the employee's name, job classification, test dates, and results, each audiometric test record is also required to show the examiner's name, the date of the audiometer's most recent acoustic or exhaustive calibration, and the date of the employee's last noise exposure assessment. Noise exposure measurements have to be retained for 2 years and audiometric records are kept for the entire duration of employment for each employee.

Employees (or their representatives) must be allowed to observe the measurements, and to have access to the noise standard and related information, training materials, and records.

PROGRAM EFFECTIVENESS

The effectiveness of a hearing conservation program might be addressed in many different ways, each providing different kinds of information. For example, one might determine how many standard threshold shifts have occurred. Another approach might be to determine the degree of employee compliance for ear protection use, or even for keeping appointments for scheduled hearing tests or training sessions. However, a different approach has been selected as the most appropriate by ANSI draft standard S12.13 (1991b). This method is a statistical procedure called **audiometric database analysis (ADBA)** (e.g., Royster & Royster, 1986, 1999). The basic concept of ADBA is to monitor the effectiveness of a hearing conservation program by evaluating audiometric findings on a group basis. This approach makes it possible to identify undesirable trends that can be alleviated by program-wide changes in policies and procedures. Instead of comparing threshold shifts between audiograms, audiometric data base analysis looks at the *variability* between sequential pairs of audiograms (e.g., between the first and second annual audiograms, the second and third, etc.). This variability is compared to criterion ranges to determine whether it is acceptable, marginal, or unacceptable. Marginally or unacceptably high variability indicates the possibility that a problem exists that needs to be addressed. For example, the hearing conservation program may be failing to provide an adequate degree of protection from on-the-job noise exposure. This might be due to poor utilization of hearing protectors, the need for engineering and/or administrative controls, deficiencies in the educational program or motivation, etc. However, other factors may also account for the variability. The most likely ones involve deficiencies in the audiometric testing program, and often have to do with inadequate audiometer calibration, acoustical test environments, and test methods.

Controlling Noise and Noise Exposure

Administrative Controls

Administrative controls involve modifications of scheduling and other policies that effectively reduce employees' exposures to excessive noise levels. For example, instead of having one group of employees working an 8-hour shift in a high-noise area exceeding the PEL, two smaller groups could be rotated between work assignments in high-noise and low-noise areas so their TWA exposures are all below the PEL. However, approaches of this type are rarely used because they present untenable practical problems for the employer and are often just as objectionable to employees and labor unions.

Engineering Controls

Numerous engineering approaches can be used to control noise exposure by reducing noise at its *source* and/or by modifying its transmission path to or at the *receiver* (i.e., the listener). Many of the major considerations have been reviewed by Bruce and Toothman (1986) and Erdreich (1999), and a clearly illustrated outline of noise control methods may be found in Bruel and Kjaer (1986). One approach that addresses the noise source is the *replacement* of noisier equipment, processes, and materials with quieter ones. Several examples include the replacement of gear drives with belt drives, compressed-air driven (pneumatic) tools with electric ones, riveting with welding or bolts, and steel wheels and gears with rubber or plastic ones. Another approach involves *modifications* of the sound sources. For example, industrial processes that involve impacts on vibrating surfaces can be made less noisy by reducing the driving force. This can be accomplished by decreasing the speed of repetitive impacts, keeping the equipment well balanced, and placing a vibration isolator (e.g., a rubber lining) at the point of impact. Vibratory responses can be reduced by adding damping materials, or by adding stiffness or mass to change the resonance of the vibrating surface. The amount of noise radiated by a vibrating surface can be diminished by reducing its area, which can be accomplished by decreasing its overall size or by adding perforations. Noises produced by flowing fluids or a turbulent stream of air (e.g., air ejection systems and high pressure vents) can be abated by reducing the speed of fluid flow and the amount of turbulence. Mufflers and wrapping with sound-absorbing materials are also used.

Modifying the acoustical path may be accomplished by placing enclosures around the offending equipment, using shields or barriers between the source and the listener, using acoustically lined ducts and mufflers, and sometimes by providing sound-isolating control rooms for workers (i.e., an enclosure around the listener). In effect, hearing protectors modify the acoustical path at its far end by obstructing the transmission of noise just before it is picked up by the ear. Noise levels are also reduced by using acoustically absorptive materials on room surfaces (ceilings, walls, etc.), which is particularly important in reverberant environments. Active noise control methods have also been developed that use advanced signal processing methods to produce a sound that cancels all or part of the original noise (e.g., Nelson & Elliot, 1992; Ericksson, 1996; Kuo & Morgan, 1996).

Towne (1994) has provided advice about noise considerations when choosing a place to live, including practical applications of noise control principles in the home. A few examples are quite instructive: Floors should be carpeted except in the kitchen, where a resilient mat should separate vinyl or linoleum floor coverings from the subflooring, especially in multistory dwellings. The entrance door should have a heavy, solid core with minimal spaces around its perimeter, and a rubber bumper to reduce noise when slammed. Similarly, sliding doors should have rubber wheels and resilient bumpers.

Hearing Protectors

Hearing protection devices (HPDs) include a variety of ear plugs and muffs used to reduce the amount of sound reaching the wearer's ears (Berger, 1986a). Hearing protectors are generally categorized as ear muffs, ear plugs, and canal caps or semiaural plugs. **Ear muffs** are rigid plastic cups or shells with soft plastic cushions that completely enclose the ears (Fig. 16–16a). The shells are filled with sound-attenuating material and the cushions are filled with foam or liquid so they fit snugly against the sides of the head, sealing off the sound path to the ears. The cups are held firmly against the head by a spring headband. The effectiveness of ear muffs is reduced by about 5 dB when eyeglasses are worn (Royster et al, 1996). Ear muffs are also available in combination with hard hats for use in jobs where head protection is also needed (Fig. 16–16b).

Ear plugs are inserted snugly into the ear canals (Fig. 16–17). *Premolded* plugs are made of flexible plastic, silicone, or similar materials that have one or more flanges that provide a snug fit when placed into the ear canal. They usually come in several sizes, although some premolded plugs are made with several tapered flanges so that "one size fits all." *Formable or user-molded* plugs are made of pliable materials that form to the size and shape of the ear canal when they are inserted. The most common materials are expandable polymer foam, silicon putty, wax-impregnated cotton, and fiberglass down or "wool." The latter type of material should be encapsulated within a plastic membrane to protect the ear canal from direct contact with the fiberglass.

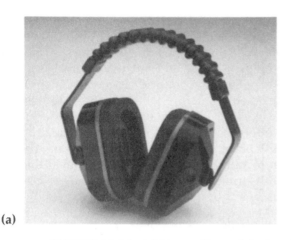

(a)

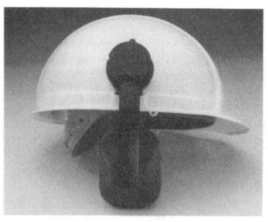

(b)

FIGURE 16–16   (a) Ear muffs used for hearing protection. (b) Ear muffs in combination with a hard hat. Courtesy of E-A-R.

The expandable foam material is compressed by rolling it between the fingers before being inserted into the ear canal. After being inserted, the foam expands and snugly seals the ear canal. Inserting balls of untreated absorbent cotton (the type commonly sold in health and beauty aid stores) into the ears provides little if any attenuation and should not be used for hearing protection. *Custom-molded* ear plugs can also be made from ear impressions like those used to make hearing aid earmolds and swim molds. In spite of the fact that they are custom-made, the amount of attenuation provided by individually molded ear plugs varies widely.

Semi-aural hearing protectors are modified ear plugs held in place by a lightweight plastic headband (Fig. 16–18). The *canal cap* variety of semiaural devices cover the entrance to the ear canal, and generally provide

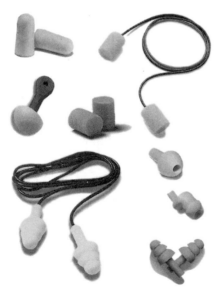

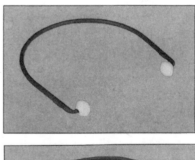

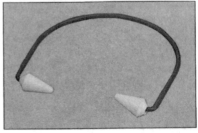

FIGURE 16–17   Examples of ear plugs used for hearing protection. Formable plugs are shown above and preformed plugs are shown below. Courtesy of E-A-R.

FIGURE 16–18   Examples of semi-aural hearing protectors: canal cap type above; pod type below. Courtesy of E-A-R.

less attenuation than *pod-type* tips, which insert part of the way into the ear canal. Semiaurals are easily and conveniently put on and taken off, but they provide the least amount of attenuation among the different types of HPDs. For these reasons, they are best suited for individuals who need hearing protection for short-duration, intermittent exposures.

Compared to ear plugs, ear muffs generally provide somewhat more attenuation, except for the expandable foam plugs; are well suited for situations where HPDs must be put on and removed frequently; provide somewhat more consistent amounts of attenuation in actual field use; are more comfortable in cold environments; and can be easier to fit regardless of head sizes or shape. Ear muffs are also quite noticeable, so their use is easier to monitor. Ear muffs have several disadvantages as well. For example, headband pressure causes discomfort particularly with longer durations of use, they are uncomfortable and promote perspiration in hot environments, and they can be problematic when the user is also wearing protective glasses and other kinds of safety devices. Although ear muffs interfere with the use of regular hard hats, this problem can be alleviated by using hard hats with built-in muffs.

In contrast to muffs, ear plugs are more comfortable when they are being worn for longer periods of time, are somewhat less expensive at least on an individual unit basis, and they do not interfere with the use of safety goggles, hard hats, or other safety gear. With the noteworthy exception of the expandable foam variety, most types of ear plugs provide somewhat less attenuation than ear muffs. The amount of attenuation actually provided by ear plugs depends on how deeply and securely they are inserted. (Using both muffs and plugs together typically provides roughly 5 to 10 dB more attenuation than either one alone.) Ear plugs are more difficult to put on than muffs, and, once inserted, many plugs often work themselves loose over the course of the workday, especially when there is jaw movement asso-

ciated with talking and chewing. Cleanliness becomes an important issue when plugs must be reinserted during the day, especially with dirty hands and in work environments where there is a lot of dust, metal shavings, or other splintering materials. Because they are less visible than muffs, it can be a bit harder to monitor employee compliance with plugs. While it is true that plugs are easier to lose than muffs, they are also available with strings that minimize loss and are certainly less trouble to carry.

Many HPD users are concerned that hearing protectors might interfere with the ability to hear speech. In addition, industrial employees are equally concerned about the ability to hear warning signals and potentially important changes in equipment sounds, and musicians are concerned about interference with the accurate perception of music. In general, it appears that HPDs do not interfere with the speech reception of normal hearing persons (and may even improve it) as long as the noise levels exceed about 85 dBA; but speech interference is a problem in low and moderate noise levels and in quiet (e.g., Berger, 1986a). Speech intelligibility is adversely affected by HPDs when the wearer has a sensorineural hearing loss or is not a fluent speaker of the language (e.g., Abel, Alberti, Haythornthwaite, & Riko, 1982a; Abel, Alberti, & Riko, 1982b; Bauman & Marston, 1986). The degree to which HPDs interfere with the reception of desired signals is minimized by the use of special kinds of HPDs that use acoustical and/or electronic methods to make the amount of attenuation provided dependent on the noise level, or so that its frequency response is similar to that of an unoccluded ear (e.g., Maxwell, Williams, Robertson, & Thomas, 1987; Killion, DeVilbiss, & Stewart, 1988; Berger, 1991).

EFFECTIVENESS OF HEARING PROTECTORS

The effectiveness of an HPD is determined by how much attenuation it provides, which can be measured in several ways (Berger, 1986b; Berger, Franks, & Lindgren, 1996; ANSI S12.6-

1984, R1990). The two principal techniques are **real ear attenuation at threshold (REAT)**, which is a behavioral method, and the **microphone in real ear (MIRE)** approach, which involves physical measurements. In the REAT method, thresholds are obtained for the same ear with and without an HPD. The amount of attenuation provided by the HPD is the difference between the two thresholds. For example, if a subject's threshold is 10 dB with the ear open and 33 dB with an ear plug, then the ear plug has provided $33 - 10 = 23$ dB of attenuation. The MIRE approach uses a tiny probe microphone located inside of the ear behind the HPD and another microphone located outside of the hearing protector. Test sounds are thus monitored on both sides of the hearing protector, and the amount of attenuation is the difference between the sound levels picked up inside and outside of the HPD. It appears that the amount of attenuation measured for an HPD is slightly larger when it is based on MIRE compared to REAT measurements (Casali, Mauney, & Burks, 1995).

The Environmental Protection Agency (1979) requires HPDs to be labeled according to the amount of attenuation they provide, expressed in terms of octave-band levels or a **noise reduction rating (NRR)**. The NRR combines the attenuation in each of the octave-bands into a single number. The NRR is the difference between the overall noise level of the "unprotected" exposure in dBC and the noise level under the HPD (the "protected" exposure) in dBA, along with a 3-dB adjustment for "spectral variations"; or

$$NRR = dBC_{unprotected} - dBA_{protected} - 3 \text{ dB}$$

The attenuation values are obtained by testing a group of subjects in the laboratory, and would typically be expressed in the form of a mean. However, the *average* amount of attenuation theoretically represents the protection provided to only *half* the population who would be using a particular kind of HPD. For this reason, two standard deviations are subtracted from the mean amount of attenuation found in the laboratory, so that the NRR theoretically represents the attenuation that would

be afforded to about 98% of the population who use that hearing protector. The **single number rating (SNR)** (ISO, 1994) is a similar system for describing HPD attenuation, and tends to estimate attenuation values that are about 3 dB larger than the NRR.

Recall that the purpose of a hearing protector is to reduce an employee's effective exposure to noise down to an acceptable maximum level. The amount of noise exposure effectively experienced by a worker while using a particular HPD (the "protected" exposure) in dBA is estimated by subtracting the NRR provided by the hearing protector from the noise level in dBC, or

$$dBA_{protected} = dBC_{unprotected} - NRR$$

This is one of the reasons it is desirable to measure noise levels in both dBA and dBC, even though damage risk and compliance are usually viewed in terms of just dBA. (Remember that all of these values are really time-weighted averages.) What if the dBC levels are not known? Under these circumstances, OSHA permits HPD effectiveness to be based on unprotected noise levels in dBA, but the NRR is reduced by 7 dB:

$$dBA_{protected} = dBA_{unprotected} - [NRR - 7]$$

The labeled attenuation values of HPDs represent the results of carefully executed laboratory measurements, but do they really predict the amount of attenuation experienced in the field, that is, by those who actually wear HPDs under normal working conditions? Comparisons of laboratory versus field data and studies involved with the development and verification of the ANSI-1997 standard (described below) have shown that *all* HPDs provide substantially less attenuation in actual (field) use compared to the laboratory-based NRRs on their labels (Berger, 1993; Berger, Franks, & Lindgren, 1996; Royster et al, 1996; Berger et al, 1998). This point is revealed in Figure 16–19, which summarizes the findings of many studies that compared the attenuation provided by various kinds of HPDs in the laboratory (as labeled on the HPD package) and in the field

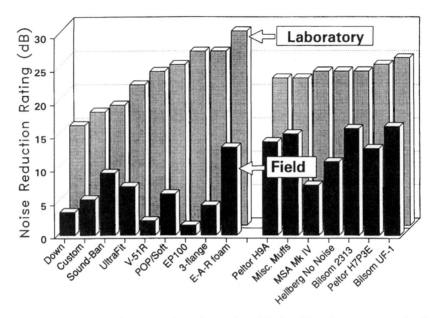

FIGURE 16–19   Noise reduction ratings for various kinds of hearing protectors in the laboratory (as labeled) versus in the field (in actual use in the field). The group on the left are ear plugs, the group on the right are ear muffs. From Berger (1993) with permission of the author and E-A-R.

(Berger, 1993; Berger et al, 1996).[7] The figure also shows that the relative rankings of HPDs from lowest to highest laboratory NRRs are not maintained in actual use. The graph suggests that most ear plugs can be expected to provide most wearers with at least 5 to 10 dB of attenuation in actual use compared to 10 to 15 dB for expandable foam plugs and ear muffs. This is not a problem because more than 90% of noise-exposed workers need only 10 dB of attenuation to bring their exposures down to acceptable levels (Royster, 1995).

In light of the foregoing discussion, it should not be surprising that authorities in the field have recommended replacing the

current NRR with a new value called the **subject-fit noise reduction rating [NRR(SF)]** (Royster, 1995; Royster et al, 1996; ANSI, 1997; Berger, 1999). The NRR(SF) is determined by subtracting one standard deviation from the mean attenuation values obtained when *naive subjects insert their own HPDs according to the manufacturer's instructions* (hence, "subject-fit"). Hence, the NRR(SF) should more closely approximate the actual attenuation expected for 84% of actual users in the field. In addition, the NRR(SF) is intended to be subtracted from the unprotected noise level in dBA to arrive at the user's protected noise exposure in dBA. The validity of the subject fit method was established by Berger et al (1998).

Until HPDs are tested and labeled according to the subject-fit approach, NIOSH (1998) has proposed that the expected amount of actual protection provided by HPD should be estimated by **derating** (i.e., reducing) the NRRs on the manufacturers' labels by 25% for ear muffs, 50% for formable ear plugs, and 70% for other types of ear plugs. These values are based on comparisons between NRRs and

---

[7] The NRRs in the graph apply to 98% of the lab population and 84% of the field population because the mean attenuation is reduced by two standard deviations in the lab and one standard deviation in the field data to keep the values realistic. Thus, the amounts of attenuation shown in the figure apply to about 98% of laboratory subjects and 84% of HPD wearers in the field, which is *less than the average* (mean) amount of attenuation that would occur in both situations.

actual attenuation values for the various kinds of HPDs (e.g., Berger, Franks, & Lindgren, 1996), and are superior to a single 50% derating for all HPDs, which has been used by OSHA inspectors for quite some time.

Occupational Hearing Loss and Workers' Compensation

People who have sustained occupational hearing losses may be entitled to payments under workers' compensation programs, although the details vary widely among states and other kinds of jurisdictions. In addition, the terms **impairment**, **handicap**, and **disability**, which are used almost interchangeably in daily clinical discourse, actually have different meanings that become important when employment-related compensation issues are involved. The generally accepted definitions of these terms are as follows (AMA, 1979, p. 2055, emphasis added):

Impairment: A change for the worse in either structure or function, *outside the range of normal.*
Handicap: The disadvantage imposed by an impairment *sufficient to affect a person's efficiency* in activities of daily living. Handicap implies a *material* impairment.
Disability: An actual or presumed inability to remain *employed at full wages.*

Notice that any deviation from the normal range can be an impairment, but an impairment is not considered to be a handicap unless it interferes materially with the ability to engage in daily activities. Finally, a handicap is not a disability until it affects compensable employment. These distinctions are very important because hearing impairments are often handicapping but are infrequently disabling according to these definitions. In fact, it was not until a 1948 New York court decision that hearing impairments became compensable in spite of the fact that it might not cause lost wages. On the other hand, the Maryland courts took the opposite point of view in 1961, and it took legislative action in 1967 to make occupa-

tional hearing impairments compensable regardless of disability in that state.

The amounts of compensation awarded for hearing loss and the duration of the payments vary from jurisdiction to jurisdiction, as do waiting periods, corrections for age (presbycusis),[8] prior losses, etc. In general, there is some maximum amount of compensation, and a proportion of these maximum compensation benefits will be awarded depending on the percentage of the hearing impairment. The arduous task of determining the occupational hearing loss compensation practices from state to state was addressed by ASHA (1992) and is summarized in Table 16–6.

Compensation methods or **formulas** are used to convert the degree of hearing loss into a *percentage* of impairment for these purposes. Before reviewing the major compensation formulas, it is worthwhile mentioning that they reflect economic, social, and political considerations as much as clinical judgments about the extent to which a hearing loss is handicapping.

Several characteristics are common to just about all of the compensation formulas in current use. Only certain frequencies are considered by each formula, and the amount of hearing loss is averaged across these frequencies separately for each ear. There is a certain minimum amount of hearing loss that must be present before a loss is potentially compensable. (This notion is the same as the criterion for what constitutes a material hearing impairment when estimating the risks of noise exposure.) This border is called the **low fence**, and it constitutes a 0% impairment. If the low fence is 25 dB, then only the part of a hearing loss above 25 dB would be considered in determining the amount of impairment. There is also a **high fence**, which constitutes a 100% impairment. If the high

---

[8] The **allocation** of part of an individual patient's hearing loss to age and part of it to noise exposure is a topic with considerable legal ramifications. Dobbie (1993, 1996) proposed an approach to doing this, although it is not without controversy (Lipscomb, 1999).

TABLE 16–6   Workers' compensation methods for hearing loss by state (based on ASHA, 1992)

State	Method	Presbycusis Correction	Tinnitus Considered	Prior Loss Considered
Alabama	Medical evidence	No	Unknown	Yes
Alaska	AAO 1979	Yes	Yes	Yes
Arizona	AAO 1979/Medical evidence	No	No	Yes
Arkansas	Medical evidence	Possibly	Possibly	Yes
California	AAO 1979	No	Yes	Yes
Colorado	AAO 1979[a]/Medical evidence	No	Yes	No
Connecticut	Medical evidence	No	Yes	Yes
Delaware	AAO 1979	No	No	No
Florida	AAO 1979[a]/Medical evidence	No	No	Possibly
Georgia	AAOO 1959 (1971)	No	No	Yes
Hawaii	Medical evidence	Yes	Yes	Yes
Idaho	AAO 1979[a]	Yes	No	Yes
Illinois	Illinois formula	No	Yes	No
Indiana	Medical evidence	Yes	Yes	Yes
Iowa	AAO 1979	No	No	Yes
Kansas	AAO 1979	No	No	Yes
Kentucky	AAO 1979[a]/Medical evidence	No	No	Yes
Louisiana	AAO 1979[a]	No	No	No
Maine	AAOO 1959 (1971)	Yes	No	Yes
Maryland	AAOO 1959 (1971)	Yes	No	Yes
Massachusetts	Medical evidence[b]	No	No	No
Michigan	(Medical expenses and wage loss for hearing loss injury)			
Minnesota	AAO 1979	No	No	Yes
Mississippi	Medical evidence	No	Yes	No
Missouri	AAOO 1959 (1971)	Yes	No	No
Montana	AAOO 1959 (1971)	No	No	Yes
Nebraska	AAO 1979/Medical evidence	No	No	No
Nevada	AAO 1979	No	No	Yes
New Hampshire	AAO 1979/Medical evidence	No	Yes	Yes
New Jersey	New Jersey formula	No	Yes	Yes
New Mexico	AAO 1979/Medical evidence	No	No	Yes
New York	AAO 1979	No	No	No
North Carolina	AAO 1979	No	No	Yes
North Dakota	AAO 1979	No	No	Yes
Ohio	AAO 1979	No	Yes	No
Oklahoma	AAO 1979	No	Yes	No
Oregon	Oregon formula	Yes	No	Yes
Pennsylvania	Medical evidence	Possibly	Possibly	Yes
Rhode Island	AAO 1979	Possibly	No	No
South Carolina	AAO 1979	No	No	Yes
South Dakota	AAO 1979	Yes	No	Yes
Tennessee	AAO 1979/Medical evidence	No	No	Yes
Texas	AAO 1979/Medical evidence	No	No	Yes
Utah	AAO 1979/Medical evidence	Yes	No	Yes
Vermont	AAO 1979	No	No	Yes
Virginia	AAOO 1959 (1971)	No	No	Yes
Washington	AAO 1979	No	Yes	Yes
Washington, D.C.	AAO 1979	No	No	Yes
West Virginia	West Virginia formula	Possibly	No	Yes
Wisconsin	Wisconsin formula	No	Yes	Yes
Wyoming	AAO 1979	No	No	Yes

[a] Reported by state but not confirmed by statutory review (ASHA, 1992).
[b] Awards for total losses (in one or both ears) only.

fence is 92 dB, then any loss of 92 dB or more would count as a 100% impairment. The range of decibels between the low fence and the high fence corresponds to the range of impairments from 0% to 100%. In our example, this range is 92 − 25 = 67 dB wide, so each decibel of hearing loss above 25 dB contributes 1.5% toward the percentage of impairment. These principles are illustrated on the left side of Figure 16–20.

After averaging the losses for the appropriate frequencies in a given ear, this average loss is compared to the low and high fences. In Figure 16–20, the average loss in case A is 23 dB. This value is less than the 25 dB low fence, so this ear has a 0% impairment. Case B has an average loss of 33 dB, which is above the low fence and under the high fence. Only the decibels above the low fence count toward the percentage of impairment, which is 33 − 25 = 8 dB. Because each decibel above the low fence counts for 1.5%, the impairment for this ear is 8 × 1.5% = 12%. Case C has an average loss of 97 dB, which is automatically considered a 100% impairment because it exceeds the 92 dB high fence.

The patient's final (binaural) percentage of impairment is arrived at by combining the percentages of impairment for the two ears, but this is done in a special way that gives the better ear substantially more weight than the poorer ear. The better ear in this context means the ear with a lower percentage of impairment. The procedure is to average the percentages of impairments of the two ears in a way that reflects the greater weighting of the better ear, and is easily understood by considering an example. Suppose that the impairments were found to be 12% for the right ear and 29% for the left ear, and that the better ear must be counted five times more than the poorer ear. Here, the better ear would be multiplied by 5, and this product would be added to the poorer ear:

$$(12\% \times 5) + 29\% = 60\% + 29\% = 89\%$$

Notice that this sum of 89% is the result of adding six values, five from the better ear and one from the poorer ear. Hence, the average value is found by dividing the sum by 6:

$$87\% \div 6 = 14.8\%$$

Consequently, this patient's overall or binaural impairment is 14.8%, which would normally be rounded to 15%. The procedural principles just illustrated are essentially the same for all of the compensation formulas in current use. We will review some of the more well-known and interesting formulas. A reasonably complete listing of the available

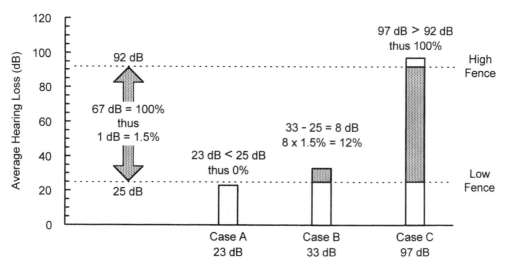

FIGURE 16–20 Illustrative examples of the low fence, high fence, and percentage of impairment for each decibel of hearing loss above the low fence (see text).

hearing loss compensation formulas is given in Table 16–7.

Early Methods One occasionally comes across references to the early compensation formulas developed by Fletcher (1929) and the American Medical Association (AMA, 1942, 1947) even though they are no longer used. The Fletcher method is often called the *point-eight rule* because it converted a range of losses from 0 dB to 128 dB into percentages, so each decibel was worth 0.8%. The early AMA approaches applied value weightings to the amount of hearing loss at each frequency considered, and the 1947 version is also known as the Fowler-Sabine method.

AAOO 1959/1971 Method The most well-known compensation formulas are those developed by the American Academy of Otolaryngology–Head and Neck Surgery (AAO), formerly known as the American Academy of Ophthalmology and Otolaryngology (AAOO), and the AMA. The AAOO introduced a compensation formula in 1959 that was updated in 1971 for use with the current ANSI standards for audiometers. This method involves the average of 500, 1000, and 2000 Hz; a low fence of 25 dB HL (ANSI, 1969), a high fence of 92 dB HL; 1.5% per decibel; and counts the better ear five times more than the poorer ear. It was proposed that these criteria reflect the ability to hear and repeat sentences, which was in turn supposed to reveal "correct hearing for everyday speech," although this contention was not supported with research evidence. The appropriateness of the 1959/1971 AAOO formula as a measure of impairment is questionable because it ignores the frequencies above 2000 Hz that are important for everyday speech understanding; sentence reception in quiet is a poor representation of real-life speech recognition ability; and a 25-dB low fence based on the 500 to 2000 Hz average is unfairly high. Suter (1985) demonstrated that the AAOO formula fails to reflect the actual speech recognition problems of hearing impaired subjects.

AAO-AMA 1979 Method The formula subsequently recommended by the AAO and the AMA addressed the issues just described by changing the frequencies that are averaged to include 500, 1000, 2000, and 3000 Hz (AMA, 1979). The fences, better ear weighting, and percentage per decibel are the same as in the earlier formula. As a result, the 1979 AAO method accounts for the high frequency nature of many occupational losses, at least to the extent that 3000 Hz is involved in the hearing loss. The 1979 AAO method is widely used, as suggested in Table 16–6. Kry-

TABLE 16–7 **Major characteristics of various methods ("formulas") used for determining the percentage of hearing impairment for workers' compensation**

Method ("Formula")	Frequencies Averaged (Hz)	Low Fence (dB)	High Fence (dB)	Percent Per dB	Better Ear Weighting
AAOO 1959/1971	500, 1000, 2000	25	92	1.5	× 5
AAO/AMA 1979	500, 1000, 2000, 3000	25	92	1.5	× 5
NIOSH 1972	1000, 2000, 3000	25	92	1.5	× 5
CHABA 1975	1000, 2000, 3000	35	92	1.75	× 4
ASHA	1000, 2000, 3000, 4000	25	75	2.0	× 5
Illinois	1000, 2000, 2000	30	85	1.82 (computed monaurally)	
New Jersey	1000, 2000, 3000	30	97	1.75	× 5
Oregon	500, 1000, 2000, 3000, 4000, 6000	25	92	1.5	× 7
West Virginia	500, 1000, 2000, 3000	27.5	92	1.6	× 5
Wisconsin	500, 1000, 2000, 3000	30	92	1.6	× 4

ter (1998) suggested modifying the 1979 AAO-AMA method by reducing the low fence to 15 dB and the high fence to 75 dB, adjustment of the values for presbycusis, and changing the better ear weighting to three instead of five.

NIOSH and CHABA Methods Similar to the AAO-AMA methods, the **1972 NIOSH formula** uses the same fences, percentages per decibel, and five-times weighting for the better ear. However, it applies these criteria to the average of 1000, 2000, and 3000 Hz, making it one of the most generous compensation formulas. The **1975 CHABA formula** also uses a 1000, 2000, and 3000 Hz average, but its low fence is raised to 35 dB, and a four-times better ear weighting is used. The low fence was elevated so that compensation awards would be the same as they would have been using the 500, 1000, and 2000 Hz average with a 25-dB low fence.

ASHA 1981 Method The method proposed by a task force of the American Speech-Language-Hearing Association (ASHA, 1981) is based on notions consistent with the following revised definitions of hearing impairment, handicap, and disability (ASHA, 1981, p. 297, emphasis added):

Hearing Impairment: a deviation or change for the worse in either auditory structure or auditory function, *usually outside the range of normal.*

Hearing Handicap: the disadvantage imposed by a hearing impairment on a person's communicative performance in the *activities of daily living.*

Hearing Disability: the determination of a financial reward for the actual or presumed loss of ability to perform *activities of daily living.*

These definitions focus on the nature of auditory disorders, how they are experienced by the patient with a hearing loss, and how they interfere with communication. Consequently, it is not surprising to find that they diverge in several ways from the more general notions embodied in the AMA definitions described earlier: Changes for the worse do not always have to be outside the normal range to constitute an impairment. A handicap does not necessarily imply a material degree of impairment. Compensable disability is tied to activities of daily living rather than to lost income. In light of these considerations, the ASHA method involves the average of 1000, 2000, 3000, and 4000 Hz; a 25-dB low fence; a 75-dB high fence; 2% per decibel; and a five-times weighting for the better ear. There is growing support for the 1000–4000 Hz average (Phaneuf, Hétu, & Hanley, 1985; Prince et al, 1997; NIOSH, 1998), and it has been adopted with a 25-dB low fence as the criterion for material hearing impairment by NIOSH (1998). Of course, the ASHA method provides larger estimates of compensable impairment than the other formulas, and has not been adopted for compensation purposed by any jurisdictions to the author's knowledge.

VA Method An interesting approach for determining the percentage of impairment for compensation purposes is used by the Department of Veterans Affairs. In this method, each ear is categorized into one of 11 categories (I to XI) based on both its speech recognition score and the average pure-tone hearing loss for 1000, 2000, 3000, and 4000 Hz. These categories are shown in Table 16–8. For example, if one of a patient's ears has an average loss of 59 dB and a speech recognition score of 58%, it would be placed into category VII. If his other ear has an average loss of 39 dB and a speech recognition score of 74%, then it would be placed into category IV. The percentage of impairment is then obtained using Table 16–9. Notice that the better ear is more heavily weighted than the poorer ear, analogous to what we have seen in the formula methods. The patient in our example has a better ear in category IV and a poorer ear in category VII. According to Table 16–9, he would have a 20% hearing impairment for compensation purposes.

TABLE 16–8 (a) Numerical hearing impairment categories used by the Department of Veterans Affairs for each ear according to the average hearing loss at 1000, 2000, 3000, and 4000 Hz combined with the speech recognition score. (b) Categories based on just the pure-tone average (under special circumstances, e.g., unreliable speech recognition due to foreign accent)

(a)

Numeric Designation of Hearing Impairment (I–XI)
Average Pure-Tone Loss in Decibels

Speech Recognition Score in Percent	0–41	42–49	50–57	58–65	66–73	74–81	82–89	90–97	98+
92–100	I	I	I	II	II	II	III	III	IV
84–90	II	II	II	III	III	III	IV	IV	IV
76–82	III	III	IV	IV	IV	V	V	V	V
68–74	IV	IV	V	V	VI	VI	VII	VII	VII
60–66	V	V	VI	VI	VII	VII	VIII	VIII	VIII
52–58	VI	VI	VII	VII	VIII	VIII	VIII	VIII	IX
44–50	VII	VII	VIII	VIII	VIII	IX	IX	IX	X
36–42	VIII	VIII	VIII	IX	IX	IX	X	X	X
0–34	IX	X	XI	XI	XI	XI	XI	XI	XI

(b) *Average Pure-Tone Loss in Decibels*

0–41	42–48	49–55	56–62	63–69	70–76	77–83	84–90	91–97	98–104	105+
I	II	II	IV	V	VI	VII	VIII	IX	X	XI

Numeric Designation of Hearing Impairment (I–XI)

Adapted from Tables VI and VIa, *Federal Register*, 52, 222, 44120.

TABLE 16–9 Percentage of hearing impairment used by the Department of Veterans Affairs, based on the numerical categories of each ear obtained from the previous table

Better ear

	XI	X	IX	VIII	VII	VI	V	IV	III	II	I
XI	100										
X	90	80									
IX	80	70	60								
VIII	70	60	50	50							
VII	60	60	50	40	40						
VI	50	50	40	40	30	30					
V	40	40	40	30	30	20	20				
IV	30	30	30	20	20	20	10	10			
III	20	20	20	20	20	10	10	10	0		
II	10	10	10	10	10	10	10	0	0	0	
I	10	10	0	0	0	0	0	0	0	0	0

Poorer ear

Adapted from Table VII, *Federal Register*, 52, 222, 44121.

REFERENCES

Abel SM, Alberti PW, Haythornthwaite C, Riko K. 1982a. Speech intelligibility in noise: Effects of fluency and hearing protector type. *J Acoust Soc Am* 71, 708–715.

Abel SM, Alberti PW, Riko K. 1982b. Speech intelligibility in noise with ear protectors. *J Otolaryngol* 9, 256–265.

American Medical Association (AMA). 1979. Guide for the evaluation of hearing handicap. *JAMA* 241, 2055–2059.

American National Standards Institute (ANSI). S3.5-1969 (R1986). *American National Standard Methods for the Calculation of the Articulation index.* New York: ANSI.

American National Standards Institute (ANSI). ANSI-S1.4-1983 (R1997). *American National Standard Specification for Sound Level Meters.* New York: ANSI.

American National Standards Institute (ANSI). S3.5-1997. *American National Standard Methods for the Calculation of the Speech Intelligibility Index.* New York: ANSI.

American National Standards Institute (ANSI). ANSI S12.6-1984 (R1990): *American National Standard Method for the Measurement of Real-Ear Attenuation of Hearing Protectors.* New York: ANSI.

American National Standards Institute (ANSI). ANSI S3.6-1969 (R1989): *American National Standard Specifications for Audiometers.* New York: ANSI.

American National Standards Institute (ANSI). 1977. ANSI S3.14-1977 (R1997): *American National Standard for Rating Noise with Respect to Speech Interference.* New York: ANSI.

American National Standards Institute (ANSI). ANSI S3.1-1991a: *Maximum Permissible Ambient Noise Levels for Audiometric Test Rooms.* New York: ANSI.

American National Standards Institute (ANSI). ANSI S12.13-1991b: *Draft American National Standard: Evaluating the Effectiveness of Hearing Conservation Programs.* New York: ANSI.

American National Standards Institute (ANSI). ANSI S3.44-1996: *American National Standard Determination of Occupational Noise Exposure and Estimation of Noise-Induced Hearing Impairment.* New York: ANSI.

American National Standards Institute (ANSI). ANSI S12.6-1997: *American National Standard Methods for Measuring Real-Ear Attenuation of Hearing Protectors.* New York: ANSI.

American Speech-Language-Hearing Association (ASHA). 1981. On the definition of hearing handicap. *ASHA* 23, 293–297.

American Speech-Language-Hearing Association (ASHA). 1992. A survey of states' worker's compensation practices for occupational hearing loss. *ASHA* 34 (suppl 8), 2–8.

Anderson BW, Kalb JT. 1987. English verification of the STI method for estimating speech intelligibility of a communication channel. *J Acoust Soc Am* 81, 1982–1985.

Bauman KS, Marston LE. 1986. Effects of hearing protection on speech intelligibility in noise. *Sound Vib* 20, 12–14.

Beranek LL. 1954/1986. *Acoustics.* New York: Acoustical Society of America.

Beranek LL. 1957. Revised criteria for noise control in buildings. *Noise Control* 3, 19–27.

Beranek LL. 1989. Balanced noise-criterion (NCB) curves. *J Acoust Soc Am* 86, 650–664.

Berger EH. 1986a. Hearing protection devices. In Berger EH, Ward WD, Morrill JC, Royster LH (Eds.): *Noise and Hearing Conservation Manual,* 4th ed. Fairfax, VA: American Industrial Hygiene Association, 319–381.

Berger EH. 1986b. Methods for measuring the attenuation of hearing protection devices. *J Acoust Soc Am* 79, 1655–1687.

Berger EH. 1991. Flat-response, moderate-attenuation, and level-dependent HPDs: How they work, and what they can do for you. *Spectrum* 8 (suppl 1), 17.

Berger EH. 1993. *The naked truth about NRRs. EARLog 20.* Indianapolis: Cabot Safety Corp.

Berger EH. 1999. So, how do you want your NRRs: Realistic or sunny-side up? *Hear Rev* 6, 68–72.

Berger EH, Franks JR, Behar A, Casali JG, Dixon-Ernst C, Kieper RW, Merry CJ, Mozo BT, Nixon CW, Ohlin D, Royster JD, Royster LH. 1998. Development of a new laboratory standard protocol for estimating the field attenuation of hearing protection devices. Part III. The validity of using subject-fit data. *J Acoust Soc Am* 103, 665–672.

Berger EH, Franks JR, Lindgren F. 1996. International review of field studies of hearing protector attenuation. In Axelsson A, Borchgrevink H, Hamernick RP, Hellstrom P, Henderson D, Salvi RJ (Eds.): *Scientific Basis of Noise-Induced Hearing Loss.* New York: Thieme, 361–377.

Berger EH, Ward WD, Morrill JC, Royster LH (Eds.). 1986. *Noise and Hearing Conservation Manual,* 4th ed. Fairfax, VA: American Industrial Hygiene Association.

Boettcher FA, Henderson D, Gratton MA, Danielson RW, Byrne CD. 1987. Synergistic interactions of noise and other ototraumatic agents. *Ear Hear* 8, 192–212.

Botsford JH. 1967. Simple method for identifying acceptable noise exposures. *J Acoust Soc Am* 42, 810–819.

Bruce RD, Toothman EH. 1986. Engineering controls. In Berger EH, Ward WD, Morrill JC, Royster LH (Eds.): *Noise and Hearing Conservation Manual,* 4th ed. Fairfax, VA: American Industrial Hygiene Association, 417–521.

Bruel & Kjaer. 1985. The Modulation Transfer Function in Room Acoustics. RASTI: A Tool for Evaluating Auditoria. Technical review no. 3-1985. MA: Bruel & Kjaer.

Bruel & Kjaer. 1986. *Noise Control: Principles and Practice.* MA: Bruel & Kjaer.

Campo P, Subramaniam M, Henderson D. 1991. Effect of "conditioning" exposures on hearing loss from traumatic exposure. *Hear Res* 55, 195–200.

Canlon B, Borg E, Flock A. 1988. Protection against noise trauma by preexposure to a low level acoustic stimulus. *Hear Res* 34, 197–200.

Casali JG, Mauney DW, Burks JA. 1995. Physical vs. psychophysical measurements of hearing protector attenuation—a.k.a. MIRE vs. REAT. *Sound Vib* 29, 20–27.

Clark WW. 1991a. Recent studies of temporary threshold shift (TTS) and permanent threshold shift (PTS) in animals. *J Acoust Soc Am* 90, 155–163.

Clark WW. 1991b. Noise exposure from leisure activities: A review. *J Acoust Soc Am* 90, 175–181.

Clark WW, Bohne BA. 1984. The effects of noise on hearing and the ear. *Med Times* 122, 17–22.

Clark WW, Bohne BA, Boettcher FA. 1987. Effect of periodic rest on hearing loss and cochlear damage. *J Acoust Soc Am* 82, 1253–1264.

Cohen A. 1977. Extraauditory effects of noise on behavior and health. In Lee DK, Falk HL, Murphy SD, Geiger SR (Eds.): *Handbook of Physiology: Reactions to Environmental Agents*, sec. 9. Baltimore: Williams & Wilkins.

Cohen S, Weinstein N. 1981. Nonauditory effects of noise on behavior and health. *J Soc Issues* 37, 36–70.

Coles RRA, Garinther GR, Rice CG, Hodge DC. 1968. Hazardous exposure to impulse noise. *J Acoust Soc Am* 43, 336–343.

Davis AC, Fortnum HM, Coles RRA, Haggard MP, Lutman ME. 1985. Damage to hearing from leisure noise: A review of the literature. MRC Inst. Hear Res. Nottingham, UK: University of Nottingham.

Department of Labor (DOL). 1969. Occupational noise exposure. *Federal Register* 34, 7946–7949.

Dobbie RA. 1993. *Medico-Legal Evaluation of Hearing Loss*. New York: Van Nostrand Reinhold.

Dobbie RA. 1996. Estimation of occupational contribution to hearing handicap. In Axelsson A, Borchgrevink H, Hamernick RP, Hellstrom P, Henderson D, Salvi RJ (Eds.): *Scientific Basis of Noise-Induced Hearing Loss*. New York: Thieme, 415–422.

Environmental Protection Agency (EPA). 1973. *Public Health and Welare Criteria for Noise* (EPA 550/9-73-002). Washington, DC: EPA.

Environmental Protection Agency (EPA). 1974. *Information on Levels of Environmental Noise Requisite to Protect Public Health and Welfare with an Adequate Margin of Safety* (EPA 550/9-74-004). Washington, DC: EPA.

Environmental Protection Agency (EPA). 1979. Noise labeling requirements for hearing protectors. *Federal Register* 42:190, 40 CFR, Part 211, 56139-56147.

Erdreich J. 1999. Engineering controls for noise abatement. *Hear Rev* 6, 42–46.

Ericksson LJ. 1996. Active sound and vibration control: A technology in transition. *Noise Control Eng J* 44, 1–9.

Federal Register. 1983. §1910.95 Occupational noise exposure. *Federal Register*, 48:46:9776–9785, March 8, 1983/Rules and regulations.

Fields JM. 1993. Effect of personal and situational variables on noise annoyance in residential areas. *J Acoust Soc Am* 93, 2753–2763.

Fields JM. 1998. Reactions to environmental noise in an ambient noise context in residential areas. *J Acoust Soc Am* 104, 2245–2260.

Florentine M., Hunter W, Robinson M, Ballou M, Buus S. 1998. On the behavioral characteristics of loud-music listening. *Ear Hear* 19, 420–428.

French NR, Steinberg GC. 1947. Factors governing the intelligibility of speech sounds. *J Acoust Soc Am* 19, 90–119.

Gasway DC. 1985. *Hearing Conservation: A Practical Manual and Guide*. Englewood Cliffs, NJ: Prentice-Hall.

Hamernick RP, Ahroon WA, Hsueh KD. 1991. The energy spectrum of an impulse: Its relation to hearing loss. *J Acoust Soc Am* 90, 197–208.

Hamernick RP, Hsueh KD. 1991. Impulse noise: Some definitions, physical acoustics and other considerations. *J Acoust Soc Am* 90, 189–196.

Henderson D, Subramaniam M, Boettcher FA. 1993. Individual susceptibility to noise-induced hearing loss: An old concept revisited. *Ear Hear* 14, 152–168.

International Electrotechnical Commission (IEC). 1987. Publ. 268: Sound system equipment part 16: Report on the RASTI method for objective rating of speech intelligibility in auditoria.

International Standards Organization (ISO-1999). 1990. *Acoustics—Determination of Occupational Noise Exposure and Estimation of Noise-Induced Hearing Impairment*. Geneva: ISO.

International Standards Organization (ISO-4869-2). 1994. *Acoustics-Hearing Protectors, Part 2: Estimation of Effective A-Weighted Sound Pressure Levels When Hearing Protectors Are Worn*. Geneva: ISO.

Killion M, DeVilbiss E, Stewart J. 1988. An earplug with uniform 15-dB attenuation. *Hear J* 41, 14–17.

Kryter KD. 1962. Methods for the calculation and use of the articulation index. *J Acoust Soc Am* 34, 1698–1702.

Kryter KD. 1985. *The Effects of Noise on Man*, 2nd ed. Orlando: Academic Press.

Kryter KD. 1998. Evaluating hearing handicap. *J Am Acad Audiol* 9, 141–146.

Kryter KD, Ward WD, Miller JD, Eldredge DH. 1966. Hazardous exposure to intermittent and steady-state noise. *J Acoust Soc Am* 39, 451–464.

Kuo SM, Morgan DR. 1996. *Active Noise Control Systems*. New York: Wiley.

Lazarus H. 1987. Prediction of verbal communication in noise: A development of generalized SIL curves and the quality of communication, Part 2. *Appl Acoust* 20, 245–261.

Lempert BL, Henderson TL. 1973. *Occupational Noise and Hearing 1968 to 1972: A NIOSH Study*. Cincinnati: NIOSH.

Lipscomb DM. 1988. *Hearing Conservation in Industry, Schools and the Military*. Boston: Little, Brown.

Lipscomb DM. 1999. Allocation among causes of hearing loss: The concept, its pros and cons. *Hear Rev* 6, 48–64.

Maxwell DW, Williams CE, Robertson RM, Thomas GB. 1987. Performance characteristics of active hearing protection devices. *Sound Vib* 21, 14–18.

Melnick W. 1991. Human temporary threshold shift (TTS) and damage risk. *J Acoust Soc Am* 90, 147–154.

Miedema HME. 1992. Response functions for environmental odour in residential areas. TNO-PG report, Liden.

Miedema HME, Vos H. 1998. Exposure-response relationships for transportation noise. *J Acoust Soc Am* 104, 3432–3445.

Miedema HME, Vos H. 1999. Demographic and attitudinal factors that modify annoyance from transportation noise. *J Acoust Soc Am* 105, 3336–3344.

Miller JD. 1974. Effects of noise on people. *J Acoust Soc Am* 56, 729–764.

Miller MH, Silverman CA. 1984. *Occupational Hearing Conservation*. Englewood Cliffs, NJ: Prentice-Hall.

National Institute for Occupational Safety and Health (NIOSH). 1972. *Criteria for a Recommended Standard: Occupational Exposure to Noise*. Publication no. HSM 73-11001. Cincinnati: NIOSH.

National Institute for Occupational Safety and Health (NIOSH). 1990. *A Practical Guide to Effective Hearing Conservation Programs in the Workplace*. Publication no. 90-120. Cincinnati: NIOSH.

National Institute for Occupational Safety and Health (NIOSH). 1996. *Preventing Occupational Hearing Loss—A Practical Guide*. Publication no. 96–110. Cincinnati: NIOSH.

National Institute for Occupational Safety and Health (NIOSH). 1998. *Criteria for a Recommended Standard: Occupational Noise Exposure—Revised Criteria 1998*. Publication no. 98-126. Cincinnati: NIOSH.

Nelson PA, Elliot SJ. 1992. *Active Control of Sound*. London: Academic.

Occupational Safety & Health Administration (OSHA). 1983. §1910.95 Occupational noise exposure. 29 CFR 1910.95 (May 29, 1971) *Federal Register* 36:10466–10466, Amended (March 8, 1983) Federal Register 48:9776–9785.

Odess JS. 1972. Acoustic trauma of sportsman hunters due to gun firing. *Laryngoscope* 82, 1971–1989.

Orfield SJ. 1987. The RASTI method of testing relative intelligibility. *Sound Vib* 21(12), 20–22.

Passchier-Vermeer W. 1974. Hearing loss due to continuous exposure to steady-state broad-band noise. *J Acoust Soc Am* 56, 1585–1593.

Pavlovic CV. 1987. Derivation of primary parameters and procedures for use in speech intelligibility predictions. *J Acoust Soc Am* 82, 413–422.

Pavlovic CV. 1991. Speech recognition and five articulation indexes. *Hear Instr* 42, 20–23.

Pavlovic CV, Studebaker GA, Sherbecoe RL. 1986. An articulation index based procedure for predicting the speech recognition performance of hearing-impaired individuals. *J Acoust Soc Am* 80, 50–57.

Phaneuf R, Hétu R, Hanley JA. 1985. A Bayesiam approach for predicting judged hearing disability. *Am J Ind Med* 7, 343–352.

Prince MM, Stayner LT, Smith RJ, Gilbert SJ. 1997. A reexamination of risk estimates from the NIOSH occupational noise and hearing survey (ONHS). *J Acoust Soc Am* 101, 950–963.

Rösler G. 1994. Progression of hearing loss caused by occupational noise. *Scand Audiol* 23, 13–37.

Royster JD, Berger EH, Merry CJ, Nixon CW, Franks JR, Behar A, Casali JG, Dixon-Ernst C, Kieper RW, Mozo BT, Ohlin D, Royster LH. 1996. Development of a new laboratory standard protocol for estimating the field attenuation of hearing protection devices. Part I. Research of working group 11, Accredited Standards Committee S12, Noise. *J Acoust Soc Am* 99, 1506–1526.

Royster JD, Royster LH. 1986. Audiometric data base analysis. In Berger EH, Ward WD, Morrill JC, Royster LH (Eds.): *Noise and Hearing Conservation Manual*, 4th ed. Fairfax, VA: American Industrial Hygiene Association, 293–317.

Royster JD, Royster LH. 1990a. *Hearing Conservation Programs: Guidelines for Success*. Chelsea, MI: Lewis.

Royster JD, Royster LH. 1999. How can we evaluate the effectiveness of occupational hearing conservation programs? *Hear Rev 6*, 28–34.

Royster LH. 1995. Recommendations for the labeling of hearing protectors. *Sound Vib 29*, 16–19.

Royster LH, Royster JD. 1990b. Employment related exposure to noise and its effect on hearing. *Hear Instr* 41, 17–18.

Steeneken HJM, Houtgast T. 1983. A physical method for measuring speech-transmission quality. *J Acoust Soc Am* 67, 318–326.

Subramaniam M, Campo P, Henderson D. 1991a. The effect of progressive resistance to noise. *Hear Res* 52, 181–188.

Subramaniam M, Campo P, Henderson D. 1991b. Development of resistance to hearing loss from high frequency noise. *Hear Res* 56, 65–68.

Subramaniam M, Henderson D, Campo P, Spongr VP. 1992. The effect of "conditioning" on hearing loss from a high frequency traumatic exposure. *Hear Res* 58, 57–62.

Suter AH. 1984. Noise sources and effects: OSHA's Hearing Conservation Amendment and the audiologist. *ASHA* 26, 39–43.

Suter AH. 1985. Speech recognition in noise by individuals with mild hearing impairments. *J Acoust Soc Am* 78, 887–900.

Suter AH. 1992a. Noise sources and effects—a new look. *Sound Vib* 26, 18–38.

Suter AH. 1992b. *The Relationship of the Exchange Rate to Noise-Induced Hearing Loss*. NTIS no. PB93-118610. Cincinnati: Alice Suter & Assoc.

Suter AH. 1993. *Hearing Conservation Manual*, 3rd ed. Milwaukee: Council for Accreditation in Occupational Hearing Conservation.

Suter AH, vonGierke HE. 1987. Noise and public policy. *Ear Hear* 8, 188–191.

Taylor W, Pearson, J, Mair A. 1965. Study of noise and hearing in jute weavers. *J Acoust Soc Am* 38, 113–120.

Towne RM. 1994. An acoustical checklist for multi-family housing units. *Sound Vib* 28, 28–32.

Ward WD. 1991. The role of intermittence in PTS. *J Acoust Soc Am* 90, 164–169.

Webster JC. 1969. Effect of noise on speech intelligibility. In Ward WD, Fricke JE (Eds.): *Noise as a Public Health Hazard* (ASHA report 4). Rockville, MD: American Speech-Language-Hearing Association, 49–73.

Webster JC. 1978. Speech interference aspects of noise. In Lipscomb DM (Ed.): *Noise and Audiology*. Baltimore: University Park Press, 193–228.

Appendix A

This appendix gives examples of how to combine octave-band levels (OBLs) in dB into overall sound pressure level (dB SPL) and A-weighted sound level (dBA). Correction values for A-weighted OBLs are in Table 1–4. The same procedures can be used with third-octave-band levels except that an appropriate (different) set of A-weightings would have to be used. The OBLs of the noise being used in these examples are as follows:

Frequency Hz	OBLs (dB)
31.5	85
63	80
125	77
250	76
500	74
1000	68
2000	60
4000	57
8000	55

Combining OBLs into dB SPL: Simplified Method

The octave-band levels are listed from highest to lowest to simplify the procedure. Then, they are combined in successive pairs based on the increments given in Table 1–3.

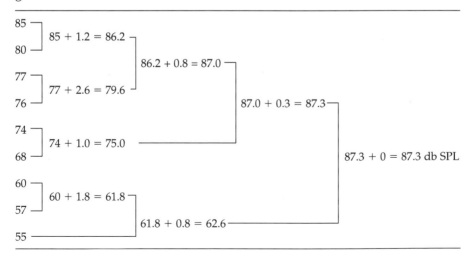

Combining OBLs into dB SPL: Formula Method

The OBLs are summed logarithmically according to the formula:

$$L = 10 \log \sum_{i=1}^{n} 10^{L_i/10} \, ,$$

where L is the overall (combined) level in dB SPL, n is the number of bands, i is the ith band, and L_i = is the OBL of the ith band. The formula calls for calculating $10^{L_i/10}$ for each octave-band level:

Frequency Hz	OBL or L_i	$10^{L_i/10}$
31.5	85	316,227,766.0
63.0	80	100,000,000.0
125.0	77	50,118,723.36
250.0	76	39,810,717.06
500.0	74	25,118,864.32
1000.0	68	6,309,573.445
2000.0	60	1,000,000.0
4000.0	57	501,187.2336
8000.0	55	316,227.766

Next, the values of $10^{L_i/10}$ are added, and their sum (Σ) is found to be: 539,403,059.2. At this point, the formula says

$$L = 10 \log 539{,}403{,}059.2 \, .$$

The logarithm of 539,403,059.2 is 8.731913405, so that we now have

$$L = 10 \times 8.731913405 \, .$$

Hence, the overall level of this sound is

$$L = 87.3 \text{ db SPL} \, .$$

Combining OBLs into dBA: Simplified Method

The corrected A-weighted OBLs are obtained from Table 1–4.

Frequency (Hz)	OBL (dB)	dBA Corrections	Corrected OBLs
31.5	85	−39.4	45.6
63.0	80	−26.2	53.8
125.0	77	−16.1	60.9
250.0	76	−8.6	67.4
500.0	74	−3.2	70.8
1000.0	68	0.0	68.0
2000.0	60	1.2	61.2
4000.0	57	1.1	58.1
8000.0	55	−1.1	53.9

The A-weighted corrected OBLs are listed from highest to lowest to simplify the procedure. Then they are combined in successive pairs based on the increments given in Table 1–3. (For simplicity, the corrected OBLs shown here have been rounded to the nearest whole number.)

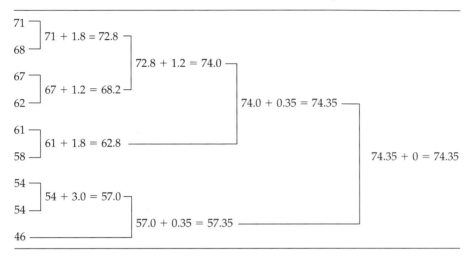

Combining OBLs into dBA: Formula Method

The OBLs are summed logarithmically according to the formula:

$$L_A = 10 \log \sum_{i=1}^{n} 10^{(L_i + k_i)/10},$$

where L_A is the overall (combined) level in dBA, n is the number of bands, i is the ith band, L_i is the OBL of the ith band, and k_i is the dBA correction value for each OBL. The correction is accomplished by adding the correction factor to the OBL ($L_i + k_i$). Adding a negative correction value is the same as subtracting.

The corrected A-weighted OBLs are obtained from Table 1–4: The formula calls for calculating $10^{(L_i + k_i)/10}$ for each octave-band level.

Frequency (Hz)	OBL (dB) (or L_i)	dBA Corrections or (k_i)	Corrected OBLs or ($L_i + k_i$)	$10^{(L_i + k_i)/10}$
31.5	85	−39.4	45.6	36,307.80548
63.0	80	−26.2	53.8	239,883.2919
125.0	77	−16.1	60.9	1,230,268.771
250.0	76	−8.6	67.4	5,495,408.739
500.0	74	−3.2	70.8	12,022,644.35
1000.0	68	0.0	68.0	6,309,573.445
2000.0	60	1.2	61.2	1,318,256.739
4000.0	57	1.1	58.1	645,654.229
8000.0	55	−1.1	53.9	245,470.8916

Next, the values of $10^{(L_i + k_i)/10}$ are added, and their sum (Σ) is found to be: 27,543,468.26. At this point, the formula says:

$$L_A = 10 \log 27,543,468.26 .$$

The logarithm of 27,543,468.26 is 7.440018625, so that we now have

$$L_A = 10 \times 7.440018625 .$$

Hence, the overall level of this sound is

$$L_A = 74.4 \text{ dBA} .$$

Appendix B

Spondaic Words in Alphabetical Order[a,b]

AIRPLANE[c]	drawbridge	hot dog	PADLOCK
ARMCHAIR	DUCK POND	ice cream	pancake
BACKBONE	eardrum	inkwell	playground
baseball	EARTHQUAKE	MOUSETRAP	RAILROAD
BIRTHDAY	EYEBROW	mushroom	STAIRWAY
BLACKBOARD	GREYHOUND	NORTHWEST	sunset
COOKBOOK	hardware	nutmeg	TOOTHBRUSH
cowboy	headlight	OATMEAL	WHITEWASH
DOORMAT	HORSESHOE	outside	woodwork

[a] From ASHA (1979, 1988), with permission.

[b] The ASHA spondee list is a revision of the CID W-1 (Hirsh et al, 1952) list that emphasizes the word selection criteria of dissimilarity and homogeneous audibility. The following words shown here do not appear on the CID W-1 list: backbone, birthday, blackboard, cookbook, doormat, earthquake, eyebrow, ice cream, nutmeg, and outside. The following words on the CID W-1 spondee list do not appear here: birthday, daybreak, doormat, farewell, grandson, hothouse, iceberg, schoolboy, sidewalk, and workshop.

[c] The 20 capitalized spondaic words were found to have the most similar audibility when presented by both recorded and monitored live voice (Rourke-Cullen, Ninya, & Nerbonne, 1955). Relative intelligibility of the revised CID W-1s as presented via MLV and Auditec recordings, *J Am Acad Audiol* 6, 183–186.

Appendix C

Spondaic Word Half-Lists

List A		List B	
airplane	ice cream	armchair	headlight
baseball	mousetrap	backbone	inkwell
blackboard	northwest	birthday	mushroom
cowboy	oatmeal	cookbook	nutmeg
drawbridge	pancake	doormat	outside
duck pond	playground	earthquake	padlock
eardrum	railroad	eyebrow	stairway
horseshoe	sunset	greyhound	toothbrush
hotdog	whitewash	hardware	woodwork

From ASHA (1979, 1988), with permission.

Appendix D

Streamlined Spondaic Word Lists for Adults

inkwell	woodwork	grandson	mousetrap
playground	baseball	eardrum	drawbridge
sidewalk	workshop	toothbrush	padlock
railroad	doormat	northwest	

Based on Young, Dudley, and Gunter (1982) and ASHA (1988), with permission.

Appendix E

Children's Picture Spondaic Word List

cupcake	toothbrush	popcorn	flashlight
airplane	bathtub	fire truck	bluebird
baseball	ice cream	mailman	toothpaste
cowboy	shoelace	snowman	reindeer
hotdog	football	sailboat	seesaw

Based on Frank (1980) and ASHA (1988), with permission.

Appendix F
CID Auditory Test W-22 Word Lists (Alphabetical Order)[a]

List 1	List 2	List 3	List 4
ace	ail	add	aid
ache	air	aim	all
an	and	are	am
as	bin	ate	arm
bathe	by	bill	art
bells	cap	book	at
carve	cars	camp	be
chew	chest	chair	bread
could	die	cute	can
dad	does	do	chin
day	dumb	done	clothes
deaf	ease	dull	cook
earn	eat	ears	darn
east	else	end	dolls
felt	flat	farm	dust
give	gave	glove	ear
high	ham	hand	eyes
him	hit	have	few
hunt	hurt	he	go
isle	ice	if	hang
it	ill	is	his
jam	jaw	jar	in
knees	key	king	jump
law	knee	knit	leave
low	live	lie	men
me	move	may	my
mew	new	nest	near
none	now	no	net
not	oak	oil	nuts
or	odd	on	of
owl	off	out	ought
poor	one	owes	our
ran	own	pie	pale
see	pew	raw	save
she	rooms	say	shoe
skin	send	shove	so
stove	show	smooth	stiff
them	smart	start	tea
there	star	tan	than
thing	tear	ten	they
toe	that	this	through
true	then	though	tin
twins	thin	three	toy
yard	too	tie	where
up	tree	use	who
us	way	we	why
wet	well	west	will
what	with	when	wood
wire	your	wool	yes
you	young	year	yet

[a]From Hirsh et al (1952), with permission.

Appendix G

Northwestern University Auditory Test No. 6 (NU-6) in alphabetical order[a]

List 1	List 2	List 3	List 4
bean	bite	bar	back
boat	book	base	bath
burn	bought	beg	bone
chalk	calm	cab	came
choice	chair	cause	chain
death	chief	chat	check
dime	dab	cheek	dip
door	dead	cool	dog
fall	deep	date	doll
fat	fail	ditch	fit
gap	far	dodge	food
goose	gaze	five	gas
hash	gin	germ	get
home	goal	good	hall
hurl	hate	gun	have
jail	haze	half	hole
jar	hush	hire	join
keen	juice	hit	judge
king	keep	jug	kick
kite	keg	late	kill
knock	learn	lid	lean
laud	live	life	lease
limb	loaf	luck	long
lot	lore	mess	lose
love	match	mop	make
met	merge	mouse	mob
mode	mill	name	mood
moon	nice	note	near
nag	numb	pain	neat
page	pad	pearl	pass
pool	pick	phone	peg
puff	pike	pole	perch
rag	rain	rat	red
raid	read	ring	ripe
raise	room	road	rose
reach	rot	rush	rough
sell	said	search	sail
shout	shack	seize	shirt
size	shawl	shall	should
sub	soap	sheep	sour
sure	south	soup	such
take	thought	talk	tape
third	ton	team	thumb
tip	tool	tell	time
tough	turn	thin	tire
vine	voice	void	vote
week	wag	walk	wash
which	white	when	wheat
whip	witch	wire	wife
yes	young	youth	yearn

[a]From Tillman and Carhart (1966), with permission.

Appendix H

Boothroyd Isophonemic Word Lists[a]

List 1	List 2	List 3	List 4	List 5
ship	fish	thug	fun	fib
rug	duck	witch	will	thatch
fan	patch	teak	vat	sum
cheek	cheese	wrap	shape	heel
haze	race	vice	wreath	wide
dice	hive	jail	hide	rake
both	bone	hen	guess	goes
well	wedge	shows	comb	shop
jot	log	food	choose	vet
move	tomb	bomb	job	June

List 6	List 7	List 8	List 9	List 10
fill	badge	bath	hush	jug
catch	hutch	hum	gas	latch
thumb	kill	dig	thin	wick
heap	thighs	five	fake	faith
wise	wave	ways	chime	sign
rave	reap	reach	weave	beep
got	foam	joke	jet	hem
shown	goose	noose	rob	rod
bed	not	pot	dope	vote
juice	shed	shell	lose	shoes

List 11	List 12	List 13	List 14	List 15
math	have	kiss	wish	hug
hip	wig	buzz	dutch	dish
gun	buff	hash	jam	ban
ride	mice	thieve	heath	rage
siege	teeth	gate	laze	chief
veil	jays	wife	bike	pies
chose	poach	pole	rove	wet
shoot	rule	wretch	pet	cove
web	den	dodge	fog	loose
cough	shock	moon	soon	moth

[a] Used with permission.

Appendix I

Lexical Neighborhood Test (LNT; Kirk, Pisoni, & Osberger, 1995)[a]

List 1 (Easy Words)	List 1 (Hard Words)	List 2 (Easy Words)	List 2 (Hard Words)
juice	thumb	down	ear
good	pie	truck	hand
drive	wet	mouth	dry
time	fight	pig	zoo
hard	toe	give	goat
gray	cut	school	toy
foot	pink	boy	call
orange	hi	put	sing
count	song	three	cut
brown	fun	farm	wrong
home	use	fish	bed
old	mine	green	fat
watch	ball	catch	man
need	kick	break	run
food	tea	house	hot
dance	book	sit	read (/rid/)
live (/lɪv/)	bone	friend	grow
stand	work	jump	bag
six	dad	bird	cake
cold	game	swim	seat
push	lost	hold	nine
stop	cook	want	sun
girl	gum	snake	bath
hurt	cap	more	ten
cow	meat	white	ride

[a] © Indiana University. Reproduced by permission of the authors and Indiana University. (Test recording available from Auditec of St. Louis.)

Appendix J

Multisyllabic Lexical Neighborhood Test (MLNT); Kirk, Pisoni, & Osberger, 1995)[a]

List 1 (Easy Words)	List 1 (Hard Words)	List 2 (Easy Words)	List 2 (Hard Words)
children	butter	water	puppy
animal	lion	banana	pickle
monkey	money	glasses	button
finger	jelly	airplane	summer
pocket	yellow	window	bottom
apple	purple	tiger	finish
morning	hello	cookie	bunny
sugar	carry	again	belly
alright	corner	another	couple
about	heaven	almost	under
because	measles	broken	naughty
crazy	ocean	china	really

[a] © Indiana University. Reproduced by permission of the authors and Indiana University. (Test recording available from Auditec of St. Louis.)

Appendix K

PBK-50 (PB Kindergarten) Words Lists in Alphabetical Order[a]

List 1	List 2	List 3	List 4
are	and	all	ache
bad	ask	as	air
bath	ball	ax	black
bead	barn	bee	blind
beef	best	bet	bounce
box	calf	bless	bug
bus	chew	bud	bush
cart	closed	cage	cab
class	cloud	camp	case
did	crack	cat	choose
dish	day	crab	clown
end	dime	darn	cost
fed	each	fair	dad
few	feel	falls	drop
five	flag	fat	else
fold	food	feed	fit
great	forth	find	frog
hit	front	freeze	grade
hot	glove	fresh	had
hunt	good	got	hurt
is	guess	grab	if
lay	gun	gray	jay
me	hook	grew	leave
mouth	kept	his	low
neck	left	knee	may
need	look	knife	most
no	ma	laugh	nest
own	new	lip	nuts
pants	night	loud	pass
pinch	off	next	press
pink	pick	on	purse
please	pig	page	quick
pond	reach	park	raw
put	rest	paste	rich
rag	rode	path	room
rat	rope	peg	seed
ride	shoe	plow	sell
scab	sick	race	set
shop	slide	rose	sheep
sled	south	sack	ship
slice	this	sing	that
slip	thread	splash	them
smile	three	suit	thick
such	toe	tray	those
take	tongue	turn	tire
teach	trade	wait	true
thank	wake	waste	vase
tree	wash	weed	white
use	wave	wreck	wide
ways	wood	yes	you

[a] From Haskins (1949), with permission.

Appendix L

Word Intelligibility by Picture Identification (WIPI) Test Word Lists[a]

List 1	List 2	List 3	List 4
school	broom	moon	spoon
ball	bowl	bell	bow
smoke	coat	coke	goat
floor	door	corn	horn
fox	socks	box	block
hat	flag	bag	black
pan	fan	can	man
bread	red	thread	bed
neck	desk	nest	dress
stair	bear	chair	pear
eye	pie	fly	tie
knee	tea	key	bee
street	meat	feet	teeth
wing	string	spring	ring
mouse	clown	crown	mouth
shirt	church	dirt	skirt
gun	thumb	sun	gum
bus	rug	cup	bug
train	cake	snake	plane
arm	barn	car	star
chick	stick	dish	fish
crib	ship	bib	lip
wheel	seal	queen	green
straw	dog	saw	frog
pail	nail	ail	tail

[a] From Ross and Lerman (1971), with permission.

Appendix M

Northwestern University Children's Perception of Speech (NU-CHIPS) Test Word Lists (Alphabetical Order)[a]

ball	horse
bear	house
bike	juice
bird	light
boat	man
bus	meat
cake	milk
clock	mouth
coat	nose
comb	purse
cup	school
dog	shirt
door	shoe
dress	sink
duck	smile
food	snake
foot	soap
frog	spoon
girl	teeth
gum	tongue
gun	train
hair	tree
ham	truck
hand	watch
head	witch

[a] From Elliott and Katz (1980), with permission.

Appendix N

High-Frequency Word Lists in Alphabetical Order[a]

Gardner (1971) List 1		Pascoe (1975) List 2	
1. fit	1. fist	1. boat	26. pip
2. fixed	2. fits	2. chick	27. pit
3. hick	3. fix	3. chip	28. poke
4. hicks	4. hip	4. coat	29. Pope
5. hiss	5. hips	5. coke	30. Rhine
6. hit	6. hissed	6. folk	31. rhyme
7. hits	7. its	7. goad	32. road
8. kick	8. kicked	8. goat	33. robe
9. kiss	9. kicks	9. grime	34. rope
10. kit	10. kissed	10. grind	35. row
11. kits	11. pick	11. hick	36. ship
12. picks	12. picked	12. hip	37. sick
13. pit	13. pits	13. hiss	38. sift
14. sip	14. sick	14. hit	39. sip
15. sipped	15. sips	15. hits	40. sipped
16. sis	16. sit	16. hope	41. sis
17. six	17. sits	17. lime	42. sit
18. skips	18. skip	18. line	43. skip
19. skit	19. skipped	19. load	44. skit
20. skits	20. spits	20. low	45. soak
21. spit	21. stick	21. mime	46. soap
22. ticked	22. stiff	22. mine	47. thick
23. ticks	23. thick	23. nine	48. tip
24. tip	24. tick	24. oak	49. wine
25. tipped	25. tips	25. oat	50. wrote

[a]Used with permission.

Appendix O
Spanish Bisyllabic Words for Speech Recognition Testing (Alphabetical)[a]

List 1	List 2	List 3	List 4
Agua (water)	Abril (April)	Actriz (actress)	Algo (some)
Baile (dance)	Alma (soul)	Ambos (both)	Aqui (here)
Blusa (blouse)	Astro (star)	Ayer (yesterday)	Banco (bank)
Boca (mouth)	Barca (boat)	Barba (beard)	Blanco (white)
Bosque (forest)	Bolsa (bag)	Beso (kill)	Boda (wedding)
Broma (joke)	Bravo (brave)	Brazo (arm)	Breve (short)
Brusco (rough)	Calle (street)	Brisa (breeze)	Buscan (search)
Burro (donkey)	Camas (beds)	Cabra (goat)	Calor (heat)
Carta (letter)	Casa (house)	Calma (calm)	Casta (breed)
Caso (case)	Centro (center)	Campo (field)	Chiste (joke)
Cestos (baskets)	Claro (clear)	Casi (almost)	Cita (appointment)
Cinco (five)	Contra (against)	Cesta (basket)	Compra (purchase)
Clima (weather)	Donde (where)	Choclo (galosh)	Cristal (crystal)
Costa (coast)	Fecha (date)	Clavo (nail)	Dentro (inside)
Culpa (guilt)	Flete (freight)	Corta (short)	Dolor (pain)
Doce (twelve)	Funda (cover)	Dicha (happiness)	Edad (age)
Finca (farm)	Ganga (bargain)	Filtro (filter)	Falta (missing)
Frente (front)	Gastar (spend)	Fonda (inn)	Fruta (fruit)
Galgo (greyhound)	Golpe (blow)	Fusil(rifle)	Gancho (hook)
Granja (farm)	Grifos (faucets)	Ganso (geese)	Grasa (grease)
Guerra (war)	Hilo (thread)	Gasto (spent)	Gratas (pleasant)
Hambre (hunger)	Horno (oven)	Guante (glove)	Gustar (like)
Hombro (shoulder)	Igual (same)	Gusto (taste)	Hijo (son)
Huevo (egg)	Kilo (kilo)	Hombre (man)	Hora (hour)
Joven (young)	Leal (loyal)	Hueso (bone)	Jardin (garden)
Lado (side)	Lila (lilac)	Isla (isle)	Jugo (juice)
Lengua (tongue)	Madre (mother)	Leche (milk)	Libros (books)
Luna (moon)	Marca (brand)	Lugar (place)	Lunes (Monday)
Mano (hand)	Mismo (same)	Malo (bad)	Manta (blanket)
Mesa (table)	Motor (engine)	Martes (Tuesday)	Metal (metal)
Modo (way)	Nariz (nose)	Mitad (half)	Mosca (fly)
Multa (fine)	Nombre (name)	Mucho (much)	Mundo (world)
Once (eleven)	Oro (gold)	Nido (nest)	Noche (night)
Ostras (oysters)	Pais (country)	Ocho (eight)	Orden (order)
Pasta (paste)	Peso (weight)	Osos (bears)	Padre (father)
Pipas (pipes)	Plato (plate)	Papel (paper)	Pelo (hair)
Queso (cheese)	Rama (branch)	Queja (complaint)	Pisos (floors)
Rancho (ranch)	Rico (rich)	Ranas (frogs)	Quince (fifteen)
Regla (ruler)	Roncar (snore)	Ropa (clothes)	Rasgos (features)
Rosca (thread)	Rostro (face)	Rumor (rumor)	Resto (rest)
Salsa (salsa)	Salud (health)	Sangre (blood)	Rosa (rose)
Sano (healthy)	Sastre (tailor)	Siglo (century)	Saltar (jump)
Sombra (shadow)	Sordo (deaf)	Tanto (much)	Santo (saint)
Tanque (tank)	Techo (ceiling)	Tela (fabric)	Sopa (soup)
Tema (theme)	Templo (temple)	Tinta (ink)	Tasa (cup)
Trampa (trap)	Torta (cake)	Total (total)	Temor (fear)
Tretas (tricks)	Trece (thirteen)	Trenza (plait)	Toro (bull)
Turno (turn)	Tronco (trunk)	Vapor (steam)	Vaca (cow)
Veinte (twenty)	Valor (price)	Verbo (verb)	Venta (sale)
Verdad (truth)	Visa (visa)	Visto (seen)	Vino (wine)

[a] With permission of Auditec of St. Louis.

Author Index

Numbers in italics indicate figure references.

Subject Index

Tympanometric width, 228–230, 233, 409–411 (*see also* Tympanometric gradient)
Tympanometry, 223–237, 386, 393, 394, 409, 410
Tympanometry procedure, 223–225
Tympanoplasty, 196, 199
Tympanosclerosis, 188, 191, 193, 196
Tympanotomy, 206
Tympanum (*see* Middle ear)
Type I auditory neurons, 68
Type II auditory neurons, 68

UCL (*see* Uncomfortable loudness level)
Umbo, 43
Uncomfortable loudness level (UCL; *see also* Loudness discomfort level and tests), 96, 266
Uncrossed acoustic reflex (*see* Ipsilateral acoustic reflex)
Uncrossed olivocochlear bundle (UOCB; *see* Olivocochlear bundle)
Undermasking, 305–306, 307
Unilateral weakness, 373
University of Oklahoma Closed Response Speech test (OUCRST), 282
Unmasked threshold, 108, 151, 294, 297
Up-5-down-10 technique, 146, 147
Upper limits of hearing, 95, 96
Upward spread of masking, 110, 417
Use gain, 454
Usher syndrome, 185
Utley lipreading test, 485, 486
Utricle, 39, 69, 71
Utriculofugal flow, 70
Utriculopedal flow, 70

VA method, 537–538
Validity, 91, 161
Valsalva maneuver, 194, 236
Valsalva test, 236
van der Hoeve's syndrome, 196
Variable intensity pulse count method, 424
Vascular loop, 209
Vascular pulsing, 201, 232
VCN (*see* Cochlear nuclei)
Vector quantities, 1
Velocity, 2
Ventilation tubes (*see* Pressure-equalization (PE) tubes)
Ventral Cochlear nucleus (*see* Cochlear nuclei)
Vents, 464
Verbal agnosia, 210
Vertigo, 180, 203, 204, 369–370, 372 (*see also* Dizziness)
Vestibular evaluation (*see* Electronystagmography)
Vestibular hair cells, 69–71
Vestibular Meniere's disease, 203
Vestibular nerve, 68, 85, 206 (*see also* Auditory nerve; Eighth cranial nerve; Statoacoustic nerve)
Vestibular neurectomy, 204
Vestibular neuronitis, 209
Vestibular neurons, 69–71, 85
Vestibular nuclei, 38, 85
Vestibular schwannoma (*see* Acoustic tumors)
Vestibular system, 59, 69–71, 85
Vestibule, 39, 57, 69, 71, 87
Vestibulocerebellar ataxia (*see* Usher syndrome)
Vestibulospinal tracts, 85
Vestibulotoxicity (*see* Ototoxicity)

Vibration, 133, 202, 502, 511
Vibro-tactile aids (*see* Tactile aids)
Vibro-tactile responses (*see* Tactile responses)
VIDSPAC test, 390
Visemes, 486
Visual reinforcement audiometry (VRA), 381–383, 386, 394
Visual Reinforcement Infant Speech Discrimination (VRISD) Test, 389–390
Visual reinforcement operant conditioning audiometry (VROCA), 383, 386, 394
Visual training (*see* Auditory and visual training)
Volley principle, 72
Volume control, 444
Von Recklinghausen's disease (*see* Neurofibromatosis type I)
VRA (*see* Visual reinforcement audiometry)
VRISD (*see* Visual Reinforcement Infant Speech Discrimination (VRISD) Test)
VROCA (*see* Visual reinforcement operant conditioning audiometry)
VU meter, 130, 257–258

W-1 (*see* CID W-1 and W-2 tests)
W-2 (*see* CID W-1 and W-2 tests)
W-22 (*see* CID W-22 test)
Waadenberg syndrome, 186
Walsh-Healey Act, 514, 522, 526
Warble-tone, 120, 379
Watt, 2, 6
Wave I, 351, 355–358, 359
Wave III, 351, 355–358, 359
Wave V, 351, 355–359
Waveform, 10
Wavelength, 12, 17, 52, 53, 162
Waves, 10–24
Weber fraction, 97, 98
Weber test, 165, 167, 298 (*see also* Audiometric Weber test)
Weber's law, 97, 98
West Virginia method, 534, 536
White noise, 21, 297
Whole-nerve action potential (*see* Compound action potential)
Whole-word scoring, 275–276 (*see also* Phonemic scoring)
Wiley-Lilly modified tone decay test, 323–324
WIPI (*see* Word Intelligibility by Picture Identification (WIPI) test)
Wisconsin method, 534, 536
Word deafness, 210
Word discrimination score (*see* Speech recognition score)
Word familiarity, 268, 273
Word frequency, 273
Word Intelligibility by Picture Identification (WIPI) test, 388, 391, 394, 554
Word recognition score (*see* Speech recognition score)
Work, 2, 5, 6
Worker's compensation (*see* Compensation for hearing loss)

X-linked dominant inheritance (*see* X-linked inheritance)